ABDOMINAL
MAGNETIC
RESONANCE
IMAGING

ABDOMINAL MAGNETIC RESONANCE IMAGING

PABLO R. ROS, MD, FACR

Professor of Radiology
Director, Divisions of Abdominal Imaging and MRI
University of Florida College of Medicine
Gainesville, Florida

W. DEAN BIDGOOD, JR., MD

Assistant Professor of Radiology
University of Florida College of Medicine
Director of MRI
Gainesville VA Medical Center
Gainesville, Florida

With 1086 Illustrations

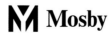

St. Louis Baltimore Boston Chicago London Philadelphia Sydney Toronto

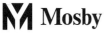
Mosby

Dedicated to Publishing Excellence

Publisher: George S. Stamathis
Editor: Anne S. Patterson
Developmental Editor: Maura K. Leib
Assistant Editor: Dana Battaglia
Project Manager: Peggy Fagen
Designer: David Zielinski
Manufacturing Supervisor: Betty Richmond

Printed in the United States of America

Mosby–Year Book, Inc.
11830 Westline Industrial Drive
St. Louis, Missouri 63146

International Standard Book Number 0-8016-6310-5

93 94 95 96 97 CL/MY 9 8 7 6 5 4 3 2 1

DEDICATION

To my wife, Ana
To my children, Pablo and Cristina
To my parents, Juan and Maria Mercedes
Thanks to their sacrifices this book is possible.

PRR

To my father, Willis D. Bidgood,
  and my mother, Betty Butler Bidgood,
  for inspiration and constant encouragement
To my children, Sara, Lee, Emily, and Grace, for sharing their Dad
To my wife, Diane, for protecting my time as if it were hers
  and for keeping our family going
Knowledge passes away, but love like this is eternal.

WDB

Contributors

Deborah A. Allen, MD
Fellow in MRI
Department of Radiology
University of Florida
Gainesville, Florida

J. Ray Ballinger, MD
Staff Radiologist
Gainesville VA Medical Center
University of Florida College of Medicine
Gainesville, Florida

Mary Ellen Bentham, RT(R)
Supervisor, MRI
Shands Hospital at the University of Florida
Gainesville, Florida

W. Dean Bidgood, Jr., MD
Assistant Professor of Radiology
University of Florida College of Medicine
Director of MRI
Gainesville VA Medical Center
Gainesville, Florida

Richard W. Briggs, PhD
Associate Professor of Radiology
University of Florida College of Medicine
Gainesville, Florida

Sharon S. Burton, MD
Assistant Professor of Radiology
University of Florida College of Medicine
Gainesville, Florida

Eugenio Erquiaga, MD
Senior Resident
Department of Radiology
University of Florida College of Medicine
Gainesville, Florida

Jeffrey R. Fitzsimmons, PhD
Associate Professor of Radiology
University of Florida College of Medicine
Gainesville, Florida

Cynthia L. Janus, MD
Associate Professor of Radiology
University of Virginia Medical Center
Charlottesville, Virginia

Juri V. Kaude, MD, PhD
Professor of Radiology
University of Florida College of Medicine
Gainesville, Florida

Stephen J. Kennedy, MD
Senior Resident
Department of Radiology
University of Florida College of Medicine
Gainesville, Florida

Paula J. Keslar, MD
Chief of Pediatric Radiology
Armed Forces Institute of Pathology
Washington, DC

Barry B. Kraus, MD
Fellow in MRI
Department of Radiology
University of Florida College of Medicine
Gainesville, Florida

Lisa M. Langmo, MD
Senior Resident
Department of Radiology
University of Florida College of Medicine
Gainesville, Florida

Jintong Mao, PhD
Assistant Research Professor of Radiology
University of Florida College of Medicine
Gainesville, Florida

David S. Mendelson, MD
Associate Professor
The Mount Sinai Hospital
New York, New York

Luis H. Ros Mendoza, MD
Research Fellow in MRI
Department of Radiology
University of Florida College of Medicine
Gainesville, Florida;
Staff Radiologist
Hospital Miguel Servet
Universidad de Zaragoza
Zaragoza, Spain

Pablo R. Ros, MD, FACR
Professor of Radiology
Director, Divisions of Abdominal Imaging and MRI
University of Florida College of Medicine
Gainesville, Florida

Mark L. Schiebler, MD
Associate Professor of Radiology
University of Pennsylvania
Philadelphia, Pennsylvania

Ali Shirkhoda, MD
Clinical Professor of Radiology
Wayne State University School of Medicine
Detroit, Michigan;
Director, Division of Diagnostic Imaging
William Beaumont Hospital
Royal Oak, Michigan

Christophoros Stoupis, MD
Fellow in MRI
Department of Radiology
University of Florida College of Medicine
Gainesville, Florida;
Staff Radiologist
Department of Radiology
University of Bern
Bern, Switzerland

Gladys M. Torres, MD
Assistant Professor of Radiology
University of Florida College of Medicine
Gainesville, Florida

Foreword

Of the major organ systems, the abdomen is the last frontier for magnetic resonance imaging (MRI). The capabilities of MRI to provide exquisite contrast resolution, multiplanar examination, and tissue characterization were rapidly applied to the central nervous system, spine, and extremities, and now after a more prolonged development cycle, are being applied with success to the abdomen.

Although considerable experience has now been accumulated, there is no comprehensive collection of data, using state-of-the-art instrumentation, dedicated to MRI of the abdomen. With the advent of faster pulsing sequences, motion reduction techniques, and a gamut of intraluminal contrast agents for the gastrointestinal (GI) tract and specific vascular agents for abdominal organs such as the liver, MRI is becoming a valid alternative to computed tomography (CT) and, in some cases, the technique of choice to study abdominal disease.

The abdomen is the growth area in MRI since its use in other areas has been maximized. This was expected since abdominal radiology is one of the main pillars of diagnostic radiology. Currently, abdominal MRI is one of the most fascinating areas of research within our specialty. There is practically not an issue of our major journals in which a new application or innovation for abdominal MRI is not present. It is ironic that abdominal MRI also constitutes one of the major challenges for us as consultants in radiology, since its high cost limits its use only to those cases in which it is clearly justified as an appropriate and informative imaging technique.

This textbook is primarily the result of the effort of radiologists and physicists from the University of Florida. Our team has accumulated data via three MRI units from two major manufacturers (Siemens and General Electric). Members of our basic science and clinical faculty, leaders in the disciplines of MRI physics, coil development, and contrast agent research, work in close cooperation to conduct our clinical practice.

Dr. Ros is the Director of the Division of Abdominal Imaging and the Division of Magnetic Resonance Imaging of Shands Hospital at the University of Florida. He came to us from the Armed Forces Institute of Pathology in Washington, DC, where he was Chief of the Gastrointestinal Radiologic-Pathologic Section. His broad experience with radiologic-pathologic correlation strengthens his interest in MRI. He has led our clinical and research efforts in abdominal MRI, receiving in 1990 the Research Award of the Society of Gastrointestinal Radiologists for his work on MRI gastrointestinal contrasts.

Dr. Bidgood is the Director of MRI at the Gainesville VA Medical Center, affiliated with the University of Florida. His interest in the technical aspects of MRI and his extensive past experience in the private practice of general radiology are apparent in the practical approach and the clear expository style of this textbook. His input on physical principles and abdominal MRI techniques is very refreshing and understandable. In addition to his clinical and research activities he has become a leader in the development of the ACR-NEMA DICOM standard for electronic communication of medical images.

This textbook summarizes for the reader the experience at the University of Florida, where two different manufacturers have provided excellent units that are kept up to date with frequent hardware and software changes. The support received from our university hospital administration in this regard is gratefully acknowledged. Our experience in clinical abdominal MRI benefits from the efforts of our MRI physicists and basic scientists who have worked for a decade on National Institutes of Health–funded research on MR spectroscopy and imaging. Their assistance to our radiologists to provide enough data, coil design, and pulsing sequences has been invaluable. I must emphasize also that the work of our physicists and physicians could not have been performed without the efforts of our industrious and creative technologists and research assistants who have provided the ideal complement to perform superb abdominal MRI.

Our Department of Radiology is primarily organized into sections by organ systems. Therefore, the authors are abdominal radiologists who perform MRI with more emphasis on clinical applications than on technical nuances. This point of view should be refreshing for the majority of clinical radiologists who are the primary targeted audience for this textbook.

With the growth of abdominal MRI, abdominal imaging is becoming an ideal field to experiment with communication of images. I hope that in subsequent editions the authors will be able to discuss the merits of a comprehensive picture archiving and communication system (PACS) that is being introduced at the University of Florida. The abdomen with multiple organs and applications for all imaging modalities should become one of the more rewarding areas of the body for electronic reading stations and PACS.

In summary, the time has come for a comprehensive text in abdominal imaging with MRI. The last organ system frontier for MRI is being conquered, and this book offers a guide to the general radiologist who needs a read-able and practical reference text in order to venture into this arena. For these reasons, I believe that this textbook will be very useful to the radiology community as a whole.

Edward V. Staab, MD
Professor and Chairman
Department of Radiology
University of Florida
College of Medicine

Preface

This book presents the current state of magnetic resonance imaging (MRI) applied to the abdomen. Of all the areas of the body, the abdomen has elicited the most expectation for the application of MRI. To conquer the intricacies of all abdominal organs with so many pathologies and encompassing two organ systems (gastrointestinal and genitourinary) has been one of the major challenges for radiologists interested in MRI. It appears now that abdominal MRI is coming of age, and it may be necessary to have in one volume a review of the current knowledge of this area.

This book represents primarily the effort of one group of abdominal radiologists working at the University of Florida, although excellent and very important contributions are presented from radiologists working in other institutions. Our goal in writing this textbook is to provide a systematic way of approaching MRI of the abdomen, rather than a ranbow of disparate protocols and styles.

The University of Florida is a center with a long tradition of excellence in MRI. The physics group at our center has excelled in coil development, and imaging applications of magnetic resonance spectroscopy. Their contributions to our clinical practice have been spectacular. In our center, a more recent tradition has been development and clinical testing of GI and hepatic contrast agents. We have a busy service in abdominal MRI with one of the largest proportions of abdominal MRI in academic centers.

However, this book has been written having in mind the mainstream radiologist and offers a general but focused overview of the current state-of-the-art of abdominal MRI. Although we try to present a sneak preview of the future techniques, our emphasis is to present the major indications for abdominal MRI with the current tools. We try to highlight what is available to all, since one of the objectives of this book is to become a practical guide to radiologists who are interested in abdominal MRI and are also interested in increasing the number of abdominal MRI studies that can be done with their units. That emphasis on a practical approach can be seen throughout the book with a large number of tables, protocols, and imaging tips.

We have been fortunate to use three scanners made by two manufacturers: General Electric and Siemens. In the course of our clinical experience with magnets of 1.0 and 1.5 Tesla, we have learned the major advantages and disadvantages of each system and the potential benefits of various imaging software features.

The textbook is divided into three parts. The first part is on basic principles and techniques, beginning with a brief review chapter on basic MRI physics in understandable terms and a chapter on the major considerations for abdominal MRI technique. Chapters on abdominal coils, contrast agents, and the principles of abdominal MR angiography follow.

The second part is dedicated to the upper abdomen, and the third part is dedicated to the pelvis. They both begin with overview chapters presenting the major applications and limitations of MRI. The introductory overviews are followed by chapters on anatomy and then by chapters organized according to individual organs and regions. The liver chapter, the most extensive, has been divided into sections. Each section is devoted to major application of MRI to the liver.

Our focus is on the needs of the general radiologist or abdominal radiologist who is interested in MRI, rather than on the MRI specialist whose interest is primarily in the new technical developments in the modality. The point of view is that of the abdominal radiologist who on a daily basis performs in addition to MRI barium studies, ultrasound, and computed tomography (CT). The entities presented frequently have the counterbalance of the findings seen by other imaging modalities, and MRI is seen not in isolation but in conjunction with all the other tools of the trade. Therefore, we hope that general radiologists will be able to enjoy and to collect the "pearls" that will allow them to improve the applications of MRI of the abdomen in their practice.

The reader needs to know that this book has been possible thanks to the effort of many people.

First and foremost, we want to highlight the effort of the entire team of abdominal imagers at the University of Florida. Many of them are direct contributors of this textbook, such as Drs. Torres, Burton, Kaude, and Keslar. Other members of our team, such as Dr. Patricia Abbitt and many of our Abdominal Imaging fellows, including Danny Rappaport, Jennifer Hamrick-Turner, John Panaccione, Tina Hendrix, and Steve Frazier, who did not write any chapters, warrant our gratitude for their continuous help and ideas to improve our approach to abdominal imaging.

Special acknowledgment is due to the many clinicians of the University of Florida College of Medicine who have believed for many years in the benefits of abdominal magnetic resonance imaging (MRI). We have been blessed with a team of surgeons, urologists, gynecologists, oncologists, etc., in our center that has provided the bulk of the clinical material that we offer in this textbook, in particular, Drs. Stephen Vogel and Kirby Bland of the Department of Surgery, Dr. Zev Wajsman of the Department of Urology, and Drs. James Cerda, Philip Toskes, Gary Davis, and Chris Forsmark of the Department of Gastroenterology.

At a personal level (PRR), I must recognize Dr. Manuel Viamonte, Professor of Radiology at the University of Miami and Chairman of the Department of Radiology at Mount Sinai Medical Center, Miami Beach, Florida, since he had the foresight to direct my career toward body MRI, involving me in this area since I was a resident in his department.

With warm thanks (WDB), I recognize Dr. James H. Scatliff, professor and former chairman of Radiology at the University of North Carolina, Chapel Hill, for exemplifying the highest ideals of academic teaching, while always encouraging a warm and productive working relationship among the staff of our department. I also gratefully recognize here the influence of the late Dr. George M. Himadi, who taught me by his own example that one can return to academic medicine after private practice, and the late Dr. J. Maxie Dell, Jr., of the Gainesville Radiology Group, who brought the best of academics to the private practice environment.

In a very special way, we are also indebted to our Chairman, Dr. Edward V. Staab, who not only encouraged us from the very beginning to put in black and white what we were doing but also supported our research efforts.

Credit needs to be given to our superb team of MRI technologists led by Mary Ellen Bentham, MRI Supervisor at Shands Hospital, and including Cleatis Chewning, Pam Darnell, Chrissy Meyer, Eric Johns, Cathy Jerkins, and Holly Stephens. Thanks to their patience in allowing us to perform additional sequences and creative innovations, we can offer superb images in this textbook. Thanks also to the technologists of the Gainesville VA Medical Center—Bill Bell, Larry Hoyle, Michelle Werner, and David Damm—for their loyal assistance and for their professional dedication to the care of our patients.

However, this book would not have been possible without the guidance of the entire group of editors at Mosby–Year Book headed by Anne Patterson and Maura Leib. A very particular note of appreciation is also due to Ms. Linda Pigott, our editorial assistant of the Department of Radiology, and to the medical illustrations staff of The Learning Resources Center of the University of Florida Health Science Center.

Pablo R. Ros

W. Dean Bidgood, Jr.

Contents

ABDOMINAL MAGNETIC RESONANCE IMAGING

Part I

BASIC PRINCIPLES AND TECHNIQUES

Chapter 1

BASIC PHYSICAL PRINCIPLES

W. Dean Bidgood, Jr.

Every day clinical decision making in magnetic resonance imaging (**MRI**)[*] requires a working knowledge of the effects of **electromagnetic fields** on the behavior of the fundamental **particles** of matter. The clinical chapters of this book assume that the reader has a basic understanding of MRI physics. Explanation of the fundamentals of tissue magnetization, resonance, dephasing, signal formation, decay constants, and pulse sequences is provided here as a convenient reference for those readers who need a brief review. A detailed, cross-referenced glossary of the terms introduced in this chapter is appended at the end of this chapter. Because the glossary entries contain substantial information not covered in the text, you are encouraged to review it carefully. Those who already understand the basics are invited to begin reading at Chapter 2.

HYDROGEN PROTON INTERACTIONS WITH OTHER PARTICLES

Atoms and subatomic particles are in constant motion whenever their surrounding temperature is above absolute zero. The outcome of their interactions (collisions and near-misses) is described statistically by the disciplines of **quantum** physics and thermodynamics. As illustrated by Fig. 1-1, the behavior of subatomic particles cannot be predicted by ordinary experience (**classical mechanics**) alone.

When groups of particles interact with each other over time, their properties (such as velocity) approach an intermediate state called equilibrium. According to the first law of thermodynamics, no **energy** or **mass** is lost in any sort of particle interaction. In MRI, we are most interested in the energy exchanges that result from proton-proton inter-

---

[*] As new terms are introduced, they are highlighted in **boldface.** A glossary of the highlighted words is provided at the end of the chapter for definitions and further explanation. Related formulas and quantities, historical notes, and cross references are provided.

Cartoon illustrations drawn by A.J. Meder. Thanks, Art.

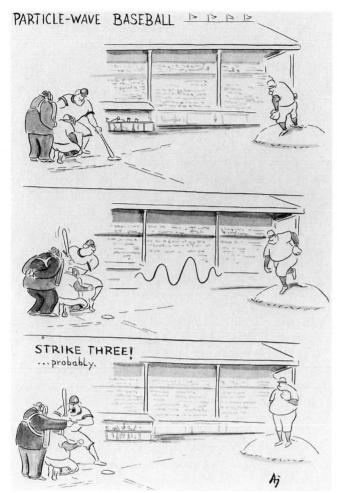

PARTICLE-WAVE BASEBALL

STRIKE THREE! ...probably.

Fig. 1-1. The behavior of subatomic particles cannot be predicted by ordinary experience alone. (From Meder AJ: Physics Today, Aug 1990, p 94.)

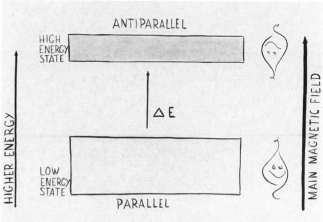

Fig. 1-2. Protons align either parallel or antiparallel to an external magnetic field. The population of higher-energy antiparallel spins *(upper rectangle)* is considerably smaller than the population of lower-energy parallel spins *(lower rectangle)*. ΔE is the energy difference between the two spin states.

teract randomly until we somehow perturb their equilibrium with energy from an external source.

We observe the motion of protons and other particles indirectly through manifestations such as heat, pressure, and radio noise, depending on what instrument we use to make our measurements. In MRI we place a sample of protons in a strong magnetic field and observe their energy states as we expose them to controlled quantities of **radiofrequency** energy.

PROTONS AND ELECTROMAGNETISM

Because protons are charged particles with the property of spin, they essentially are small electromagnets. In any spin-spin and spin-lattice interactions, their intrinsic electromagnetic field subjects protons to a force called a **magnetic moment.** In fact, magnetic moments result not only from near-collisions but from interaction with any magnetic field the proton encounters, whether produced by another proton, a group of molecules, or the MRI electromagnet coils.

Spin orientation and energy states

When in a strong, uniform magnetic field, protons (small magnets with north and south poles) must line up either in the parallel spin state (for example, north-south) or in the antiparallel spin state (south-north). It is highly improbable that any protons would remain very long in an orientation perpendicular to a strong outside field (Fig. 1-3). According to the second law of thermodynamics, the lowest possible energy state is favored. The proton experiences a lower magnetic moment in the parallel spin state than in the the antiparallel spin state. In either the parallel or the antiparallel state, the magnetic moment of the proton is substantially less than in any other orientation. The

actions (**spin-spin** interactions) and from the interactions of protons with their environment (**spin-lattice** interactions). By **protons,** I am referring to hydrogen atoms, which have only one unpaired proton in their nucleus. Only hydrogen, sodium, phosphorus, and a few other elements have an unpaired **nucleon** (unpaired proton or neutron in the nucleus of the atom), which allows them to exhibit the magnetic resonance phenomenon. Protons have an attribute called **spin,** which is present in quantum amounts. Only two proton spin states exist, according to quantum mechanics. The states (which can be measured while protons are in a magnetic field) correspond to energy levels (Fig. 1-2).

According to the second law of thermodynamics, protons are more likely to convert from a high energy spin state to a low energy spin state (by releasing a quantum of energy) than to do the opposite (by absorbing energy). The natural tendency is toward disorder—to release stored energy down to the point of thermal equilibrium. Protons in-

proton's energy level (when aligned either parallel or antiparallel to an external magnetic field) is so much lower than in any other orientation that the small energy difference between the two preferred states is nearly negligible in comparison. Even so, the difference is significant. It is enough to produce a slight surplus population of parallel spins, on the order of one in a million, whenever a sample of protons is placed into a uniform magnetic field (Fig. 1-2).

Population statistics. How can we make use of such a small difference? We must deal with the entire population of protons rather than with individual particles. Even a proportion of one in a million adds up to a large **number** when the total population is over 1,000,000,000,000,000,000,000,000,000 protons (Fig. 1-4).

Net magnetization

Under ordinary conditions, the magnetic moments of protons with parallel and antiparallel spins cancel each other. However, when a volume of tissue containing fat or water protons is placed in a strong, uniform magnetic field, an excess population of parallel spins is created. The magnetic moments of these uncancelled protons add up to

produce the *net magnetization* of the tissue. Once this initial reorganization has occurred, we observe no further (global, statistical) change in net magnetization until the protons are removed from the steady magnetic field (unless we disturb them in some other way).

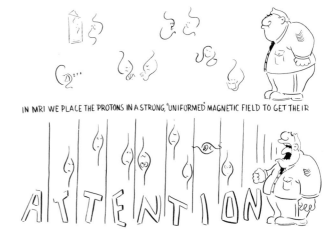

IN MRI WE PLACE THE PROTONS IN A STRONG, "UNIFORMED" MAGNETIC FIELD TO GET THEIR ATTENTION

Fig. 1-3. In a strong magnetic field, protons line up either in the parallel or the antiparallel spin state; they cannot remain very long in a perpendicular orientation.

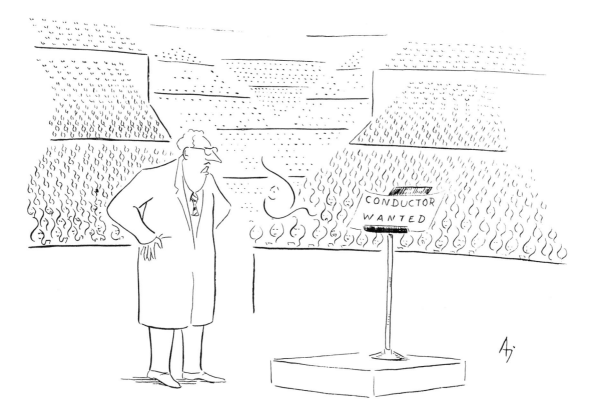

"Now let me get this straight: you have a chorus of gazillions, they each know a couple of notes which they sing as they please, and you expect me to make music?!"

Fig. 1-4. "MRI symphony orchestra."

MAGNETIC RESONANCE

What is resonance? A group of protons in a strong magnetic field, when stimulated with an excess of the right-sized energy quanta, exchange the quanta at a stereotyped rate. They continue to do so until other forces intervene (and the quanta are lost to the surrounding environment). The rate, or frequency, of the exchange is determined by the **flux density** of the magnetic field in which the proton resides (see below). The unique frequency at which this phenomenon occurs is called the **resonant frequency** (the **Larmor frequency**) (Fig. 1-5).

Wine glass example. The combined effect of all the quantum exchanges is something like rhythmic vibration. The process continues until all of the excitation energy (received from an outside source) has been expelled (following the first and second laws of thermodynamics). An everyday example of the resonance phenomenon is the musical tone produced when a moistened finger is lightly rubbed along the rim of a drinking glass. The tone of the resonant note varies with the level of water in the glass, just as the resonant frequency of protons varies with the flux density of an imposed magnetic field. A tuning fork (having the same frequency as the resonant note of the glass) causes the glass to resonate sympathetically, even without direct physical contact (Fig. 1-6). When outside energy (from the finger or the tuning fork) no longer is

available to sustain the resonance phenomenon, the sound gradually fades away. The rate at which the note subsides depends on the type of glass. (This fact also applies to the magnetic resonance phenomenon, which has different characteristics among various tissues.)

Larmor equation

Determining the size of energy quantum required to make protons resonate is relatively straightforward. Be-

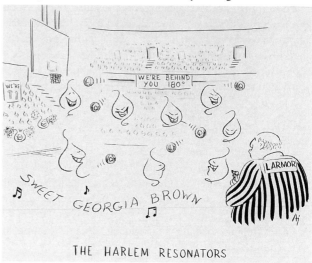

Fig 1-5. Protons are in resonance when they exchange energy quanta at a particular rate, named "Larmor frequency."

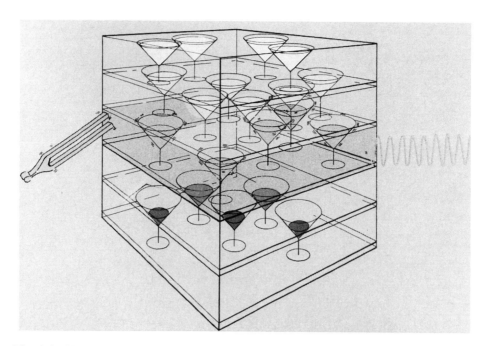

Fig. 1-6. Glasses containing the right amount of water absorb sound energy and vibrate at the same frequency as the nearby tuning fork. None of the other glasses vibrate (because they contain either more or less liquid and have resonant frequencies that do not match the frequency of the tuning fork). (Reprinted with permission of Johnson and Johnson, Inc. From Hinshaw WS, Kramer DM, Yeung HN, Hill BC: The fundamentals of magnetic resonance imaging, Solon, Ohio, 1984, Technicare Corp.)

cause our instruments are calibrated in radiofrequencies, which are proportional to energy levels, we use a formula called the **Larmor equation.** The equation requires only two parameters: the *strength* of the imposed magnetic field and a constant that describes the *responsiveness* of the protons to external magnetic and RF fields.

Flux density. The first parameter of the Larmor equation represents the density of the lines of force of the magnet. A better expression for *density of lines of force* is *flux density.* The term **field strength** is widely used when *flux density* actually is meant. Flux density is expressed in **tesla** (T). The standard international unit of measure for field strength is the Oersted (defined as an ampere of current flow per meter).

Gyromagnetic ratio. The second parameter of the Larmor equation takes into account several properties of atoms. The appropriate parameters are folded into a constant called the **gyromagnetic ratio,** which is unique for each type of atom.

The product of flux density and the gyromagnetic ratio is the resonant frequency of a particular type of atom in a magnetic field of a given flux density, that is, the Larmor frequency. The operator of the MRI scanner sets the RF transmit and receive frequencies to values determined empirically from calibration testing, and the circuits of the scanner produce RF quanta of the correct energy for induction of proton magnetic resonance.

Radiofrequency excitation pulses

To review, the protons of a sample tissue are placed inside the bore of a hollow magnet. Because of the excess of low energy parallel spins, the protons develop net magnetism, which is the key to the MRI process (see Figs. 1-2 and 1-3). This steady state of stable net magnetism continues until we disturb the system by conveying a measured amount of electromagnetic energy to the tissue from an external source. This step is accomplished by exposing the tissue to RF pulses at the Larmor frequency (Fig. 1-7).

The *radio pulses must have not only the correct energy (wavelength) but also the correct strength.* Determining the optimal RF pulse strength for various purposes is less straightforward than determining resonant frequency. The basic principles are outlined in the next section.

RF pulse strength. Absolute quantities, such as amplitude (in volts), duration (in msec), bandwidth (in kHz), and phase (in degrees or radians), are used to describe the strength and quality of RF pulses. For clinical purposes, it is usually sufficient to name the pulse according to its effect on a sample volume rather than by the exact parameters of the pulse itself. If actual values are required, they are accessible at the operator's console.

The functional names of RF pulses are derived from the pattern of proton response to increases in pulse strength. The response pattern is periodic, following the pattern of a sine wave.

90-degree RF pulse. The smallest pulse that transfers the maximum usable energy to the protons of a sample volume is called a **90-degree pulse.** Those who prefer **radians** to degrees call this a π/2 pulse. If the power of RF excitation pulses is increased gradually, the population of antiparallel (high energy) spins, steadily increases, up to the pulse strength called 90 degrees.

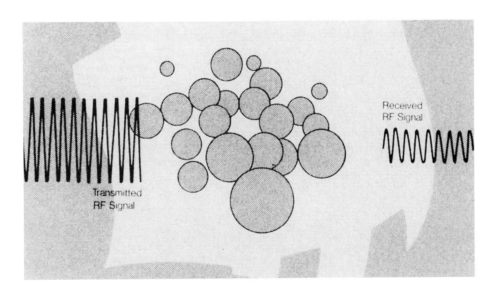

Fig. 1-7. The transmitted RF signal imparts energy to protons in the same manner that the tuning fork of Fig. 1-6 imparts sound energy to the glasses. The energy released by the resonating (vibrating) protons at the Larmor frequency is the received RF signal. This signal is analogous to the audible tone produced by the vibrating glasses in Fig. 1-6. (Reprinted with permission of Johnson and Johnson, Inc. From Hinshaw WS, Kramer DM, Yeung HN, Hill BC: The fundamentals of magnetic resonance imaging, Solon, Ohio, 1984, Technicare Corp.)

The actual voltage or power needed to reach the 90-degree level depends on many factors, which the computer programs that control the scanner consider. The actual numbers vary widely. The computer turns off the RF pulse as soon as maximum energy transfer is detected.

Beyond 90 degrees. Beyond the 90-degree power level (whatever the actual value is), the surplus of antiparallel spins drops steadily at first, as the power level of the RF transmitter is increased. On a graph, the number of high energy spins follows a sine wave pattern, with alternating maximum and minimum values. The next maximum point is designated as the 270-degree level.

Consequences of excess RF power. Beyond the 90-degree point, as fast as one proton absorbs a quantum and converts from low to high energy, another expels a packet of energy and drops back to the favored lower state. *Continuing to transmit a steady RF signal into the proton population will evoke no greater net magnetization than a 90-degree pulse.* Instead, the steady influx of RF packets results in tremendous turnover of energy from proton to proton (spin to spin) and proton to neighborhood (spin to lattice). Most of this radio energy is wasted in the form of heat. Because heat can damage tissue, the maximum amount of RF power permitted for MRI scanners is limited by law (see Chapter 3).

Steady state equilibrium

As soon as RF energy transmission begins at the Larmor frequency, some protons are promoted to the high en-ergy antiparallel state. Even though this state is inherently unstable, throughout the transmission time of the RF pulse, an artificial steady state equilibrium is maintained. A higher than usual proportion of the spins is forced to be antiparallel. Rapid toggling of individual proton spin states occurs, but the net effect is constant until the RF excitation pulse ceases.

T1 relaxation

Immediately after excitation by a 90-degree RF pulse, tissue magnetization momentarily falls to zero along the longitudinal axis (parallel to the flux lines of the magnet). The orientation of the tissue's magnetic field is rotated into the transverse plane by the energy of the RF pulse. Only during the time of this unstable (high energy state) transverse orientation RF signal produced by the excited tissue is detectable. *The energy packets released by resonating protons in the high energy state as they make the transition to the more stable lower energy state are detected by the MRI receiver as radio signals.* As the protons release the excess energy imparted by the RF pulse, the amplitude of the RF signal decays exponentially (Fig. 1-8). As the signal fades, the longitudinal magnetization of the tissue recovers (but not at the same rate at which the signal decays—see Phase Dispersion). The rate of recovery of tissue longitudinal magnetization after an RF excitation pulse is a function of the "relaxation coefficient," **T1** (Fig. 1-9). If another RF pulse follows soon after the first, the protons have time to release only a fraction of the energy absorbed

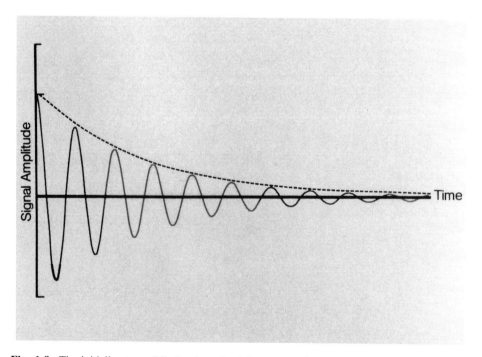

Fig. 1-8. The initially strong RF signal received from resonating protons decays **exponentially.** (Reprinted with permission of Johnson and Johnson, Inc. From Hinshaw WS, Kramer DM, Yeung HN, Hill BC: The fundamentals of magnetic resonance imaging, Solon, Ohio, 1984, Technicare Corp.)

from the first pulse before the relaxation process is truncated, and the tissue longitudinal magnetization is again obliterated. As a result, a smaller signal is produced by each RF pulse in a chain of pulses than by an isolated but otherwise similar RF pulse (Fig. 1-10).

T1-related proton saturation. Some tissues release stored RF energy more rapidly than others during excitation by a series of RF pulses. Substances that recover slowly after an RF pulse (tissues containing protons with long **T1 relaxation times**) are more adversely affected by rapid pulsing. They release only a small fraction of their surplus RF excitation energy to produce a weak radio signal between RF pulses (i.e., water). Substances that recover quickly (tissues that contain protons with short T1 relaxation times) rapidly emit a large fraction of their stored excitation energy to produce a strong radio signal between RF pulses (i.e., fat).

Factors producing T1 differences. *Each species of*

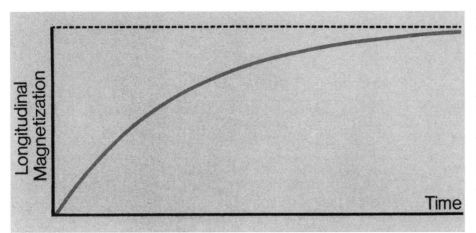

Fig. 1-9. Over time, after an RF excitation pulse that converts longitudinal magnetization to transverse magnetization, the energy-releasing ability of protons is restored. Regrowth of the longitudinal net magnetization vector of the tissue occurs at an exponential rate that has time constant T1. (Reprinted with permission of Johnson and Johnson, Inc. From Hinshaw WS, Kramer DM, Yeung HN, Hill BC: The fundamentals of magnetic resonance imaging, Solon, Ohio, 1984, Technicare Corp.)

Fig. 1-10. The first excitation pulse elicits a received signal of the highest possible amplitude. Subsequent excitation pulses evoke smaller signals if the interval between pulses is too short to allow full restoration of longitudinal magnetization along its T1 exponential recovery curve. (Reprinted with permission of Johnson and Johnson, Inc. From Hinshaw WS, Kramer DM, Yeung HN, Hill BC: The fundamentals of magnetic resonance imaging, Solon, Ohio, 1984, Technicare Corp.)

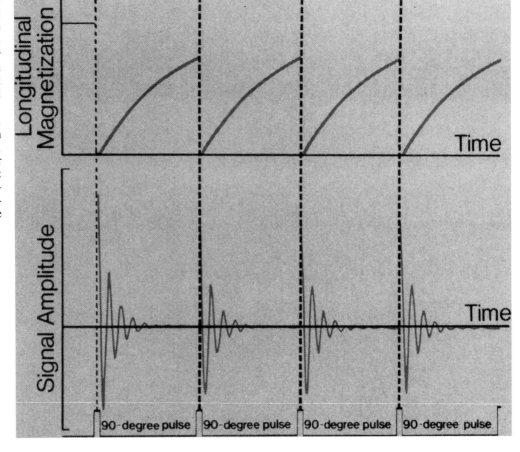

protons (for instance, protons of fat, muscle, or liver) has its characteristic T1 relaxation time, which depends on its physical composition, magnetic field strength, and temperature. All of these factors affect energy transfer (spin lattice), which is the essence of T1 relaxation. The rate of spin-lattice energy transfer is determined by the quality and quantity of interactions between protons and their environment.

Spin-lattice orientation and quantum size. Two conditions must be met for atomic particles to transfer energy. First, their magnetic fields must be perpendicular; that is, their spins must be angled 90 degrees apart. Second, the giving and receiving particles in a prospective energy exchange transaction must have the same quantum size preference. The same amount of energy released by one particle must be absorbed by another.

Spin state and phase angle. The two proton spin states have opposite energy levels. Therefore, the energy levels of the two perpendicular particles are 90 degrees out of **phase.** While one of the particles is in the higher energy state, the other is making the downward transition to the lower energy state. While one of the particles is in the lower energy state, the other is making the upward transition to the higher energy state. The pattern is similar to the sine wave described in the section on RF pulse strength.

Spin-spin energy transfer. Resonating protons toggle back and forth between the higher and lower energy states at the Larmor frequency. When they come into perpendicular orientation with each other, energy transfer is very likely, as the higher energy particle is at its most unstable state at the time its partner is ready to receive energy. Energy transfers between resonating protons are frequent. They have no effect on the net energy of the population because there is no net gain or loss.

Particle motion. To transfer energy to their environment, protons require the same perpendicular orientation with some particle in the lattice (the local environment) as they do for transfer to another proton. The transfer of energy to the lattice is a complex process because the size and speed of different species of particles may be radically different from those of the proton.

Favored frequency. Protons in a material in which the particles vibrate or rotate at frequencies near the Larmor frequency are more likely to exchange energy with their environment. These materials rapidly release stored up MR radio energy; their T1 relaxation times are short.

Particle interaction. Energy transfers are less likely to occur if the lattice particles are moving at rates far removed from the Larmor frequency. To achieve this goal, they must be in the correct orientation, and they must maintain that orientation by moving at exactly the same frequency. Once proper orientation is achieved, the likelihood of energy transfer increases with time. In this context, the quality of particle interactions is expressed indirectly by a quantity called **correlation time.**

Beyond T1: other factors. The T1 relaxation **time constant** only partially describes the behavior of protons after RF excitation in MRI. The signal from resonating protons decays at least 10 times faster than expected from the T1 constant alone.

Local magnetic environment. The unexpectedly rapid decay is due to the behavior of individual protons immediately after termination of the RF excitation pulse. In theory, the protons in a given tissue should have similar local environments and should release exactly the same quantum of energy at approximately the same time after cessation of the RF pulse. At the subatomic level, however, the magnetic environment is markedly different from one location to another within a volume of tissue. In fact, from moment to moment, the energy capacity of each proton continually changes as it moves in and out of larger and smaller magnetic fields in its local environment.

Energy proportional to flux. A proton that tumbles randomly into the field of a large protein molecule is subjected to a magnetic flux density that may be many times greater than the flux density imposed by the MRI magnet (Fig. 1-11). *The quantum size needed for resonance is proportional to magnetic field flux density.* Because energy and frequency are directly related by **Planck's constant,** the resonant frequency of a proton is proportional to its energy preference.

Random signals/random noise. Resonating protons are radio transmitters that vary in frequency from moment to moment as their preferred energy levels respond to changes in the magnetic environment. Only random noise is detectable from the disordered motion of protons outside of a magnetic field. Rapid, disorderly variation of proton transmitting frequencies within a magnetic field produces similar random noise (instead of the strong signal that would be detected if all of the protons were transmitting with the same frequency). Grasping this concept leads to an understanding of the second major **exponential decay** constant of MRI: **T2.**

Resonating protons become more and more dissimilar with time after cessation of the RF pulse (as their frequencies change due to the effect of inhomogeneity of the magnetic field in which they exist). Relatively quickly, their combined radio signal fades, even though, as individual particles, they have the capacity to produce signal for a substantially longer time. T2 describes the rate of signal loss caused by a proton's interaction with its neighbors (spin-spin interaction).

T2 decay

T2: natural magnetic field variations. Each tissue has more or less texture in its magnetic environment at the atomic and molecular levels. The **T2 decay** factor results

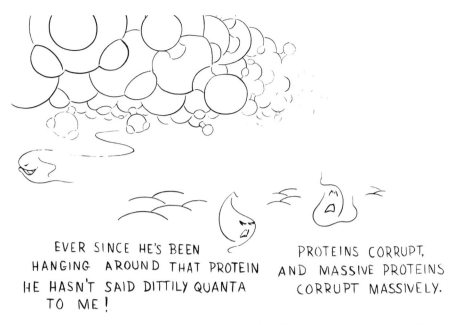

Fig. 1-11. Large proteins influence surrounding proteins. The magnetic flux density of a large protein is many times greater than that of the MRI magnet.

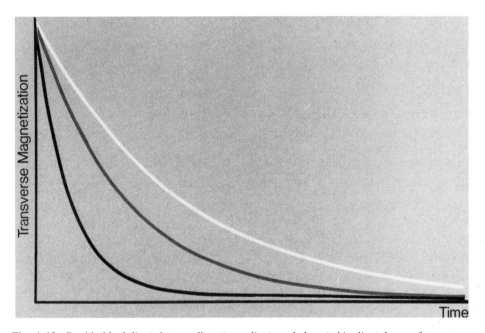

Fig. 1-12. Rapid *(black line)*, intermediate *(gray line)*, and slow *(white line)* decay of transverse magnetization. Note: The rate of decay of transverse magnetization (a function of the T2 exponential decay time constant) is not identical to the rate of recovery of longitudinal magnetization. In fact, the decay of transverse magnetization typically occurs about 10 times faster than the recovery of longitudinal magnetization. (Reprinted with permission of Johnson and Johnson, Inc. From Hinshaw WS, Kramer DM, Yeung HN, Hill BC: The Fundamentals of magnetic resonance imaging, Solon, Ohio, 1984, Technicare Corp.)

from this natural variation (Fig. 1-12).

T2*: scanner magnetic field variations. Even more significant to the proton than natural T2 decay is the effect of variations in the magnetic field of the MRI scanner. No magnetic field is perfectly homogeneous. Even though in-

homogeneity of less than 10 parts per million is considered satisfactory for routine MRI scanning, the resulting iatrogenic field variation significantly shortens the interval during which the proton signal is detectable after RF excitation. *Any irregularity of the scanner's field is magnified by*

Fig. 1-13. Three sine waves of identical frequency (period) and amplitude. They are alike in general, but, with exception of a few special points at which their curves cross, their amplitudes do not match. They are out of phase. Reading the graph from left to right, the white curve reaches maximum (at the zero time point) before either of the other two. It "leads" in phase. The others "lag." (Reprinted with permission of Johnson and Johnson, Inc. From Hinshaw WS, Kramer DM, Yeung HN, Hill BC: The fundamentals of magnetic resonance imaging, Solon, Ohio, 1984, Technicare Corp.)

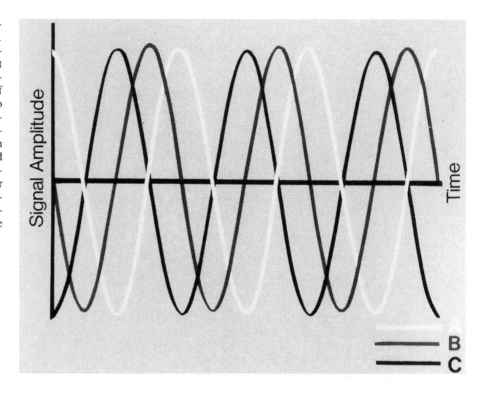

natural differences already present in the tissues. The effect increases rapidly, as the square of the magnetic field strength. This additional decay factor, T2*, is the main cause of the rapid decline of proton resonance after the RF pulse is turned off. It is also the most significant determinant of tissue contrast weighting in an MRI technique called *gradient echo,* which uses intentional variations in magnetic field strength (pulsed magnetic gradients) to produce useful signals.

Phase coherence

Any regularly recurring process is composed of lowest common denominator events (cycles), which require a certain time for completion. This time is called the *period.* The period of a radiofrequency signal is 1/frequency. For instance, the period of a 2 Hz signal (two cycles per second) is 0.50 second. The period of a 4 Hz signal is 0.25 second, and so on. Recurring processes having the same frequency also have the same period. However, even with identical periods (and amplitudes), the processes are not necessarily identical. They may differ in another property—phase (Fig. 1-13).

Phase is an attribute that conveys the relative timing of similar points among cycles in a recurring process. The implications of various phase relationships are illustrated by the following three examples:

1. Recurring (cyclical) processes that start at the same time and have identical values at *all* measurement times mutually reinforce each other (Fig. 1-14). They are in phase. In other words, their phases are coherent.

2. Similar recurring processes starting at different times only partially reinforce each other, as their maxima occur at different times. Their amplitudes partially cancel because they are out of phase (Fig. 1-15).
3. Initially, identical recurring processes that undergo dissimilar frequency changes over time eventually mutually cancel each other. Such processes, initially in phase and mutually reinforcing, become mutually destructive as they lose phase coherence (Fig. 1-16).

Recurring events (such as RF signals) with identical frequencies maintain phase coherence as long as they have the same relative amplitudes at all measurement times during a test period (see Fig. 1-14). A special case of phase coherence also must be considered. Signals of different frequencies alternately cancel and reinforce each other in a regular cyclical pattern, if the period of one signal is an integral multiple of the other. This results in periodic transient rephasing of the signals (alternating phase dispersion and phase convergence).

Loss of phase coherence. Immediately after the termination of the RF excitation pulse, all of the protons in the sample volume are in phase, relaxing to the lower energy state. At first they release identical energies; then things begin to change. *As individual protons are altered by higher or lower local magnetic fields to slightly different energy preferences, the period between packet release either shortens (higher field, higher frequency) or lengthens (lower field, lower frequency) and within a few milliseconds, phase coherence is lost entirely.* The MRI receiver senses a decaying signal that rapidly fades into the back-

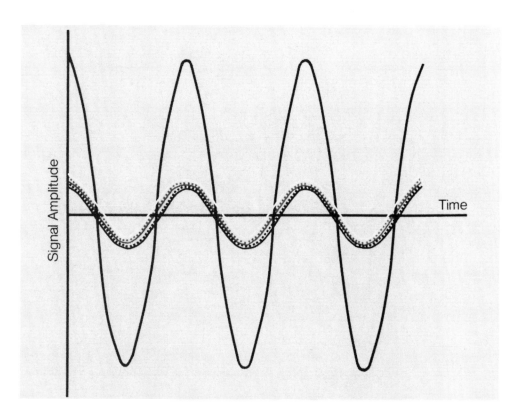

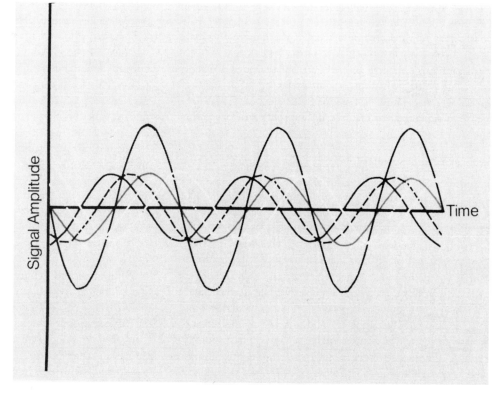

Fig. 1-16. From left to right (along the time axis) the phase difference among several otherwise identical sine waves increases rapidly. Mutual cancellation occurs to greater degree as the negative peaks of some waves begin to occur at the same time as the positive peaks of others. Although the individual waves have essentially the same amplitude at all times (in this idealized example), the net total signal of the population declines rapidly. The rapidity of signal decay is proportional to the rapidity of phase dispersion. (Reprinted with permission of Johnson and Johnson, Inc. From Hinshaw WS, Kramer DM, Yeung HN, Hill BC: The fundamentals of magnetic resonance imaging, Solon, Ohio, 1984, Technicare Corp.)

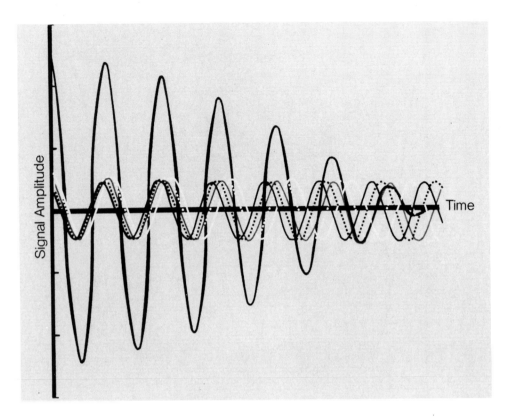

ground noise (see Fig. 1-8). Individually, the protons still are releasing RF energy (transmitting a signal) even after their combined signal fades away (see Fig. 1-16). The fade-out is not due to permanent spin-lattice energy loss but rather to random mixing and cancellation of signals due to phase dispersion (loss of phase coherence).

Latent signal. The initial short burst of signal from a population of resonating protons fades rapidly (see Fig. 1-8). Because individual protons still have energy to release, a signal can be restored if the problem of phase dispersion is overcome.

Restoring phase coherence

180-degree RF pulses. Protons respond to 180-degree RF pulses by instantly reversing their phase (Fig. 1-17). Antiparallel spins become parallel spins, and vice versa. The effect of this mirror-image phase reversal can be understood, in theory, as a temporary reversal of time. The phase-inverted waveform appears to move "backward in time," as if the clock had been reversed. If a 180-degree RF pulse follows a 90-degree pulse by time T, then phase coherence is restored momentarily, after a second interval T (Fig. 1-18). The effect is similar to the special case of phase coherence described earlier named "phase convergence." Phase convergence occurs at an integral multiple (2T) of the interval (T) between the 90- and 180-degree RF pulses. When the mirror-image period after the 180-degree pulse has elapsed, the MRI receiver detects a signal from the rephased protons (Fig. 1-19).

Magnetic field gradients. Similar phase reversal occurs when the magnetic field is intentionally altered so that proton energy preferences (and therefore frequencies) are forced to change in a controlled way. Instead of maintaining uniform flux density from right to left, for example, the field is altered so that the right side has higher flux density and the left side has lower flux density temporarily. This temporary inequality is called a magnetic field gradient (Fig. 1-20). The protons in the right side of the field advance in phase (because their frequency increases). The protons in the left side of the field resonate at lower frequency and lag in phase. Reversal of the gradient, so that the right side experiences low flux density and the left side experiences high flux density, causes a reversal of the initial phase relationships. After a few milliseconds, all of the protons momentarily converge again into phase. The end result is a temporary restoration of phase coherence after a mirror-image time period, similar to the 180-degree pulse example.

Spin echo and gradient echo. The rephased (formerly hidden but recoverable) signal is called either a spin echo or a gradient echo, depending on whether it was evoked by an RF pulse or by the application of magnetic field gradients. *The process of dephasing and rephasing can be repeated by a series of mirror-image pulses or magnetic field gradients.* However, the amplitude of each succeeding echo is smaller (Fig. 1-21). This loss of echo amplitude over time is evidence of the previously mentioned T2 decay process.

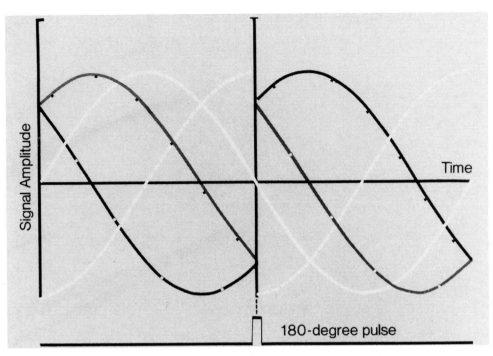

Fig. 1-17. Phase reversal by 180-degree shifting of sine waves along the x-axis. Amplitude advances instantaneously in response to a 180-degree pulse. In essence, a small time warp occurs. For instance, the white-dashed curve is transformed by the pulse instantly from maximum to mimimum peak value. Its phase is advanced by one-half cycle (180/360 degrees = 1/2 cycle). Its amplitude at the peak of the 180-degree pulse is the same as it was one-half cycle earlier, at the zero time point of this plot. Notice that the solid white curve is unchanged in phase by the 180-degree pulse, as its amplitude is zero at the instant of the pulse. All of the other curves flip in amplitude to the mirror-image (positive or negative) value across the x-axis at the peak of the 180-degree pulse. (Diagram modified from an original in Hinshaw WS, Kramer DM, Yeung HN, Hill BC: The fundamentals of magnetic resonance imaging, Solon, Ohio, 1984, Technicare Corp.)

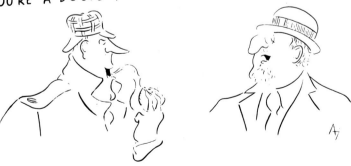

Fig. 1-18. If a 180-degree pulse follows a 90-degree pulse, then phase convergence is restored.

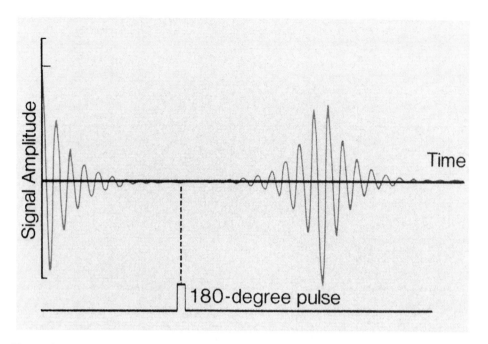

Fig. 1-19. Once phase reversal has been accomplished, either by a 180-degree pulse or by reversal of a magnetic field gradient, the trend toward increasing phase dispersion is converted to a trend toward phase coherence. If the rate of phase change (regardless of its direction) is constant throughout the experiment, then the rate of phase restoration after phase reversal equals the rate of phase dispersion before phase reversal. Thus, after an interval equal to the time between excitation pulse and phase-reversal, an echo occurs. (Reprinted with permission of Johnson and Johnson, Inc. From Hinshaw WS, Kramer DM, Yeung HN, Hill BC: The fundamentals of magnetic resonance imaging, Solon, Ohio, 1984, Technicare Corp.)

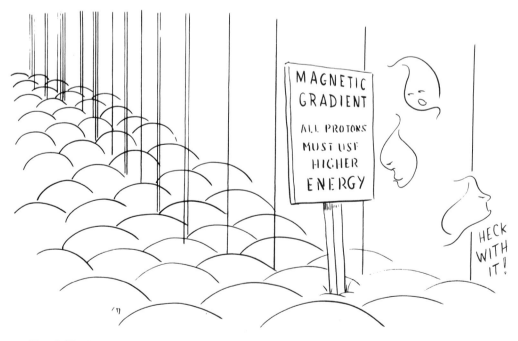

Fig. 1-20. A magnetic field gradient forces protons to alter their energy and, therefore, frequency.

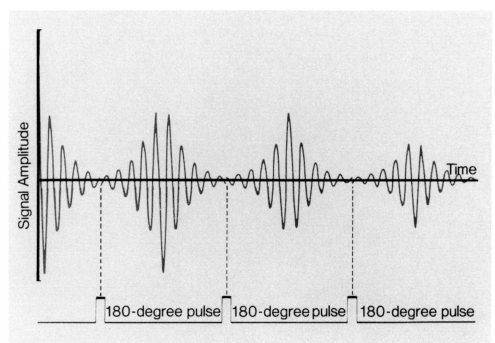

Fig. 1-21. Because the rate of phase dispersion is not constant for every proton in a sample of tissue throughout an MRI pulse sequence, full restoration of phase coherence is not achievable in a real-world experiment. Decay of maximum (echo signal) amplitude occurs at the T2 rate. The maximum amplitude of the echoes in this diagram decreases from left to right (the trailing echoes of the series show the effect of accumulating irreversible phase dispersion). (Reprinted with permission of Johnson and Johnson, Inc. From Hinshaw WS, Kramer DM, Yeung HN, Hill BC: The fundamentals of magnetic resonance imaging, Solon, Ohio, 1984, Technicare Corp.)

Reversible and irreversible phase dispersion

Dispersion proportional to time. The sequence of pulses and gradients used to produce multiple mirror-image echoes requires careful timing. The more echoes, the longer the duration of the entire sequence. The longer the time from the 90-degree pulse to an echo, the greater the diversity of phase among the population. Some of this phase dispersion is reversible; correcting it produces an echo. However, part of the phase dispersion is irreversible.

Stable differences in magnetic flux. The flux density of an imaging magnet varies slightly in different regions, but these variations are constant over time. The 180-degree spin-echo pulse is effective in dealing with the dephasing produced by such stable variations. Stable field variations produce reversible phase dispersion. The dephasing before the 180-degree pulse is the mirror image of that occurring after the pulse. Phases eventually realign, and an echo is formed (Fig. 1-19).

Variable local magnetic flux. At the level of the proton, even if the field imposed by the imaging magnet is stable at any one location, the local magnetic field nevertheless constantly changes as moving particles exert varying forces on each other (see Fig. 1-11). Depending on the magnetic "texture" of a particular material, the fluctuations vary in significance over time. Changes in the local magnetic environment of the proton before and after the 180-degree spin-echo pulse (or refocusing gradients) distort mirror image, which is the basis of phase restoration. Because perfect magnetic field symmetry is *not* present in the environment of the proton before and after attempted phase reversal, some of the potential signal is not recov-

ered (Fig. 1-21). In summary, irreversible phase dispersion results from rapid small variations in local magnetic fields, which transiently alter the energy (and, therefore, the frequency) of resonating protons in a random pattern.

T2: irreversible dephasing. Thus, each succeeding echo in a train of multiple echoes has smaller and smaller amplitude due to accumulation of irreversible phase dispersion. Decrease of peak signal amplitude in a train of echoes occurs at the T2 decay rate (Fig. 1-21).

T2: fat and water. Rapid T2 decay (rapid irreversible dephasing of transverse magnetization) leads to rapid irreversible loss of signal. For example, *the protons in fat tissue rapidly dephase; their T2 decay time is short. On the other hand, the protons of water dephase slowly; they have a long T2 decay time (Fig. 1-22).* Water still produces enough signal to be detectable long after the fat signal has vanished (see Fig. 1-12).

TISSUE CONTRAST PRINCIPLES
T1-weighting

As a general rule, *protons with long T2 decay times also have long T1 relaxation times.* In fact, the T1 time is always longer than (or at least equal to) the T2 time. Water has both long T1 and T2 decay times. Scanning sequences having rapidly repeating RF pulses represent water as an area of low signal strength. Sequences of this type are said to be **T1-weighted (T1W),** as the time between 90-degree pulses is short enough to bring out differences among tissues with various T1 relaxation rates. On the computer monitor or on a sheet of film, *water is usually depicted as a dark region on a T1W pulse sequence (Fig. 1-23).*

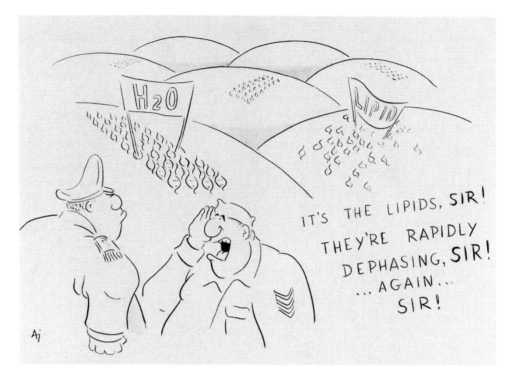

Fig. 1-22. Protons in fat rapidly dephase (short T2 decay time), while those in water dephase slowly (long T2 delay time).

Fat has short T1 and T2 times. Its protons recover quickly (release their stored energy quickly) after each 90-degree pulse. *On T1W sequences, fat is represented as an area of high signal strength,* which is usually depicted as a bright region on the computer monitor or on film (Fig. 1-23).

Pulse sequence parameters

TR and TE. *The time between 90-degree RF pulses is called the* **repetition time (TR)**. *The time delay between the 90-degree RF pulse and its echo is called the* **echo time (TE)** *(Fig. 1-24).*

Flip angle. *The angle of the RF excitation pulse is called the Ernst angle, tip angle, or* **flip angle.** Gradient-echo sequences can use flip angles of less than 90-degrees. Because less energy is carried by an RF pulse of less than 90 degrees, the effect on T1W contrast is similar to using a longer TR. The protons recover more easily from a milder pulse than from the full 90-degree pulse.

T2-weighting

Scanning sequences having long TE favor materials that have long T2 decay times. Sequences of this type are said to be **T2-weighted (T2W)** *because their TEs are long enough to bring out differences among tissues with various T2 decay rates. On the computer monitor or on a sheet of film,* water *is usually depicted as a bright region on a T2W pulse sequence (Fig. 1-25, B). The signal intensity of*

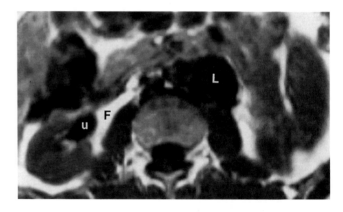

Fig. 1-23. Transaxial T1W MRI. Iatrogenous lymphocele. A lymphocele, containing primarily aqueous fluid *(L)*, has low intensity similar to urine in the right renal pelvis *(u)*. Retroperitoneal fat *(F)* has markedly higher intensity on this sequence.

fat decreases gradually versus the signal of water on each successive echo in a series of echoes (Fig. 1-25). Each echo is more heavily T2-weighted than the one that preceded it.

T2*-weighting

Gradient-echo sequences can be used to emphasize differences in the T2* relaxation rate of tissues. Heavy T2*-dephasing is represented as an area of very low signal intensity on gradient echo sequences. Deposits of hemosi-

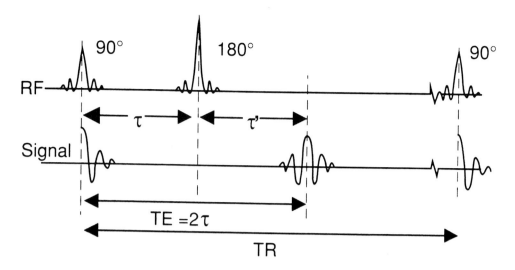

Fig. 1-24. Spin-echo pulse sequence diagram. The interval *(T)* between the 90-degree pulse and 180-degree pulse is equal to the interval *(T′)* between the 180-degree pulse and the echo. (Courtesy of Siemens Medical Systems.)

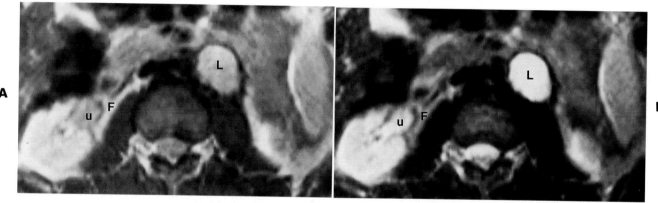

Fig. 1-25. Transaxial T2W MRI. Same case as Fig. 1-23. Iatrogenous lymphocele. **A,** The signal intensity of fat *(F)* is only slightly greater than the intensity of lymphocele fluid *(L)* and urine *(u)* on this first echo of a dual echo T1-weighted sequence (TE = 45 msec). **B,** The signal intensity of fat *(F)* is less than lymphocele fluid *(L)* and urine *(u)* on the second echo (TE = 90 msec). As measurements are made at longer TEs, the absolute signal intensity of water decreases very slowly. The signal intensity of fat drops quickly, however, as expected from its steep T2W decay curve. Thus, the relative hyperintensity of water on an image with TE = 90 msec is not due to the signal of water increasing in any way. Compared to other substances in the field of view that have undergone rapid signal decay between 0 and 90 msec, the small remaining signal of water is relatively hyperintense.

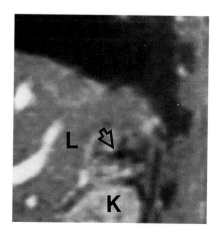

Fig. 1-26. Gradient echo sagittal MRI. Melanoma metastasis to the adrenal gland. Central low intensity *(open arrow)* has been produced by hemosiderin (residual product of an old hemorrhage) or by deposition of paramagnetic pigment material (such as melanin). Kidney *(K)*. Liver *(L)*.

derin (long after an episode of bleeding) have high **susceptibility** to T2* dephasing. Hemosiderin and other paramagnetic substances usually are depicted as a dark region on the computer monitor or on film (Fig. 1-26).

GLOSSARY

angular momentum (L) measures a rotational property of motion. $L = mv_pr$ where m = mass of the moving object, v_p = the component of velocity perpendicular to the line between the moving object and the reference point, and r is the distance from object to reference point.

atomic mass units (a.m.u.) the mass of one proton or neutron. 1.6726×10^{-24} g.

Avogadro's number (N_o) the number of particles in one mole of a substance; the number of **atomic mass units** in 1 unit of a substance. $N_o = 6.0225 \times 10^{23}$ particles/mole or a.m.u./g.

charge (+ or −) K.W. Ford[5] defines charge "as being like French perfume. It is that certain something worn by particles which makes them attractive . . ."

classical mechanics physics according to Newton. His laws describe ordinary observations, but break down for special cases such as objects traveling near the speed of light and certain properties and behaviors of microscopic particles.

computed tomography (CT) cross-sectional imaging modality using an x-ray source rotating around an object to produce a two-dimensional record of x-ray attenuation values.

correlation time (τ_c) the time for one rotational or translational unit of motion of a particle. It is used indirectly as an index of the quality of interaction between moving particles; it is the reciprocal of the frequency of particle motion. Ian Young (citing Bloembergen, Purcell, and Pound's work) reminds us that relaxation times are a complex function of τ_c and ω_o (resonant frequency).[12]

cross-sectional imaging the process of making images of an object, which are bounded by the intersection of the perimeter of the object with any plane passing through its volume. See **computed tomography** and **magnetic resonance imaging.**

echo time (TE) the delay between an RF excitation pulse and the resulting MR signal. Measurement is from the midpoint of the pulse to the midpoint of the RF echo. Typical values range from 8 to 30 msec for T1W spin-echo sequences and 60 to 120 msec for T2W sequences. See **repetition time.**

electromagnetic field Halliday and Resnick[6] define a field as "any physical quantity which can be specified simultaneously for all points within a given region of interest." Ford[5] calls a field a "nebulous physical substance . . . that can propagate as a wave through space and that can carry energy and momentum and mass and **charge** and other measurable quantities . . ." He continues, saying "it has a definite mass associated with it." In quantum mechanics, all types of particles are "regarded as the quantum lumps of an underlying field."

electron (e^-) negatively charged particle with mass of 5.4860×10^{-4} **a.m.u.** Identified as such by J.J. Thompson in 1897, who found it to be the smallest unit of negative charge. Murray Gell-Mann proposes a family of "subparticles" carrying fractional electric charges. If he is correct, these particles, called "quarks," would become the "new" unit of charge (until the next layer is uncovered?). An electron, according to quantum theory, can possibly be located outside the atom or inside the nucleus but is far more likely to be found in the atom, outside the nucleus.

energy (E) "the capacity to do work." In relativistic terms is equal to $-Dm_oc^2$ where $-Dm_o$ is the difference in mass observed after atomic fission versus before fission and c is the speed of light (3×10^8 meters/sec). Energy is conserved. Although it may be transformed into any of its various forms (such as heat, kinetic energy, potential energy, sound, light, electricity, magnetism), none is destroyed or created.

energy states the proton exists in either of two energy states. Think of them not as high or low, but as low and nearly as low. . . . because every other possible energy state is very much higher (and therefore much less probable). The probability of finding a proton in the lowest energy state is the highest. It is just a squeak more probable than the lowest state, however. (By very slim odds; only a 1,000,001:1,000,000 advantage; that is the same as saying "one in a million excess").

exponential decay (e^{-kt}) the decrease of a quantity over time as a function of the number e (2.71828, approximately). Where k is a decay constant which is characteristic of a given system under given conditions and t is the time elapsed since the beginning of the decay process. Three decay constants used frequently in MRI are T1, T2, and T2*. In this chapter, the "T's" signify relaxation times. The inverse of relaxation time is relaxation rate. A short T1 relaxation time yields a high T1 relaxation rate (rapid relaxation; rapid recovery of longitudinal magnetization). Incidentally, the slope of the exponential function e^{-kt} is proportional to the value of the function at any given point t. In other words, the instantaneous rate of decay at any given time after the start of a decay process is equal to the population remaining in the sample at that time.[5] Example from MRI: the rate of decrease in signal strength at any time (TE) after the 90-degree pulse is proportional to the remaining signal amplitude at that TE. In general: the stronger the signal, the faster the rate of decay. No other mathematical function links sample size and decay rate in this way; the relationship is unique to functions of the number "e."

field strength (T) common name for the flux density of a magnetic field; the density of the lines of force. The unit of magnetic flux is the Weber (Wb). Flux density is stated as Wb/meter^2 and expressed as the units gauss (G) or tesla (T). The earth's magnetic field is approximately 0.5 to 1.0 gauss on the surface. 1 T = 10,000 G. 1 mT (1 millitesla) = 10 G. The actual SI units for "field strength" are amperes/meter.

flip angle (θ) the phase angle of the sine function which determines the amplitude of an MR signal as a function of RF pulse strength. RF pulse strength is the product of pulse amplitude times pulse duration. In practice, amplitude usually is constant and pulse strength is modulated by lengthening or shortening the pulse. A 90-degree pulse contains the smallest amount of energy sufficient to induce maximum MR response from a sample. In the **vector,** rotating frame-of-reference model of MR, θ is the angle of the **net magnetization vector (M)** with respect to the Z-axis, following an RF excitation pulse. Rotation to angle θ occurs because of the precession of M about longitudinal axis of the B_1 magnetic field, which is produced by the RF excitation pulse. The B_1 field must be perpendicular to the B_0 field in order to be effective.

frequency (Hz) the number of occurrences of an event per unit of time. 1 Hz = 1 cycle per second. 1000 Hz = 1 kHz. 1,000,000 Hz = 1 MHz (1 megahertz). See **Hertz, Heinrich R.**

gyromagnetic ratio (γ) a constant that uniquely links the magnetic resonance frequency of an atom to a magnetic field strength. The relationship is expressed by the Larmor equation: $f_{resonance} = \gamma \times B_o$, where $f_{resonance}$ is the resonant frequency in megahertz, γ is the gyromagnetic ratio in MHz/T, and B_o is the flux density of the main magnetic field in T. See **Larmor equation.**

Hertz, Heinrich R Dr. Hertz (1857-1894), a German physicist, developed sending and receiving devices for electromagnetic waves, which he used to verify Maxwell's theoretical work. The unit of frequency now bears his name. See **frequency.**

imaging modality type of diagnostic radiology examination such as **CT,** ultrasonography, plain film radiography, nuclear medicine, angiography, or MRI.

ionizing radiation high energy electromagnetic radiation consisting of photons with energy of ≤15 eV (electron volts). This is sufficient to separate the electrons and protons of atoms or molecules to produce charged ions. Diagnostic x-rays, radiation for cancer therapy, and cosmic radiation are examples of ionizing radiation, in order of increasing energy (and frequency). $E = h\nu$, where E = photon energy, h = Planck's constant $(6.63 \times 10^{-34}$ J·sec), and ν = frequency.

Larmor equation Sir Joseph Larmor (1857-1942) found that the frequency of precession of a charged particle placed in a magnetic field is equal to the electronic charge times the strength of the magnetic field divided by 4π times the mass. [8] Expressed in other terms, the relationship between the frequency of resonance (frequency of precession) and magnetic field strength is $f_{resonance} = \gamma \times B_o$, where $f_{resonance}$ is the frequency of resonance in megahertz, γ is the gyromagnetic ratio in MHz/T, and B_o is the strength of the main magnetic field in T. See **particles** for more about Joseph Larmor.

Larmor frequency (f_{Larmor}) the frequency of resonance of the protons of a particular element in a magnetic field of any given strength. The frequency is calculated by using the **Larmor equation.**

macroscopic domain, macroscopic world the world of objects and forces that is the context of our everyday existence.

magnetic moment (μ) the force arising from interaction of a single particle's magnetic field with another field. An indirect indicator of the strength of a particle's magnetic field.

magnetic resonance (MR) sometimes used as an abbreviation for magnetic resonance imaging (MRI). Also the phenomenon of field strength-dependent resonance of particles that is the basis of the signals detected by MRI scanners. Dr. FW Wehrli describes it this way: "In MR, resonance occurs when radiofrequency (RF) energy is applied at the Larmor frequency, flipping the **magnetic moments** from their m = +1/2 (lower energy) to their m = −1/2 (higher energy) states."

magnetic resonance imaging (MRI) a diagnostic imaging modality by which cross-sectional and volume images of objects are obtained by sampling radio signals from protons that are "under the influence" of magnetic fields.

mass (m) quantity of matter. Note that mass is not equivalent to weight. Weight is a force. In ordinary circumstances, weight is mass times gravity.

nanosecond (nsec) one billionth of a second. If this seems like a long time, either you are a subatomic particle or your watch is fast.

net magnetization vector (M) the sum of all the magnetic forces of the protons in the scanned volume. The individual magnetic moments (μ) are considered mathematically to be vectors (magnetic forces with specific directional orientation at any given time). By the rules of vector arithmetic, the multitude of tiny individual forces sum up to the whole.

neutron (n) a **nucleon** having no charge, but having spin and a mass of 1.00867 **a.m.u.** $(1.6750 \times 10^{-27}$ kg).

nucleon subatomic particle existing in the nucleus except when the rules of probability in quantum mechanics allow its location to be elsewhere temporarily. Examples include **protons, neutrons,** neutrinos, mesons, baryons.

number of protons in the body a 70 kg person with 70% of body weight as water would contain 49 liters of water. 49 liters is (49000 g/18 g/mole) or 2722 moles of water. Each mole of water contains 2 moles of hydrogen, for a total of 4744 moles of hydrogen. $4744 \times (6.0225 \times 10^{23}$ particles/mole) = 2.857×10^{27}. The protons of fat raise the number significantly higher yet.

packet a quantum of energy. Essentially a "bundle"; a particle; a photon.

particles Democritus (c. 470 BC) imagined all matter to be composed of eternal, unchangeable tiny particles, which he called "atoms." The word in Greek means "indestructible." J.J. Thompson in 1897 described a specific particle—the electron—as the smallest unit of negative charge. An unsung hero in the story of particles is Sir Joseph Larmor (1857-1942), who in 1894 and 1895 published articles proposing discrete charged particles as centers of "rotational strain in the ether." According to A.E. Woodruff, Larmor also discussed the relation between a microscopic theory treating the dynamics of the electron and a macroscopic theory in which the current and other variables are treated as statistical averages. He published these thoughts 2 years before Thompson described the electron. Both men were on the Cambridge faculty.[12]

phase (ϕ) the relative positions of identical portions of two waveforms. Two sine wave signals of equal frequency beginning at the same time are identical at all measurement times. Slight decrease or increase of the period of one of the signals (slight increase or decrease of the frequency) causes it to lead or lag the other signal with respect to phase. Engineers express phase differences as the angle f, which lies in the range of 0 to 360 degrees. Two equal sine wave signals 180 degrees apart exactly cancel each other, so that when added continuously over time, the output is always zero. Two equal sine wave signals 0 or 360 degrees apart exactly reinforce each other when added, so that the output is two times the amplitude of either one. The output of adding two equal sine wave signals separated by any other phase angle is a periodic function (the output varies from maximum to minimum repetitively with a constant period between identical states).

phase coherence signals in phase; their amplitudes add arithmetically. No canceling of signal due to phase dispersion. Restoration of phase coherence is the object of refocusing gradients and 180-degree refocusing pulses.

photon a particle of energy. A photon has quantum spin but has no mass and no charge. The energy content of a photon is proportional to the frequency of the electromagnetic energy which it contains. $E = hv$ describes the relationship, in which: E = energy, h = **Planck's constant,** and v = frequency.

Planck's constant (h) called by its discoverer, the "elementary **quantum** of action," h has a value of 6.626×10^{-34} joule-seconds. Max Planck, a German physicist at the turn of the twentieth century, tackled the problem of describing the behavior of black-body radiators. He brilliantly reconciled the existing theories of his day, and then broke through to an entirely new understanding of energy, which is the foundation of quantum theory. In the process, he made the remarkable discovery that $E = hv$, where E is energy and v is frequency.

proton (p) the hero of this saga. Stalwart nucleon and resonant protagonist of the highest order. Charge (in coulombs) = 1.60×10^{-19} C. Mass (at rest) = 1.67×10^{-27} kg—a ratio of 1836.15152 times the mass of an electron.[6] Spin quantum number (I) = 1/2. Magnetic quantum numbers (m) = +1/2 and −1/2.

proton density (PD) an MRI scan sequence in which the contrast between tissues depends only on the relative abundance of mobile hydrogen atoms. Ideally, a PD sequence would be obtained with an infinitely short **TE** and an infinitely long **TR**. In practice, the first echo of a dual echo T2W sequence is often substituted for the ideal sequence. Thus, the "so-called" proton density scan usually is a lightly T2-weighted scan. Gradient-echo sequences with small **flip angles** (θ) superficially resemble T2-weighted contrast but actually are closer to PD (combined with **T2***).

quantum an indivisible particle of something. A unit of energy or spin, for instance. In Latin, the word "quantum" means: "How much?"

quantum mechanics a system of mathematical analysis involving quanta. Max Planck (1858-1947) worked out the conversion factor between frequency and energy while solving a problem concerning the light emitted by a heated metal object.[6] Einstein and Bohr followed close behind, using Planck's theory to explain other phenomena that could not be explained by classical mechanics (in which energy is infinitely divisible, rather than in particles). All of modern physics is built on quantum mechanical principles.

radians (R) a unit of arc of a circle. 2π radians of arc equal 360 degrees. One radian is $360/2\pi$, or approximately 57 degrees.

radiofrequency (RF) the range of frequencies in the electromagnetic spectrum from approximately 10 kHz to 300 gHz (10 kHz to 300 gHz; 10,000 to 300,000,000,000 cycles per second) is the radiofrequency region. In clinical MRI, the resonant frequency of hydrogen protons ranges from approximately 4.2 to 197.4 mHz in 0.1 T to 4.7 magnets.

repetition time (TR) the time between successive RF excitation pulses. Measurement is from midpoint to midpoint of each pulse. Typical values range from 300 to 1000 msec for T1W spin-echo sequences and over 2000 for T2W sequences. See **echo time.**

resonant frequency see **Larmor frequency** and **magnetic resonance.**

spin (m_s) a quantum number. A variable of the motion of a particle, which can be thought of as rotation. A concept introduced to explain changes in the electromagnetic spectra of electrons, known as the Zeeman effect.

spin-lattice interactions the transfer of energy to or from a particle to its environment. T1 relaxation occurs by loss of proton energy to the surrounding lattice of molecules.

spin-spin interactions the transfer of energy between protons. This is the mechanism of T2 decay.

submicroscopic domain the world of molecules, atoms, and subatomic particles.

susceptibility (χ_m) a constant describing the tendency of a substance to be magnetized by an applied field. $\chi_m = \mu/(1+4\pi)$, where μ designates permeability. Variations in susceptibility of adjacent tissue volumes lead to clinically significant local magnetic field inhomogeneity. For example, bowel gas magnetizes far less than adjacent water-containing structures, leading to field inhomogeneity, which produces a low intensity artifact due to irrecoverable phase dispersion.

T1 relaxation time (T1R) the time constant describing the rate of energy loss by antiparallel (high energy) protons to their environment (the lattice). In the vector, rotating frame-of-reference model of MR, this is the time constant of recovery of the Z-axis component of magnetization after a 90-degree RF pulse.

T2 decay time (T2R) the time constant describing the rate of MR signal decay as energy is shared by antiparallel (high energy) protons with other protons. This time describes the effect of increasing phase dispersion, which destroys the coherence of the proton signals. They eventually cancel out each other. In the vector, rotating frame-of-reference model of MR, this is the time constant of disappearance of the transverse component of magnetization.

T2* decay (T2*) the time constant describing the rapid loss of phase coherence brought about by inhomogeneity of the magnetic field. Roughly a factor of 10 shorter than T2.

TE see **echo time.**

tesla (T) the unit of magnetic flux density. 1 T = 10,000 gauss. The tesla is often inaccurately called the unit of magnetic field strength. Nikola Tesla (1856-1943) made alternating current practical for widespread use by electric power companies by developing transformers and inventing the A.C. motor. He did all of this in spite of the virulent opposition of Thomas Edison. He earned the honor of this "unit" fair and square.

time constant the time at which a value has increased to within $(1 - e^{-1})$, or approximately 63%, of its maximum value (or the time at which a value has decreased by 63% from its maximum value).

TR see **repetition time.**

vector ($\longrightarrow$) an entity having both magnitude and direction. Its symbol is an arrow whose length signifies its magnitude and whose orientation signifies its direction. Simplified vector models of MRI portray as stationary vectors, forces which actually are rotating at the **Larmor frequency.**

velocity (V) speed in a certain direction. V = dT (where d = distance and T = time).

wave (~) PCW Davies defines an electromagnetic wave as an "undulation of electric and magnetic force . . . a moving and changing field." Imagine, for a moment, that you are at the beach . . .

REFERENCES

1. Asimov I: Asimov's biographical encyclopedia of science and technology, Garden City, NY, 1972, Doubleday.

2. Curry TS, Dowdey JE, Murry RC Jr: Christensen's physics of diagnostic radiology, ed 4, Philadelphia, 1990, Lea & Febiger.

3. Davies PCW: The search for gravity waves, New York, 1980, Cambridge University Press.

4. Edelman RR, Hesselink JR: Clinical magnetic resonance imaging, Philadelphia, 1990, WB Saunders.

5. Ford KW: Basic physics, Waltham, Mass, 1968, Blaisdel Publishing.

6. Halliday D, Resnick R: Fundamentals of physics, New York, 1981, John Wiley.

7. Harms SE, Morgan TJ, Yamanashi WS, et al: Principles of nuclear magnetic resonance imaging, Radiographics 4:26-43, 1984.

8. Hinshaw WS, Kramer DM, Yeung HN, Hill BC: The fundamentals of magnetic resonance imaging, Solon, Ohio, 1984, Technicare Corp.

9. Stein J, Urdang L, editors: Random House dictionary of the English language, Unabridged Edition, New York, 1969, Random House.

10. Saini S, Frankel RB, Stark DD, Ferrucci JT: Magnetism: a primer and review, Am J Roentgenol 150:735-743, 1988.

11. Wehrli FW: Principles of magnetic resonance. In Stark DD, Bradley WG, editors: Magnetic resonance imaging, St Louis, 1988, Mosby–Year Book.

12. Woodruff AE: Joseph Larmor. In Gillispie CC, Lane JH, Macquer PJ, editors: Dictionary of scientific biography, New York, 1973, Charles Scribner's Sons.

13. Young IR: Special pulse sequences and techniques. In Stark DD, Bradley WG, editors: Magnetic resonance imaging, St Louis, 1988, Mosby–Year Book.

14. FLASH and FISP Gradient Echo Pulse Sequences, Publication No. MG/5000-217-121, Siemens Medical Systems, Inc.,Iselin, NJ.

Chapter 2

TECHNIQUE

W. Dean Bidgood, Jr.
Barry B. Kraus

Attention to technique is essential to perform clinically useful abdominal MRI studies. We consider this chapter "compulsory" reading to master daily abdominal MRI protocols. The sections of this chapter—covering plane and pulse selection, signal-to-noise ratio optimization, artifacts (recognition and control), special techniques, and coil selection—provide a guide to navigate through abdominal MRI technique.

SCAN PLAN SELECTION
CT and MRI comparison

Since the late 1970s, computed tomography (CT) has set the standards for cross-sectional imaging of the abdomen and pelvis. CT image contrast depends on differences in electron density among body tissues. Because this value, for most tissues, falls in a relatively narrow range, the soft tissue contrast resolution, contrast-to-noise ratio (CNR), of CT is limited. CT provides clinically satisfactory spatial resolution in the axial plane while maintaining good signal-to-noise ratio (SNR). However, the transaxial plane is the only orientation available for scanning of the abdomen. Reformatting of other planes introduces imprecision in spatial resolution due to the thickness of slices in the longitudinal direction. Although slip ring (spiral) scanning improves this limitation of CT, spatial resolution in CT always will be limited by hardware.

Magnetic resonance imaging (MRI) provides superior tissue contrast in multiple imaging planes, allowing for detection of lesions which are below the contrast-to-noise threshold of CT. However, the MRI operator must contend with numerous artifacts and must compromise on spatial resolution, as compared to CT, for large fields of view. To maximize image quality and minimize artifacts, proper choice of pulse sequence parameters is necessary. A broad variety of scan acquisition options demand careful consideration to produce optimal SNR and CNR. Special imaging techniques and radiofrequency (RF) coil designs are available to enhance specific applications.

Principles of scan plane selection

The ability to freely select cross-sectional orientation is a significant contribution of MRI to large field-of-view

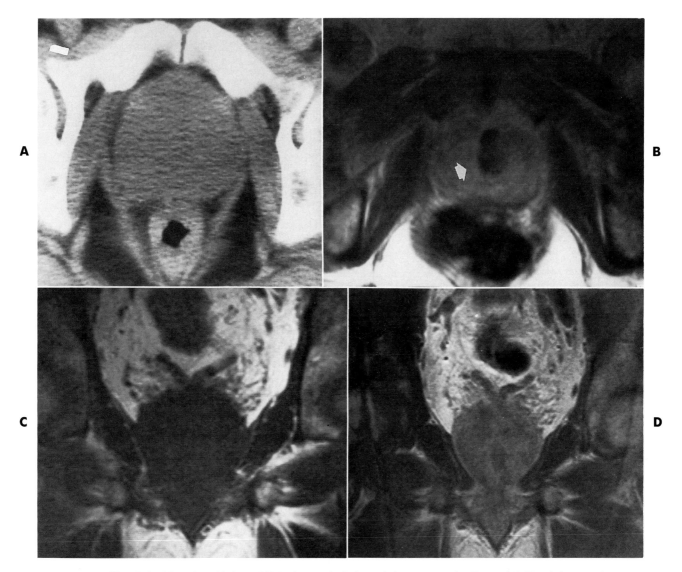

Fig. 2-1. CT and multiplanar MRI of a cystic lesion of the prostate. **A,** Transaxial CT of the prostate, with iodine contrast. **B,** T1W MRI with IV gadolinium contrast clearly depicts a cystic lesion *(white arrow).* **C,** Coronal T1W MRI with no IV contrast. Seminal vesicles, retroperitoneal vessels, and floor of pelvis demonstrated. Cystic lesion is not visible. **D,** T1W MRI with gadolinium. Retroperitoneal fat and vessels, prostatic tissue, cystic lesion, and pelvic side walls are well demonstrated. *Continued.*

(FOV) abdominal imaging (Fig. 2-1). The first section of this chapter reviews the principles of scan plane selection. CT examinations facilitate planning of MRI, as time and throughput considerations limit the complexity of a given MRI examination. Correlation with prior CT studies defines the area of interest to better advantage and focuses the application of the more versatile MRI to the significant clinical questions.

Transverse plane. Familiarity with transverse ana-

tomic relationships from experience with CT scanning allows the radiologist to make an easy transition to transverse MR images. The transverse plane is standard for nearly all abdominal and pelvic MR examinations; CT and MR transverse sections are directly comparable (Figs. 2-1, *A* and *B,* and 2-2, *A* and *B*). Because the abdominal diameter generally is greater in the craniocaudad dimension than in the transverse dimension, a relatively smaller field of view can be used to include the entire abdomen in the

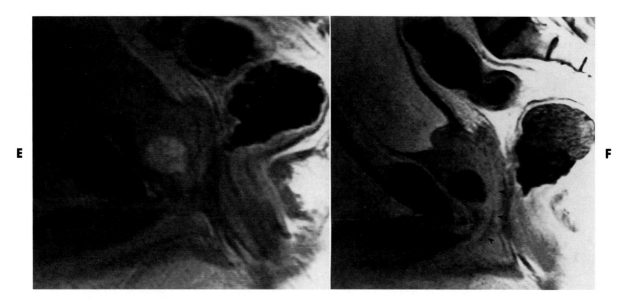

Fig. 2-1, cont'd. E, T2W sagittal MRI reveals the heterogeneous character of the cystic lesion. **F,** T1W sagittal section with gadolinium. Relationship of the prostate to the bladder base and rectum demonstrated well. Cystic lesion displaces the urethra *(arrowheads)* posteriorly.

transverse plane than in either the sagittal or coronal planes. Use of a relatively smaller field of view allows for better spatial resolution. In order to include the requisite number of sections to survey the entire abdomen and pelvis in one scan, however, TR must be prolonged versus comparable volume coverage with coronal sections.

Coronal plane. Coronal images clearly display anatomic relationships that transverse images cannot display (Figs. 2-1, *B* and *C,* and 2-2, *B* and *C*). This plane may help determine the origin and relationships of large masses in the upper abdomen. Coronal imaging is especially useful for interpreting subdiaphragmatic pathology; disease in the dome of the liver; and pathology affecting the aorta, inferior vena cava, hepatic veins, portal vein, and superior mesenteric vessels. Also well depicted are the kidneys, adrenals, psoas muscles, other retroperitoneal structures, and the genitourinary system. A large field of view may be used to cover the entire abdomen and pelvis in one set of images, thereby reducing scan time at the expense of spatial resolution. However, the smaller anteroposterior distance (relative to the superoinferior distance covered with transverse images) allows one to obtain more, thinner slices in the same scan time. This increases resolution in the slice-selection direction.

Sagittal plane. Sagittal images enhance the evaluation of pathology near the dome of the liver and the diaphragm (Fig. 2-3). They are also useful in the pelvis, where many structures lying in or near the midline may be viewed entirely within one image (Fig. 2-1, *E* and *F*). These structures include the bladder, prostate, urethra, penis, uterus, rectum, retropubic space, rectovesical space, and rectouterine space. The parasagittal plane displays the seminal vesicles, testes, spermatic cord, and ovaries. Adequate imaging of the pelvis must include sagittal images from the top of the bladder to the rectum and from hip joint to hip joint.

Oblique plane. Used less commonly than they probably should be, oblique images are reserved for specific indications. An oblique sequence oriented parallel or perpendicular to the course of the portal vein may facilitate examination of hepatic hilus pathology. Oblique sections of the pancreas prevent the foreshortening, which plagues CT assessment of that organ (Fig. 2-4). Assessment of masses near the lumbar vertebrae may require oblique images oriented parallel to the intervertebral disk space. Oblique coronal sections are useful for demonstrating the uterus, broad ligaments, and ovaries. Optimal orientation of oblique scan planes must be tailored individually.

PULSE SEQUENCE SELECTION

Current MRI technology uses one of two basic paradigms for producing signals for diagnostic imaging: the spin-echo and gradient-echo techniques. The clinical utility of each will be examined in the following sections.

Principles

Spin echo. Long the standard imaging sequence in clinical use, spin echo uses a 180-degree RF pulse at time

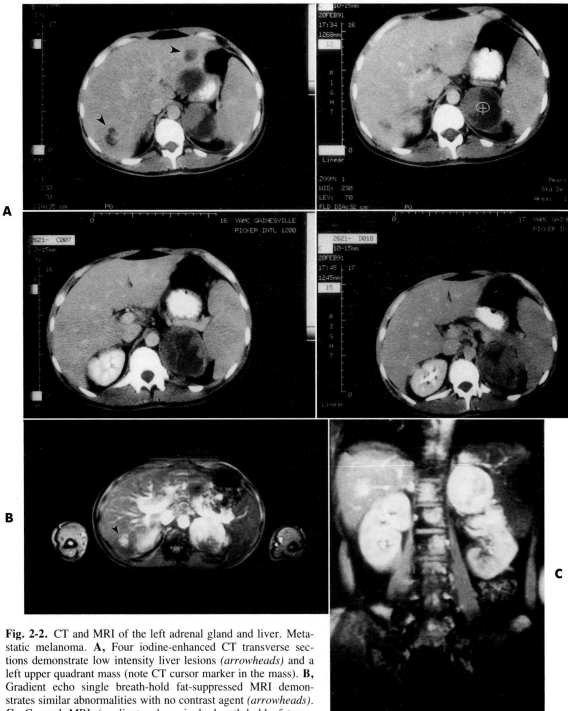

Fig. 2-2. CT and MRI of the left adrenal gland and liver. Metastatic melanoma. **A,** Four iodine-enhanced CT transverse sections demonstrate low intensity liver lesions *(arrowheads)* and a left upper quadrant mass (note CT cursor marker in the mass). **B,** Gradient echo single breath-hold fat-suppressed MRI demonstrates similar abnormalities with no contrast agent *(arrowheads)*. **C,** Coronal MRI (gradient echo, single breath-hold, fat-suppressed) demonstrates the relationships of the mass to better advantage, allowing precise localization to the adrenal gland. Liver metastasis also visible.

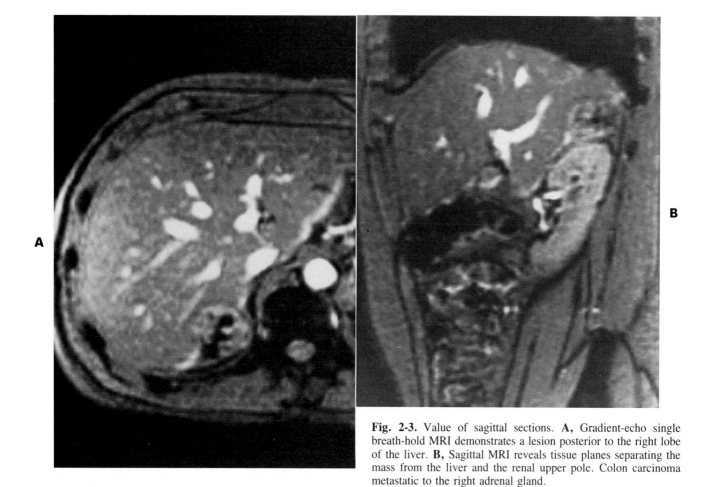

Fig. 2-3. Value of sagittal sections. **A,** Gradient-echo single breath-hold MRI demonstrates a lesion posterior to the right lobe of the liver. **B,** Sagittal MRI reveals tissue planes separating the mass from the liver and the renal upper pole. Colon carcinoma metastatic to the right adrenal gland.

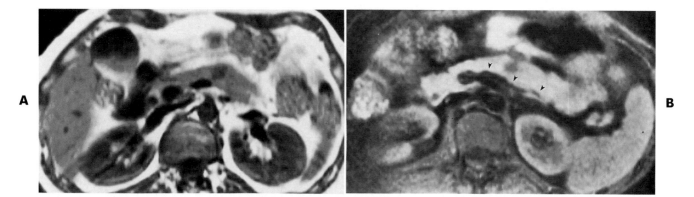

Fig. 2-4. Oblique section of the pancreas. **A,** Transverse T1W MRI of the pancreas. Conventional orientation. **B,** Oblique T1W MRI of the pancreas. On this fat-suppressed image, the intensity of the pancreas is greater with respect to the surrounding fat. The full length of the gland is appreciated on a single section. Note the visibility of a longer segment of the splenic vein than in Fig. 2-4, *A (arrowheads).*

T to rephase the proton spins in the transverse plane at time 2T after the initial 90-degree RF pulse (Fig. 2-5, *A*). Spin-echo sequences provide reliable tissue contrast and good SNR. Drawbacks include unreliable blood-pool signal and long scan times (Fig. 2-6). To exploit the differences in relaxation rates of various normal and pathologic tissues, one should obtain both T1-weighted and T2-weighted spin-echo images (Fig. 2-7).[5,10,86]

Because each organ has a characteristic range of T1 and T2 values, optimum imaging might seem to require choosing the repetition time (TR) and echo time (TE) to best image each tissue; however, neither is practical nor necessary for several reasons. First, the tissue type of interest is often not known before the scan is performed (for example, the patient referred to evaluate "abdominal pain"). Second, abnormalities often affect many tissues within the abdomen and pelvis, making it necessary to choose a set of parameters that would provide nearly optimal contrast in all tissues. Third, many choices for TR and TE would make sequence setup more difficult and increase study time, thereby reducing patient throughput.

To obtain T1-weighted spin-echo images, a TR of 300 to 1000 msec is a good compromise range for all tissues within the abdomen and pelvis. The longer values are used when examination requires a large number of sections.

The TE should be as low as possible to ensure strong T1 weighting. The receiver sampling time and the rate of switching of encoding gradients limit the minimum obtainable TE with the spin-echo technique. Many currently used systems can attain a TE of approximately 15 msec.

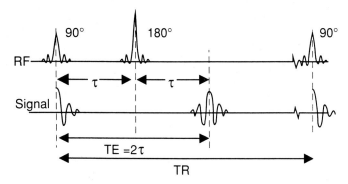

Fig. 2-5. Spin echo pulse sequence diagram. The echo returns at time = 2T. The 180-degree pulse is exactly at the midpoint of the TE interval. The next excitation by a 90-degree pulse begins after a delay, at repetition time TR. (From FLASH and FISP gradient echo pulse sequences, Publication No MG/5000-217-121, Siemens Medical Systems, Inc, Iselin, NJ.)

Fig. 2-6. MRI of pancreatitis with biliary obstruction. **A,** Axial T1W. Bile has low intensity signal. The spleen and kidneys are hypointense to the liver. **B,** Axial T2W. Reversal of spleen/kidneys versus liver intensities. Bile ducts have high intensity. The heterogeneous signal of the inflamed pancreas is slightly hypointense to the spleen. **C,** Single breath-hold, fat-suppressed gradient echo MRI with flow compensation. Consistently bright vessels. Note the visibility of portal vein branches, better than on spin-echo sequences. Fatty replacement of left lobe of liver enhanced by fat-suppression *(small arrowheads)*. Varices *(large arrow)* are distinctly visible left of the aorta.

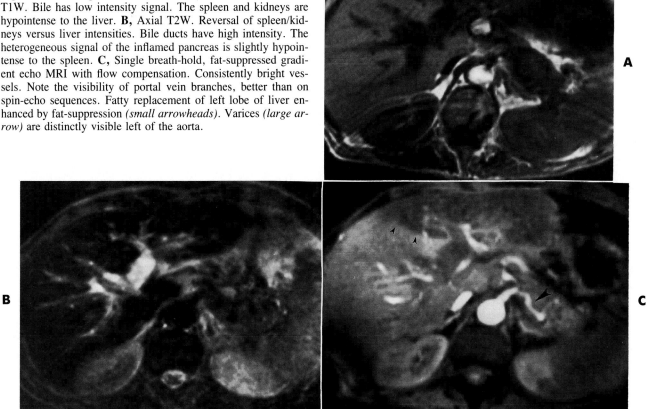

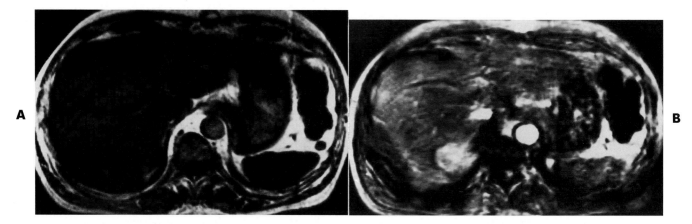

Fig. 2-7. T1W and T2W scans are effective in pairs. **A,** Axial T1W. The right lobe of the liver has nearly homogeneous low intensity. **B,** Axial T2W. A high intensity mass is present in the posterior right hepatic lobe. However, motion artifact is greater on this long TR, long TE scan than on the T1W scan (**A**).

TEs in the range of 30 msec or shorter ensure strong T1 weighting.

To obtain T2 weighted spin-echo images, a long TE is used. A TE of 45 to 60 msec provides moderate T2 weighting; a TE of 80 to 120 msec ensures strong T2 weighting. A TR of approximately 2000 msec is preferred for the upper abdomen. This represents a compromise among tissue contrast, SNR, and reduction of artifacts. On occasion, a TR of up to 3000 msec is used, but the resultant images are degraded by motion artifacts. A TR of 2500 msec typically is adequate for the pelvis, where motion artifact is less troublesome. Variable bandwidth dual echo T2-weighted sequences are available to optimize SNR for the second echo while still reserving time in the sequence for collection of an adequate first echo (a discussion on bandwidth follows later in this chapter).

T1-weighted spin-echo images provide excellent spatial resolution and SNR with minimal artifacts (Fig. 2-6, *A*). These images are used to examine anatomic detail but often provide inadequate contrast between normal and pathologic tissue. T2-weighted spin-echo images provide excellent contrast between tissue and water at the expense of spatial resolution, SNR, and increased artifacts (Fig. 2-7, *B*). Because most masses and infiltrative processes in the abdomen alter the water content of the affected tissue, T2 weighting is appropriate. These images should be used to evaluate areas of pathology that require improved CNR.

For evaluation of anatomic variations (when anatomic detail is more important than tissue contrast), one may obtain sufficient information from just T1-weighted images. For evaluation of any suspected pathology, both T1- and T2-weighted sequences are recommended.

Gradient echo. Gradient-echo sequences use symmetric pulsed gradient fields to rephase the proton spins in the transverse plane after the initial RF pulse (Fig. 2-8).[10,33,37]

The initial RF pulse uses a flip angle of less than or equal to 90 degrees. Smaller flip angles allow the longitudinal component of the signal to make a full recovery faster. Elimination of the 180-degree refocusing pulse also reduces greatly the RF deposition to the patient (by a factor of 5 or greater).[31] Gradient-echo images provide reliable blood pool signal (especially when used in combination with gradient moment nulling) and fast scan times (Fig. 2-9). Compared to spin echo, gradient echo provides better SNR at very short TR (less than 50 to 100 msec) but significantly worse SNRs at TRs in the range of standard spin-echo imaging. Because they use additional refocusing gradients rather than 180-degree RF pulses to evoke usable signal echoes, gradient-echo sequences are more susceptible to fixed magnetic field inhomogeneities, which manifest as artifacts due to chemical shift, differences in magnetic susceptibility, and high sensitivity to ferromagnetic objects.

Several eponyms have been created to describe the various gradient echo sequences now commercially available. These include FLASH, SPGR, MPGR, FISP, GRASS, and SSFP.[31,60] All represent gradient-echo sequences that use partial flip angles and refocusing gradients.

FLASH (fast low angle shot) (Figs. 2-10, *A* and *B* and 2-9, *C* and *D*) and SPGR (spoiled gradient recalled acquisition) (Fig. 2-11, *A* and *B*) use "spoiler" or "rewinding" gradients to eliminate the transverse magnetization that remains before the next echo.[26,27,31,33,34,60] Thus, signal intensity depends only on longitudinal magnetization and not on steady-state magnetization in the transverse plane. Short TR imaging permits breath-hold image acquisition, which eliminates respiratory motion artifacts (Fig. 2-9, *C* and *D*).

Rather than use spoiler gradients, MPGR (multi-planar GRASS) uses a long TR to effectively eliminate the residual transverse magnetization.[60] At low flip angles, an

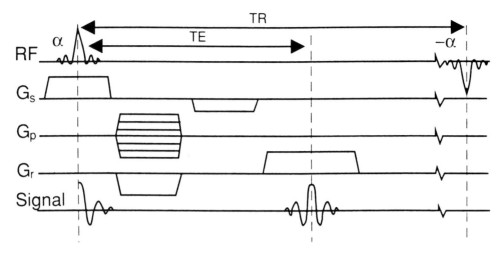

Fig. 2-8. Gradient echo pulse sequence diagram. *RF,* Radiofrequency excitation pulse. *Gs,* Slice selection gradient. *Gp,* Composite representation of multiple phase encoding gradient steps, which increase incrementally throughout the sequence from zero to a defined maximum amplitude. *Gr,* Readout gradient. Recalls the echo in a manner similar to the 180-degree RF pulse of a spin-echo sequence. Signal is produced immediately after the excitation pulse and at during the second occurrence of Gr. (From FLASH and FISP gradient echo pulse sequences, Publication No MG/5000-217-121, Siemens Medical Systems, Inc, Iselin, NJ.)

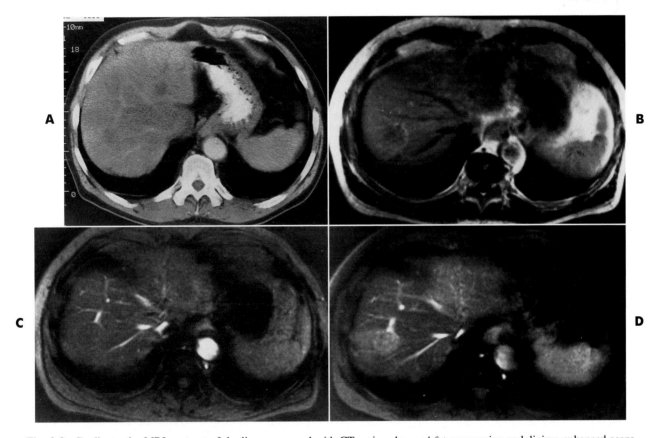

Fig. 2-9. Gradient echo MRI contrast of the liver compared with CT, spin echo, and fat-suppression gadolinium-enhanced scans. **A,** CT demonstrates two colon carcinoma metastases in the liver and fatty replacement of much of the right lobe. **B,** T1W spin echo with gadolinium reveals one of the lesions. **C,** Gradient echo reveals splaying of vessels by one lesion, but the low intensity mass is lost in the low intensity of the background fatty-replaced liver tissue. **D,** Gradient echo with fat suppression and gadolinium demonstrates the same mass to better advantage after suppression of the fatty liver tissue. However, the second mass in the left lobe is not detectable by this sequence. Its intensity nearly matches the normal nonfatty hepatic tissue.

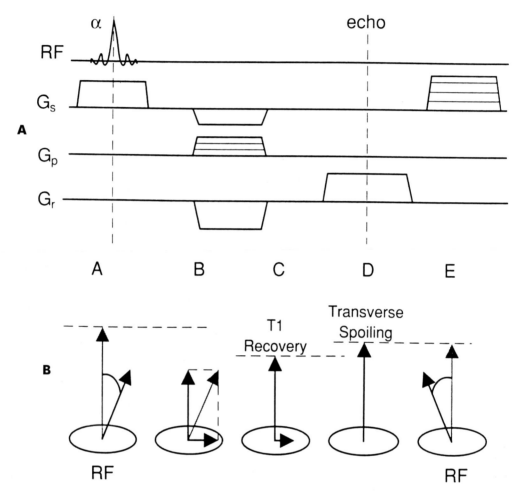

Fig. 2-10. FLASH gradient-echo sequence. **A,** FLASH pulse sequence diagram. *RF*, Radiofrequency excitation pulse. *Gs*, Slice selection gradient. *Gp*, Phase encoding gradient. *Gr*, Frequency readout gradient. Not shown is a spoiler gradient, which is applied after each excitation to eliminate residual in-phase magnetization in the transverse plane. **B,** Diagram of longitudinal and transverse magnetization vectors during a FLASH sequence. *A,* RF excitation. *B,* Longitudinal and transverse components of the magnetization vector. *C,* After partial recovery of longitudinal magnetization, some transverse component remains. *D,* The spoiler gradient has dephased the residual transverse magnetization, producing cancellation of residual signal. *E,* Excitation for the next phase step in the sequence. (From FLASH and FISP gradient echo pulse sequences, Publication No MG/5000-217-121, Siemens Medical Systems, Inc, Iselin, NJ.)

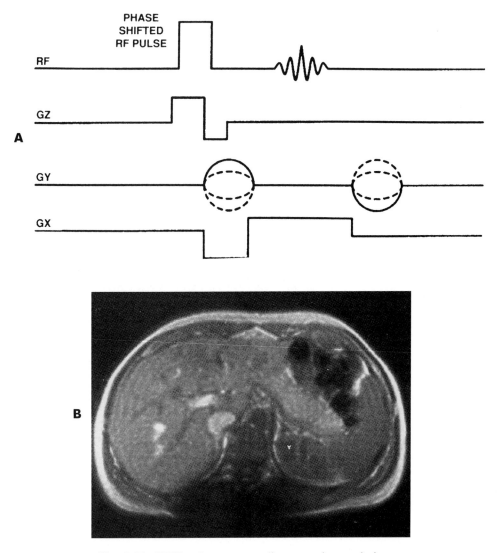

PHASE
SHIFTED
RF PULSE

RF

GZ

A

GY

GX

B

Fig. 2-11. SPGR pulse sequence diagram and example image. **A,** Sequence diagram. *RF,* Radiofrequency pulse. *Gz,* Slice selection gradient. *Gy,* Phase encoding gradient. *Gx,* Frequency readout gradient. **B,** Note bright vessels. Tissue intensity pattern similar to FLASH. (From Prorok RJ: Signa applications guide, vol 2, Milwaukee, 1989, General Electric Medical Systems.)

MPGR sequence provides images similar to FLASH and SPGR (Fig. 2-12). In MPGR, slice acquisition is multiplexed rather than sequential. Therefore, scan time is independent of the number of slices acquired. However, because scan times in general are longer than for GRASS and FLASH, breath holding is not practical. In the abdomen, this results in significant respiratory motion artifacts.

FISP (fast imaging with steady-state precession) and GRASS (gradient recalled acquisition in steady state) use gradients that maintain the transverse magnetization (Fig. 2-13).[13,60,84] Thus, signal intensity depends on both the longitudinal and transverse components of magnetization. The signal behavior of these images approaches that of the

"spoiled" gradient-echo sequences as the transverse magnetization approaches zero. Short TR imaging with FISP and GRASS allows for breath-hold imaging, thereby eliminating respiratory motion artifacts.

SSFP (steady state free precession) imaging represents a newer fast scanning technique whose physical basis differs from other gradient-echo sequences.[60] Each excitation pulse (corresponding to the 90-degree RF pulse in a spin-echo sequence) is also the refocusing pulse (corresponding to the 180-degree RF pulse in a spin-echo sequence) for the prior excitation. Because one cannot apply a pulse and listen for an echo at the same time, gradients are applied to shift the refocusing a few milliseconds before the next ex-

Fig. 2-12. MPGR sequence. Series of abdominal coronal images with flip angle decreasing from 90 degrees (upper left image) to 10 degrees (lower right image) in 10-degree steps. Note the high intensity of fat in the high flip angle images, which have greater T1 dependence. With lower angles, the contrast is predominantly proton density weighted. (From Field SA, Wehrli FW: Signa applications guide vol 1, Publication Number E8804CA, Milwaukee, 1990, General Electric Medical Systems.)

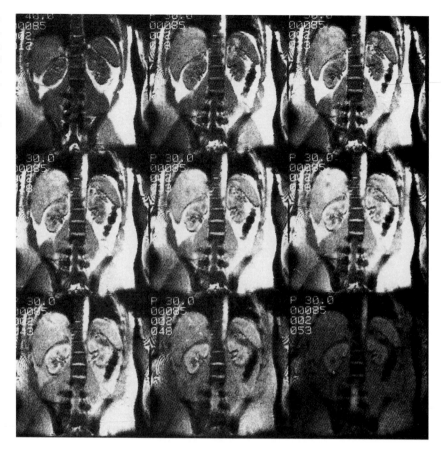

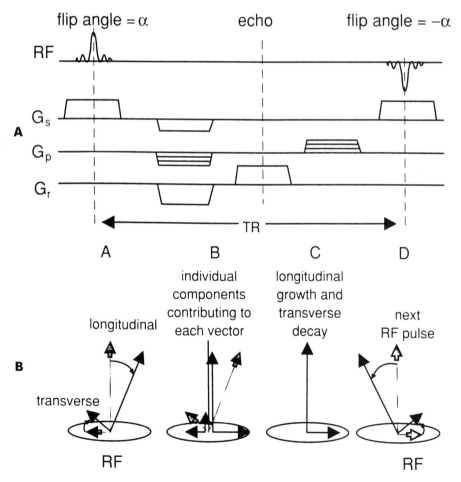

Fig. 2-13. FISP sequence. **A,** Pulse sequence diagram. *RF,* Radiofrequency pulse. *Gs,* Slice selection gradient. *Gp,* Phase encoding gradient. *Gr,* Frequency readout gradient. No spoiler gradient is used. **B,** Vector diagram of longitudinal magnetization. *A,* immediately after RF excitation, the longitudinal magnetization is rotated partially into the transverse plane. *B,* Longitudinal and transverse components of the tissue magnetization vector. *C,* The longitudinal component of the residual transverse magnetization of *A* has added to the longitudinal component of the tissue magnetization vector to reinforce the signal strength. *D,* Rotation of the vectors by the next RF pulse. Steady state magnetization is present in transverse plane. (From FLASH and FISP gradient echo pulse sequences, Publication No MG/5000-217-121, Siemens Medical Systems, Inc, Iselin, NJ.)

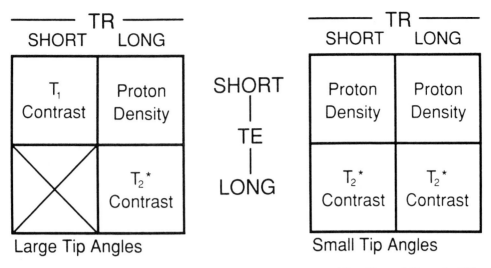

Fig. 2-14. Tissue contrast characteristics of the FLASH sequence. The effects of flip angle, TE, and TR are demonstrated. For example: large tip angles, short TR, and short TE produce T1W contrast. (From FLASH and FISP gradient echo pulse sequences, Publication No MG/5000-217-121, Siemens Medical Systems, Inc, Iselin, NJ.)

citation. SSFP images use short TR and longer TE (for example, TR of 25 msec and TE of 40 msec) to obtain heavily T2-weighted images. SSFP images suffer from low SNR (due to the long TE) and variable flow signal.

With FLASH and GRASS sequences, T1-weighting increases as the flip angle approaches 90 degrees. At small flip angles, the contrast pattern most resembles proton density (Fig. 2-14).[60] FLASH, FISP, and SPGR images may be obtained within a breath-hold. Due to the absence of 180-degree pulses, all gradient-echo sequences depend heavily on T2*. The relative significance of T1, T2*, and proton density contrast depends on TR, TE, and tip angle (Fig. 2-15 D).

TurboFLASH and related sequences (snapshot FLASH, segmented turboFLASH) are short-TR gradient echo sequences that use one or more RF presaturation pulses to modify tissue contrast.[19] The simplest variation produces single sections in a breath-hold sequence. Tissue contrast response is controlled by varying the timing of a 180-degree presaturation pulse. Variations of the turboFLASH sequence may use a series of prepulses to alter contrast weighting. The segmented turboFLASH sequence, in addition to providing flexible control of tissue contrast by RF presaturation pulses, also provides a multislice examination within a single breath hold, through efficient reordering of data acquisition (see the section on reordered and segmented phase decoding, below).[19]

Optimization of signal-to-noise ratio

Bandwidth. Bandwidth in MRI is defined as a range of frequencies. Most commonly it refers to the frequency range of the signals making up the image dataset. In the MRI literature, the term also is used to describe other frequency ranges, such as the spectrum of frequencies produced by a 90-degree pulse.

Bandwidth may be calculated by several approaches. The most direct approach is subtraction of the lowest from the highest frequencies in the passband. (The passband is the set of frequencies contained in a given bandwidth.) A typical value is 32,000 Hz (also expressed as plus or minus 16,000 Hz) (Fig. 2-16).

Another approach to bandwidth calculation is division of the number of frequency-encoding steps by the readout sampling time. For example, 256 readout samples divided by 8 msec readout time equals 32,000 Hz (Fig. 2-17).[69] This calculation converts *samples per 8 msec* into *samples per second*, which is expressed in Hz.

The x-axis (frequency readout) gradient slope determines the maximum gradient amplitude. The zero-crossing point is at the magnet isocenter (Fig. 2-18); therefore, the maximum amplitudes are expressed as positive and negative values. The field strengths at the edges of the FOV are as follows:

$$\text{Maximum field strength at one edge of the FOV} = B_o + G_{pos}$$
$$\text{Minimum field strength at the other edge} = B_o - G_{neg}$$

where G_{pos} and G_{neg} are maximum gradient amplitudes and B_o is the main magnetic field strength. These values, through the Larmor equation, provide the maximum and minimum frequencies contained in the FOV. Given a fixed number of frequency-encoding samples across the FOV, one observes that the *bandwidth per pixel increases as to-*

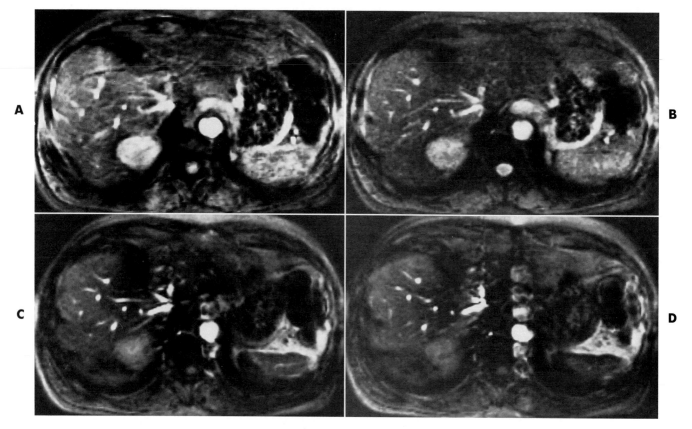

Fig. 2-15. Dependency of FLASH tissue contrast on flip angle setting. **A,** Single breath-hold FLASH image with 10-degree flip angle. Tissue contrast is predominantly density weighted. Flow compensation is on. **B,** Flip angle 30 degrees. Better SNR. Good compromise for liver and vessels. **C,** 60-degree flip angle. Increased pulsation artifact from aorta. Vascular signals are more intense. **D,** 90-degree flip angle. Increased vascular pulsation artifact. Note also the increased intensity of the subcutaneous fat.

Fig. 2-16. A 32,000 Hz (32 kHz) bandwidth is demonstrated, with a center frequency of 100 kHz, which could represent the frequency offsets produced by the x gradient field along the readout axis of a spin-echo image. The offsets range from 84 to 116 kHz greater than the baseline resonant frequency due to the fixed field. Their difference (116 − 84) in kHz is the bandwidth of the image. (From Prorok RJ: Signa applications guide, vol 2, Milwaukee, 1989, General Electric Medical Systems.)

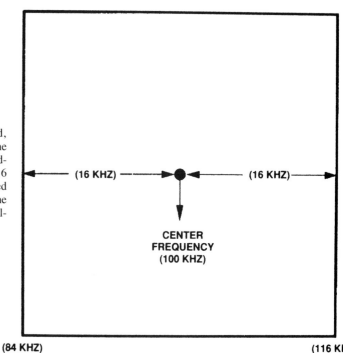

ASSUME 256² MATRIX RECEIVER BANDWIDTH	IMAGE WIDTH	HZ/ PIXELS	CHEMICAL SHIFT IN PIXELS	READOUT TIME	% INCREASE IN SNR
± 16 KHZ	32 KHZ	125	1.8	8 msec.	—
± 13 KHZ	26 KHZ	94	2.2	10 msec.	12%
± 8 KHZ	16 KHZ	62.5	3.5	16 msec.	40%
± 4 KHZ	8 KHZ	31	7.0	32 msec.	100%
± 2 KHZ	4 KHZ	16	14.0	64 msec.	180%

Fig. 2-17. Effect of decreasing receiver bandwidth on chemical shift, readout time, and SNR. A 256 × 256 matrix is assumed. Narrow bandwidths produce improved SNR at the expense of increased chemical shift artifact. SNR increases as the square of the increase in readout time. Readout time varys inversely with changes in bandwidth. (From Prorok RJ: Signa applications guide, vol 2, Milwaukee, 1989, General Electric Medical Systems.)

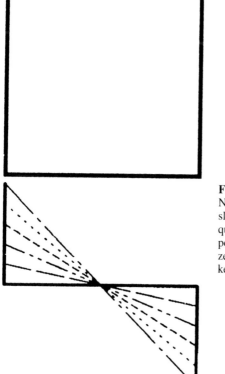

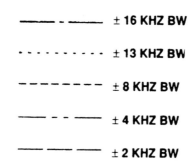

——— - ——— ± 16 KHZ BW

· · · · · · · · · ± 13 KHZ BW

— — — — — ± 8 KHZ BW

——— - - ——— ± 4 KHZ BW

——— —— ——— ± 2 KHZ BW

Fig. 2-18. Gradient amplitude is plotted versus x axis position. Narrow bandwidth is produced by a relatively small gradient slope. Steeper slopes produce larger bandwidth (greater frequency difference from left to right). Note the central crossover point, at which the frequency offset due to the gradient field is zero. (From Prorok RJ: Signa applications guide, vol 2, Milwaukee, 1989, General Electric Medical Systems.)

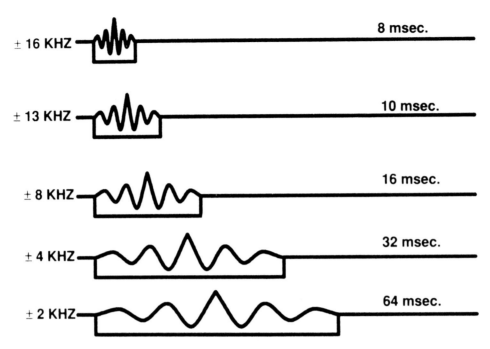

Fig. 2-19. Sampling time is inversely proportional to bandwidth. With wide bandwidth, gradient amplitude is high. Strong gradient fields accellerate dephasing of transverse magnetization and reduce the duration of the echo. The weaker gradients used for narrow bandwidth sequences produce prolonged echos. Longer echos can be sampled more precisely. An inverse effect is observed in relation to the duration of RF pulses. Soft RF pulses are long-duration pulses that excite a narrow bandwidth of tissue. Hard pulses are short duration events that excite a wide bandwidth. (From Prorok RJ: Signa applications guide, vol 2, Milwaukee, 1989, General Electric Medical Systems.)

tal bandwidth increases (Fig. 2-17). Two additional facts are relevant here:

1. Background noise is proportional to bandwidth. A broad bandwidth system admits a wide range of noise frequencies to the image data. Narrowing the bandwidth reduces the number of noise frequencies that are admitted through the passband of the MRI receiver.

2. T2* decay rate is proportional to gradient amplitude. As the gradient slope increases, for a given field of view, the bandwidth broadens (Figs. 2-18 and 2-21). The steeper the gradient slope, the more extreme the variation in magnetic field strength from pixel to pixel. Therefore, the inhomogeneity of the magnetic field, due to the imposed gradient, becomes more significant at increasing gradient amplitudes. This increasing inhomogeneity produces increasingly rapid dephasing of transverse magnetization (T2* decay)

Three clinically useful principles are derived from these fundamentals:

1. SNR increases as bandwidth decreases.
2. Echoes have longer duration as bandwidth decreases.
3. Chemical shift artifact increases as bandwidth decreases.

Doubling the bandwidth increases the SNR by 40%

(Fig. 2-17), as a smaller range of background noise frequencies is contained in the smaller bandpass. Lower bandwidth sequences use lower gradient amplitudes, which produce less phase dispersion of the echo. The resulting longer duration of the echo allows the use of longer sampling time, if indicated (Fig. 2-19).

The bandwidth is inversely proportional to frequency sampling time is the basis for the dual-echo reduced bandwidth T2-weighted sequences, which are in common clinical use (Fig. 2-20). Sampling time is increased for the second echo readout, improving substantially the SNR. A shorter sampling time is used for the first echo because a longer readout time would overlap the times of the spatial localization and motion correction gradients.

Narrow bandwidth sequences produce greater misregistration of fat- and water-containing pixels (see Fig. 2-38). The fixed water-fat difference is allocated over a larger number of pixels at narrow bandwidth (Fig. 2-21).

SNR versus time. For practical purposes, the sampling rate of MR systems is unlimited in the frequency encoding direction. One must consider the effect of frequency readout sampling rate along with the gradient amplitude slope and sampling time, both of which affect bandwidth and SNR.

In the phase encoding direction, the sampling rate is

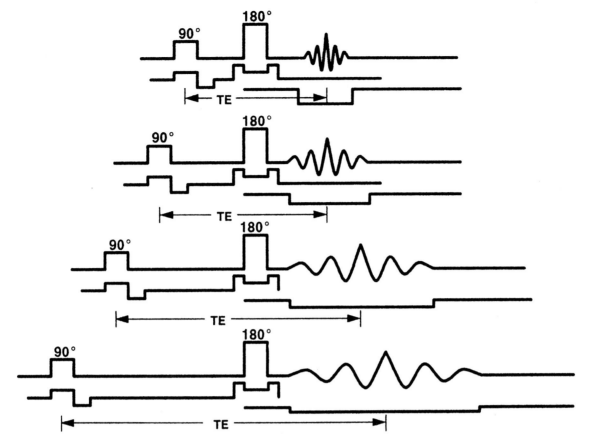

Fig. 2-20. A narrow bandwidth sequence improves SNR. Maximum permissable sampling time increases with TE. Long sampling time is impossible at short TEs due to conflict with the timing of the 180-degree pulse; however, at long TEs, the center point of the 180-degree pulse and the echo are widely separated (by TE/2). (From Prorok RJ: Signa applications guide, vol 2, Milwaukee, 1989, General Electric Medical Systems.)

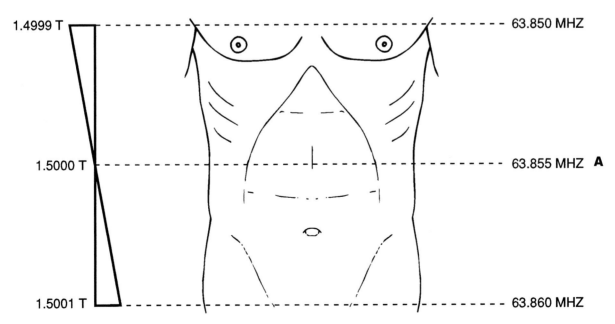

Fig. 2-21. Narrow versus wide bandwidth. **A,** At narrow bandwidth, the frequency range is only 63.850 to 63.859 mHz across this FOV. *Continued.*

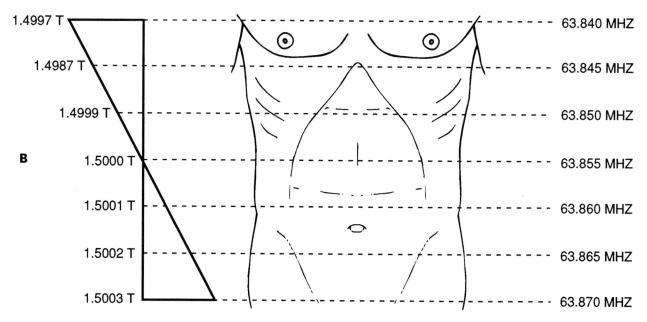

Fig. 2-21, cont'd. B, With wide bandwidth, the frequency range of **A** is confined only to the central zone of the imaging volume. Thus, the number of Hz per pixel is greater with wide bandwidth. Because the offset between fat and water is fixed for a given field strength, the chemical shift effect is more pronounced at narrow bandwidth.

equal to the TR. Thus, imaging time depends strongly on the number of phase-encoding samples and on the TR. Samples along the phase-encoded axis also are called phase steps, phase lines, y-axis samples, y-gradient steps, lines in "k space," or simply k-lines.

As a general rule, whenever a time parameter is changed, the SNR changes by a square root factor. For example, doubling the number of phase-encoding steps from 128 to 256, doubling the frequency readout sampling window from 8 to 16 msec, or doubling the number of excitations (also known as acquisitions) averaged together (NEX; see p. 42) results in a 40% (square root of 2) SNR improvement (Fig. 2-22).

Field of view and matrix size. A large FOV is required to depict the entire abdomen in a rapid survey examination (Fig. 2-23). Smaller FOVs may be used to evaluate localized abnormalities. However, very small FOV imaging may be hampered by unacceptable reductions in SNR. Remember that signal strength is proportional to the number of protons in the sample. The smaller the pixel, the better the spatial resolution, the lower the number of protons represented by each pixel, and the worse the SNR.

The scan matrix divides an imaging plane into picture elements (pixels) (Fig. 2-24). Thus, the scan plane of a digital imaging modality is similar to a checkerboard. The number of "squares" along one side is equal to the number of frequency-encoding steps (along the x axis). The number of "squares" along the other edge is equal to the number of phase-encoding steps (along the y axis). The matrix size is expressed not in terms of physical dimensions but in numbers of sampling steps. FOV is given in centimeters or millimeters. Sequence acquisition time is proportional to the number of phase encoding steps, but is unaffected by the size of the FOV.

If the number of pixels is held constant (i.e., if the number of phase-encoding and frequency-encoding steps is held constant) and the FOV is reduced by 50%, the pixels become smaller by a factor of 2 in both dimensions of the scan plane, and the area of each pixel decreases by a factor of 4. Therefore, *increased spatial resolution is obtainable by reducing the FOV at the expense of SNR.* If the resulting SNR is marginal, one must then compensate for the loss of signal strength by other means.

If the FOV is reduced by 50% and the number of both the x and y sampling steps (the matrix dimensions) are also halved along both axes, then the volume of each pixel and the number of sampling steps *per pixel* are constant. Total scan time is divided by 2, since its value is directly proportional to the decrease in the number of y steps. The time gained may be invested in doubling the NEX, which results in a 40% SNR improvement at no net increase from the original examination time. Where spatial resolution is adequate and SNR is marginal, even a 10% improvement in net signal strength is noticeable. *By equal reductions of FOV and matrix dimensions, one can improve the SNR significantly (40%) at the expense of the FOV.* This is often not a bad tradeoff; it is analogous to "coning-down" on small objects with videofluoroscopy by changing the magnification factor of the image intensifier.

Sampling 192 phase lines in the craniocaudal z axis and

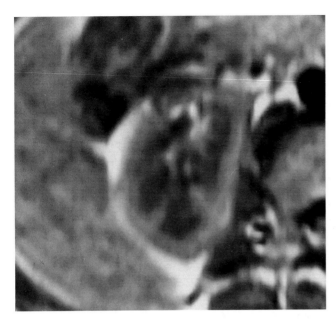

Fig. 2-22. T1W image of the right kidney with matrix of 128 × 256, TR 888, TE 15, and four averages (NEX). Acquisition time is 6:02, SNR is improved by 40% over a 2 NEX image. Decreasing the matrix from 256 × 256 to 128 × 256 shortens imaging time by 50%, saving 6 minutes in this case, in return for increased SNR. Note the good corticomedullary contrast of this image.

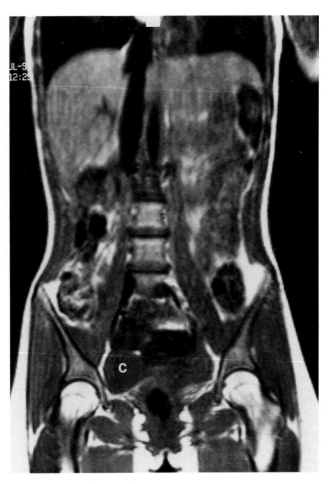

Fig. 2-23. T1W coronal with 50 cm FOV, 4 NEX and TR of 450. Survey of entire abdomen with high SNR. An incidental right ovarian cyst is visible (white "C"). A 192 × 256 matrix has reduced total scan time by 25%.

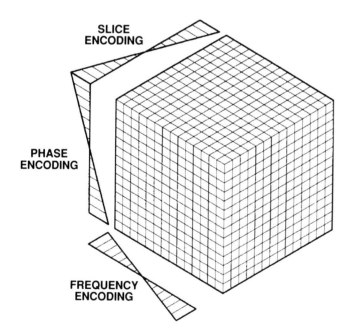

Fig. 2-24. Pixels (picture elements) divide a plane into a matrix. Mapped onto a volume, with the added dimension of depth, they become voxels (volume elements). This cube is divided into multiple slices that contain voxels of equal dimensions. The voxels are indistinguishable, one from another, except by the frequency and phase properties that mark their "address" and their signal amplitude, which is a function of proton density and contrast weighting. (From Prorok RJ: Signa applications guide, vol 2, Milwaukee, 1989, General Electric Medical Systems.)

256 frequency-encoding steps in the transverse axis matches the matrix to the rectangular configuration of the abdomen (Fig. 2-23). This strategy directly reduces scan time by reducing the number of phase-encode steps by a factor of 192/256 and minimizes flow-ghost artifacts from the great vessels (which propagate in the direction of the phase-encoding axis).

Another strategy for scan time reduction and SNR improvement is balanced reduction in the number of phase-encoding steps matched by a proportionate reduction of field of view in the phase-encoding dimension. This technique produces rectangular pixels with twice the volume as the original 256 × 256 array, but provides adequate coverage for many abdomens in the transverse and sagittal planes (Fig. 2-25).

For coronal and sagittal imaging, an FOV ranging from approximately 24 to 50 cm is used. For transverse imaging, a FOV large enough to display the entire cross section on the image is used. Smaller FOVs can be used with suc-

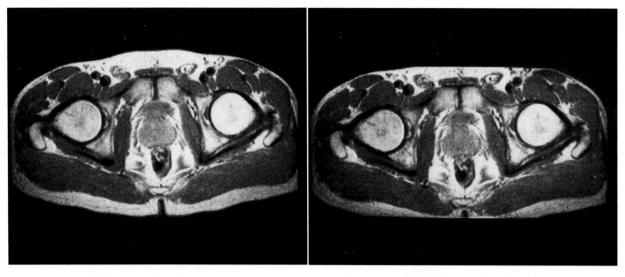

Fig. 2-25. Rectangular FOV. **A,** T1W 256 × 256 matrix. Acquisition time 8:54. **B,** Rectangular field of view, using a 128 × 256 matrix. Acquisition time cut by nearly 50% to 4:38. No significant information is lost; only a thin section of subcutaneous fat is excluded from view. (From FLASH and FISP gradient echo pulse sequences, Publication No MG/5000-217-121, Siemens Medical Systems, Inc, Iselin, NJ.)

cess during imaging with surface coils. The higher SNR inherent in these coils allows for reduction in pixel size while maintaining adequate signal. Such imaging can be used to evaluate the scrotum, prostate, rectum, and other localized areas.

Matrix size and number of acquisitions. Choice of matrix size and number of acquisitions (NEX) depends on the area of interest. Matrix size (along with the field of view) determines pixel size and thus factors into spatial resolution as well as SNR (Fig. 2-26). The NEX also is a factor in SNR. Each directly affects scan time. The scan time is directly proportional to the number of phase-encoding steps (which is one dimension of the matrix size) and to the NEX. However, the increase in SNR is proportional only to the square root of the NEX.[74] Reducing the number of y steps by 50% cuts the scan time in half. If constant FOV is maintained, SNR increases by 40%, as pixel size is doubled in the y dimension. Doubling the NEX doubles scan time but only increases SNR by 1.4 (the square root of 2). Thus, doubling NEX alone is an inefficient maneuver. If coupled with another strategy to compensate for the added scan time, however, increasing NEX can be an effective clinical tool (Fig. 2-27).

The upper abdomen suffers more from respiratory motion artifact than the pelvis. To minimize motion-induced blurring of the upper abdomen by ghost artifacts, one can decrease the TR and increase the NEX (see Fig. 2-23). This strategy is more likely to be effective when NEX is increased to 4 or greater. If total imaging time is held constant, cutting the TR by 50% allows for doubling of the

NEX. *Balanced reduction of TR and increase of NEX reduces motion artifact and increases SNR by 40% at the cost of decreased number of sections per multislice sequence and some increased T1 contrast weighting.* Because respiratory motion causes less artifact in the pelvis, fewer NEX (1 to 2) may be used with success. Reducing the NEX can reduce imaging time or provide time for additional parameter changes such as increased matrix size (increased resolution) with no net increase in imaging time.

Slice thickness and interslice gap. Pixels have only two dimensions. Cross-sectional images actually have a third dimension, which is equal to the thickness of the cross section (slice thickness). Three-dimensional picture elements are called volume elements (voxels). The signal strength of one voxel depends directly on the number of protons in the voxel. Noise is random; it is independent of the number of protons in the voxel. As slice thickness increases, signal amplitude increases arithmetically and noise amplitude remains constant. Therefore, SNR is directly proportional to slice thickness.

Choice of slice thickness is limited by SNR and the size of the region of interest. Typically, for screening the abdomen and pelvis, a slice thickness of 7 to 10 mm is used. This amount provides adequate resolution in the slice-selection direction, covers large areas in acceptable scan times, and produces excellent SNR. If the volume of interest is small, 4 to 7 mm slices can be used. However, slices less than 7 mm on T2W spin-echo images or less than 5 mm on T1W images may yield suboptimal SNR, unless

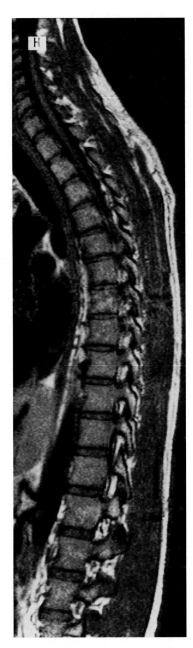

Fig. 2-26. The frequency readout matrix dimension has been increased to 512 to provide a high resolution T1W scout image of the entire spine with no increase in imaging time.

decreased voxel volume is balanced by increased NEX (Figs. 2-27 and 2-28).

A gap (skip) between slices may be desirable.[43,68,74] Interslice gaps increase the volume coverage of a series of sections. The maximum number of possible MR slices possible in a given pulse sequence is roughly proportional to the TR. Where time and other parameters permit either long TR or acquisition of multiple sets of slices, contiguous sections usually are preferable; however, interslice gaps can increase the scan volume for a given number of slices at no penalty in imaging time or slice thickness. Slice acquisition most frequently is interleaved, allowing sequential excitement of widely separated regions rather than contiguous regions in anatomic order. Interslice gaps are mandatory in noninterleaved pulse sequences to avoid excessive background noise due to unintentional interference from the signal of adjacent sections (Fig. 2-29).

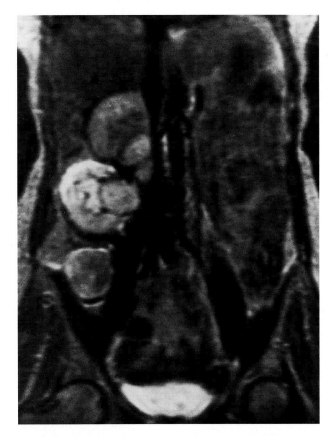

Fig. 2-27. T2W, TR 2535, TE 80, and 128 × 256 matrix. Retroperitoneal sarcoma; renal displacement. Slice thickness 5 mm. In spite of the thin sections, SNR is adequate because of doubling the NEX to 2. Scan time has been maintained at 11:21 by compensating the NEX increase with balanced reduction in phase encoding steps from 256 to 128.

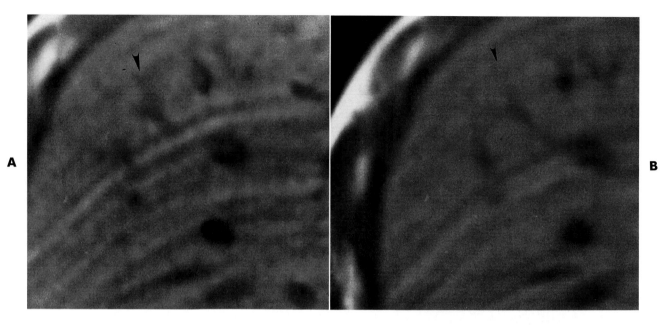

Fig. 2-28. Effect of slice thickness on SNR and spatial resolution. **A,** T1W scan of the liver with 5 mm slice thickness. Branching vessels more clearly depicted than in **B** *(arrowhead)*. However, random variation of the liver parenchymal intensity is more apparent, due to the reduced SNR with small voxels. **B,** Smoother image with 10 mm slice thickness. The number of protons sampled in each voxel has increased by 100%. This image has 40% better SNR than **A,** but less spatial resolution. The small vessel branches are less distinct *(arrowhead)*.

Fig. 2-29. The bandwidth of this RF pulse at one half of its maximum amplitude is equal to the nominal bandwidth of the slice *(dashed lines)*. However, low intensity sidebands extend both higher and lower in frequency—beyond the specified thickness of the slice. These sidebands would introduce spurious responses (noise artifact) in the receiver if the adjacent slices were sampled while this section still was producing a coherent signal. (From Hinshaw WS, Kramer DM, Yeung HN, Hill BC: Fundamentals of magnetic resonance imaging, Solon, Ohio, 1984, Technicare Corp.)

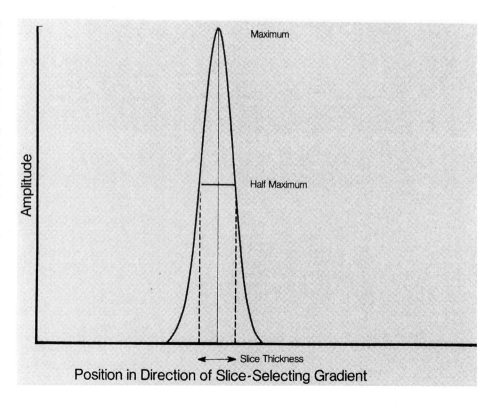

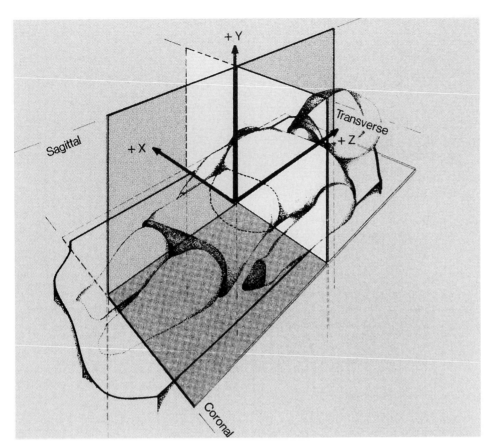

Fig. 2-30. The three orthogonal imaging planes: transverse, sagittal, and coronal. Each plane is defined by a pair of gradient coordinates: xy (transverse), xz (coronal), and yz (sagittal). (From Hinshaw WS, Kramer DM, Yeung HN, Hill BC: Fundamentals of magnetic resonance imaging, Solon, Ohio, 1984, Technicare Corp.)

MRI SPATIAL LOCALIZATION
Frequency encoding

MRI spatial encoding depends entirely on the linear relationship between proton resonant frequency and magnetic field strength (see Chapter 1). Imaging magnets are constructed with sets of electromagnet coils positioned to produce controlled variations of magnetic field strength independently along the x, y, and z axes (Fig. 2-30). These variations are called magnetic field gradients; the coils that produce them are the gradient coils. They are designed to produce linear increases in magnetic flux density in any given direction. Gradient strength varies positively and negatively on each side of the zero point (see Fig. 2-18).

Linear increase of magnetic field strength from right to left (x axis), anterior to posterior (y axis), or head to foot (z axis) produces a linear distribution of proton resonant frequencies along the desired axis or combination of axes (Figs. 2-31 and 2-32). MRI radio receivers collect the signals of all frequencies within a selected bandwidth and pass them on to the processing circuits (Fig. 2-33). The computer breaks down the complex time-varying signal into set of numbers that represent the amplitude of each individual frequency component of the whole (Fig. 2-34). If set for a matrix size of 256 × 256, the computer produces 256 values in the frequency-readout (frequency-encoding)

direction. These values are assigned to a row of voxels along one axis (typically the x axis for the transverse plane of section).

By assigning each voxel a different field strength, we have provided for the decoding of signals arising from a column of tissue 1 voxel wide by 256 voxels long (using the x axis dimension of the preceding example). To sample the amplitude of all the other columns of tissue making up a cross-sectional plane of tissue, we must use another property of signals—phase—in addition to frequency.

Phase encoding

Phase encoding can be used in one or both of the remaining dimensions of a scan volume, depending on whether planar or volume imaging is being performed. In a typical planar image acquisition (slice-by-slice scan), only one dimension is phase-encoded. For this example, we will assign phase-encoding to the y axis of a transverse section.

The concept of phase is reviewed in Chapter 1. Phase shifts of controlled increments can be introduced in the voxels along the y axis by momentarily applying a magnetic field gradient (Fig. 2-35). Protons in voxels at the extremes of the y axis advance in phase, both negatively and

Fig. 2-31. The linear distribution of radiofrequencies produced by the x axis gradient field is represented by the the gray scale shading of the body, from black (low frequency) to white (high frequency) across this transverse section. (From Hinshaw WS, Kramer DM, Yeung HN, Hill BC: Fundamentals of magnetic resonance imaging, Solon, Ohio, 1984, Technicare Corp.)

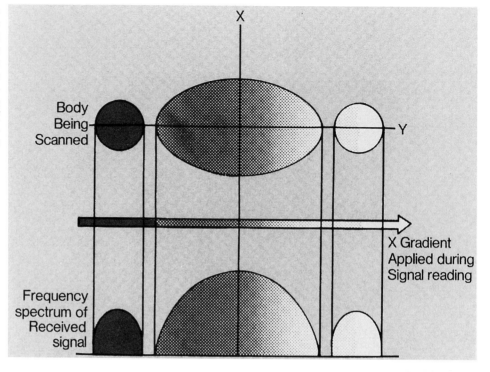

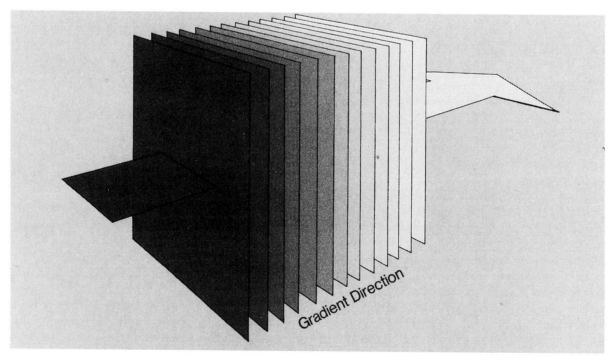

Fig. 2-32. The smooth, unbroken slope of the gradient flux density across the FOV in Fig. 2-31 is translated by the slice selection process into a discontinuous series of cross-sections having finite thickness. In this simplified diagram, each section is represented as having single average frequency. More precisely, however, each section has a bandwidth of its own, which is a small fraction of the full bandwidth of the FOV. (From Hinshaw WS, Kramer DM, Yeung HN, Hill BC: Fundamentals of magnetic resonance imaging, Solon, Ohio, 1984, Technicare Corp.)

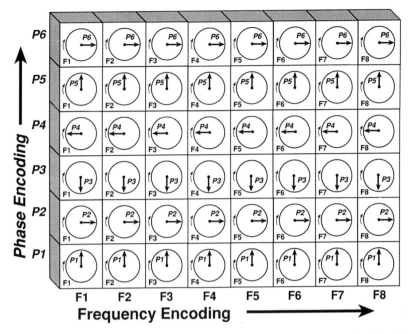

Fig. 2-33. Schematic representation of a 6 × 8 scan matrix. 48 voxels are contained in this slice. Heavy arrows in each voxel represent the average phase angle of its protons. Small curved arrows indicate the direction of vector rotation in the transverse plane. The phase angle is same within each row. The frequency is the same within each column. Note that the difference in phase angles between vertically contiguous voxels is 90 degrees. (In a 256 × 256 matrix, the angle is approximately 2 degrees). The sequence of phase angles in column F1 from voxel F1,P1 to voxel F1,P6 is: 0, 90, 180, 270, 360, 450. The voxels located farthest from the zero line (farthest from the x axis) have the largest phase angle shift. This property distinguishes them from the centrally located voxels. In a strong y gradient field, the P6 voxels are far ahead of the P1 voxels in phase. In a weak gradient field, they are only slightly ahead (but they are ahead still).

positively, more rapidly than those located more centrally (Fig. 2-33). The protons precisely at the zero-crossing point of the gradient undergo no phase shift (see Fig. 2-18).

Referring again to the previous example, 256 lines perpendicular to the y axis are acquired by the imaging system, after each line has been encoded with a unique phase offset from the (central) zero-crossing line. State-of-the-art digital receivers and signal processing boards have the ability to **lock on** to signals of any given phase relative to the signal of the zero line. Thus, the phase encoding can be recovered with high accuracy automatically by the equipment. Unique phase encoding of each of the 256 lines requires a separate pulse sequence (duration of each sequence = TR) for each scan line. Thus, total scan time equals the number of phase steps multiplied by the repetition time TR (and multiplied again by the number of scan averages NEX).

Frequency decoding is performed rapidly during the acquisition window (at the time of the echo) of each phase line. In the preceding example, 256 different batches of

signal data are passed to the computer for processing. The end result is a signal amplitude value for every voxel in the plane of section (Fig. 2-34).

In conventional spin-echo imaging, slice selection is accomplished by transmitting an excitation RF pulse while a magnetic field gradient is applied in the z-axis direction (Figs. 2-30 and 2-32). Depending on the flux density at any point (just as in the case of the frequency readout axis), the proton resonant frequency varies. The only transverse section having the same resonant frequency both before and during application of the slice selection gradient is the one located at the zero-crossing point of the gradient (see Fig. 2-18). All other sections are exposed to either higher or lower flux density once the z gradient has been applied. The frequency of the 90-degree pulse is chosen to match the resonant frequency of one section. No other slice has the same field strength (under normal conditions); therefore, no other slice resonates. (For a review of the proton magnetic resonance phenomenon and the relationship of frequency to changing field strength, see Chapter 1.) Each of the 256 phase line data acquisitions of

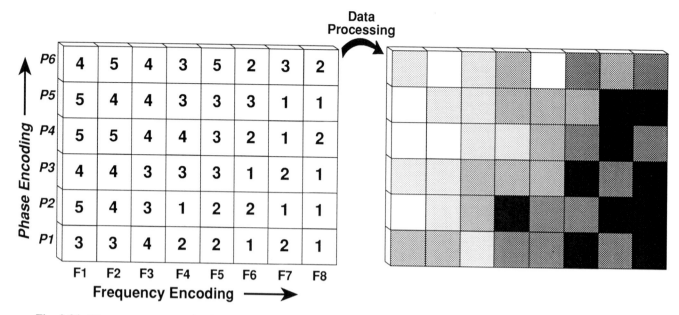

Fig. 2-34. The array processor circuit calculates pixel intensity values by applying Fourier transforms to the frequency and phase values of each pixel. A matrix of intensity numbers results. This is stored by the computer for future reference (as the image dataset) and is printed on film or displayed on a CRT screen for our immediate use. High intensity values translate to bright pixels on the display medium. Software converts the large range of data numbers into the relatively narrow range of CRT or film brightness through a translation table.

the preceding example requires at least one z-axis gradient pulse and an RF excitation pulse.

Volume scan acquisitions encode both the y-axis and z-axis information by phase modulation of the signal. Transient magnetic field gradients are applied in an orderly sequence, which uniquely tags the y lines for each section. The z-axis gradient amplifiers and their coils are turned on momentarily to produce incremental field strength variations at appropriate times during the data collection so that z-axis phase information is intercalated with the y-axis data.

Summary of spatial localization

Four physical principles apply to MRI spatial localization:

1. Voxel resonant frequency depends on magnetic field strength. Proceeding along the frequency readout axis from right to left, the magnetic field flux density increases or decreases linearly at a constant slope, as long as a stable gradient field is applied (see Fig. 2-21). The gradient essentially maps frequency to a location along a line.

2. Gradients cause voxel resonant frequencies to increase along any axis. The thickness and orientation of MRI slice sections is controlled by software and generated through the combination of x, y, and z gradient fields (see Fig. 2-30). CT slice thickness and section orientation are completely dependent on the configuration of the mechanical collimators of the scan beam. The patient must be repositioned if other than transverse sections are desired.

3. Simultaneous RF excitation pulses and z-axis gradi-

ents select slices. The resonant frequency of only one slice within a series of contiguous slices along the z-axis gradient is matched by the frequency of the RF excitation pulse (see Figs. 2-31 and 2-32).

4. Transiently applied gradients alter the phase of resonating voxels. While protons are in the resonant condition, increased flux density immediately boosts their frequency, causing their phase angle to advance prematurely, as if an interval of time had passed (Fig. 2-35). Increased gradient flux density produces dephasing equivalent to a proportionate increase in gradient pulse duration (Fig. 2-36).

Three practical engineering principles can be applied to MRI spatial localization:

1. Frequency decoding is nearly instantaneous for each resonating line. Microsecond sampling intervals are sufficient; 256 frequency-encoding samples are accomplished within an 8 msec sampling window with time to spare (see Fig. 2-19).

2. Phase decoding requires repetitive sampling of many lines per plane. Phase expresses the relationships among constantly changing signals. A single sample (one phase step) of the data is practically meaningless. The precision of phase measurement increases with an increasing number of samples.

3. Phase samples are taken at intervals equal to the TR of the sequence. Unlike frequency samples, which are processed in microseconds, phase samples require repetitive measurements. If the TR = 2 seconds, then a scan sequence of 256 phase steps requires 512 seconds (8 minutes

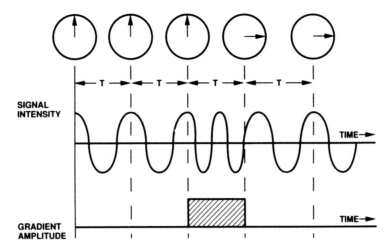

Fig. 2-35. While a gradient field is present, the frequency of this voxel is increased. Thus, its phase is advanced after the gradient is removed. The vector advances immediately upon application of the gradient, but does not fall back after cessation of the gradient. This property is known as "phase memory". (From Turshi P et al: Vascular magnetic resonance imaging, signa applications guide, vol 3, Publication No E8804DB, Milwaukee, 1990, General Electric Medical Systems.)

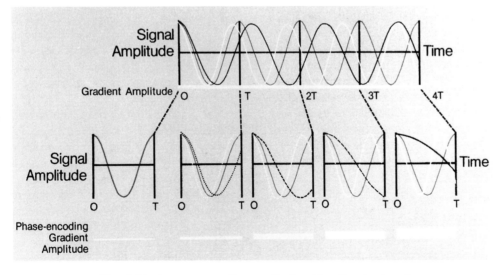

Fig. 2-36. A constant gradient amplitude with a flux density of 0.1 unit, applied constantly for 4 msec produces the same phase shift as a brief gradient pulse having an amplitude of 4 units and a duration of 0.1 msec. Note the relative positions of the three RF signal sine curves (white, gray, and black) at the dashed vertical lines marked 0, 1T, 2T, 3T, and 4T. These mark equal intervals. Gradient amplitude and duration are represented by the white bars beneath the curves. (From Hinshaw WS, Kramer DM, Yeung HN, Hill BC: Fundamentals of magnetic resonance imaging, Solon, Ohio, 1984, Technicare Corp.)

and 32 seconds), not including any additional data processing time, to acquire a single image.

Three imaging principles follow:

1. Slice thickness depends on the shape of the RF excitation pulse and the rate of increase (slope) of gradient amplitude along the slice-selection axis. A real-world RF pulse and a real section of tissue of a given thickness both actually contain (or respond to) a band of frequencies rather than a single pure frequency (see Fig. 2-29). Therefore, the pulse must be shaped electronically to excite a nearly rectangular section of tissue, and its bandwidth must be controlled to match the range of frequencies of the desired slice. Compared to weak gradient fields, strong gradient fields produce a larger separation of frequencies between neighboring pixels within a slice. Therefore, an RF pulse of a certain bandwidth excites a thicker slice of pixels in a low amplitude gradient field than in a high amplitude gradient field (and a narrow bandwidth pulse excites a thinner slice than a wide bandwidth pulse).

2. Chemical shift artifacts appear along the frequency-encoding axis and the slice-selection axis, but not along the phase-encoding axis (see Fig. 2-38). Chemical shift artifacts are produced by the frequency offset between protons of fat and water. Phase encoding is independent of frequency. No frequency offset is generated along the phase-encoding axis.

3. Motion artifacts appear in the phase-encoding axis regardless of the orientation axis of the motion itself. Because individual frequency readout samples are fast enough to stop physiologic motion, no degradation is perceived in the axes that are dependent on frequency encoding. Each phase-encoded view of the data contains information about all of the pixels in the slice. Any physical change within the scan volume during acquisition of a set of related phase steps degrades the phase-encoded component of the image data (which is displayed along the phase-encoding axis) (see Fig. 2-41).

ARTIFACT RECOGNITION
Chemical shift misregistration

Chemical shift.[1,7,73,89] Water protons and fat protons precess at different frequencies, owing to differences in their local environments. This difference is about 220 Hz in a 1.5 T magnetic field. This corresponds to approximately 3.5 parts per million (Fig. 2-37). Depending on the magnetic field strength, the gyromagnetic ratio, and the bandwidth per pixel, the difference corresponds to a shift in image position by a given number of pixels.

The signal of water has a higher frequency than that of fat. Thus, a 1 mm cube of water is located by the scanner slightly farther toward the high-frequency edge of a given imaging plane than a 1 mm cube of fat in the same actual physical location. If the fat happens to be located immediately adjacent to and on the higher frequency (stronger gradient amplitude) side of the water, the water signal is

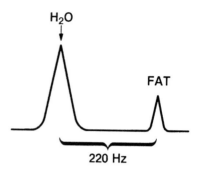

Fig. 2-37. Water protons resonate at a higher frequency than fat protons in the same magnetic flux density. The difference is due to intrinsic properties of the molecules themselves, not to any outside influence. This natural chemical shift is the basis for separation of the two populations for imaging purposes. A 220 Hz separation is significant at narrow bandwidths, as several pixels are spanned by that frequency difference. Even if located in the same voxel with fat, water appears to be located several pixels toward the high end of the gradient field because of its naturally higher resonant frequency. (From Prorok RJ: Signa applications guide, vol 2, Milwaukee, 1989, General Electric Medical Systems.)

depicted artifactually as originating from the fat pixel. Because the water signal is spatially misregistered toward the higher gradient amplitude side of the image, a signal void remains on the lower gradient amplitude side. In the abdomen, this effect is typically most noticeable along the interface of the renal cortex and the perirenal fat (Fig. 2-38). Fat and water signals arising from the same pixel may cancel on a gradient echo scan, depending on the TE (see Fat Suppression).

The chemical shift misregistration artifact is most pronounced on long TR, long TE (that is, T2-weighted) spin-echo imaging, and gradient-echo imaging. Narrow bandwidth imaging magnifies the appearance of the artifact because the absolute frequency difference between water and fat is fixed for a given field strength regardless of the bandwidth of the MR system. Narrow bandwidth simply means less Hz/pixel; therefore, more pixels are spanned by the misregistered water signal at low bandwidth than at high bandwidth (see Fig. 2-17).

Aliasing

Wrap-around.[36,58,61] If regions of anatomy extend outside of the field of view, the MR machine may misregister signal from these regions, resulting in wrap-around or aliasing—projection of the misregistered regions onto the images. For example, a small field of view may project the left hip onto the right side of the resultant image, obscuring detail in the region of interest. Aliasing can occur in either the phase-encoding or frequency-encoding direction (Fig. 2-39). Aliasing is a form of undersampling artifact, which may occur in any digital system. Samples must be obtained at intervals of less than one half the period of the

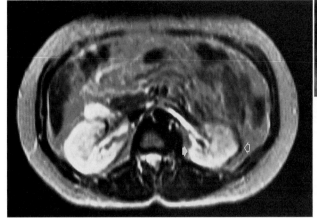

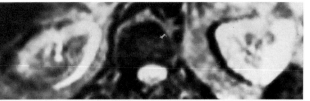

Fig. 2-38. Chemical shift artifact. **A,** Axial T2W spin echo. Signal void *(hollow arrow)* at the lateral margin of the left kidney occurs because the water signal of the renal cortex is misregistered toward the high end of the gradient field (the right side of the patient). The intense signal at the right margin of the kidney *(solid white arrow)* results from the summation of the misregistered water signal with the signal of the fat which is actually present in these voxels. **B,** In this example, also a T2W-spin echo scan, the gradient direction has been reversed. The signal voids are located on the right side of the kidneys. The water signal is displaced toward the left.

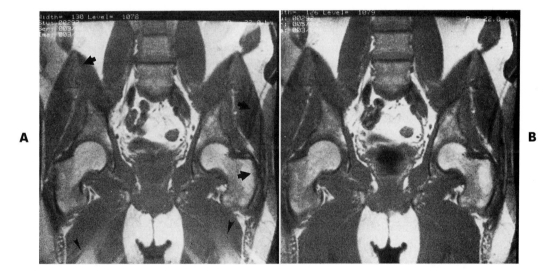

Fig. 2-39. Aliasing due to undersampling of frequency and phase information. **A,** Coronal T1W. The upper portion of the abdomen is misregistered and superimposed on the adductor muscles of the thighs *(arrowheads)* due to undersampling in the frequency encoding direction. The soft tissues of the hips wrap around in the phase encoding axis *(arrows)*. **B,** Coronal T1W (same position as **A**). Frequency axis wrap-around corrected by software. Aliasing persists in the phase encoding direction. *Continued.*

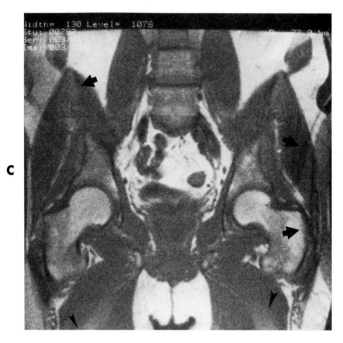

Fig. 2-39, cont'd. C, Coronal T1W (same position as **A** and **B**). Both phase and frequency wraparound artifacts have been corrected. This software requires at least 2 NEX of data to perform aliasing correction. No imaging time is lost. (From Field SA, Wehrli FW: Signa applications guide, vol 1, Publication No E8804CA, Milwaukee 1990, General Electric Medical Systems.)

measured signal to avoid aliasing (Fig. 2-40). In MRI, the frequency sampling period is inversely proportional to the bandwidth of the measurement. For a fixed receiver sampling time, the likelihood of aliasing increases as bandwidth increases. For example, a 32 kHz signal must be sampled more than 64,000 times per second to avoid aliasing (wrap-around) artifact.

Ghosting artifacts. Motion, whether from respiration, vessel pulsation, peristalsis, or random patient movement, causes the most troublesome of all artifacts in the abdomen.[13,36,56,58,59] When an echo is sampled, the receiver and array processor record the signals from all voxels simultaneously. Each line of *k* space contains information from the entire scan volume. Conventional spin-echo and gradient-echo MRI image reconstruction algorithms assume that each gradient step is measured under identical conditions. However, motion defeats this condition. Because an interval of TR exists between each of the *k* lines, physiologic motion often occurs between *k* line samples, changing the configuration of the tissue being examined, and presenting invalid data to the image reconstruction software. Spurious signals, therefore, are combined with the image dataset. Regardless of the direction of the motion, the artifact is superimposed on the image along the y

axis (the phase-encoding axis) (Fig. 2-41).

Movement of the voxels during imaging creates blurring of the image and ghost shadows. If the signal of the moving tissue is high intensity, the ghosts are also high intensity, making the artifact worse. This effect frequently is seen in the upper abdomen, especially on transverse images, where high intensity fat in the abdominal wall moves with respiration. Variations in blood flow may also cause ghosting, especially true on the arterial side, where pulsations create variations in intravascular signal intensity and vessel position (see Fig. 2-15, *D*). Several methods have been devised to reduce or eliminate ghosting artifacts (see below).[2,17,53,55,63]

Flow phenomena. The physical basis for the appearance of intravascular blood on MRI is complex. Likewise, a wide spectrum of artifacts is produced by flow.[57] See Chapter 7 for a detailed description of flow phenomena.

ARTIFACT CONTROL

Optimal MRI examinations are designed with these goals: maximization of tissue contrast, minimization of artifacts, and efficient use of time. The MRI operator has a number of options to improve image quality.

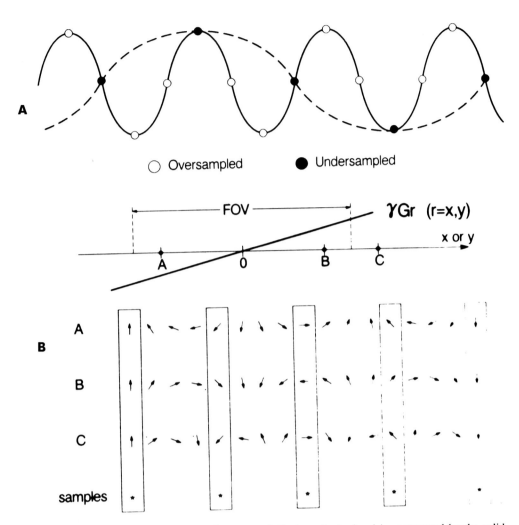

Fig. 2-40. Undersampling error—the cause of aliasing. **A,** A signal is represented by the solid line passing through the hollow dots. The signal is sampled at the points marked by black dots. The samples are taken at intervals of more than one half of the period of the signal. The dashed line drawn through the sampling points is a poor approximation of the original signal (actually, the approximation is the third harmonic of the signal). In order to arrive at an accurate representation of a sine wave through intermittent sampling, the sampling frequency must be greater than half of the signal frequency. Otherwise, the sampling results are ambiguous and likely to be inaccurate. These errors produce artifacts when they occur in digital sampling equipment such as oscilloscopes, compact disc players, and Doppler ultrsound machines, as well as MRI scanners. **B,** Region C is outside the FOV; regions A and B are within. Below the gradient diagram is a vector representation of the phase angles of regions A, B, and C, sampled successively during data acquisition. Reading horizontally from left to right in row A, notice that the pattern of arrows within the rectangular sampling windows is identical to the pattern of row C, observed at the same points. Because their phase readings are identical, their locations are ambiguous. Region C is misregistered to the location of region A (inside the FOV because the computer is not aware of the existance of any points outside of the FOV). More frequent sampling would have corrected the ambiguity. After comparing rows A and C closely, point by point, it becomes evident that the only points at which the two rows match are the points fortuitously chosen for sampling within the vertical rectangles. (From Wehrli FW: Advanced MR imaging techniques, Publication No 7513, Milwaukee, 1988, General Electric Medical Systems.)

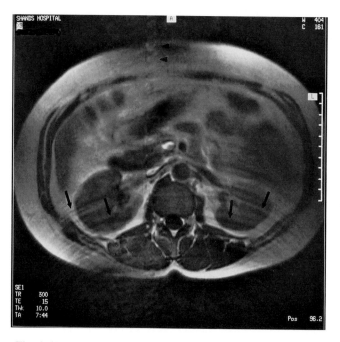

Fig. 2-41. Respiratory motion, primarily in the z and y axes, results in multiple replicas of the high intensity anterior abdominal wall being displayed along the y axis *(black arrows)*. The ghosts of the aorta and inferior vena cava *(arrowheads)*, also projected along the y axis, are due to blood flow and pulsatile motion of the vessel wall.

Controlling sampling artifacts

One may eliminate aliasing by using options called *no phase wrap* and *no frequency wrap* (Fig. 2-39). The computer collects twice the number of views (for example, 256 instead of 128), doubles the field of view in the selected direction, and halves the number of acquisitions. In this way, pixel size, SNR, and imaging time are maintained. After data acquisition, the first and last quarters of the data are discarded, leaving only the desired field of view. Note that each phase encoding step is a view of the entire dataset (not just a representation of one linear strip of the image). Therefore, discarding data is not the same as truncating the boundaries of the displayed image. Note also that the maximum resolution along the frequency-encoding axis depends on the maximum gradient amplitude within the FOV boundaries, not on the number of frequency sampling steps. Thus, extremes of the combined data can be discarded because data from the 256 centrally located readout samples are preserved. Other than the requirement to use at least 2 NEX, there is no penalty for using these options. They are helpful when parts of the anatomy extend outside the selected FOV.

Controlling motion artifacts

Abdominal compression band. An effective means of reducing respiratory motion artifacts is mechanical compression of the abdomen using a wide belt. This belt is strapped tightly over the patient's abdomen and limits the excursion of the abdominal wall during respiration, thereby reducing the extent of ghosting. It often works well but may yield unreliable suppression of artifact. As it does not lengthen imaging time, this technique can be routinely used in abdominal imaging. Because respiratory motion artifact has a minimal effect in the pelvis, respiratory compression is not routinely necessary there.

Respiratory gating. Respiratory gating was developed to reduce the most troublesome artifact in abdominal imaging (due to respiratory motion). It consists of gating image acquisition according to the respiratory cycle.[63] Gating is achieved by placing a flexible strap over the patient's abdomen. This strap contains a sensor that, when compressed or stretched during abdominal expansion, sends a signal to the machine. In theory, images may be acquired at the same point in the respiratory cycle. However, gating is often unreliable, causing less than satisfactory suppression of artifact. Because images are gated to the respiratory cycle, which in the average patient lasts 3 to 5 seconds, the primary drawback to this technique is the extremely long acquisition time. Thus, respiratory compensation at present is cumbersome and generally should not be used.

Respiratory ordering of phase encoding. Respiratory gating reduces artifacts by limiting data collection to one relatively motion-free part of the respiratory cycle. However, this technique wastes data collection time. Respiratory ordering of phase encoding (ROPE or EXORCIST) is

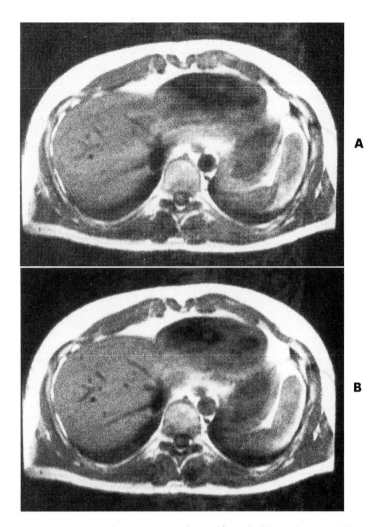

Fig. 2-42. Respiratory compensation reduces motion artifact. **A,** Phase ghosts and blurring due to respiratory motion. **B,** Hepatic vessels sharply displayed in contrast to **A.** Beneficial effect of respiratory compensation by reordered phase step encoding. (From Field SA, Wehrli FW: Signa applications guide, vol 1, Publication No E8804CA, Milwaukee, 1990, General Electric Medical Systems.)

a more efficient algorithm.[2,47] The order of phase line acquisition is linked to the degree of expansion of the chest or upper abdomen. Under software control, gradient steps are sampled at similar relative points during the respiratory cycle throughout the study. Some artifact results from variations in breathing depth and timing, but the intensity of the image distortion is significantly less than occurs with no respiratory compensation (Fig. 2-42).[2,47]

Single breath-hold imaging

Gradient echo. With conventional spin-echo MRI, the shortest possible TR is used with multiple acquisitions. This situation is at best a compromise that may limit difficult examinations to T1 sequences. Even with relatively short TR, scan times are longer than with CT. Because of the adverse effects of respiratory motion and other motion

on image quality, investigators have developed gradient-echo acquisition sequences to produce images with suitable tissue contrast within a single breath-hold (Fig. 2-43).[18,19,90] Some other sequences fast enough for breath-hold imaging are hybrid spin echo (RARE) and echo planar imaging (EPI).* The development of flexible-contrast, fast (1 sec or less) scan sequences will make breath holding the standard technique for MRI of the abdomen.

Half-Fourier reconstruction. Imaging time can be cut by an additional 50% by using a reconstruction technique known as half-Fourier reconstruction (also called half-NEX). Image data in *k space* (the mathematical domain

---

*References 20, 23, 32, 38, 39, 42, 46, 64-66, 75, and 76.

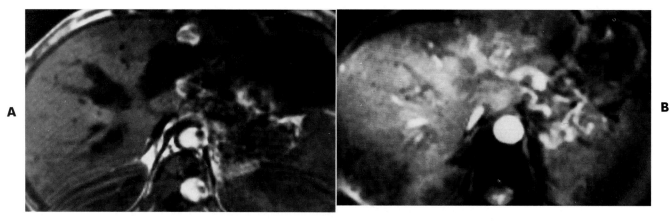

Fig. 2-43. Rapid gradient echo imaging can capture anatomic detail and record the presence of blood flow, which is obscured on conventional spin-echo sequences. **A,** T1W spin-echo image. Poor definition of small vessels. Respiratory motion artifact. Acquisition time 3:34. **B,** Gradient echo, single breath-hold, fat-suppressed image with flow compensation. Visibility of collateral vessels is markedly improved.

containing the data of the phase-encoding lines) has a significant redundancy, which can be exploited to clinical advantage. Mirror-image symmetry is present between two halves of the image data. The image data are contained in the array of phase-encoding lines. Each phase-encoding line is acquired after a short y-axis gradient pulse. The pulse amplitudes increase in equal-amplitude steps until the entire family of phase-encoding lines for one sequence has been acquired. If the number of steps is 256, then 256 different gradient amplitudes are used to form the image dataset. Half of these have a negative phase shift with respect to a zero line (The zero line is the k line for which the y-gradient amplitude is zero). The other half of the lines have a positive phase shift with respect to the zero line (the central line). In a half-Fourier sequence, only half of the dataset is acquired. The missing half set is generated mathematically by mirror-image duplication of the actually sampled half-dataset. The SNR is 40% less than a full dataset, due to the reduction of samples (and imaging time), but the spatial resolution is not diminished.

Reordered and segmented phase decoding. These techniques for reducing imaging time address the inefficiency of phase encoding with standard spin-echo sequences. Modifications are based on the mathematics of complex numbers and differential equations, carried out in a domain mathematicians refer to as *k-space*. Theoretical mathematical concepts can be applied easily to MRI, as most of the really difficult work is calculated by software.[19,51]

The most significant phase lines of the image dataset are known mathematically to be those acquired at and near zero amplitude of the y-gradient pulses. These lines contribute most heavily to the low spatial frequencies of the reconstructed image. The phase lines acquired with larger y-gradient pulses contribute to the higher spatial frequencies. If optimal tissue contrast is expected at a given TE value, then the pulse designer can manipulate the order of phase sampling so that the most significant lines are acquired in a cluster about the target echo time. The usual number of phase lines is acquired. Only the acquisition timing or the steps is altered. This effect is known as reordering of phase encoding.[19,23,39]

Hybrid spin echo. The FSE technique is a variety of the RARE method.[38,39] FSE uses a spin-echo technique, with 90-degree and 180-degree refocusing pulses, to obtain images.[20,42] In a traditional spin echo, only one phase encoding step is performed per slice per repetition time (TR). Since 64 to 512 steps are needed to form a diagnostic image, the scan time extends to 64 to 512 times the TR (several minutes). Rather than acquire several slices per TR, one may perform several phase encoding steps per TR. Fewer slices are obtained as more scan time is used to perform the phase encodes. This sequence allows for breath-hold T1- and T2-weighted imaging and the use of a 512 matrix within acceptable scan times. Costly system upgrades, differences in contrast (as compared to standard spin-echo imaging), and increased radiofrequency power deposition are the most significant drawbacks to this technique.

Echo planar imaging. With echo planar imaging (EPI), data for an entire image are collected in less than a 0.1 second (<100 msec). The sequence uses rapidly oscillating readout and phase encoding gradient pulses to sample the refocused echo (Fig. 2-44). Consider the following example of an EPI sequence with a TE of 40 msec and a readout sampling time of 32 msec (similar to Fig. 2-44). To collect a typical dataset of 64 phase encoding steps, the x gradient is activated at the beginning of the readout pro-

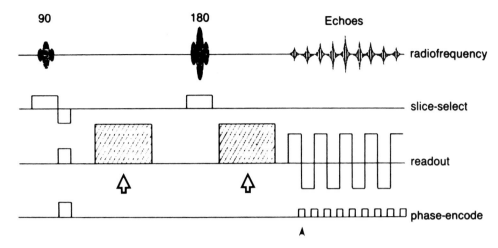

Fig. 2-44. Diffusion echo-planar imaging sequence. In this echo-planar sequence, all of the phase encoded data for an image is collected within one acquisition window after a single 90-degree RF pulse. An oscillating readout gradient transforms the spin echo into a series of gradient echoes. Phase encoding is accomplished by brief gradient pulses *(arrowhead)* of progressively increasing amplitude. The sequence illustrated in this figure is used for diffusion measurements. Diffusion sensitivity is achieved by the activation of large gradients *(open arrows)* before and after the 180-degree RF pulse. The EPI technique for single-shot imaging can be combined with a variety of pulse sequences to provide practically any pattern of tissue contrast weighting. (Courtesy of D. Le Bihan, NIH.)

cess and oscillated continuously between positive and negative at a rate of at least 1600 cycles/second. This pulse rate allows 64 positive-negative gradient cycles to occur during the sampling window. Individual samples are taken during microsecond intervals within the positive half of each x gradient oscillation. Immediately before each sampling interval, the y gradient field is pulsed on for a period of microseconds. With each succeeding sample, the amplitude of the y gradient is gradually increased. Thus, an entire dataset of 64 phase lines is acquired within 56 msec (TE plus one half of the sampling time). The TR essentially is infinite for a single acquisition, as no further RF excitation pulses follow the first one). Therefore EPI can produce heavily T2-weighted images with good SNR. Image contrast can be modified flexibly by additional pulses or gradients applied immediately before or after signal acquisition to provide more or less T1-weighting, T1-selective suppression, or fat-water selective suppression. Either spin-echo or gradient-echo techniques may be used to provide signal for rapid echo-planar sampling. Just about any tissue contrast pattern that can be obtained with other MRI sequences can be obtained with EPI by encapsulating the EPI sampling window within the appropriate pulse and gradient train (Fig. 2-44). A number of implementations and variations of the basic EPI technique have been developed (Fig. 2-45).[23,32,41,46,62,64-66,76]

Fat suppression. In addition to respiratory cycle gating, acquisition sequencing, and various types of rapid imaging, one other major strategy in motion artifact control is the suppression of the unwanted high intensity signal of fat present incidentally in the scanning volume. The reason for the success of fat suppression in the realm of artifact control is not intuitive and is discussed in detail here.

Principles. Software limits the magnitude of intensity values displayable in each phase encode step of an MRI dataset. The high amplitude of the signal from omental, mesenteric, retroperitoneal, and subcutaneous fat disproportionately weight the reconstruction algorithm so that low contrast regions may not be depicted to best advantage. Therefore, one can improve the effective dynamic range of the image data by attenuating the fat signal. This technique allows one to enhance indirectly the weaker signals from water protons. The desired anatomic details also become more conspicuous due to the reduction of motion artifacts brought about by fat suppression. Movement of a low intensity object within the imaging volume is barely perceived, whereas the same movement of a high intensity object may deface the image entirely.[70]

Techniques. With the gradient-echo technique, some degree of fat suppression is observed in a cyclical pattern, which depends on the TE.[45] Amplitude modulation of the MR signal by the difference frequency between fat and water protons (about 220 Hz at 1.5 T) produces variations with a period of approximately 4.5 msec (Fig. 2-46). As the flip angle of a spoiled gradient-echo sequence increases, the contrast weighting changes from proton density to become more dependent on T1. Therefore, the signal of fat increases significantly with respect to water and artifact due to moving high intensity tissues is markedly more evident (see Figs. 2-15, *D,* and 2-52, *A*).

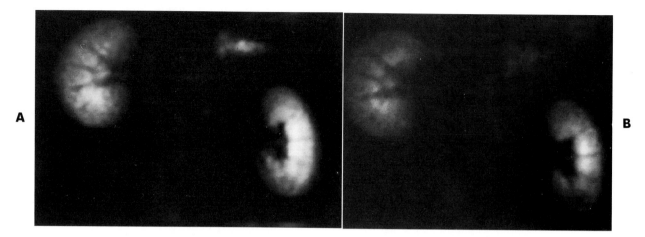

Fig. 2-45. MRI renal diffusion imaging. **A,** Control image (b = 0) for a series of EPI diffusion-sensitized images of rabbit kidneys at 1.5T. TR 4000 msec, TE 80 msec, 50 msec acquisition time per image, 5 mm thickness, 128 × 64 matrix. Note the relatively uniform signal intensity of the renal cortex and medulla. **B,** Diffusion weighted image of rabbit kidneys at 1.5T (b = 550 s/mm*2). No motion artifact or blurring is visible. The cortical signal is attenuated more than the medulla, due to the higher diffusion/perfusion rate of the cortex. (Courtesy of D. Le Bihan and R. Turner, NIH.)

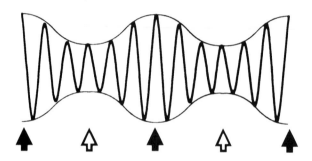

Fig. 2-46. In the body, the signals from water and fat mix, and combine in all possible ways to produce sum and difference products. Their difference frequency, approximately 220 Hz at 1.5 T, mixes with the primary signal (approximately 63 mHz) and modulates it as if it were an AM carrier wave. Because the period of a 220 Hz sine wave is approximately 4.5 msec, the mixed signals of fat and water protons have a regular pattern of alternating minima (*open arrows:* water and fat signals out of phase) and maxima (*solid arrows:* water and fat signals in phase), at 2.25 msec intervals. This effect can be seen on gradient echo scans, as TE is varied slightly. (Modified from Wehrli FW: Advanced MR imaging techniques, Publication No 7513, Milwaukee, 1988, General Electric Medical Systems.)

The STIR (short tau inversion recovery) technique uses an inversion recovery (IR) sequence to suppress the signal from fat (Fig. 2-47).[92] IR sequences use a 180-degree inverting pulse before the standard 90-degree, 180-degree spin-echo sequence. The inversion time (the time TI between the first 180-degree pulse and the 90-degree pulse) becomes the major determinant of T1-weighting, with the TR playing a minimal role. For any value of TI, there is a

T1 for which the signal is zero.[92] The STIR sequence takes advantage of this fact. By selecting an appropriate TI and TR, the signal from fat may be suppressed. Unfortunately, these times are usually long, which results in prolonged acquisition times. Tissues enhanced by paramagnetic contrast agents (which shorten the T1-relaxation time) also undergo undesired suppression by STIR. Until recently, STIR was the primary fat suppression technique used clinically.

The Dixon method and variations of it have been used primarily in the laboratory. This technique requires two separate data acquisition sequences to produce a fat suppressed image.[15] Acquisition 1 is a standard spin-echo sequence, which evokes echoes from both water and fat in phase, without preference. In acquisition 2, the spin-echo refocusing pulse is advanced in phase by 90 degrees (approximately 1 msec in a 1.5 T magnet), so that only the water signal is fully refocused. The out of phase fat signal is partially canceled. Pixel-by-pixel combination of the data from acquisitions 1 and 2 produces either a water- or a fat-suppressed image. Any motion occurring between acquisitions markedly degrades the composite image, as accurate summation of the two datasets is highly dependent on accurate pixel alignment. Furthermore, the method requires careful shimming of the magnetic field for each patient to achieve a higher than usual level of field homogeneity. Due to these constraints, the Dixon method is not used routinely for clinical fat suppression imaging.

More recently, selective chemical presaturation (fat saturation, CHESS, chem-sat) techniques have been developed to suppress the signal from fat.[7,49,50,70] These tech-

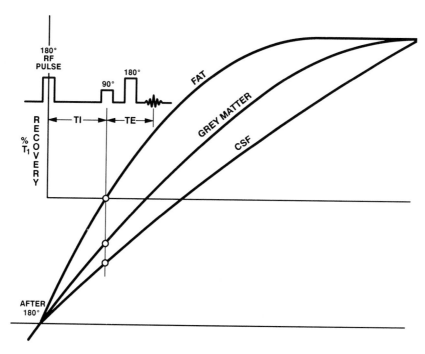

Fig. 2-47. Inversion recovery sequences enhance the T1 relaxation time differences between tissues. A 90-degree excitation pulse follows a 180-degree prepulse. The rate of recovery of longitudinal magnetization and the separation of the 90- and 180-degree pulses (interval TI) determine the appearance of the tissues. The technique can provide lipid suppression, but other substances (such as contrast agents) that have similar relaxation times are also suppressed. (From Prorok RJ: Signa applications guide, vol 2, Milwaukee, 1989, General Electric Medical Systems.)

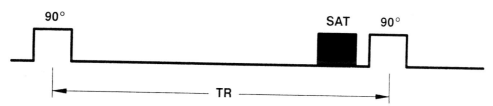

Fig. 2-48. Simplified presaturation pulse sequence. For elimination of blood signal (spatial presaturation), wide bandwidth pulses are used outside the imaging FOV. For selective presaturation of fat (or water), narrow bandwidth pulses are tuned to the resonant frequency of the target substance. The pulse is placed immediately before the 90-degree excitation pulse of the imaging sequence. (From Prorok RJ: Signa applications guide, vol 2, Milwaukee, 1989, General Electric Medical Systems.)

niques employ a tuned 90-degree pulse and a spoiler gradient before the imaging sequence to eliminate the signal from fat (Fig. 2-48). Hydrogen protons precess at varying frequencies, depending on their local environment and the magnetic field strength. Because the resonant frequency of fat is about 3.5 parts per million lower than that of water, at 1.5 T their frequency difference is approximately 220 Hz (see Fig. 2-37).[1,7,73,89] Presaturation techniques exploit this difference: A narrow bandwidth presaturation pulse, at the resonant frequency of fat protons, is used just before

the spin-echo sequence. The longitudinal magnetization vector of fat is rotated into the transverse plane and dephased by a spoiler gradient (Fig. 2-49).[60] Being thus saturated, approximately 66% of the protons in adipose tissue are unable to emit a spin-echo signal when excited by the 90-degree pulse of the imaging sequence that follows shortly thereafter.[4] The scan time of a CHESS sequence closely approaches that of a standard spin-echo sequence (which is significantly less than a STIR sequence). It is compatible with short TR, short TE imaging.

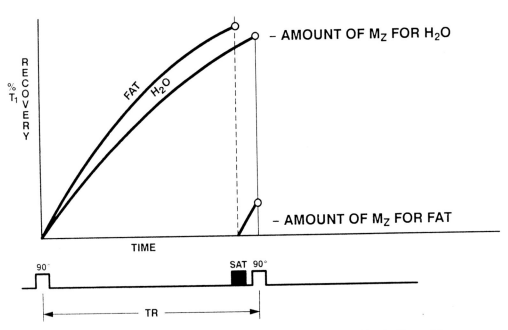

Fig. 2-49. Only the protons of fat respond to a properly tuned pulse. No significant T1 recovery occurs in the interval between the presaturation pulse and the 90-degree excitation pulse. The effectiveness of fat suppression by the CHESS (presaturation) technique is highly dependent on the shape of the presaturation pulse. (From Prorok RJ: Signa applications guide, vol 2, Milwaukee, 1989, General Electric Medical Systems.)

Conventional CHESS fat saturation imaging requires homogeneous static and RF magnetic fields.[7,71] Because field homogeneity decreases at points progressively farther from the isocenter of the magnet, saturation is less effective in the periphery of the bore. Therefore, most implementations of the CHESS technique have been effective only with limited FOVs and small volumes. In addition, each patient's inherent magnetic susceptibility contributes to uneven suppression.[49,50] Hybrid fat suppression sequences have been invented in an attempt to improve on the CHESS method. These sequences combine the Dixon and CHESS techniques. However, uniformity of fat suppression is poor over a large FOV, and setup time is prolonged due to the need for re-shimming of the magnet.[54,78,79]

The homogeneity of CHESS fat suppression depends strongly on the shape of the presaturation pulse. Mao et al.[49,50] designed an improved presaturation pulse that allows the CHESS method to be used successfully in the abdomen. Homogeneous suppression is routinely achieved in clinical imaging with this improved pulse across any projection of the abdomen with no need for special shimming of the magnet (Fig. 2-50, A).[49]

Fat suppression techniques, in combination with intravenous administration of paramagnetic contrast agents, have been shown to increase the rate of detection of renal lesions.[71] Even without contrast agents, the conspicuity of pathology may be improved by fat suppression (Fig. 2-50, B).

Controlling cardiac motion. Although pulse gating is useful for suppression of pulsatile motion artifact, it prolongs scan times. Gating is triggered from an optical transducer linked to the scan controller by fiber optic cable (peripheral pulse), or from the electrocardiogram (ECG). It is often impractical for reducing vascular pulsations (i.e., takes too long relative to the diagnostic yield) but may be useful to eliminate cardiac ghosting in the extreme upper abdomen (i.e., for looking at lesions in the liver dome). In addition, ECG gating can be unreliable on some MRI units due to interference from the strong transient electromagnetic fields.

Controlling body motion. Highly significant artifact arises from any bulk physical motion in the scan volume. Placement of the arms extended along the abdomen is a setup for phase misregistration artifact due to movement. This motion is irregular and cannot be nulled prospectively. Routine scanner software offers little for postprocessing jerky spontaneous motion. Prevention is the key. Reconstruction of images from serially acquired phase lines of data is based on the assumption of symmetry of background throughout the acquisition. Movement of spins in and out of the sensitive volume heavily distorts the mathematical computations of image processing (Figs. 2-51, A, and 2-52, A). Proper explanation of the scanning procedure to the patient, and orientation to the noises and sensations of the scanner bore are essential to motion control.

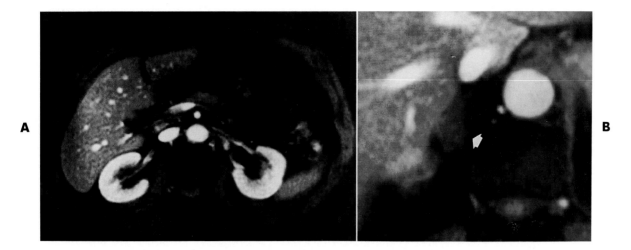

Fig. 2-50. CHESS (Chemical shift selective) fat suppression with an optimized presaturation pulse. **A,** Uniform fat suppression has been achieved across the full diameter of the abdomen with this optimized gradient echo, single breath-hold fat suppression sequence.[68,70] This patient was allergic to iodine contrast agent and was suspected of having renal carcinoma. **B,** Same patient as **A.** An incidental mass is present in the right adrenal gland *(arrow).* No renal mass is present.

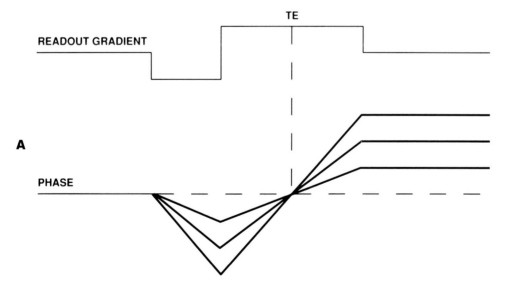

Fig. 2-51. Flow compensation by gradient moment nulling. **A,** Stationary protons are rephased by the readout gradient of a gradient echo sequence. Constant velocity motion through a gradient field introduces a steady phase shift that defeats the rephasing gradient. The phase plots for three different velocities are demonstrated. Failure of the lines to return to the zero axis is a representation of residual dephasing, which attenuates signal.

Continued.

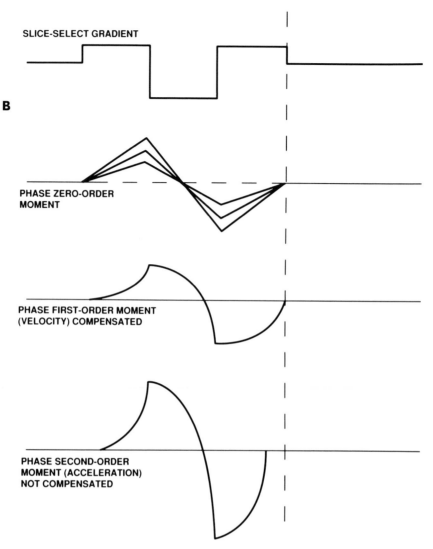

SLICE-SELECT GRADIENT

B

PHASE ZERO-ORDER
MOMENT

PHASE FIRST-ORDER MOMENT
(VELOCITY) COMPENSATED

PHASE SECOND-ORDER
MOMENT (ACCELERATION)
NOT COMPENSATED

Fig. 2-51, cont'd. B, Effect of flow compensation gradients. Stationary tissue (zero order moment) rephases properly in a flow compensation gradient sequence. First order motion dephasing (due to constant velocity) is corrected. Second order motion dephasing (due to acceleration) is only partially corrected by flow compensation. (From Turshi P et al: Vascular magnetic resonance imaging, Signa applications guide, vol 3, Publication No E8804DB, Milwaukee, 1990, General Electric Medical Systems.)

Controlling flow artifacts

Gradient moment nulling. Also called gradient motion rephasing or flow compensation, this technique uses additional gradients to correct phase errors resulting from flowing blood (Figs. 2-51, *B,* and 2-52, *B*).[30] Gradients that correct first order motion effects can recover signal from excited protons moving at constant velocity. Second order motion correction addresses acceleration. Third order and fourth order correction algorithms are for regular (rhythmic pulsation) and irregular (intermittent jerk) motions. Flow compensation or gradient moment nulling as it is most commonly used in standard clinical MRI units is first order correction.

Because blood velocity varies with the cardiac cycle (especially in arteries), blood signal also varies. Pulsatility may produce unreliable blood signal intensity and create ghosts of vessels along the phase encoding direction. Note that the artifact is depicted in the phase encoding direction regardless of the direction of the motion (Fig. 2-52, *A*).

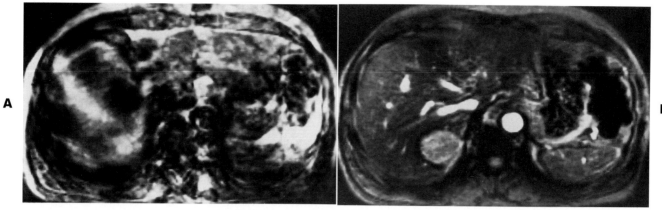

Fig. 2-52. Combined effect of flow compensation and optimal flip angle on motion artifact. **A,** Gradient echo single breath-hold scan with flip angle of 90 degrees. Substantial artifacts from moving fat. Vascular pulsation ghosts. Flow compensation disabled. **B,** With flow compensation enabled, high intensity vascular signals are restored. Reduction of artifacts versus **A** is primarily due to reduction of the flip angle to 30 degrees. Motion of low intensity structures has negligible artifact-producing effect. In this sequence, the intensity of fat in the abdominal wall is significantly lower than in **A.**

Gradient moment nulling corrects for some of the effects of pulsatile flow. Clinically, this results in dependable high signal intensity for flowing blood and a reduction in ghosting artifacts. Because the vascular signal is so bright, however, nearby pathology may be obscured, especially when one must evaluate isolated lesions in the liver, where high signal in the intrahepatic vessels may be confused for pathology on T2-weighted images.

Flow rate and direction are important variables, particularly in the sections that lie at the extreme margins of the imaging volume. The entry slice phenomenon is caused by unsaturated blood responding with a vigorous echo to the first few pulses it encounters on entering the imaging volume. Higher velocity propels the high amplitude signal deeper into the volume before saturation and signal loss occur (see Chapter 7) (Fig. 2-53).

Spatial presaturation. This technique uses a 90-degree pulse at the resonant frequency of water placed just outside the FOV. Such pulses effectively saturate all protons in the selected zones, including those flowing in vessels. The presaturation pulse destroys the longitudinal magnetization so that when blood flows into the FOV it cannot emit a signal.[21] This technique produces a reliable signal void within blood vessels containing flowing blood. A presaturation pulse must be placed upstream from the area of interest to achieve the desired effect. For example, saturation of the abdominal aorta may be accomplished by placing a presaturation pulse above the diaphragm (Fig. 2-54). Saturation of the intrahepatic inferior vena cava may be accomplished by placing the presaturation pulse caudal to the inferior margin of the liver. Presaturation eliminates ghosting artifacts and artifactual variations in intraluminal signal intensity.

SPECIAL IMAGING TECHNIQUES
MR angiography

This technique uses gradient echo acquisition with gradient moment nulling and a postprocessing algorithm to produce angiograms without using intravenous contrast agents. Although this technique is currently used most commonly for evaluation of the head and neck vasculature, it may be used in certain instances to evaluate the vessels of the abdomen and pelvis. MR angiography (MRA) can be used to assess the abdominal aorta, the inferior vena cava, the portal and hepatic veins, the renal arteries and veins, and many other vessels in the abdomen and pelvis (see Chapter 7).

MR cineangiography

This technique also uses gradient-echo acquisition but yield information different from MRA; it exploits the cyclical nature of cardiac motion and blood flow to produce images. Electrocardiogram-gated spin-echo acquisition yields images of the heart or vasculature at a given point in the cardiac cycle, effectively eliminating motion artifact due to the beating heart. Rather than acquire many slices at one point in the cycle, MR cine acquires one or two slices at many points in the cycle. A postprocessing algorithm plays the images back rapidly, in a cinematic loop, to create motion in the same manner as a movie reel.[27,83]

In the heart, MR cine provides valuable information regarding wall motion and thickness, ejection fraction, and valve function.[9,12,16,24,69,77,80,82,85] However, MR cine may also be quite useful in the abdomen and pelvis. Sites of turbulence create spin dephasing and signal loss within flowing blood. Thus, at areas of stenosis, one may see a signal void the size of which varies during the cardiac cy-

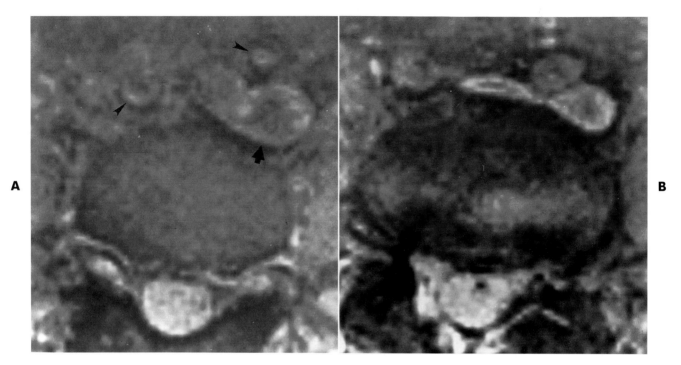

Fig. 2-53. Entry slice phenomenon. A cause of paradoxical high intensity in vessels. **A,** Left-sided inferior vena cava. Gradient-echo sequence. Intensity of venous blood *(arrow)* similar to arterial blood *(arrowheads)*. **B,** Caudal to **A.** High intensity of inflowing blood was the clue to the correct diagnosis of the venous anomaly.

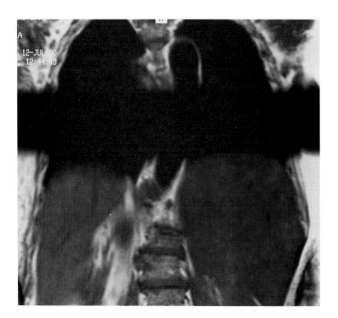

Fig. 2-54. Spatial presaturation. An RF pulse of appropriate frequency and bandwidth, transmitted immediately before the imaging pulse series, produces a horizontal band of hypointensity which, in this case, includes the heart. The protons of rapidly flowing arterial blood do not have a sufficient recovery time to reconstitute their longitudinal magnetization before entering the abdominal aorta. Therefore, they produce no undesirable signals in response to the imaging pulse sequence.

cle. MR cine best shows the nature and extent of this flow abnormality.

MR cine may be used to evaluate the extent of tumor thrombus in the inferior vena cava and right atrium in patients with renal cell carcinoma. However, a conventional MRI sequence can provide the information needed for clinical diagnosis even if one is not equipped with special cine-angiographic software (Fig. 2-55).

COIL SELECTION

Until recently, only the body coil could be used for abdominal imaging. Although this large-volume coil can provide sufficient fields of view to demonstrate the entire abdomen or pelvis, it has a relatively poor SNR (which limits spatial resolution). For most MR examinations of the abdomen and pelvis, the body coil provides diagnostic quality images. However, for small regions of interest, where pathology may be subtle and high SNR high resolution scans are needed, other coils should be used.[44] These alternatives include the body Helmholz coil (for regional imaging, especially of the liver and pelvis) (Fig. 2-56), an endorectal coil (for prostate and rectum imaging), and surface coils (for scrotal imaging) (Fig. 2-57). All provide higher SNR than the body coil but limit the available field of view. Much investigation continues in an effort to develop coils of specialized size and geometry (see Chapter 5).

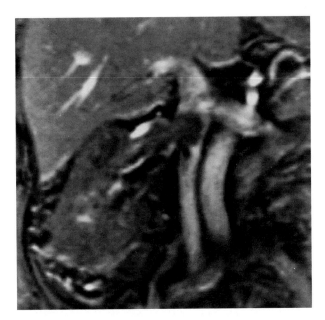

Fig. 2-55. Single breath-hold optimized CHESS fat suppression sequence. Tumor thrombus partially occluding the inferior vena cava is demonstrated to good advantage.

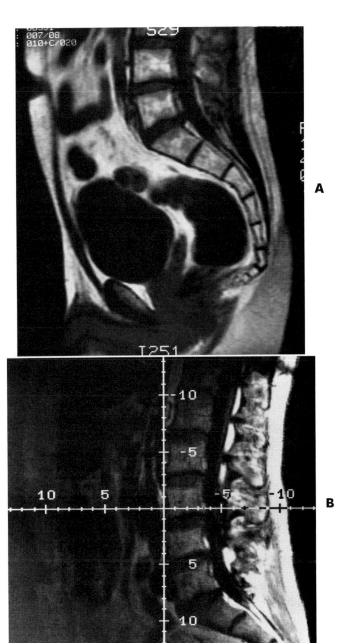

A

B

Fig. 2-57. Surface coil examination of the scrotum. The epididymis, blood vessels, corpora cavernosa, and a hydrocele are well demonstrated.

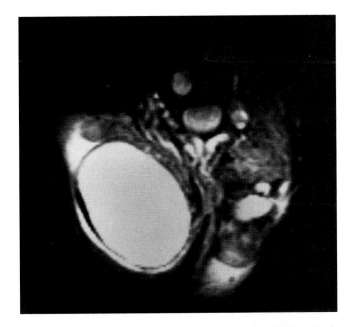

Fig. 2-56. Coil selection for uniform SNR. **A,** T1W sagittal MRI. Uniform high SNR is obtained throughout the pelvis. **B,** The rapid fall-off of field intensity in this surface coil sagittal image is a marked contrast to the uniformity of the Helmholz pair. Surface coils can be used to good advantage, however, for regions near the skin surface.

SPECTROSCOPY

MR spectroscopy (MRS) has been used experimentally for evaluation of the liver,[3,28] prostate,[72,67] and other regions of the genitourinary tract.[8,11,29] Spectra have been obtained from three naturally occurring nuclei: hydrogen (^{1}H), phosphorus (^{31}P), and carbon (^{13}C).[3,11,28,72] Changes are observed during the infusion of naturally occurring substances, (such as fructose, glucose, and L-alanine) and synthetic substances (such as ^{19}F perfluorochemicals and 5-fluorouracil).[52,91] Technical challenges limit spectroscopy to experimental use at the time of this writing. Even at 1.5 T, MRS of low-abundance nuclei (such as ^{31}P and ^{13}C) is complicated by extremely poor SNR, which mandates custom shim adjustment for every experiment, large voxels, and signal averaging. SNR can be increased with stronger magnets (flux density of 4T and greater). The greatly increased cost and the increased risk of biologic side effects limit the potential for use of magnets greater than 2T in the clinical practice of abdominal MRI (see Chapter 3).

FUTURE TECHNICAL DEVELOPMENTS

Rapid changes in abdominal MRI techniques are occurring in the areas of coil design, pharmaceutical contrast agents, pulse sequences, and fast scanning. Multielement surface coils and improved insertable microcoils will be standard equipment for abdominal MRI examinations. Oral ferromagnetic contrast agents will have wide applicability. Intravenous superparamagnetic contrast agents for MRI lymphangiography are expected in the future. Magnetization transfer and diffusion-weighted pulse sequences will be released for general use to allow demonstration of previously undetectable contrast differences among tissues (see Fig. 2-45). Finally, as improvements in gradient systems become widely available, echoplanar imaging will provide motion-free images and dynamic sequences that will revolutionize the clinical practice of abdominal MRI (see Figs. 2-44 and 2-45).

ACKNOWLEDGMENTS

Raymond Ballinger, MD, reviewed MR spectroscopy and provided all of the annotated bibliographic material for the preparation of the spectroscopy section. Jintong Mao, PhD, wrote the single breath-hold modified-CHESS fat suppression pulse sequences used for most of the cases in this chapter.[49,50]

REFERENCES

1. Babcock EE, Brateman L, Weinreb JC: Edge artifacts in MR images: chemical shift effect, J Comput Assist Tomogr 9:252, 1985.
2. Bailes DR, Gilderdale DJ, Bydder GM, et al: Respiratory ordered phase encoding (ROPE): a method for reducing respiratory motion artifacts in MR imaging, J Comput Assist Tomogr 9:835, 1985.
3. Barany M, et al: High resolution proton magnetic resonance spectroscopy of human brain and liver, Magn Reson Imaging 5:393-398, 1987.
4. Booth RFG, Honey AD, Martin JF, et al: Lipid characterization in an animal model of atherosclerosis using NMR spectroscopy and imaging, NMR Biomed 3:95, 1990.
5. Bottomly PA, Hardy CJ, Argersinger RE, et al: A review of 1H nuclear magnetic resonance relaxation in pathology: are T1 and T2 diagnostic? Med Phys 14:1, 1987.
6. Bottomly PA: NMR imaging techniques and applications: a review, Rev Sci Instrum 53:1319, 1982.
7. Brateman L: Chemical shift imaging, AJR 146:971, 1986.
8. Bretan PN, et al: Assessment of testicular metabolic integrity with P31 MR spectroscopy, Radiology 162:867-871, 1987.
9. Buckwalter KA, et al: Gated cardiac MRI: ejection fraction determination using the right anterior oblique view, AJR 147:33, 1986.
10. Buxton RB, Edelman RR, Rosen BR, et al: Contrast in rapid MR imaging: T1- and T2-weighted imaging, J Comput Assist Tomogr 11:776, 1987.
11. Chew WE, Hricak H, Carroll PR: The study of testicular pathologies with an integrated 1H MRI and 31P MRS examination (abstr), In Book of abstracts: Society of Magnetic Resonance in Medicine 1991, San Francisco, 1991, Society of Magnetic Resonance in Medicine.
12. Chiles C, et al: Evaluation of congenital absence or stenosis of a pulmonary artery: new techniques, Annual Meeting of the Radiology Society of North America, Chicago, November, 1986, p 257.
13. Clark JA II, Kelly WM: Common artifacts encountered in magnetic resonance imaging, Radiol Clin North Am 26:893, 1988.
14. Czervionke LF, Daniels DL, Wehrli FW, et al: Magnetic susceptibility artifact in gradient recalled echo MR imaging, Am J Neuroradiol 9:1149, 1988.
15. Dixon WT: Simple proton spectroscopic imaging, Radiology 153:189-194, 1984.
16. Dodge JT, Sheehan FJ: Quantitative contrast angiography for assessment of ventricular performance in heart disease, J Am Coll Cardiol 1:73, 1983.
17. Edelman RR, Atkinson DJ, Silver MS, et al: FRODO pulse sequence: a new means of eliminating motion, flow, and wraparound artifact, Radiology 166:231, 1988.
18. Edelman RR, et al: Rapid MR imaging with suspended respiration: clinical application in the liver, Radiology 161:125-132, 1986.
19. Edelman RR, et al: Segmented TurboFLASH: method for breathhold MR imaging of the liver with flexible contrast, Radiology 177:515-521, 1990.
20. Egerter DE, Jones-Bey H: Fast spin-echo, MRA alters disease diagnosis, Diagn Imaging, 125, 1991.
21. Felmlee JP, Ehman RL: Spatial presaturation: a method for suppressing flow artifacts and improving depiction of vascular anatomy in MR imaging, Radiology 164:559, 1987.
22. Field SA, Wehrli FW: Signa applications guide, vol 1, Publication Number E8804CA, Milwaukee, 1990, General Electric Medical Systems.
23. Finn JP: Fast MR imaging: MRI decisions May/June, pp 23-27, 1991.
24. Fisher MR, Von Schulthess GK, Higgins CB: Multi-phasic cardiac magnetic resonance imaging with normal regional left ventricular wall thickening, AJR 145:27, 1985.
25. FLASH and FISP Gradient Echo Pulse Sequences, Publication Number MG/5000-217-121, Siemens Medical Systems, Inc, Iselin, NJ.
26. Frahm J, Haase A, Matthaei D, et al: FLASH MR imaging: from images to movies, Presented at the 71st Annual Meeting of the Radiological Society of North America, Chicago, Nov, 17-22, 1985.
27. Frahm J, Haase A, Matthaei D: Rapid NMR imaging of dynamic processes using the flash technique, Magn Reson Med 3:324, 1986.
28. Glazer GM, et al: Image localized 31P magnetic resonance spectroscopy of the human liver, NMR Biomed 1(4):184-189, 1989.
29. Grist TM, Charles HC, Sostman HD: Renal transplant rejection: diagnosis with 31P MR Spectroscopy, AJR 156(1):105-112, 1991.
30. Haacke EM, Lenz GW: Improving MR image quality in the presence of motion by using rephasing gradients, AJR 148:1251, 1989.

31. Haacke EM, Hausmann R, Laub G, et al: MR angiography: Magnetom SP, Erlangen, Germany, 1990, Siemens Aktiengesellschaft.

32. Haacke EM, Tkach JA: Fast MR imaging: techniques and clinical applications, Radiology 155:951, 1990.

33. Haase A, Frahm J, Matthaei D, et al: FLASH imaging, Rapid NMR imaging using low flip angle pulses, J Magn Reson 67:258,1986.

34. Haase A, Frahm J, Matthaei D, et al: Rapid images and NMR movies, Proceedings of the Fourth Annual Meeting of the Society of Magnetic Resonance in Medicine, London, August 19, 1985.

35. Hahn EL: Spin echoes, Physiol Rev 80:580, 1950.

36. Hahn FJ, Chu W-K, Coleman PE, et al: Artifacts and pitfalls on magnetic resonance imaging: a clinical review, Radiol Clin North Am 26:717, 1988.

37. Hendrick RE, Kneeland JB, Stark DD: Maximizing signal-to-noise and contrast-to-noise ratios in FLASH imaging, Magn Reson Imaging 5:117, 1987.

38. Hennig J, Friedburg H: Clinical applications and methodological developments of the RARE technique, Magn Reson Imaging 6:391, 1988.

39. Hennig J, Nauerth A, Friedburg H: RARE Imaging: fast imaging method for clinical MR, Magn Reson Med 1986;3:823-833.

40. Hinshaw WS, et al: Fundamentals of magnetic resonance imaging, Solon, Ohio, 1984, Technicare Corp.

41. Housman JF et al: Improvements in snapshot NMR imaging, Br J Radiol 61:822, 1988.

42. Jolesz FA, et al: Fast spin echo technique, Presented at Society of Magnetic Resonance in Medicine Annual Meeting, August, 1990.

43. Kneeland JB, Shimakawa A, Wehrli FW: Effect of intersection spacing on MR image contrast and study time, Radiology 158:819, 1986.

44. Kneeland JB: Instrumentation. In Stark DD, Bradley WG, editors: Magnetic resonance imaging, ed 1, St Louis, 1988, Mosby–Year Book.

45. Lang P, et al: Hematopoietic bone marrow hyperplasia of the knee: use of out-of-phase gradient-echo MR imaging. In Lemke HU, editor: Computer assisted radiology, New York, 1991, Springer-Verlag.

46. LeBihan D: Molecular diffusion nuclear magnetic resonance imaging, Magn Reson Q 7:1, 1991.

47. Li KCP, Ho-Tai P: MR imaging of the liver: technique considerations, Appl Radiol 10, 1990.

48. Mansfield et al: Biological and medical imaging by NMR, J Magn Reson 29:355, 1978.

49. Mao J, Bidgood WD Jr, Ang GP, et al: A clinically available technique of fat suppression for abdomen and pelvis, Magn Reson Med, 21:320-326, 1991.

50. Mao J, Yan H, Bidgood WD Jr.: Fat suppression with an improved selective presaturation pulse, Magn Reson Imaging 10: 49-53, 1992.

51. Martin JF, Edelman RR, Fast MR: Imaging. In Edelman RR, Hesselink JR, editors: Clinical magnetic resonance imaging, Philadelphia, 1990, WB Saunders.

52. Mason RP, et al.: Perfluorocarbon imaging in vivo: a 19F MRI study in tumor-bearing mice, Magn Reson Imaging 7:475-485, 1989.

53. Mitchell DG, Vinitksi S, Burk DL Jr et al: Motion artifact reduction in MR imaging of the abdomen: gradient moment nulling versus respiratory-sorted phase encoding, Radiology 169:155, 1988.

54. Mitchell DG, Vinitsky S, Saponaro S, et al: Liver and pancreas: improved spin-echo T1 contrast by shorter echo time and fat suppression at 1.5 T, Radiology 178:67, 1991.

55. Pattany PM, Phillips JJ, Chin LC, et al: Motion artifact suppression technique (MAST) for MR imaging, J Comput Assist Tomogr 11:369, 1987.

56. Patton JA, Kulkarni MV, Craig JK, et al: Techniques, pitfalls and artifacts in magnetic resonance imaging, Radiography 7:505,1987.

57. Perman WH, Moran PR, Moran RA, et al: Artifacts from pulsatile flow in MR imaging, J Comput Assist Tomogr 10:473,1986.

58. Porter BA, Hastrip W, Richardson ML, et al: Classification and investigation of artifacts in magnetic resonance imaging, Radiography 7:271, 1987.

59. Powers T, Lum A, Patton JA: Abdominal MRI artifacts, Semin Ultrasound CT MR 10:2, 1989.

60. Prorok RJ: Signa applications guide, vol 2, Milwaukee, 1989, General Electric Medical Systems.

61. Pusey E, Yoon C, Anselmo ML, et al: Aliasing artifacts in MR imaging, Comput Med Imaging Graph 12:219, 1989.

62. Pykett IL, Rzedzian RR: Instant images of the body by magnetic resonance, Magn Reson Med 5:563, 1987.

63. Runge VM, Clanton JA, Partain CL: Respiratory gating in magnetic resonance imaging at 0.5 Tesla, Radiology 151:521,1984.

64. Rzedzian RR, Pykett IL: Instant images of the human heart using a new, whole-body MR imaging system, AJR 149:245, 1987.

65. Rzedzian RR, Doyle M, Mansfield P, et al: Echo planar imaging in pediatrics: real-time nuclear magnetic resonance, Radiology 153:566, 1984.

66. Saini S, Stark DD, Rzedzian RR, et al: Forty-millisecond MR imaging of the abdomen at 2.0 T, Radiology 173:111, 1989.

67. Scheibler M, et al: In-vitro high resolution proton spectroscopy of the human prostate: benign prostatic hyperplasia and adenocarcinoma (abstract). In Book of abstracts: Society of Magnetic Resonance in Medicine 1991, San Francisco, 1991.

68. Schwarghofer BW, Yu KK, Mattrey RF: Diagnostic significance of interslice gap and imaging volume in body MR imaging, AJR 153:629, 1989.

69. Sechtem UP, et al: Assessment of regional left ventricular wall thickening by MRI, (abstract), Annual Meeting of the Society of Magnetic Resonance in Medicine, Montreal, Canada, August 1986.

70. Semelka RC, Chew W, Hricak H, et al: Fat-saturation MR imaging of the upper abdomen, AJR 155:1111, 1990.

71. Semelka RC, Hricak H, Stevens SK, et al: Combined gadolinium-enhanced and fat-saturation MR imaging of renal masses, Radiology 178:803, 1991.

72. Sillerud LO, et al: In vivo 13C NMR spectroscopy of the human prostate, Magn Reson Med 8(2):224-230, 1988.

73. Soila KP, Viamonte M Jr, Starewicz PM: Chemical shift misregistration effect in magnetic resonance imaging, Radiology 153:819, 1984.

74. Sprawls P: Spatial characteristics of the MR image. In Stark DD, Bradley WG, editors: Magnetic resonance imaging, ed 1, St Louis, 1988, Mosby–Year Book.

75. Stehling MK, Evans DF, Lamont G, et al: Gastrointestinal tract: dynamic MR studies with echo-planar imaging, Radiology 171:41, 1989.

76. Stehling MK, Howseman AM, Ordidge RJ, et al: Whole-body echo-planar MR imaging at 0.5 T, Radiology 170:257, 1989.

77. Stratmeier EJ, et al: Ejection fraction determination by MR imaging: comparison with left ventricular angiography, Radiology 158:755, 1986.

78. Szumowski J, Simon JH: Fat suppression improves contrast-enhancing imaging, Q Magazine Magn Reson 47, 1991.

79. Szumowski J, Eisen JK, Vinitski, et al: Hybrid methods of chemical shift imaging, Magn Reson Med 9:379, 1989.

80. Thompson R, et al: Accurate determination of left ventricular ejection fraction and regional wall motion in man from contiguous short axis magnetic resonance tomograms: comparison with angiography, (abstract). Annual Meeting Society of Magnetic Resonance in Medicine, Montreal, Canada, August 1986.

81. Turshi P, et al: Vascular magnetic resonance imaging, Signa Applications Guide vol 3, Publication Number E8804DB, Milwaukee, General Electric Medical Systems, 1990.

82. Utz JA, et al: Rapid dynamic MR imaging of the heart in the evaluation of valvular function, (abstract). Annual Meeting of the Radiological Society of North America, Chicago, November, 1986.

83. Utz JA, et al: Rapid dynamic NMR imaging of the heart, (abstract). Annual Meeting of the Society of Magnetic Resonance in Medicine, Montreal, Canada, August 1986.

84. Utz JA, Herfkens MD, Glover G, et al: Three-second clinical NMR images using a gradient recall acquisition in a steady-state mode (GRASS), (abstract). Magn Reson Imaging 4:106, 1986.

85. Utz JA, Herfkens RJ, et al: CINE MRI determination of left ventricular ejection fraction, AJR 148:839, 1987.

86. Wehrli FW, MacFall J, Newton TH: Parameters determining the appearance of NMR images. In Newton TH, Potts DG, editors: Advanced imaging techniques, vol II, San Francisco, 1983, Clavadel Press.

87. Wehrli FW: Principles of magnetic resonance. In Stark DD, Bradley WG, editors: Magnetic resonance imaging, ed 1, St Louis, 1988, Mosby–Year Book.

88. Wehrli FW: Advanced MR imaging techniques, Publication Number 7513, Milwaukee, 1988, General Electric Medical Systems.

89. Weinreb JC, Brateman L, Babcock EE, et al: Chemical shift artifact in clinical magnetic resonance images at 0.35 T, AJR 145:183, 1985.

90. Winkler ML, et al: Hepatic neoplasia: breath-hold MR Imaging, Radiology 170:801-806, 1989.

91. Wolf W, et al.: Fluorine-19 NMR spectroscopic studies of the metabolism of 5-fluorouracil in the liver of patients undergoing chemotherapy, Magn Reson Imaging 5:165-169, 1987.

92. Young IR: Special pulse sequences and techniques. In Stark DD, Bradley WG, editors: Magnetic resonance imaging, ed 1, St Louis, 1988, Mosby–Year Book.

Chapter 3

EQUIPMENT, OPERATION, AND SAFETY

W. Dean Bidgood, Jr.
Jeffrey R. Fitzsimmons

Equipment
    System design
    Magnet
    Control and display
    Software
Operation
Safety
    Main magnetic field effects
    Radiofrequency energy effects
    Biomagnetic effects

EQUIPMENT

A magnetic resonance imaging (MRI) system is composed of major modular subsystems. These subsystems include magnet, gradient amplifiers and coils, radio transmitter, radio receiver, patient table, power supply, line conditioning unit, radiofrequency (RF) shielding, and magnetic shielding. For practical purposes, these use stable, well-developed technology, although incremental improvements are being continually developed (Fig. 3-1).

Advances in magnet design allow installation in as little as 250 to 500 sq ft. More efficient designs and new strong, lighter materials have reduced some superconducting systems to approximately 13,000 lb.[7] Improved refrigeration for superconducting magnets reduces the consumption of cryogens. Linear, high output digital gradient amplifiers and shielded gradient coils support rapid scanning and special techniques, such as diffusion imaging.[2,4,5]

Digital RF transmitters offer superior precision over analog devices in timing and shaping of pulses. Digital modules offer equivalent advantages in the receiver system. Direct digital frequency synthesizers combine a microprocessor, a digital-to-analog (D/A) converter, and digitally designed low-pass filters to produce signals with arbitrarily fine frequency resolution. For practical purposes, RF equipment is no longer a limiting factor in clinical MRI.[6]

Postprocessing (3D reconstruction and image enhancement), archiving (electronic filing), and image transmission (networking) are bringing entirely new capabilities to the MRI system. The most frequent MRI hardware upgrades concern the main central processing unit (CPU) and its image processing boards. The upgrades provide increased speed, capacity, and simultaneous processing for operations such as image reconstruction, preparation of finished copy for interpretation, special image processing, reformatting of arbitrary planes of view, angiography, and phase/motion displays. Some designs embody open system concepts, which facilitate connectivity and compatibility with electronic networks, external display monitors, and image processing subsystems.

System design

Fixed versus transportable systems. Transportable MRI units offer the advantage of multisite coverage at less expense than building a series of underused fixed units. Transportable units are providing relatively economical and reliable service at numerous installations of all descriptions. A typical nonsuperconducting mobile MRI unit can deliver service up time in the high 90% range. Special problems must be considered, however. Buildings and

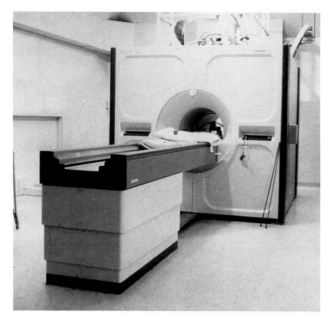

Fig. 3-1. Super conducting 1.5 T MRI scanner. This scanner is in service 18 hours per day. Its up-time reliability has been greater than 95%.

utility service at each site must be planned carefully to maximize convenience and privacy of patients, while maximizing safety to passers-by and minimizing the effect of objects in the vicinity of the scanner on the uniformity of its magnetic field.

Mobile installations require special attention to the quality of the electrical power provided at "docking pads" (Fig. 3-2). Power line surges are frequent causes of component failures and excessive down time. Power outages due to lightning strikes and transient line voltage drops (brownouts) take a heavy toll of circuit boards, not to mention the number of partially completed studies that must be repeated. A power conditioning unit provides some protection. Technical anomalies, such as undetected reversal of three phase power feed lines, can cause chronic equipment failures that are difficult to diagnose in spite of well-intentioned maintenance efforts.

MRI installations in a large medical center may require a long cable run with significant voltage drop. The most direct route to the public utility service connection point should be specified. Circuits shared with heating, air conditioning, elevators, or other machinery are a potential source of problems. Therefore, power conditioning is ben-

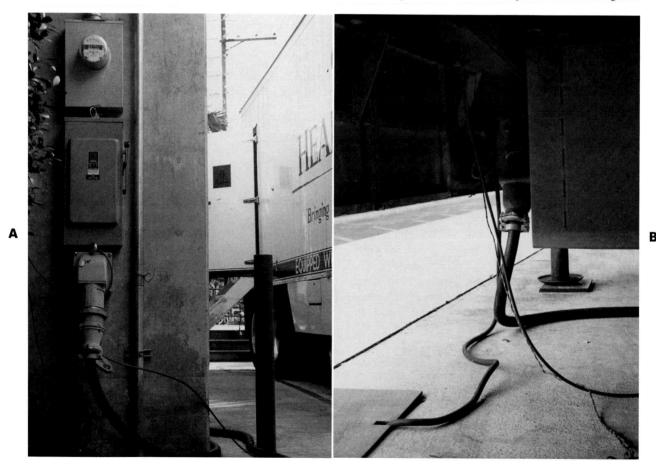

Fig. 3-2. Transportable MRI installation. **A,** A disconnect box provides a safe termination for line voltage when the scanner is located else where. **B,** At the scanner end of the mobile installation, the heavy power cable, a ground wire, a fiber optic cable for a remote view station, and a twisted pair phone line are connected. (Courtesy of Santa Fe Healthcare System Inc.)

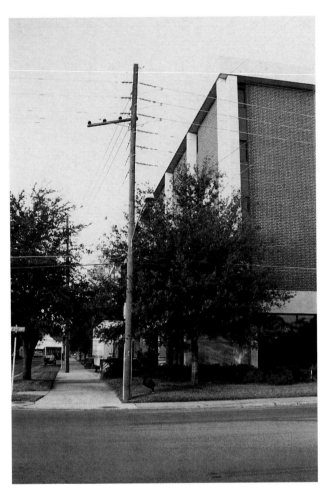

Fig. 3-3. Although open to view, the transportable scanner is well camouflaged by landscaping. This is a simple but effective installation. (Courtesy of Santa Fe Healthcare System Inc.)

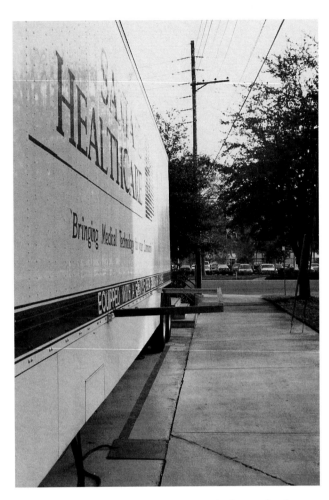

Fig. 3-4. A shield formed of angle iron indicates the 5 gauss line. Note the covered access to the ground wire termination. (Courtesy of Santa Fe Healthcare Inc.)

eficial for fixed sites as well as for transportable units.

Architecture. Although both permanent and transportable units must plan for magnetic field safety, the portable installation has the special problem of creating (attractive) access for a large tractor-trailer (Fig. 3-3). Often the only available space is already encumbered by surrounding buildings. Some sites integrate the mobile unit with a permanent building by way of a permanent passageway or a flexible structure, such as an awning, to give a sense of permanency. This approach also avoids compromise of personal modesty (while the patient moves from the dressing room to scan area) and protects patients and staff from the weather. One's options are limited by local zoning and traffic laws. The prevailing regulations must be investigated thoroughly, as appropriate rezoning or granting of special use permits might come only after a long and costly delay.

If the best compromise location places the magnet in a position allowing dangerously close approach by cardiac pacemaker users and others at risk from magnetic fields, remov-

able cordons or gates may be used to protect passersby (Fig. 3-4). Warning signs frequently are overlooked either carelessly or intentionally (Fig. 3-5). Strategically placed landscaping features can be more effective than signage for preventing exposure to the fringe magnetic field of the MRI scanner (Fig. 3-6).

Outpatient appeal versus inpatient convenience. A new freestanding magnetic imaging center can be a powerful marketing tool for a radiology group or hospital. The examinations are amenable to off-site supervision, and complications are rare. However, transport of inpatients to a freestanding center is awkward and inconvenient, even in good weather. Transportation (whether by ambulance, car, stretcher, or wheelchair) may be a major obstacle to use of outpatient MRI facility by hospital inpatients. Hospitals often balk at having their inpatient care personnel transport inpatients anywhere outside of the hospital itself, even if the unit is owned by a related company or subsidiary. Medical liability is the primary issue. Emergency coverage responsibility is problematic. In some cases, the

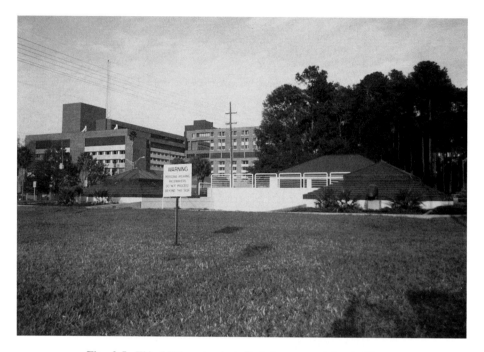

Fig. 3-5. This MRI center is built below ground level. The 5 gauss line is approximately at the visible concrete border. Located in this wide open lawn, a small warning sign is virtually ineffective.

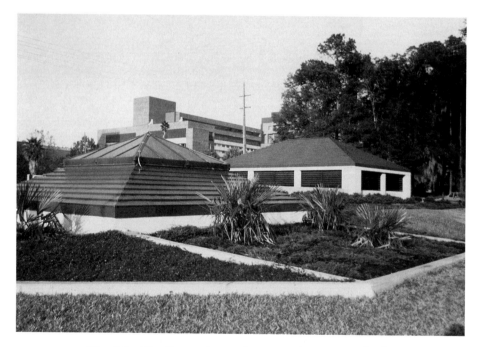

Fig. 3-6. Attractive vent ground cover and a concrete border foundation are effective deterrents to casual violation of the 5 gauss line.

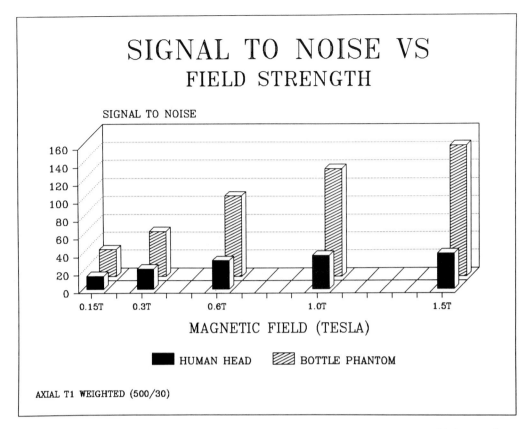

Fig. 3-7. SNR for T1W measurement of the human head increases only slightly with increased flux density from 0.6 to 1.5 T. The improvement is greater for a bottle phantom then for a person's head.

only alternative might be public 911 ambulance service to the hospital emergency room. Thus, particularly for patients with abdominal disease, direct access to a permanently installed hospital MRI scanner has advantages.

Magnet

Field strength. The issue of field strength has proven to be relatively minor in the clinical practice of MRI. Excellent diagnostic quality scans of the abdomen may be obtained from mid-field (up to about 0.5 T) and high-field strength (approximately 1.0 to 1.5 T and stronger) magnets (Fig. 3-7). Because signal strength is proportional to magnetic field strength, it is necessary in some cases for the lower-field units to compensate by increasing scan time. In many cases, even though the image obtained at low magnetic flux density may have some "noise" (similar to the "quantum mottle" effect of conventional radiography), the diagnostic quality may be equal to the "smoother" image of the high-field scanner (Fig. 3-8).

Throughput of patients is enhanced by increased field strength. A typical T2-weighted spin-echo sequence on a 1.5 T magnet takes about 8 minutes (range: 6 to 11 minutes), a 0.3 T magnet performs a similar sequence in roughly 14 to 16 minutes. These figures provide only a

rough index of throughput, as numerous variable parameters must also be considered. Rapid imaging for dynamic studies of vascular structures, phase imaging of fluid flow, angiography, or single breath-hold examinations to overcome respiratory motion artifact are difficult or impossible to obtain (with equal tissue contrast characteristics) on lower-field units. The significant trade-off of field strength is cost, which is considerably higher for system components, installation, and daily operation of the high-field superconducting units versus the lower-field units.[1] Satisfactory compromise techniques are likely to be developed for low-field units as coil, gradient system, computer hardware, and software technology improves.

The appearance of blood is markedly different between high and low-field scanners. The physical characteristics of hemoglobin in various stages of clot formation make it strikingly visible on high-field scans; however, hematoma signal appearance patterns on low-field scans also have been worked out. Knowing the limitations of the low-field unit, one can avoid clinical errors by supplementing the evaluation with computed tomography (CT) or other examination, as indicated.

Radiofrequency shielding. RF shielding involves both the isolation of the MRI scanner from potential RF inter-

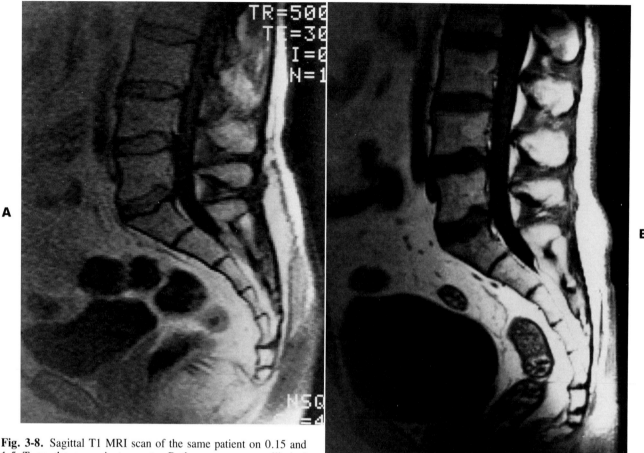

Fig. 3-8. Sagittal T1 MRI scan of the same patient on 0.15 and 1.5 T on the same instruments. Both scans use an elliptical curve. **A,** The 0.15 T grainy image provides essentially as much clinical information as the smoother image. **B,** Scan at 1.5 T. Better SNR. No significant new findings.

ference and the containment of the RF energy produced by the scanner itself (Fig. 3-9). Local broadcasting stations, various communications services, and other electronic equipment produce signals that could completely obscure the weak magnetic resonance signal if RF shielding were not present. Conversely, the MRI radio pulse transmitter could interfere with devices in the outside world. To prevent RF interference, the scan room typically is contained within a thin sheath of copper or other metal. The metal sheets of RF shielding must be bonded carefully to prevent mechanical movement (which would allow leakage of signal and produce electronic noise) and must be well grounded. All pipes, conduits (Fig. 3-10), ventilation ducts, doors (Fig. 3-11), vents, and windows (see Figs. 3-9, *A*, and 3-12) require special shielding techniques.

Magnetic field shielding. Magnetic field shielding may be accomplished by passive and active techniques. The simplest form of passive magnetic field shielding is empty space . . . lots of it. In some hospitals, however, the only choice is to situate the magnet in crowded quarters (Figs. 3-10 and 3-12). It is possible, although expen-

sive, to provide "brute force" magnetic shielding by wrapping the scan room with heavy steel plates, which limit the fringe field. Active shielding is a more efficient, less costly method that is increasingly common as electromagnet technology improves. The pattern of the fringe field is shaped by the orientation of the electromagnet coil windings that determine the direction and strength of current flow within portions of the coil and by the metal housing of the magnet (Fig. 3-13).

Bore. The bore of the magnet is the opening through which the patient moves in order to lie in the highest flux density region of the magnetic field for MRI examination. Although a typical whole body magnet has a bore of 1 meter, the space is encumbered by gradient and shim coils, the body send-receive coil, and protective moldings that limit the opening to about 55 cm (see Fig. 3-1). One commercially available permanent magnet has a broad rectangular bore opening, which allows comfortable positioning of the arms during an abdominal scan (Fig. 3-14). Its bore is limited in the A-P dimension, however, so that the patient's face is close to the upper lining of the space.

Text continued on p. 79.

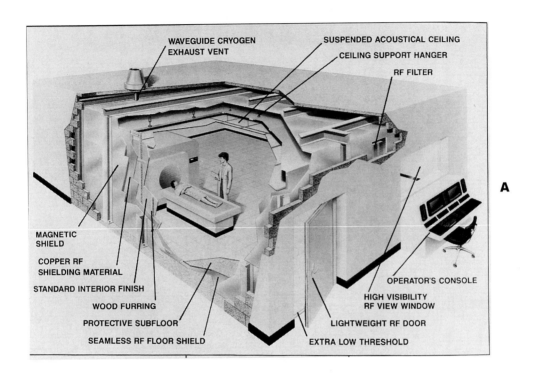

SHIELDING MATERIAL	MAGNETIC FIELD		ELECTRIC FIELD		PLANEWAVE		MICROWAVE	
	14 KHz	200 KHz	10 KHz	30 MHz	50 MHz	450 MHz	1 GHz	10 GHz
3 Ounce Copper (LT 3)	30db	50db	100db	100 db	100db	100db	100db	80/100db
24 Gauge Galvanized Steel (LT 24)	60db	100db	100db	100db	100db	80/100db	70db	60db
3 Ounce Copper & 24 Gauge Galvanized Steel (LT 324)	75db	120db	120db	120db	120db	120db	120db	112db

Fig. 3-9. A, Cut-away view of an MRI laboratory. Note structural wall and ceiling, magnetic shield, copper RF shield, subfloor space for wiring, RF shielded exhaust vent, and forced air climate control system. **B,** Comparison of magnetic and electric (RF) shielding properties of copper sheathing, galvanized steel sheathing, combination of copper and steel shielding. (Courtesy of Lindgren R.F. Enclosures, Inc.)

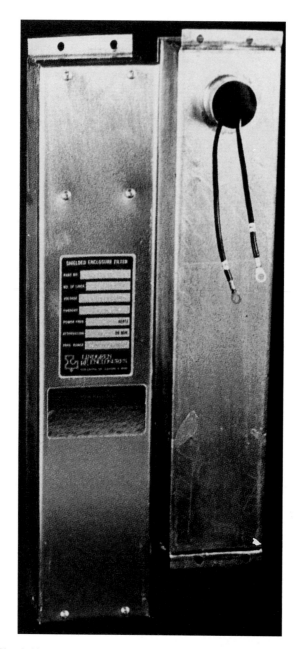

Fig. 3-10. RF baffle conduit termination for passage of cables in and out of the scan room. (Courtesy of Lindgren R.F. Enclosures, Inc.)

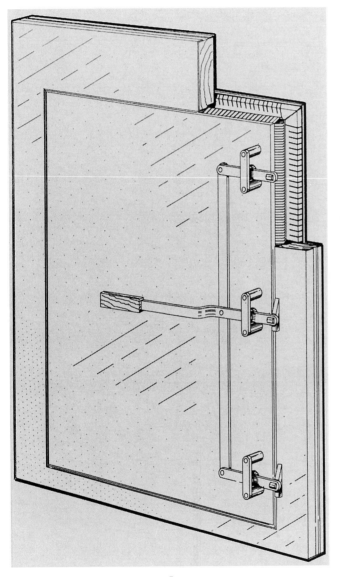

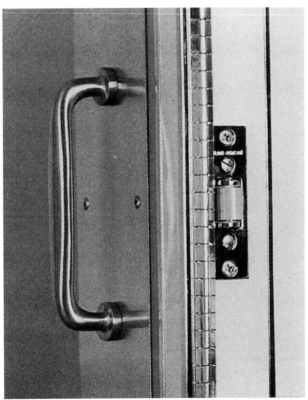

Fig. 3-11. Shielded door for MRI room. **A,** Copper "fingers" seal the gap at the door margins. Heavy positive-latching cam-system ensures no residual leakage of RF. **B,** Closeup of RF seal "finger" at door margin. (Courtesy of Lindgren R.F. Enclosures, Inc.)

A

B

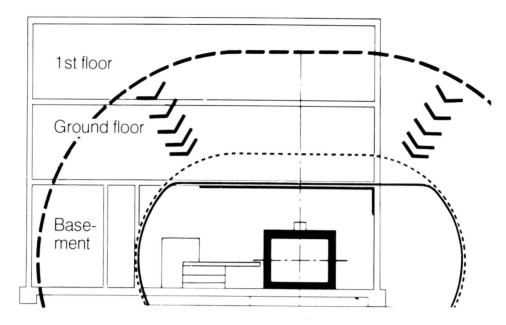

--- 0.5 mT line without shielding

····· 0.5 mT line with self-shielding

——— 0.5 mT line with self-shielding and ceiling-mounted plate

Fig. 3-12. Schematic of magnetic fringe field of a basement-located MRI scanner. Note the beneficial effect of self-shielding and passive metal-shielding (in the ceiling of the scan room). (Courtesy of Siemens Medical Systems, Inc., Iselin, N.J.)

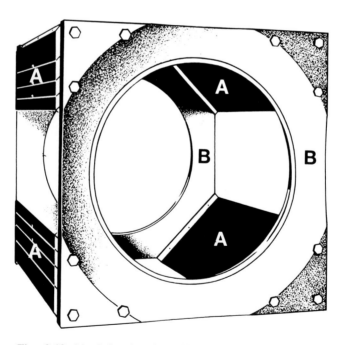

Fig. 3-13. Metal housing for self-shielding magnet. Passive shield configuration enhances field containment. (Courtesy of Siemens Medical Systems, Inc., Iselin, NJ.)

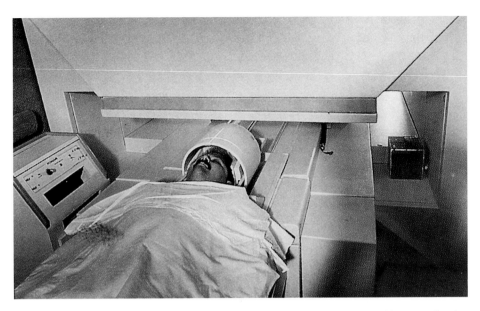

Fig. 3-14. Hybrid resistive magnet design allows a rectangular bore that provides some freedom of lateral movement. (Courtesy of Santa Fe Healthcare System Inc.)

Circular bore designs allow more clear space above the patient's face for light and circulation of air. Either design may provoke a feeling of claustrophobia, regardless of a particular manufacturer's claims.

Coils. Four classes of coils are present in an MRI system. The main field coil, shim coils, gradient coils, and various types of RF coils are used. Current flowing in the first three types produces the magnetic fields that make the magnetic resonance signal possible. The RF coils act as transmitting and receiving antennas for radiofrequency energy, which is given to and received back from the volume being studied.

The largest of these four coil sets is the main field coil. This coil carries a large current at low voltage (for instance 200 amps at 3 volts). Wire for the coil is drawn from a special alloy of niobium and titanium, which reaches superconductivity at higher temperature than ordinary copper wire. Cooled to near absolute zero (the temperature at which all molecular motion theoretically would stop), the wire of the main field coil loses electrical resistance and becomes superconductive. In practical terms, this characteristic of the system means that (1) the field engineer carefully "ramps up" the superconducting magnet by injecting current slowly over a prescribed time; (2) if the cooling system fails, resistance returns, resulting in heat generation, which damages the coil; and (3) the superconducting magnet is always "on," even during an electrical power failure.

The shim coils are adjusted to fine tune the homogeneity of magnetic field flux density throughout the scan volume. They actively supplement the effect of passive sheet metal shims placed strategically within the bore (external to the patient tube). Current flow is adjusted at installation and is changed only as required to maintain field homogeneity. Failure of the active shim circuit produces significant artifacts.

Gradient coils produce controlled variations in the strength of the main magnetic field, which are the key to spatial resolution in MRI. The rapid switching of gradient coil current also is the cause of the loud pounding noise that occurs during scanning. These are very powerful magnets; the considerable mechanical forces produced within the supporting structure by rapidly changing gradient field directions result in small but forceful movements, which are quite loud inside the scanner bore. One gradient coil set is built into the bore for each of the three main axes of the scanner: Head-to-foot (z axis), right-to-left (x axis), and front-to-back (y axis) (Fig. 3-15).

When evaluating a system for conventional diagnostic MRI, consider the maximum gradient amplitude (in G/cm or mT/m) and the minimum gradient rise time (expressed in msec or in G/msec). Good values for a 1.5 T unit are at least 10 mT/m amplitude and 1.0 msec rise time for an increase in gradient amplitude from 0 to 10 mT/m. Gradient slopes of up to 10 mT/M are common in conventional superconducting diagnostic MRI systems. Increases to 20 to 40 mT/M are desirable for diffusion imaging.[5] Higher field strength (4.7 T) and echo-planar imaging (see Chapter 2) also are advantages for applications that require maximum sensitivity and the shortest possible scanning time. Newer systems provide "shielded" gradients to reduce eddy currents. Improved gradient stabilization and reduced noise are important benefits of these improved coils. Safety limits on the strength of switched gradient magnetic fields and constant magnetic fields are presented in a later section of this chapter.

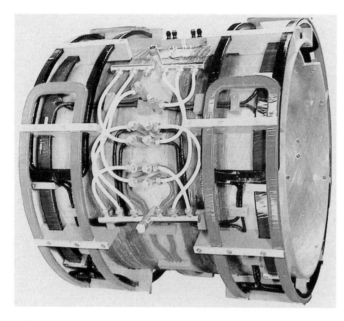

Fig. 3-15. The outer housing has been removed to expose the gradient coils of this MRI magnet. (Courtesy of Oxford Magnet Technology, Osney Med, Oxford, England.)

RF head and body coils usually are combined transmit and receive devices. Some coils are used for both transmit and receive. This simplifies the design of RF coils, but makes rapid, low loss, high isolation transmit-receive switching a necessity. RF coils must couple effectively with the molecular dipole "antennas" within patients of various sizes to bring in the greatest useful signal from the target area and reject noise from everywhere else. The variables are sufficiently complex that no one coil "does it all." See Chapter 5 for an in-depth discussion of RF coil use in abdominal imaging.

Control and display

Image processing and storage. The RF electronics, gradient amplifiers, patient support table, and all other hardware functions of the system are controlled by a CPU. Scanner software is menu driven and relatively easy to use. Scan sequence parameters may be altered by programming techniques, within system and safety limits. The importance of a full range of pulse sequences cannot be overstressed, as this software allows the examiner to use a wide variety of physical parameters in order to elicit diagnostic contrast between body tissues. Some MRI control software is conveniently easy to learn for the most frequently needed routines. Other software is more difficult, but when learned in depth, provides extensive control over the capabilities of the entire system.

MRI scanners are operated through an electronic work station, at which the user enters commands and monitors the acquired images. Local magnetic disc storage provides a temporary buffer for images until the time of permanent archiving. Hard-wired image processing boards are available to speed up 3D reformatting and complex angiographic calculations. These boards enhance the image manipulation functions available in software. The tradeoff in hardware versus software image manipulation functions is price versus speed. Hardware may be more expensive, but it is usually significantly faster.

A local permanent archival device is a valuable accessory. Even if a department has a picture archiving system with an optical disc "jukebox" or digital tape storage unit, an optical drive in the MRI system is a prudent investment in data security. Local access to old examinations is also convenient.

One may use either soft copy (electronic monitor) display of images or conventional hard copy (film) display at the time of image interpretation. Electronic displays bring useful new capabilities, such as magnification of details, electronic measurement of pixel (picture element) intensity values, electronic size measurement, and manipulation of image contrast presentation.

Film, for all its limitations, does have the advantage of high bandwidth versus the electronic display system. The eye of the trained observer rapidly scans a series of film images that would require substantial time for frame-by-frame electronic display. Although the speed and presentation of soft copy displays are improving, film is faster (Fig. 3-16). Film is a permanent archival medium. However, one sheet is visible in only one location at a time, and if it is lost, the patient record is incomplete.

Organization. Studies frequently contain more than 100 separate images. Therefore, good organization of the visual information is mandatory. *As a general rule, one should display only one projection per sheet of film.* Leave a few blanks and move to a new sheet when changing from axial to coronal views of the liver. Use explanatory text annotations liberally. A scout view demonstrating slice orientation should be placed in a constant location (such as the upper left hand corner) of the film. Special measurements of size or intensity and special magnified views may be added at the bottom of a partially used sheet or on a separate sheet. Any major technique change (i.e., contrast enhancement, fat suppression, gradient echo flow sequence, position change of the patient) requires a new sheet of film. Perhaps the most essential strategy is the placement of images of the same cross-sectional location in identical position on succeeding sheets of film. For example, the first and second echoes of a dual-echo T2-weighted sequence should be recorded on two sheets of film so that the section locations match precisely in the corresponding panels of each sheet as the case is reviewed. A strict filming protocol is justified not only by increased interpretational efficiency and accuracy of the radiologist, but by avoidance of errors by observers unfamiliar with the complexities of MRI, who might be misled inadvertently by disorganized presentation of the data (Fig. 3-17).

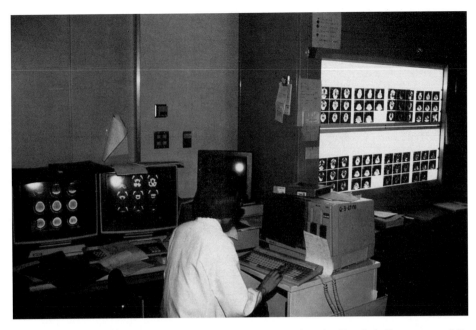

Fig. 3-16. CT and MRI reading room of East Hokkaido University Hospital, Department of Radiology. CT interpretation is accomplished from "soft reading." (Monitors on the left side of desk.) The alternator on the right is the work station for the "hard copy" MRI reading. Note the subdued room lighting. (Courtesy of Drs. Irie and Miyasaka.)

Film versus CRT monitor display

Film (hard copy display). Laser film printers with digital interfaces have supplanted analog printers for MRI. They produce a more flexible choice of output format. Multiple copies of each film are available as needed, whereas older analog cameras require tedious slice by slice refilming. Some of the newer MRI scanners accept only digital printers. With laser printers, one has the choice of translucent or opaque black background for the film. The black background increases the perceived contrast of the images by decreasing the level of stray light. Less glare from the film illuminator also reduces eye strain for the radiologist.

Viewbox versus alternator. Managing large numbers of MRI images takes practice to develop full efficiency. Because contrast and density levels typically are good, it is not necessary to handle the films during interpretation as often as one must move and touch plain radiographs. A set of viewboxes, placed as close as possible to a reading desk of typing height, can comfortably display well illuminated MRI images. Two rows of viewboxes mounted four over four handle the majority of studies. An additional set of viewboxes on another wall is useful for consultation, and for exceptionally complex cases. Because case interpretation at times is a prolonged activity, it is worthwhile to have overflow viewbox space to avoid wasted time hanging and rehanging the studies. An alternator is a compromise alternative that combines film display and short-term archiving. Advantages include efficient retrieval for fre-

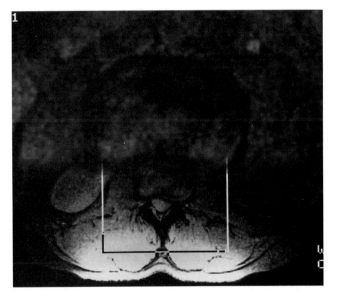

Fig. 3-17. Hard copy presentation artifact. The technologist has filmed this image of a lumbar vertebra midway through a screen point. This results in a confusing image that could be misleading to an unwary observer.

quent consultation and the ability to have studies mounted by a clerk or technologist for later interpretation. Disadvantages include suboptimal illumination, uncomfortable desk workspace with usually excessive distance from eye to film, and poor leg space.

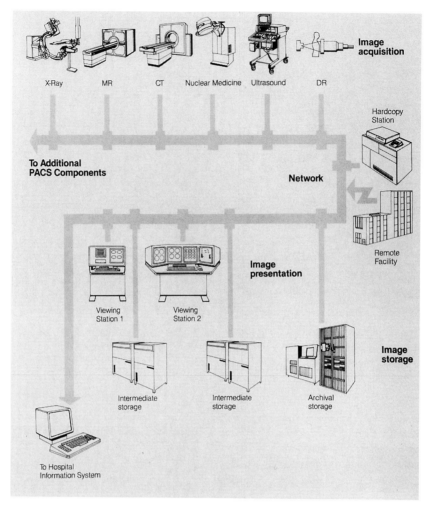

Fig. 3-18. Schematic diagram of interconnection of radiology acquisition equipment, image archives, and physician's work stations in a picture archiving and communication system (PACS). (Courtesy of Siemens Medical Systems, Inc., Iselin, NJ.)

CRT monitor (soft-copy display). MRI images of 256 × 256 pixel matrix are depicted well by electronic displays. Control console CRTs typically are capable of at least 512 × 512 display, and frequently are have 1024 × 1024 capacity. The display brightness is low compared to a viewbox. Therefore, the reading area should be designed to avoid stray light if "soft-copy" reading is planned. Glare on monitors in the scan control room is fatiguing and is an annoyance that may cause the technologist to misjudge the contrast characteristics of the images, and consequently to film them at suboptimal center and window settings.

The sheer numbers of MRI images per study present an obstacle to convenient display on computer monitors. Software must allow survey of "filmstrip" or "postage stamp" sized replicas of the images, and easy selection of the appropriate sections for full-sized display. Screen paint time and the number of images per full screen display are critical throughput factors. Selection of images for display must be very flexible, or the system will not be acceptable for use in a busy department.

Digital image management system. Picture archiving and communications systems (PACS) offer automated management of MRI studies from acquisition through final archiving to long-term storage media (Fig. 3-18). Purchase contracts for new MRI equipment should specify that the devices conform to the ACR-NEMA DICOM (digital imaging and communictions in medicine) standard to minimize the task of interfacing with other PACS components.[19,20] Previous studies are preserved in a secure archive and are available over a computer network for comparison. Referring physicians have immediate access to the images. Images can be displayed simultaneously in more than one location, facilitating consultative review.

Teleradiology. Teleradiology (sending of images from place to place for review) is a natural extension of a digital image management system. Remote reading is a benefit to outlying hospitals or offices that may be served by a mobile MRI, but do not have an on-site physician trained in MRI interpretation. Note that a relatively inexpensive tele-radiology system may be based on the technique of video frame grabbing. This technique avoids some of the complexity of acquiring compatible direct digital data for an imaging network.

Systems have been developed for routing of images to multiple laser printers and/or electronic display stations. The DuPont LINX system allows a combination of image acquisition devices to function with multiple laser printers. The system is capable of sorting films by examination type to enable automatic distribution to appropriate desti-nations. The Kodak Image Manager system combines video frame grabbing (analog to digital conversion) with intelligent distribution of films and soft copy images. These types of image management systems can reduce routine clerical duties; rapidly deliver studies to the appropriate work station for interpretation; and accelerate delivery of the final product to other offices, departments, and clinics.

Software

Control software is the lifeblood of the MRI system. Upgrades to system control software generally are distrib-uted at no charge. However, new special functions (for ex-ample, angiographic sequences and ultrafast scans) are made available at extra cost. Software upgrades can give "new life" to an aging scanner even though the hardware design may have been superseded by newer models. New functionality ranges from off-center reconstruction (of shoulders and extremities) to variable control of matrix size, fat suppression sequences, simplification of control operations, improvement of spectroscopic capability, and easier organization of images for filming. Various postpro-cessing capabilities (calculation of long-TE images, 3D re-construction, multiplanar reformatting) may be valuable. Although some software upgrades may require investment in additional memory or special processing boards for the system computer, most are as simple as loading a new pro-gram. Hardware upgrades such as gradient coils, power supplies, and digital RF modules require a more elaborate and costly installation.

OPERATION

An on-site service person provides major operational benefits to an MRI center. With some negotiation, the equipment vendor might be persuaded to use your facility as "home base" for a service engineer (who could addi-tionally be responsible for several systems in your local-ity).

Day-to-day operation of an MRI system is straightfor-ward and can be handled by any technologist competent and reliable enough to be trained for CT, ultrasonography, or nuclear medicine equipment. The user interface can be learned in a day. Basic competence can be obtained in a

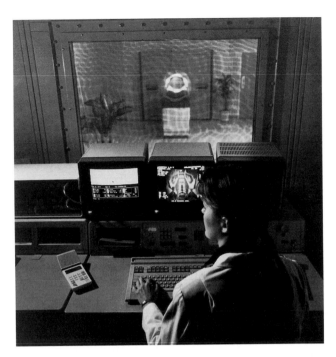

Fig. 3-19. The MRI technologist observes the patient through a shielded window and is able to communicate with the patient through an intercom.

few weeks, and sophisticated use of the equipment can be achieved in months. Mastery of the subtleties and intui-tive, efficient use of all the options takes years of experi-ence by a bright, dedicated individual (Fig. 3-19).

SAFETY
Main magnetic field effects

The main safety issue that must be addressed by every MRI system operator is the powerful attractive force of modern MRI magnets.[11] Low field magnets (0.20 to 0.3 T) do not pose as great a threat as the 1 to 1.5 T systems; however, all magnets are capable of exerting considerable attractive force on ferromagnetic objects (Table 3-1). By far the greatest source of injury for MRI users is entry into the magnet room of a ferromagnetic object (oxygen tank, stretcher), which is subsequently pulled into the magnet abruptly and seemingly without warning. Because mag-netic fields are odorless, tasteless, and invisible, it is easy for people to forget that they exist. Building workers have been known to walk into a facility (past warning signs [Fig. 3-20]) and approach a magnet with metal tools. They are frequently surprised to learn that the magnet is on even when no one is using the system. Because the magnetic field flux density tapers off at the rate of $1/r^3$ (r = radius; distance from the center of the field), very little force is exerted on an object 10 feet away from the magnet. At closer range (3 to 6 feet), however, depending on the mass of the object, the force is sufficient to pull the object and the person holding it into the magnet. This force can be so

Fig. 3-20. Although the words of this warning sign are mostly written in Japanese, the bold, simple graphics clearly convey the principal hazards of a strong magnetic field.

great that neither the object nor the individual can be extricated from the magnet without ramping down the main field. Most systems are provided with a large red emergency button that will force the collapse of the magnetic field. Its location should be known by all users of the system and by fire and safety personnel.

The obvious solution to the problem posed by the main field is to guard the door to the magnet room with high security. A lock should be installed on the magnet room door so that technologists can lock the door when the system is not in use. Install lighted signs over the doorway with a "Magnet On" message. Hold seminars to teach people magnet safety and demonstrate the pulling power of the magnet with some lightweight object (which can be controlled).

An equally important area of concern is the potential effect of the main magnetic field on objects that are in the patients body.[13,14] Each patient must be screened carefully for the presence of ferromagnetic clips, cardiac pacemakers, ferromagnetic rods, and other devices (see box). Even the eyes must be checked to be sure that no minute fleck of

Table 3-1. Biologic effects of RF and magnetic fields

Energy	Static field	Gradient field	RF field
Low	<0.2 T	0.5 G/cm	5 kW
	No effects	No effects	No effects
High	0.2-1.0 T	1 G/cm	10 kW
	Pacemakers	No effects	Modest heating
	Metal objects		
High	1.0-2.0 T	1-5 G/cm	15 kW
	Pacemakers	No effects	Heating potential
	Metal objects		Stray leads
	Implants		Exceeds SAR
Very high	>2.0 T	10-20 G/cm	20 kW
	Pacemakers	Possible	High heating
	Metal objects	peripheral nerve	Excessive SAR
	Implants	stimulation	Extreme caution
	Sensory effects		
	Nausea		
	Dizziness		

MRI safety checklist questions

What is (or was) your occupation?
  Have you ever worked with metal or machine tools?
  Have you ever served in the military?
    Were you wounded in action?
Has an injury ever caused anything to become lodged in your body?
  Have you ever been shot?
  Has a piece of metal ever gotten into your eye?
  Have you ever had a metal splinter?
Have you ever had surgery?
  Has any metal device or part ever been put in your body by a surgeon?
  Do you have a heart pacemaker?
  Have you had any type of electrical or metal device put into your ear?
  Do you have any kind of nerve stimulating device?
  Have you had brain surgery of any type?
    Have you had aneurysm surgery? Were any metal clips used in the surgery?
Are you a hunter?
  Do you eat wildfowl or game animals which someone has shot?
  Have you done so recently?

---

metal or old forgotten BB projectile is present.

Federal regulations (1992) on the composition of birdshot and other projectiles greatly increase the risk of encountering ingested steel foreign objects in the general population. Ask about consumption of wildfowl and other game animals when taking a medical history before MRI.[12,17]

A careful interview of the patient, guided by a complete checklist of common objects and situations, is mandatory (Table 3-2). In addition, a plain film should be obtained if

Table 3-2. Detection of hazardous objects

Objects that could cause problems or hazards during MRI	Question categories to discover them			
	Occupation ?	Injury ?	Surgery ?	Hunting ?
Artificial joint			✓	
BBs		✓	✓	✓
Cardiac pacemaker			✓	
Cardiac valves			✓	
Aneurysm clip			✓	
Ingested metal	✓	✓		✓
Metal splinter	✓	✓		✓
Otic implant			✓	
Orthopedic screws		✓	✓	
Orthopedic pins		✓	✓	
Orthopedic plates		✓	✓	
Orthopedic rods		✓	✓	
Projectiles	✓	✓	✓	✓
Surgical sutures		✓	✓	
Surgical hemoclips		✓	✓	
Shrapnel		✓	✓	
Wildfowl as food	✓			✓

a metal foreign object is suspected. If questions still remain, the MRI supervising physician should take necessary steps to clear all reasonable doubt before placing the patient in the magnet. A CT scan may be more sensitive to a particle of metal than a plain x-ray film. Old films may be available from a number of sources, to assist decision making without reexposure to radiation.

After metal screening has been completed, all patients should be instructed to inform the technologist of any surprise reactions while in the magnet. The technologist must be ready to abort the scan immediately if there is any sign of a possible adverse event.

Radiofrequency energy effects

In addition to the effect of the main magnetic field, one must also be aware of potential harm from wire connecting leads (ECG, Holter monitor, hearing aid, pulse oximeter or others) put into the bore in close proximity to the patient (see Table 3-1). Reports have been published of superficial burns caused by ECG leads being coiled up in the bore on the patients chest.[11,18] Similar burns have been caused by RF coil leads coming in contact with the patient during examination. Technologists should be aware that no wire leads of any kind can be coiled up on the patient's body during the MRI scan. Energy from the transmitter coil is coupled to these stray leads and may present a serious safety hazard. Optoelectronic devices and fiber optic cables offer an effective and safe alternative to conventional monitors and electrical transducers interconnected by wire leads.[18]

Another safety issue has been raised regarding the use of surface coils.[16] Surface coils must be decoupled from the transmitter coil (the body coil) to avoid energy transfer from the transmitter coil to the surface coil. If the decoupling circuits on the surface coil fail, it is possible that sufficient energy could be coupled to the surface coil to cause local tissue heating. Although this is a potential concern, well-insulated surface coils and proper design have practically eliminated this occurrence.

A more likely cause of significant energy deposition in the body is power absorption from the body coil.[8] The Federal Drug Administration (FDA) has set the specific absorption rate (SAR) limit at 4 W/kg. One watt per kilogram (W/kg) is sufficient energy to raise the temperature of 1 kg of tissue 1 degree in 1 hour. If the sequence being used (fast spin echo, for instance) has a large number of 180-degree pulses occurring at a high rate, then this limit could be exceeded. At this point, the clinician and patient must decide if the scan is worth risking possible tissue heating effects. Although studies have been performed with healthy volunteers using 8 W/kg without serious side effects, there is still reason to exercise caution beyond the FDA limit. Many MRI systems will permit the operator to exceed the limits simply by pressing the proper button. (I believe that this option is questionable, as the same scan information is likely to be obtainable without exceeding the FDA guidelines.)

Biomagnetic effects

Active research is underway concerning the nature of magnetic fields and their effect on the human body (see Table 3-1). The first conference on the bioeffects of electromagnetic fields was held in 1991 in Washington, DC. Tests are being conducted at flux densities much higher than those used in typical imaging experiments. Real concerns have been raised that at 4.0 T a number of effects become noticeable.

Switched gradient fields applied at the high rates used in echo planar imaging can cause muscle twitching to occur.[9,10] However, conventional MRI systems widely used in the field are not capable of inducing this response. Reportedly, a 4.0 T whole body magnet can induce the sensation of a metallic taste and a feeling of nausea.[15] Again, these effects are not evident at flux densities of 1.5 T and below.

RF power deposition guidelines might be exceeded with some new high speed imaging techniques (fast spin echoes); however, no detrimental effects have been reported using these techniques. In short, although concerns have been raised regarding the use of high field magnets and high power gradients and RF, no major side effects have been reported after using these techniques on typical 1.5 T MRI systems. It is prudent to exercise caution when approaching these limits. Be sensitive to a patient's reports of side effects so that scanning can be stopped immediately, before any harm occurs. See reference 11 for an excellent comprehensive review of MRI safety issues.

REFERENCES

1. Bidgood WD, Horii S: Radiographics March 1992 (in press).
2. Budinger TF: Thresholds for physiological effects due to RF and magnetic fields used in NMR Imaging, IEEE Trans Nucl Sci 26:2821-2825, 1979.
3. Budinger TF, Fischer H, Hentchel D, et al: Neural stimulation dB/dt thresholds for frequency and number of oscillations using sinosoidal magnetic field gradients, Abstracts of the Society of Magnetic Resonance in Medicine, 1990.
4. Egerter D: MR nerve stimulation: new safety concern, Diagn Imaging 127-131, 1990.
5. Freedman GS, Stephens WH: Economic considerations in magnetic resonance imaging. In Mettler FA, Muroff LR, Kulkani MV, editors: Magnetic resonance imaging and spectroscopy, New York, 1986, Churchill Livingstone.
6. Horii S, Bidgood WD: Radiographics, April, 1992 (in press).
7. Kanal E, Shellock FG, Talagbla L: Safety consideration in MR imaging, Radiology 176:593-606, 1990.
8. Lorentz CH, Pickens DR, Puffer DB, Price RR: Diffusion/perfusion phantom experiments. Syllabus of the meeting on future directions in MRI of diffusion and microcirculation. Berkeley, Calif, 1990, Society of Magnetic Resonance in Medicine.
9. Lufkin, RB: MR imaging of firearm projectiles (letter to the editor), Radiology 179:285, 1991.
10. Magnetom 63 SP Technical Data Publication, PA 6893, Siemens Medical Systems, Inc., Iselin, NJ.
11. New PF, Rosen BR, Brady TJ, Buonanno F: Potential hazard and artifacts of ferromagnetic and non-ferromagnetic surgical and dental materials and devices in NMR imaging, Radiology 147:139-143, 1983.
12. Pavlicek MS, Geisinger M, Castle L, et al: The effects of NMR on patients with cardiac pacemakers, Radiology 147:149-153, 1983.
13. Rhode UL: Digital HF radio: a sampling of techniques, Ham Radio 18-42, 1985.
14. Schenck JF, Dumoulin CL, Souza SP, et al: Health and physiology effects of human exposure to whole-body 4T magnetic field during magnetic resonance scanning, Abstracts of the Society of Magnetic Resonance in Medicine, 1990.
15. Shellock FG, Myers SM, Kimble KJ: Monitoring heart rate and oxygen saturation with a fiberoptic pulse oximeter during MR imaging, Am J Roentgenol 158:663-664, 1992.
16. Stephenson GM, Freiherr: Indifference to safety heightens MRI risks, Diagn Imaging 79-83, 1990.
17. Tampa MR/CT Newsletter, 1991, Siemens Medical.
18. Turner R, Le Bihan D, Maier J, et al: Echo-planar IVIM imaging of the body, Application to kidney, In Book of abstracts: Society of Magnetic Resonance in Medicine 1990, Berkeley, Calif, 1990, Society of Magnetic Resonance in Medicine.
19. Turner R, Le Bihan D, Maier J, et al: Echoplanar imaging of intravoxel incoherent motion, Radiology 177:407-414, 1990.
20. Williams T: Let them eat steel, Audubon 90:22-33, 1988.

Chapter 4

QUALITY ASSESSMENT AND CRYOGENS

W. Dean Bidgood, Jr.
Jintong Mao

Quality assessment
  Reference phantoms
  Standard reference measurements
  Routine performance evaluation
  Additional performance evaluation
Maintenance
  Routine preventive maintenance
  Cryogens
  Metering
  Safety procedures
  Repairs

Regular performance evaluation and routine preventive maintenance are essential for any complex electromechanical equipment. Magnetic resonance imaging (MRI) scanners are no exception. Miscalibration and malfunction of any subsystem can degrade diagnostic imaging. Because of their complexity and their high operating cost, MRI scanners must have regular preventive maintenance to optimize image quality and to minimize unexpected down time for repairs. Routine performance evaluations are designed to detect changes in key parameters even before significant artifacts are visible in clinical images. The tuning of an MRI system requires a regular protocol to control the many variables affecting image acquisition.

QUALITY ASSESSMENT

A standard set of test procedures must be defined to evaluate the performance of a clinical MRI system and to report the test results. Performance evaluation procedures are an integral part of the routine quality assurance program of an MRI facility.

The purpose of a quality assurance program is to detect changes in system performance relative to an established baseline. Six specific image parameter evaluations are described in this chapter. Potential implications of each performance area in clinical MRI of the abdomen are:

1. Resonant frequency
     Cryogen replenishment
     General system maintenance
2. Signal-to-noise ratio (SNR)
     Low contrast lesions
     Rapid imaging
     T2-weighted sequences
3. Image uniformity
     Active shim current settings
     Fat suppression
     Metallic foreign objects
     T2-weighted sequences
4. Spatial linearity
     Gradient artifacts
     Large field of view (FOV)
5. Spatial resolution
     Adenopathy
     Adrenal ovary
     Calcification
     Fascial planes
     Fibrous septa
     Small nodular lesions
     Varices

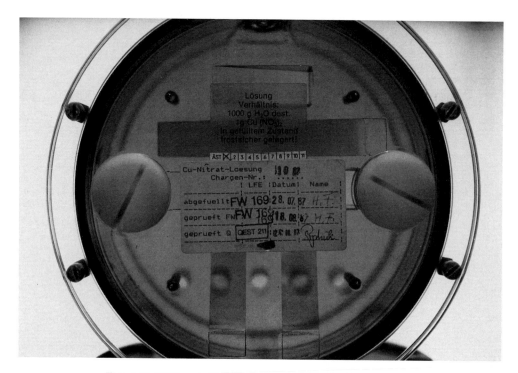

Fig. 4-1. Multipurpose MRI performance evaluation phantom. The cylindrical phantom contains copper nitrate to simulate the relaxation properties of the internal plastic parts more closely than distilled water. Subtle contrast differences can be tested.

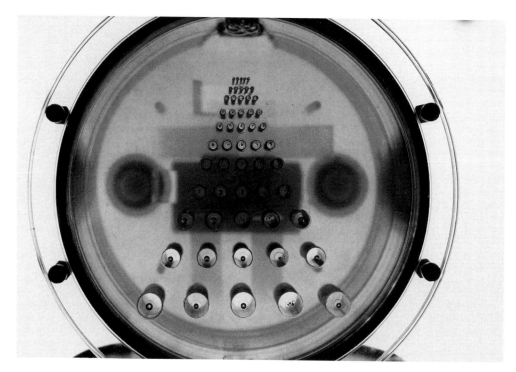

Fig. 4-2. Multipurpose phantom. Plastic rods of known size and separation provide standard scan targets for measurement of spatial resolution.

6. Phase-related artifacts
   Coil changes
   Flow, general

This set is not exhaustive and does not include procedures for assessing all possible image parameters. However, the procedures are adequate for monitoring the sensitivity and geometric characteristics of a scanner for general MRI diagnostic service.

Reference phantoms

Quality assurance phantoms must be constructed of materials having the following properties: (1) chemical and thermal stability; (2) absence of significant chemical shifts; and (3) T1, T2, and proton density values in the biologic range.

The following set of four phantoms is sufficient for routine quality assurance tests. All of them satisfy the preceding requirements. The first three are uniform cylinders. The fourth one is a multipurpose phantom (Figs. 4-1 and 4-2).

1. Diameter 7 inches; height 2.38 inches
2. Diameter 10.25 inches; height 4.0 inches
3. Diameter 10.25 inches; height 12.75 inches
4. Multipurpose phantom

Standard reference measurements

A diagnostic program supplied by the manufacturer is used to establish correctly the standard value for the transmitter RF square wave pulse voltage, the receiver gain, and the scale for image display. A standard reference measurement is obtained with the body phantom positioned in the axial direction. After successful scaling of the image, the values are recorded and used for later determinations and for future comparative measurements.

Routine perfomance evaluation

Resonant frequency. The resonant frequency is the radiofrequency (RF) that matches the static magnetic field (B_o) according to the Larmor equation: RF = (gyromagnetic ratio * B_o), where the gyromagnetic ratio is the proper one for the nuclei under study. For hydrogen protons, the Larmor frequency is 42.58 MHz/T. For a 1.5 T system, the resonant frequency of hydrogen is about 63.62 MHz. The exact value varies from magnet to magnet.

Clinical significance in abdominal MRI. It is essential to verify that the system is tuned to resonance before any scanning is performed. Off-resonance operation will result in deterioration of SNR and linearity. Reduction of SNR is most apparent in low-contrast targets, such as lymph nodes, or in long-TE T2W scans of the liver where signal strength is at a premium.

Factors affecting resonant frequency

1. Heat production by resistive magnets. Water chiller and heat exchanger function are the major factors in resistive magnet stability.

2. Room temperature and permanent magnets. Massive iron cores of permanent magnets are efficient "heat sinks," which respond to the environmental temperature. Variations in core temperature affect field strength.
3. Superconducting magnets are highly stable instruments. Cryogen boil off has little effect on field strength unless the volume falls to a dangerously low level.

Changes in the resonant frequency may be due to changes in current density because of thermal or mechanical effects, shim-coil changes, or effects of external ferromagnetic materials. Superconducting systems typically are highly stable. A resonant frequency check should be performed before each quality assurance measurement and each time a different phantom is used to ensure optimum image quality. Resonant frequency should also be recorded daily to confirm the stability of the primary magnetic field as a backup to the routine monitoring of cryogen levels. This measurement could avert costly damage to the superconducting magnet in the event of undetected failure of the cryogen fill-level transducer, circuit, or indicator.

Measurement method. A uniform cylinder phantom of appropriate diameter is selected for resonant frequency measurement to optimize the filling factor of the RF coil. The phantom is positioned in the center of the magnet with all gradient fields turned off. The RF frequency is adjusted by controlling the RF synthesizer center frequency to achieve maximum signal. This procedure is automatically controlled by manufacturer-provided software.

Signal-to-noise ratio. The signal is the mean pixel signal intensity within the region of interest minus the average pixel background intensity. Noise is the average pixel background intensity. Images with obvious artifacts are not suitable for determining the signal-to-noise ratio (SNR).

Clinical significance in abdominal MRI. As noted in the section on resonant frequency, SNR optimization is most critical for low-contrast lesions and for low-intensity signals. Detection of infiltrative lesions of solid organs may depend on slight lesion-background differences. Targets as diverse as calcifications and slightly hyperintense T2-weighted lesions may be obscured if SNR is suboptimal. Echo planar imaging (EPI) and other rapid imaging protocols demand maximum attainable SNR from the equipment, as the margins for error are small.

Factors affecting SNR

1. Calibration of the system parameters. Synthesizer frequency, transmitter power, and other operator-controllable settings must be correct.
2. Preamplifier gain. In the range of linear amplification of all signals, the gain should be as high as possible (Fig. 4-3).
3. Coil tuning. The coil must be tuned to the resonant frequency.

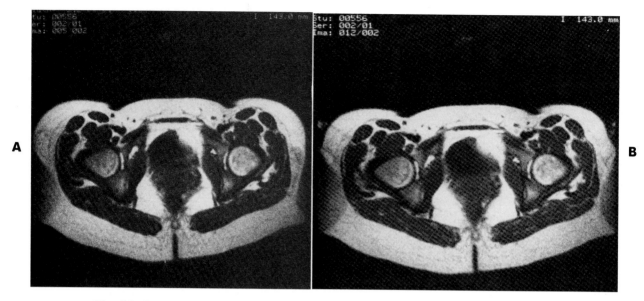

Fig. 4-3. Receiver preamplifier malfunction. Effect on SNR. **A,** Insufficient preamplifier gain. Random background noise is prominent in contrast to **B. B,** Normally functioning receiver. Note the improvement of the "grainy" appearance observed on **A.** (From Field SA, Wehrli FW: Sign applications guide, vol I, Publication No. E8804CA, General Electric Medical Systems, Milwaukee, Wis, 1990.)

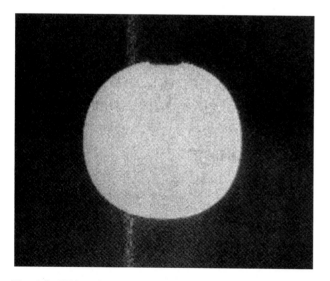

Fig. 4-4. RF interference from a steady carrier frequency source. Effect on SNR. A strong signal from the nitrogen fill-monitor circuit is detected within the passband of the MRI receiver. It is displayed as a full vertical column perpendicular to the x coordinate that corresponds to the frequency of the spurious signal. The receiver performance overall is degraded by intermodulation distortion, causing the background noise level to rise in comparison with the signal of the phantom. (From Informationen für Med-Technicker, Magnetom Trouble Shooting, Publication No. C2-010, 118.01.01.02, Siemens Medical Systems, Erlangen Germany.)

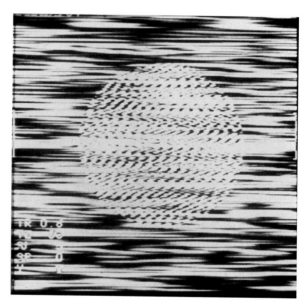

Fig. 4-5. Burst of static electricity during data acquisition. The effect of broadband RF interference is total loss of intelligibility of the desired signal. (From Famano P: MRI Artifacts slide collection, Siemens Medical Systems, Inc., Iselin, NJ.)

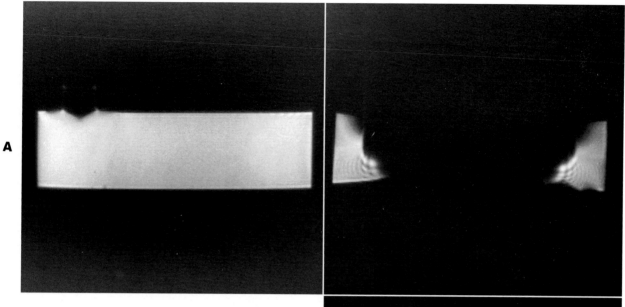

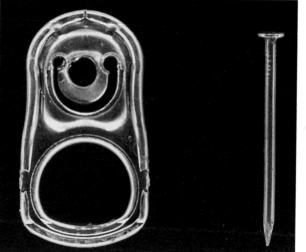

Fig. 4-6. Uniform cylindrical water phantom. Evaluation of image uniformity. **A,** A small nonferrous object placed into the bore of the scanner adjacent to the phantom produces no distortion of static magnetic field homogeneity. **B,** A steel nail heavily distorts static field uniformity and thereby distorts image uniformity severely. **C,** The aluminum "pop-top" and steel nail used in **A** and **B.**

4. RF shielding. The scanner must be isolated from external RF interference (Figs. 4-4 and 4-5).
5. Coil loading. The major noise source is from the biologic sample rather than from the coil itself (see Chapter 5).
6. Image processing. The extra noise from inappropriate processing algorithms should be eliminated during measurements.
7. Scan parameters (TE, TR, NEX, etc.). A standard evaluation sequence must be established as a routine protocol for ongoing SNR monitoring.

Measurement method. A standard uniform cylindrical phantom is used along with a standard scanning sequence to determine the SNR. An automatic program supplied by the manufacturer can be used. Alternatively, SNR can be determined manually by collecting and handling measurements according to the definition of SNR stated earlier. SNR measurement is performed every day early in the morning before routine scans begin. A log of the daily SNR values is kept for future reference.

SNR is dependent on essentially all scan parameters and test conditions. SNR values are relative numbers that vary from unit to unit. A value of 50 units is a typical minimum acceptable level for clinical scanning. The acceptance threshold for a particular unit is determined with advice from the service engineer confirmed by a review of clinical images.

Image uniformity. Image uniformity is an index of the ability of the MR imaging system to produce the same signal intensity in each voxel of a uniform test object.

Clinical significance in abdominal MRI. Extraneous metallic objects can produce a devastating effect on image quality with any MRI sequence. Selective presaturation fat suppression sequences require precise adjustment of active shim (electromagnet) settings. Relatively slight field nonuniformity can obliterate the homogeneity of fat suppression. Field uniformity is next most evident in long-TE, T2W sequences.

Factors affecting image uniformity

1. Static field inhomogeneity. Currently available MRI systems provide highly uniform magnetic fields with nonuniformities of only a few parts per million throughout the imaging volume (Fig. 4-6).

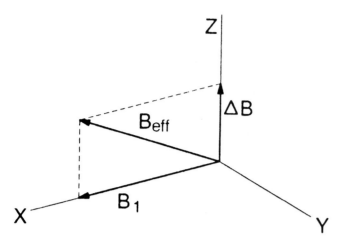

Fig. 4-7. RF field nonuniformity. Variability of RF field strength from point to point in the target tissue results in an inhomogeneous population of various flip angles rather than a nearly uniform flip angle being produced by an RF excitation pulse. The result is nonuniformity of image intensity across the FOV. (From Field SA, Wehrli FW: Sign applications guide, vol I, Publication No. E8804CA, General Electric Medical Systems, Milwaukee, Wis, 1990.)

2. RF field nonuniformity. Inhomogeneous RF fields cause unpredictable differences in the flip angles of the longitudinal magnetization vectors of various regions within the volume of interest (Figs. 4-7 and 4-8).
3. Eddy currents. Currents induced in the structure of the scanner itself and in other conducting structures (by changing gradient magnetic fields) oppose the applied fields and strongly contribute to magnetic field inhomogeneity. Such currents distort the gradient waveform and produce image artifacts.
4. Image processing. For example, software-generated truncation artifacts are rendered as periodic transitions in image intensity, which are perceived as parallel thin bands superimposed on the desired image.
5. CRT monitors. Luminance varies across the screen of the monitor. For "soft copy" interpretation from the MRI system monitor, or an off-line diagnostic console, the performance of the CRT can limit the system; frequent performance evaluation and adjustment can be necessary.

Measurement method. A uniform thin disk phantom or a phantom having discrete cylinders symmetrically distributed is used to determine image uniformity. Any typical spin-echo sequence, such as a TE 20/TR 500, can be used in the measurement process. For pixels within approximately the central 75% of the phantom area, the maximum (S1) and minimum (S2) intensities are obtained. Care is taken not to include edge truncation artifacts in the region of interest (ROI) for the disk phantom. The difference D and the average value S are calculated as follows:

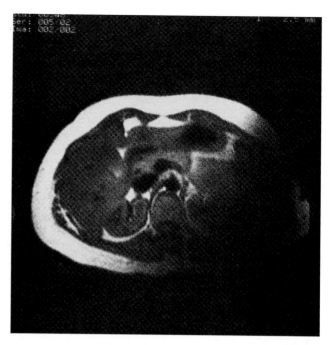

Fig. 4-8. Nonuniformity of image intensity produced by RF field inhomogeneity. Note the region of hypointensity in the left flank. The cause in this case is improper setting of active shim coil current, producing an unwanted focal gradient in the main magnetic field. (From Field SA, Wehrli FW: Sign applications guide, vol I, Publication No. E8804CA, General Electric Medical Systems, Milwaukee, Wis, 1990.)

$$D = (S1 - S2)/2$$
$$S = (S1 + S2)/2$$

The image uniformity (U) is determined by:

$$U = (1 - D/S) * 100\%$$

Perfect uniformity is U = 100%.

D values in both horizontal and vertical directions for body and head coils typically are recorded monthly. Daily measurements are not usually necessary in the majority of superconducting systems. The values of D and S can be obtained by running the manufacturers support program to determine the SNR of the appropriate regions.

The preceding quantitative measurements provide an absolute index of field uniformity. Uniformity of the images also must be evaluated qualitatively. Some of the important patterns follow:

1. *Linear artifact parallel to the phase-encoding axis.* RF interference or DC offset in the gradient circuit for the frequency-encoding axis (Figs. 4-4 and 4-9).
2. *Repeating bands parallel to the frequency-encoding axis.* Instability of the gradient amplifier for the phase-encoding axis (Figs. 4-10 to 4-12).
3. *Central hypointensity or hyperintensity.* Matching DC offsets in the x, y, and z gradient circuits simultaneously.

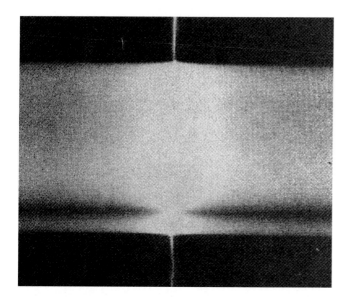

Fig. 4-9. Gradient offset. In this example, a thin vertical line is due to DC gradient offset. The broad horizontal band of intensity (extending longitudinally in the frequency-encode direction) is the result of failure of the frequency readout gradient. (From Informationen für Med-Technicker, Magnetom Trouble Shooting, Publication No. C2-010, 118.01.01.02, Siemens Medical Systems, Erlangen, Germany.)

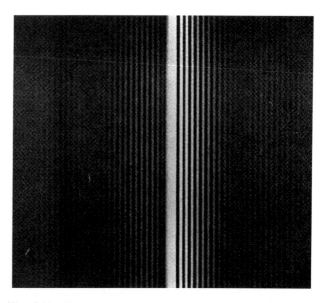

Fig. 4-10. Characteristic parallel line pattern produced by failure of the phase encoding gradient. Because all of the received signals have the same phase angle (in the absence of a functioning PE gradient source), the frequency data of every scan line accumulate in only one memory register in the display processor (instead of being distributed into the full number of available scan line memory areas). The all-or-none transition from the "full" central memory register to the "empty" adjacent registers essentially is a square wave transition, which, by Fourier transformation, becomes a sinc function (alternating high and low amplitude bands). (From Informationen für Med-Technikes, Magnetom Trouble Shooting, Publication No. C2-010.118.01.01.02, Siemens Medical Systems, Erlangen, Germany.)

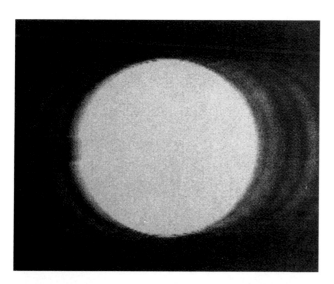

Fig. 4-11. Phase instability of a gradient amplifier. Transient abnormal variations in gradient strength result in multiple "ghost" images that resemble motion artifact. In this case, however, it is the gradient that is "moving," and not the patient. (From Informationen für Med-Technikes, Magnetom Trouble Shooting, Publication No. C2-010.118.01.01.02, Siemens Medical Systems, Erlangen, Germany.)

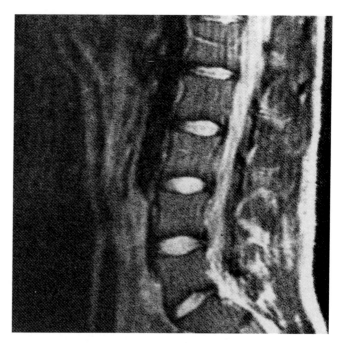

Fig. 4-12. Gradient instability. The resulting phase artifact is a series of parallel high and low intensity bands distributed along the phase encoding axis (horizontal PE axis, in this example). Image courtesy of General Electric Medical Systems, Milwaukee, Wis.[13]

4. *Focal peripheral hypointensity.* Eddy current, or ferromagnetic foreign object in the magnet bore (Fig. 4-6, *B* and *C*). Screen luminance of the monitor can be measured with a photosensitive device. An SMPTE (Society of Motion Picture and Television Engineers) test pattern is useful for qualitative evaluation of CRT uniformity. Either the SMPTE test pattern or a similar test image should be displayed daily.
5. *Global distortion of low spatial frequencies (intensity reversal or geographic regions of intensity distortion; spurious signals in the periphery of the image).* RF clipping (due to excessive transmitter power or insufficient attenuation at the receiver) or improper tuning while using a selective chemical presaturation sequence.[5]

Spatial linearity. Spatial linearity is a measurement of the system's ability to produce an image of a sample without geometric distortion.

Clinical significance in abdominal MRI. Abdominal survey examinations require large FOVs that exercise gradient linearity to the limit of specifications. Fortunately, malfunction is uncommon in clinical practice.

Factors affecting spatial linearity

1. Inhomogeneity of the main magnetic field. Because spatial localization depends entirely on the Larmor relationship, any local distortion of magnetic flux density causes some degree of spatial mismapping of the target volume (Fig. 4-6).
2. Nonlinearity of magnetic field gradients. Gradient nonlinearity is proportional to distance from the epicenter of the gradient. Artifacts are worst at FOVs > 35 cm. Coronal and sagittal planes are most troublesome due to the orientation of the gradient coils controlling these planes (Figs. 4-13 and 4-14).[8]

Adjustment of active shim coils and passive metal shims may be required from time to time as both the magnet and its environment change. For example, the authors observed a marked deterioration in the homogeneity of a portable MRI system after installing a second portable unit nearby. The newer unit, which was actively shielded, compensated for the fringe field of the original magnet. The older unit required significant shim adjustments to remain in service.

Distortion of aspect ratio can result from gradient system malfunction. Remember to investigate other common causes. Film printer and display monitor component failure or maladjustment should be considered as well (Fig. 4-16).

Methods of measurement. A large multipurpose phantom is used along with a routine multislice spin-echo sequence. The diameter of the phantom should be no less than 80% of the FOV. The image of the phantom is evaluated visually for any distortion of straight lines. The test is repeated in each of the three standard orthogonal orientations (see Fig. 4-4).

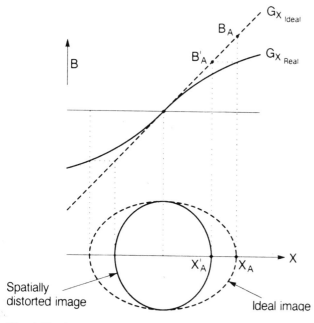

Fig. 4-13. Accurate mapping of points in the body to points on the frequency readout axis occurs only if the rise of gradient amplitude is (sufficiently) linear across the FOV. A nonlinear gradient slope produces geometric distortion in the same way that a concave or convex mirror distorts a virtual optical image. Component failure that limits gradient amplifier current to some fraction of the normal value minifies the image proportionally. (From Field SA, Wehrli FW: Sign applications guide, vol I, Publication No. E8804CA, General Electric Medical Systems, Milwaukee, Wis, 1990.)

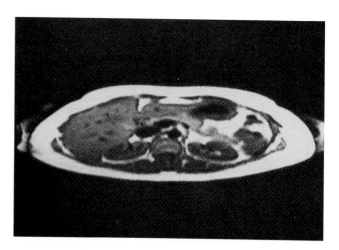

Fig. 4-14. Example of gradient amplitude falloff resulting in A-P minification of a T1W axial image of the upper abdomen. (From Field SA, Wehrli FW: Sign applications guide, vol I, Publication No. E8804CA, General Electric Medical Systems, Milwaukee, Wis, 1990.)

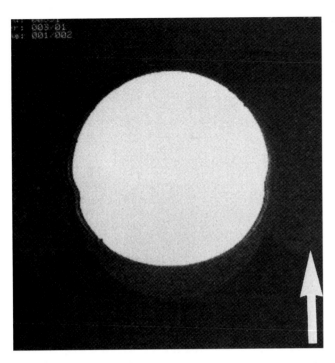

Fig. 4-15. Phase mismatch in a quadrature receiver. Properly functioning quadrature channels are locked into a 90-degree phase shift. Slight mistuning of the phase-lock circuits violates basic design assumptions and results in mathematical errors occurring in the display processor. The extraneous values are displayed as "ghost" images. (From Field SA, Wehrli FW: Sign applications guide, vol I, Publication No. E8804CA, General Electric Medical Systems, Milwaukee, Wis, 1990.)

Spatial resolution. Spatial resolution is the measurement of a system's ability to distinguish two points as being separate.

Clinical significance in abdominal MRI. The effect of spatial resolution is most evident on small objects: for example, thin fibrous septa, small calcifications, small lymph nodes, varices, and small hepatic nodules. The lower the intensity of the abnormality, the more likely it is to be hidden if spatial resolution is poor.

Factors affecting spatial resolution

1. FOV. Spatial resolution is inversely proportional to field of view. FOV depends on hardware (RF volume coil or surface coil diameter and gradient amplitude) and software factors.
2. Acquisition matrix. Assuming a fixed FOV, increasing matrix size increases spatial resolution. Resolution is inversely proportional to voxel volume.
3. Sampling time. Spatial resolution in the phase encoding direction is directly proportional to sampling time (assuming all other factors are constant). Sampling time in the frequency-encoding direction is not a limiting factor in conventional abdominal imaging.
4. Post-processing. Software filters, such as unsharp masking, markedly affect the depiction of high-spatial-frequency details.
5. CRT monitor. Monitor malfunction affects not only soft copy interpretation but also interferes with hard copy filming by misleading the technologist as to the actual appearance of the image.

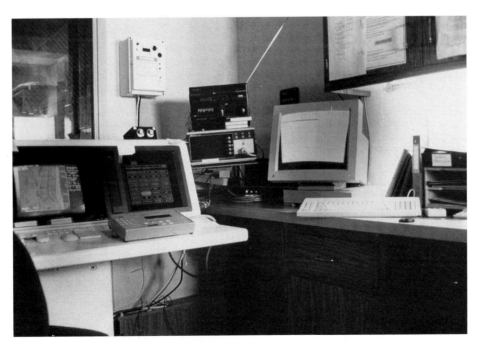

Fig. 4-16. Spatial nonlinearity of a CRT image. The magnetic field of an MRI scanner, not a gradient system malfunction, causes warping of the display of the computer monitor (right of center) in this scan control room. Note the absence of geometric distortion in the two monitors at the left. These monitors are protected by effective magnetic shielding built into their housings.

Measurement method. A multipurpose phantom is scanned, using a standard multislice spin-echo sequence. A standard FOV is used for each coil/phantom combination. For routine spatial resolution determination, images of points and lines of known size, separation, and conspicuity are evaluated visually (see Figs. 4-1 and 4-2). A multipurpose phantom image or an SMPTE test pattern is needed to determine monitor spatial resolution. Spatial resolution of high-contrast objects of 0.5 mm or less is obtainable by a state-of-the-art system.

Phase-related artifacts. Phase-related artifacts are an indication of maladjustment or component failure in the phase encoding decoding subsystem (Fig. 4-10).

Clinical significance in abdominal MRI. One source of these artifacts in clinical imaging is frequent coil changes and errors in instrument or coil set-up. Usually, however, these circuits are well protected and are stable unless a component fails in routine service.

Factors affecting phase-related artifacts

1. Phase-encoding gradient instability. Periodic variability in phase encoding gradient amplitude produces an artifact similar to that caused by pulsatile flow (Fig. 4-13).
2. Incorrect quadrature offset. When quadrature signal combination is used, the receiver and transmitter both must be adjusted to maintain a 90-degree phase angle between the two orthogonal quadrature channels (see Fig. 4-16).
3. Gradient current offset. Steady leakage of gradient amplifier current produces artifacts along one or all of the gradient axes (see Fig. 4-19).

Measurement method. A uniform cylinder phantom is examined with a standard pulse sequence (see Fig. 4-14). Images are observed for typical patterns of inhomogeneity. This observation typically takes place during routine evaluation of field homogeneity (see Factors Affecting Image Uniformity). The procedure is performed at other times to analyze or confirm artifacts observed or suspected during routine clinical imaging.

Quadrature ghosts are detected by scanning a small object placed off center in the magnet bore. To test the receiver, the object is offset from magnet isocenter along the x and y axes. To test the transmitter, the object is offset from center in all three axes. In either case, if the phase angle between quadrature channels is incorrect, a ghost will be projected to a mirror-image location on the line passing through both the center of the object and the isocenter of the magnet. For example, if the phantom is at position x = 0, y = 5, then the receiver ghost appears at position x = 0, y = −5. If the phantom is located at x = 0, y = 5, and z = 5, then the transmitter ghost image appears at position x = 0, y = −5, and z = −5. Transmitter quadrature-circuit failure or maladjustment requires a multislice sequence for detection.

Examples of phase-related artifacts are fluctuations in signal intensity in the phase-encoding direction and spurious depiction of signals from areas containing no resonating protons. Periodic variation in phase-encoding gradient amplitude produces *zebra stripes*—alternating high and low intensity bands superimposed on the image that simulate motion artifact (see Figs. 4-12 and 4-14). DC offset—steady leakage of current from a gradient amplifier—produces a band of artifact through the center of the image, parallel to the phase-encoding axis (see Fig. 4-9). Equal DC offsets simultaneously in all three gradient amplifiers produce a spot of fixed hyperintensity or hypointensity in the isocenter of the main magnetic field.

Additional performance evaluation

Measurement of slice thickness, slice position, and interslice gap is beyond the scope of this chapter. Rigorous evaluation of these parameters entails a complex protocol, which is unwarranted as a routine procedure because the parameters ordinarily are stable. Refer to reference 1 for a detailed description.

Other types of image artifacts and aspects of equipment performance are evaluated as needed during regular preventive maintenance sessions (Fig. 4-17). See Chapter 2 for more detail on other image artifacts. Additional quality assessment sources are listed in the references.

MAINTENANCE
Routine preventive maintenance

A scheduled block of approximately 2 to 4 hours/week is required to perform routine preventive maintenance. Superconducting magnets may require cryogen inspection or replenishment at this time. The technologists and clerical staff can enhance operational efficiency by working in short-notice additional preventive maintenance or minor repairs during schedule slots provided by no-shows.

Elements of the quality assessment protocol can be combined with routine preventive maintenance afternoons. Cryogen replenishment typically occurs at 1- to 2-week intervals.

A log of artifacts and screen prints is essential for documenting system performance. Actual images save valuable time in maintenance sessions (and in unexpected service encounters at odd hours) (Fig. 4-18). All error messages and performance inconsistencies of any sort should be recorded, as they provide potentially invaluable reference data.

Good, "clean" RF-free power feeds are essential. Heavy-duty power conditioning is recommended for areas having frequent power line failures and lightning storms.

Cryogens

Superconducting magnets are widely used due to their high flux density and magnetic field stability and uniformity. The superconducting magnet consists of a large coil

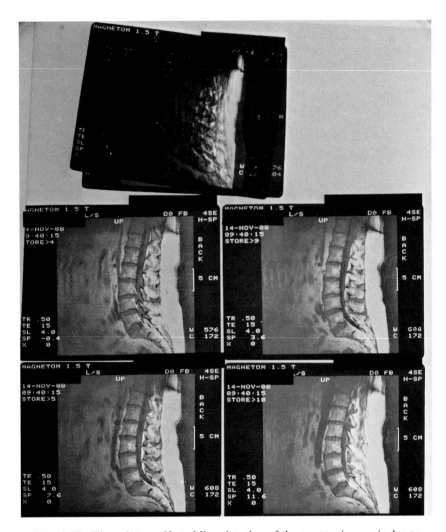

Fig. 4-17. Film printer artifact. Misregistration of the top two images is due to component failure. Any part of the MRI system could be the "weak link" in the imaging chain on a given day. Preventive maintenance significantly reduces the frequency of unexpected failures.

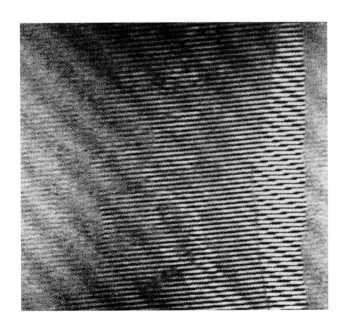

Fig. 4-18. Failure of the array processor. Events such as this should be logged for review by the service engineer, even though no problem seems to be present after software reboot. (From Field SA, Wehrli FW: Sign applications guide, vol I, Publication No. E8804CA, General Electric Medical Systems, Milwaukee, Wis, 1990.)

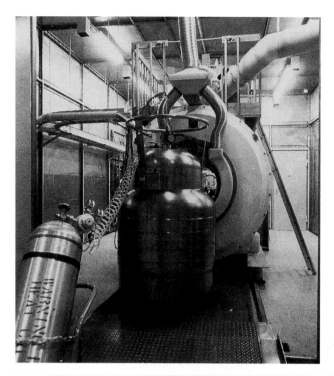

Fig. 4-19. Helium replenishment. High pressure helium gas, from the tank in the foreground, propels liquid helium from the dewar (the large tank with a circular handrail) into the cryostat. From Magnetom Brochure, MG/5000-109-121, Siemens Medical Systems, Inc, Iselin, NJ.)

of niobium-titanium alloy wire immersed in liquid helium. The boiling point of helium is 4.2° K. To keep the helium contained in a dewar, called a cryostat, in the liquid state, the heat transferred from the environment by convection, conduction, and radiation is minimized by careful design and construction. The jacket of the cryostat is vacuum insulated; the cryostat is supported by fiberglass of low conductivity, and the cryostat is shielded by insulating foil. However, no matter how sophisticated the design, there is a certain amount of heat transfer from the environment. The helium slowly vaporizes. Occasional replenishment of helium is necessary. To conserve this expensive material, the helium cryostat is suspended within a tank filled with less expensive liquid nitrogen, which boils off at a much faster rate. The boiling point of nitrogen is 77° K. The refill of liquid nitrogen typically takes place once a week, requiring approximately 230 liters (the capacity of a typical nitrogen dewar).

Replenishment of liquid helium at many MRI sites occurs at intervals of approximately 2 to 3 weeks. A typical cryostat requires about 500 liters. The helium dewar contains 250 liters (Fig. 4-19). Helium gas from a 2500 psi cylinder is used to pump liquid helium into the cryostat. The capacity of a cylinder is sufficient for approximately three weekly fills. Conservative maintenance of cryogens ensures levels above 70%. One could allow a longer interval between fills and allow the level to drop to 50% or be-

low with typically no perceptible effect on scan quality. If longer intervals are chosen between fills, however, fill levels must be monitored fastidiously.

A quench is loss of superconductivity, resulting in return of resistivity in the field coils, thermal damage to coils and other components, loss of cryogens, and damage to the cryostat and gas plumbing subsystems. To provide a conservative safety margin against a quench of the superconducting magnet, the level of liquid helium should be kept above 50%.

The magnet boil-off rate is monitored and calculated on a percent per day basis. The usual boil-off rates for a 1.5 T magnet are about 1% per day. This rate does not vary significantly with fill level (from 70 to 100 range). Note that the apparent boil-off rate, as depicted by the fill level transducer, may vary due to the shape of the helium vessel at different fill levels.

Metering

Care must be exercised in reading the volume of helium and nitrogen. Helium is measured by determination of the resistance of a segment of specially fabricated wire immersed in the liquid cryogen. A preliminary current is passed through the wire to allow conditions to stabilize for the reading. Introduction of current produces heat, which does induce some boil off. If the service person inadvertently leaves the warming current on for a prolonged period, disastrous results could follow. The safest policy is to allow intermittent heating only. Some scanners have the additional safety feature of disconnecting power to both the nitrogen and helium measuring devices during any scan. A volume meter left in the constant current mode for 3 days can generate enough heat to vaporize a substantial portion (75%) of the helium volume.

Nitrogen volume metering could remain on constantly with little effect on cryogen volume, as the device usually uses a non-heat-producing technique for measurement. Note, however, that a radiofrequency artifact is produced by some pressure monitoring devices. Therefore, measurement usually is performed only intermittently.

Safety procedures

Gloves, goggles, face protectors, and heavy clothing are recommended for cryogen handling. The helium dewar has a top fitting, which permits a long metal tube called the "stinger" to be introduced inside for tapping the contents. One should be careful of the pressure fittings that secure the stinger in the dewar. Unexpected loss of seal could result in damage to the face and upper body. Liquid helium is introduced by forced flush of helium gas from a 2500 psi cylinder (Fig. 4-19). One should exercise caution in securing fittings and handling plumbing devices.

Observe all dewars periodically to check for icing-over of the safety valves. Three safety valves typically are

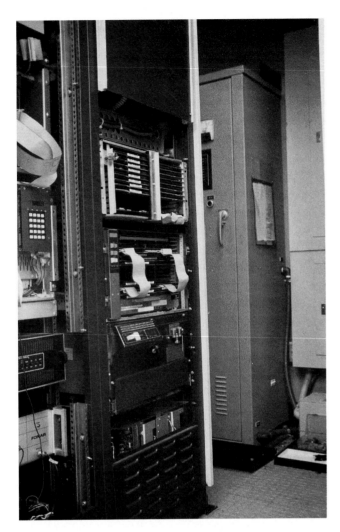

Fig. 4-20. Rack-mounted components. Edge connectors and ribbon cables allow the service engineer to replace boards quickly and easily. Vital modules and test points are exposed for maintenance access.

present. Two low-pressure valves are at the top, and one "vacuum valve bursting disk" is located at the midportion of the body of a typical dewar. Icing could lead to explosive overpressure. The bursting disk is designed as a last measure of safety, although it would waste the entire contents of the vessel.

Before filling either helium or nitrogen, the service person cools the lines first. Introduction of dead space room temperature air could result in significant loss of cryogen from the scanner. At the end of a helium refill, the service engineer listens for gas leaks. Pressure is bled off the dewar before removing the stinger. The ends of the fill tubing are capped to prevent insects and other debris from entering the line.

Dewars require no special shelter except that which provides adequate protection from damage and vandalism. They are vacuum insulated and can sustain prolonged exposure to direct sunlight without significant loss of vol-

ume. However, reasonable care must be taken to protect them well, as they and their contents are expensive.

Consider escape routes in MRI areas because rapid replacement of oxygen by expelled cryogen gases is a real hazard. Overpressure also could restrict door opening. A vent should be installed to release vaporized oxygen outside the building. A conservative margin of safety is always the best policy.

Repairs

Most repairs can be accomplished quickly by finding and replacing circuit boards rather than individual electronic components (Fig. 4-20). Repairs are accomplished with the assistance of electronic diagnostic programs running on the system control computer or on an independent diagnostic computer. Field service engineers for some vendors diagnose malfunctioning hardware or software with the aid of an analysis program running on a portable computer. Some manufacturers maintain an on-line service database accessible nationwide via telephone, allowing reference to documentation of all upgrades and software patches and review of troubleshooting and repair notes, which have been tried by others in the field.[7]

REFERENCES

1. Brice J: Vendors revamp strategy for equipment service, Diagn Imaging 65-72, 1991.
2. Dixon RL: MRI: acceptance testing and quality control, Proceeding of an AAPM Symposium, Madison, Wis, 1988, Medical Physics Publishing Corp.
3. Famano P: MRI artifacts slide collection, Siemens Medical Systems, Inc, Iselin, NJ.
4. Field SA, Wehrli FW: Signa applications guide, vol I, Publication No. E8804CA, General Electric Medical Systems, Milwaukee, Wis, 1990.
5. Haacke EM, Bellon EM: Artifacts. In Stark DD, Bradley WG, editors: Magnetic resonance imaging, St Louis, 1988, Mosby–Year Book.
6. Henkelman RL, Bronskill MJ: Artifacts in magnetic resonance imaging, New York, 1987, Pergamon Press.
7. Informationen für Med-Techniker, Magnetom Trouble Shooting, Publication Number C2-010.118.01.01.02, Siemens Medical Systems, Erlangen, Germany.
8. Johnson BA, Kelly WM: Common MRI artifacts: an overview, MRI Decisions (March/April) 17-23, 1989.
9. Magnetom Brochure, MG/5000-109-121, Siemens Medical Systems, Inc, Iselin, NJ.
10. Magnetom One Floor Installation Brochure, Magnetic Field Contour Chart, #A9001-M2221110-G545-01-7600, Siemens Medical Systems, Inc, Iselin, NJ.
11. Mao J: Quality assurance procedure and monthly report, Magnetic Resonance Imaging Center, Gainesville Veterans Affairs Hospital, Gainesville, Fla, 1990.
12. Pacs: Technology in Progress Brochure, MG/10/115/5c, Siemens Medical Systems, Inc, Iselin, NJ.
13. Partain CL, Price RR, Patton JA, et al: Magnetic resonance imaging, Philadelphia, 1988, WB Saunders.
14. Self-Shielding Magnet Enclosures Brochure, #A91001-M2210-G455-02—7600, Siemens Medical Systems, Inc, Iselin, NJ.

Chapter 5

RADIOFREQUENCY COILS

Jeffrey R. Fitzsimmons
W. Dean Bidgood, Jr.

Many factors contribute to the clinical success of an MRI examination, including some that are fixed for a particular scanner (such as the magnet field strength, gradient strength, etc.). The key to maximizing the clinical utility of magnetic resonance imaging (MRI) lies in optimizing variables that can either be programmed or easily added to the available system hardware. Among these variable factors, the application of specially designed radiofrequency (RF) coils has been one of the most powerful means for improving clinical MRI of the body.

Until recently, one's choices of coils for abdominal imaging have been very limited. However, in conjunction with simultaneous advances in other areas, such as rapid imaging, RF coils are now an area of active research and development. Vendors are marketing coil products to clinical departments for abdominal use. How good are they? When and where should they be used? In order to use RF coils to best advantage in the abdomen, one must first understand the basic principles that underlie their function and account for their success.

The MRI system is in a sense little more than a sophisticated transmitter and receiver set operating in conjunction with a large, powerful magnet (the computer only serves as a control unit and data manager). For clinical imaging, the intended audience of the scanner's transmitted signals is the population of hydrogen atoms within the sample volume. If the transmitted signal is of the right frequency, the hydrogen atoms respond by resonating (giving back energy of the same frequency). However, this response is extremely weak in amplitude. Common to both the sending and receiving links of the magnetic resonance phenomenon is an antenna (the RF coil), which is every bit as essential as its counterparts in more familiar implementations of radio communications. Without the antenna, with the wrong antenna, or with a malfunctioning antenna, signals from the hydrogen atoms cannot be detected. Fortunately, antennas are an area in which elegantly simple physical designs can achieve robust new functionality. Just as in common radio and television applications, in MRI one may use a variety of antenna designs with properties of directivity (control of the distribution of the transmitted signal or rejection of undesired interfering signals), forward gain (magnification of signal strength in a favored direction), and bandwidth (tradeoff of peak function at a design frequency versus function over an entire band of frequencies).

Historically, RF coil design dealt almost exclusively with small, nonconducting samples (5 or 10 mm diameter) placed within small-volume coils. Coil performance was largely determined by the quality factor (Q) of the tuned circuit and not by the sample contents. The introduction of living organisms of various dimensions into the tuned circuit created a new set of demands on the RF coil designer. These demands have been met by a wide range of surface, volume, and quasivolume coil geometries as well as numerous methods for tuning, matching, and decoupling these coils from unwanted interactions. The design of whole body RF coils has been particularly challenging because of problems with RF field penetration and RF eddy currents within the body at high frequencies. Designers have found ways to circumvent these problems and have succeeded in producing large (55 cm diameter) quadrature body coils for improvements of up to 40% over early linear designs. Surface coil technology has also evolved considerably since its introduction. Current development in this area is focused on customizing coils for particular organ systems including cardiac, liver, prostate, and abdomen. Quadrature arrangements of surface coil pairs have also been introduced to increase surface coil performance. More recently, surface coil arrays have been designed as a means of extending the field of view without sacrificing signal-to-noise performance. The techniques for making surface coil arrays have also found application in a new form of body coil, which may prove to be even better than the quadrature body coil.

Designers of RF coils for use in whole body MRI systems must consider that the tuned circuit is operating in an unusual environment. Circuit design must be modified to account for the effects of large conductive samples regardless of coil geometry. Therefore, we will first consider some of these problems and ways to minimize their impact before turning to particular design implementations.

The designers of MRI systems have a number of ways of maximizing available signal-to-noise ratio (SNR). The first and most expensive solution is to increase the strength of the magnetic field. Thus, going from 0.1 to 1.0 T will yield a proportional increase in the available spins.[16] This is an effective but expensive way to improve SNR. As can be seen in Fig. 5-1, a doubling of the SNR would require a doubling of the main magnetic field. This not only increases the cost of the magnet but also increases the cost of cryogens and physical site requirements.

Another popular method of maximizing spins is to design pulse sequences that optimize the trade-offs between acquisition time and SNR. This approach may yield significant results as can be seen in fast gradient echo techniques.[30] One of the most common methods of improving SNR is to use signal averaging. In clinical MRI, however, there is a practical limit for imaging time on a single patient usually set by the patient's ability to hold still. Finally, we may resort to custom designing the RF coils,

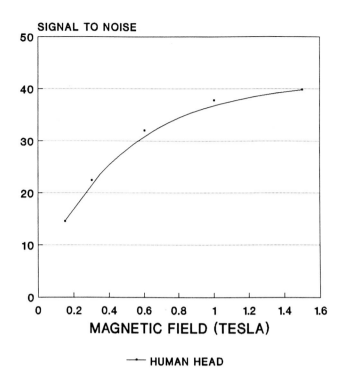

T1 weighted axial (500/30)

Fig. 5-1. Relationship between magnetic field strength and SNR. The graph is based on data from several magnets using human volunteers. All imaging parameters other than field strength were the same for each of the scans (TR,TE, slice thickness, etc.).

which are used to capture the small RF magnetic fields produced by the available spins. Careful design of these RF coils can yield improvements in SNR ranging from 40% to 100% over that which is available with conventional whole body RF coils. In addition, these gains can be applied to any imaging technique and do not increase imaging time.

One approach to improving SNR is to optimize the receiver coil physical geometry. Although early designers focused their attention on building adequate head and body coils, it quickly became apparent that one could do much better. Research has shown that by designing an MR receiver probe to fit a particular body region as closely as possible one can optimize SNR for a single coil system.[2] In many cases this means using a small coil that has higher SNR and smaller regional coverage than a larger coil. This basic concept has led to a wide variety of designs all aimed at optimizing SNR over a particular field of view (FOV).

SIGNAL-TO-NOISE RATIO

The SNR obtainable from a given coil design is determined by a number of factors, including the magnet field strength, the sample characteristic T1- and T2-relaxation times, and the pulse parameters used to acquire the data.[21] However, if the preceding variables are held constant and only those parameters that relate to the physical aspects of the coil are examined, the situation is considerably simplified. The most basic model for the RF coil is a single loop of wire in a magnetic field (see Fig. 5-2).

According to Faraday's law of induction we can expect to generate an electromotive force (EMF), which is determined by the amount of magnetic flux passing through the loop and the rate of change with respect to time:

$$emf = -d\Phi/dt \qquad \text{5-1}$$

In MRI terms we can visualize the flux (o) as being determined by the number of spins available per unit volume and the rate of change (dt) as being determined by the frequency of precession. In short, if we increase the number of spins or the frequency of precession we can expect an increase in the EMF from our simple loop coil. For an MRI experiment with spins rotating in the xy plane we can say that the signal is determined in the following way:

$$Signal = W_o\, M\, V_s\, B1_{xy} \qquad \text{5-2}$$

where W_o is the frequency of interest, M is the spin magnetization that is proportional to w and the density of spins, V is the volume from which the signal derives, and $B1$ is the magnetic field that would be present given a unit current in the coil. This last term may be viewed as a coil performance variable, which is determined by the coil geometry. The coil geometry determines the relationship between a current in the coil and the flux density present within the coil. Generally, the smaller the coil, the higher the flux density or B1 field.

The noise present in this system is a function of two basic factors. Consider first a model in which signals are represented by current (I) flowing in a conductor. Current flowing through resistance (R) produces a voltage (E) of a certain amplitude (recall Ohm's law; E=IR). Now consider a "real world" RF coil made of metal wire. Every substance at room temperature has resistance. Due to the random (Brownian) motion of electrons within the wire, a random voltage is produced at the terminals of the coil. Because this motion depends on the temperature of the wire, it is commonly called *thermal noise*. The first factor in system noise then derives from the thermal noise in the coil, which may be viewed as having a resistance Rc. This factor should be minimized by proper use of high purity copper conductors.

The second factor that generates noise is the human body itself and the random motion of electrolytes within it. This source of noise can also be viewed as having an equivalent resistance Rp. In the laboratory we could eliminate the factor of patient noise simply by cooling the person to absolute zero (this is not an option in the Radiology Department, of course) (Fig. 5-3).

In the absence of any molecular motion, and with superconductivity brought about by cooling, Rp would disappear. However, because few of us would be willing to undergo this state change for a routine diagnostic examination, we must consider both Rc and Rp in expressing system noise at comfortable room temperatures. One other important factor must be brought in at this point. Random electrical currents, such as randomly moving macroscopic particles seen through a microscope, are just as likely to move in direction −x as +x. Over time, the distance trav-

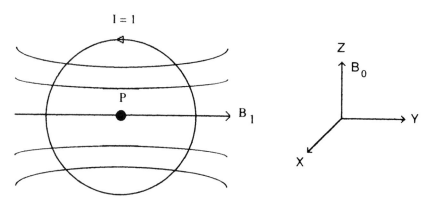

Faradays Law of Induction:

$$emf = -\frac{d\Phi}{dt} \qquad \text{where } \Phi = B \cdot A$$

Fig. 5-2. The electromotive force (EMF) induced in a loop of wire is given by Faraday's law. This calculation is accurate for direct currents and low frequencies. At high radiofrequencies the EMF is a more complex function of the coil-patient interaction.

eled (by a particle) or the amount of signal generated (the integral of the amplitude of signal over time) may be expressed as a sort of average by neutralizing the changing direction of movement by expressing it in terms of the *root mean square* (RMS) in which one considers the absolute value rather than the particular change of direction. The total noise is then:

$$\sqrt{R_c + R_p} \qquad \text{5-3}$$

In addition, we need to know what happens to these losses as we go to higher and higher frequencies (larger magnetic fields). **The Q (or quality factor of an RF coil) is a function of two properties of the coil: its resistance and its inductance. A high Q factor is a desirable property for MRI RF coils.** A high Q coil has the ability to selectively pass certain frequencies and reject others. At a given frequency, Q is proportional to the ratio of inductance to resistance. As we move to higher frequencies, however, the inductance does not change at the same rate as the resistance. As a consequence, the coil Q increases with increasing frequency until one approaches self-resonance. Self-resonance occurs because of increasing phase shift along the conductor and distributed capacitance in the inductor itself. This self-resonance condition then limits the useful frequency range of the coil. The solution to this problem is to break up the coil inductance using many capacitors. This greatly extends the operating range of a given RF coil.

Note that any physical object, including coils, in the real world also have the property of capacitance. Capacitive reactance acts like resistance in an alternating current (AC) circuit and, therefore, may be a source of noise voltage (recall Ohm's law E = IR). Stray capacitance between the coil and surrounding objects is also a source of signal loss. At higher frequencies of operation, the impedance to current flow due to capacitive reactance decreases. Higher frequencies are siphoned off into surrounding material through stray capacitance and prevented from reaching the receiver circuit. The coil designer must maximize the Q factor of the coil antenna by optimizing the inductance and minimizing stray capacitance.

The component of total resistance contributed by the coil is not a significant factor at high frequencies (high fields). In fact, the patient resistance (Rp) becomes the dominant source of noise at frequencies above about 25 MHz (0.5 T). Therefore, the overall SNR can be approximated by the following:

$$SNR = \frac{W_o\, M\, V_s\, B1_{xy}}{\sqrt{R_p}} \qquad \text{5-4}$$

As a result of the patient-induced losses (Rp), which go up dramatically with higher operating frequencies, the benefit of having higher magnet field strength is significantly reduced. In fact, a typical plot of SNR versus magnet field strength shows that such improvements do not follow the theoretical square of the field strength but rather increase at a rate which is closer to linear (Fig. 5-1).

If we now set aside the issues of field strength, patient loss Rp, and spin density M, the remaining variables of importance have to do with the relationship between the sample size (Vs) and the achievable B1 field over the region of interest. The optimized coil geometry provides the largest B1 field over the particular region of interest. Thus in practical terms, the goal is to choose a coil geometry that is not much larger than the FOV needed to capture the organ system of interest.

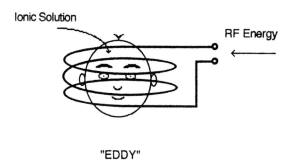

"EDDY"

NMR
- Oscillating magnetic field
- Oscillating currents in the body
- Induced currents form small loops (Eddy currents)

Electrical Resistance in Fluid
- Eddy current loss of magnetic field energy
- Loss greatest at tissue surface

Consequence of Loss
- Thermal energy available to produce random Eddy currents
- Noise induced in coil

FIELD OF VIEW

FOV is a software-determined variable in MRI. For a constant number of pixels, a large FOV is created by applying a small switched field gradient, whereas a small FOV is created by applying a large gradient. Large gradient amplitudes produce anomalies in the delicate pattern of tissue magnetization and tend to mask desired signals indirectly. Another consequence of using a large gradient is that the available signal information is spread out over a large range of frequencies leading to a reduction in SNR

Fig. 5-3. The relationship between the coil and the patient gives rise to RF eddy currents, which in turn change the performance of the coil. The higher the frequency, the more the coil performance is degraded.

per pixel. Again, the larger the gradient, the farther apart the maximum and minimum resonant frequencies of the extreme dimensions of the sampled volume. This greater spread of signal frequencies is accompanied by a broader palette of noise frequencies. There is no escaping the basic physical principle: Noise increases as the square root of the bandwidth. The result of a high-gradient-amplitude examination is a highly resolved image with poor SNR.

The RF coil designer attempts to build a coil that matches the software-selected FOV with the physical size of the coil so that one can achieve the highest possible SNR over the region of interest. It is up to the clinician, however, to determine the optimum FOV for a given organ system. Therefore, the coil designer must work closely with the clinician to optimize the FOV of the imaging technique and the FOV of the coil.

MAGNETIC FIELD CALCULATION

The magnetic field, B1xy, produced by a given coil can be determined by applying known physical principles. The law of Biot and Savart permits one to calculate the magnetic field at a given point in space resulting from a particular coil element.[5] Many coil geometries have been looked at in this way to give a visual presentation of the theoretical magnetic fields. An example of such a field plot is given below for one half of a simple surface coil, such as one could use to image the spine or kidneys. It can be seen from this plot that the field varies smoothly with distance in all directions. The contour lines represent regions with the same RF magnetic field (B1xy) (Fig. 5-4).

If the data from this plot are analyzed on axis only, it can be seen that the field intensity falls off rapidly with distance from the coil plane. This fact is of overwhelming importance in the operation and use of surface coils, as primary areas of interest in clinical imaging typically lie at some depth beneath the skin (and high amplitude signal from subcutaneous and retroperitoneal fat typically is induced in the more intense near field of the coil) (Fig. 5-5).

These same coil modeling efforts can be used for volume coils. Because the volume coil is radially symmetric, it provides much higher RF field homogeneity than the surface coil. However, there are differences between volume coils. The oldest design is the so-called saddle coil. It provides modest homogeneity and reasonably good sensitivity. The saddle coil configuration still is being used to image regions having curved contour, such as the neck. The slotted tube resonator is used at higher frequencies because of its inherently low inductance, but it provides homogeneity similar to the saddle coil. The distributed phase coil provides high homogeneity because of the equal distribution of active elements. The bird cage is similar to the distributed phase coil in this regard and provides excellent homogeneity of the entire abdomen, head, or extremities. These volume coil geometries are discussed further in the next section because of their obvious application to whole body imaging.

WHOLE BODY COILS
Development of body coils

Early attempts to image the human torso involved very large (50 cm diameter) volume coils of several designs. The saddle coil was the best known so it was the first design to find use in whole body imaging[17] (Figs. 5-6 and 5-7).

Early designers were quickly confronted with the problem of self-resonance, which occurs when a coil's self-inductance and distributed capacitance become large enough to resonate without any external components. Some workers became so pessimistic about this problem that they said that "the construction of coils above 10 MHz (0.25 T) will not be practical."[18] Breaking this barrier became a chal-

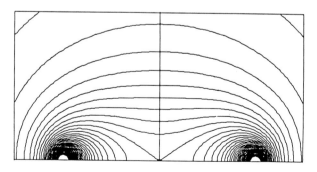

Fig. 5-4. This profile plot shows the pattern of magnetic flux lines resulting from current flowing through the wires of a loop, shown on edge. Coil measurements made in the transmission mode give a good indication of the function of the coil in the reception mode, as the two processes are reciprocal.

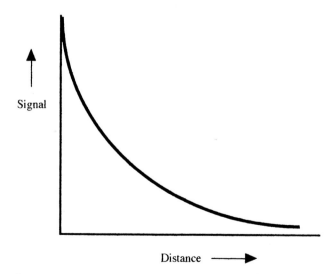

Fig. 5-5. When the field intensity is only considered on axis for surface coil, one obtains the function given above. The rapid fall-off with depth is obvious in this plot.

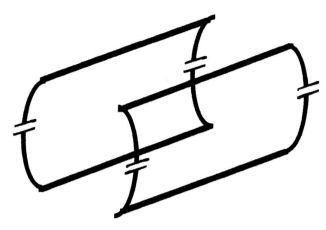

Fig. 5-6. The conventional saddle coil is a volume design with two halves. These sections are connected by wires not shown so that their outputs are combined into a single lead. This coil design yields modest homogeneity over the volume of interest.

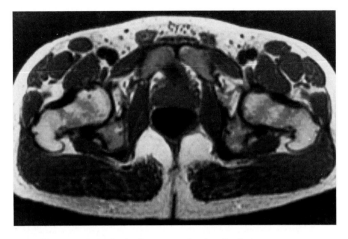

Fig. 5-7. A whole body image at the level of the greater trocanter and prostate obtained with a large volume coil.

lenge to several research and development groups. One of the pioneers in this area was Waldo Hinshaw who developed a unique distributed phase coil.[15] This coil consisted of a continuous toroid of RF transmission line, which was encased in a large cylindrical former. The outer conductor of the transmission line was separated at well-defined intervals so as to distribute the phase of currents around the cylinder, resulting in a highly homogeneous magnetic field (Fig. 5-8).

The design was successful in achieving very good homogeneity over its useful volume; however, some inherent losses (in the transmission line) prevented it from giving the optimal SNR. The first whole body coil to incorporate the distributed phase concept with high SNR was the so-called bird cage.[14] This coil is also based on transmission line theory, providing an even distribution of RF phases around the circumference of the coil. Because the number of elements may be varied from 4 to 32, the homogeneity can be easily controlled (Fig. 5-9).

This coil achieved high homogeneity, was able to operate at high frequencies (64 MHz for 1.5 T systems), and had near-optimal performance. The bird cage also used the

concept of distributed capacitance, which keeps stray capacitive losses to a minimum and practically eliminated the need for tuning the coil for each patient.

One problem that remained even in the new bird cage design was that of an asymmetric artifact in the image (Fig. 5-10). This problem was due to the linear nature of the existing coils.[10] The signal inhomogeneity, called the *quadrupole deletion artifact,* can be seen in images produced by any linearly polarized RF coil.

Other solutions to body imaging have been developed for region-specific imaging such as the abdomen, heart, and shoulder. The Helmholtz pair or simply the Helmholtz coil is configured in a vertical fashion with one loop below the torso and the other loop above (Fig. 5-11). This design has been used successfully on low- and high-field magnets.[19] The bladder, uterus, and ovaries are positioned fa-

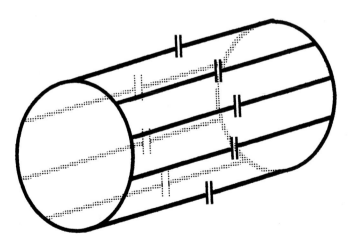

Fig. 5-9. The bird cage coil is made up of 4 to 32 elements equally spaced around the volume of interest. The number of elements determines the homogeneity of the field produced. Typically, these coils are made with 16 or 32 elements.

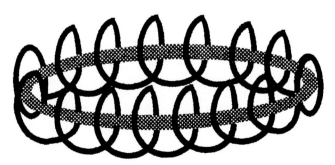

Fig. 5-8. A distributed phase coil using the toroidal design. It may be used as a volume coil with high homogeneity.

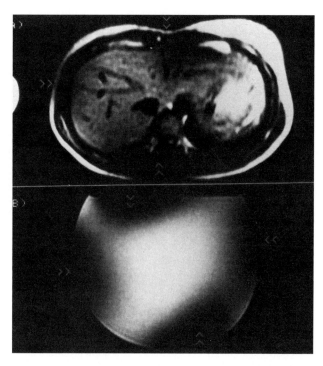

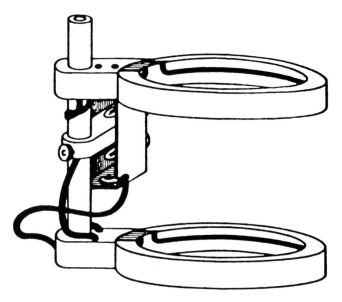

Fig. 5-11. The Helmholtz coil is made up of two opposing loops of wire. These may be configured to image a large volume or focused on a smaller region such as the bladder or right upper quadrant. These designs offer moderate homogeneity and high efficiency.

Fig. 5-10. A linear volume coil gives rise to an asymmetric artifact. This is due to RF eddy currents in the body primarily at high fields. The upper image demonstrates a loss of signal in the region of the liver simulating a low intensity infiltrating lesion. The lower image is a cross-section of a cylindrical water phantom, which should have a homogeneous circular configuration. The image demonstrates the areas of signal loss due to eddy currents in the sample. The use of quadrature drive eliminates this problem on newer systems.

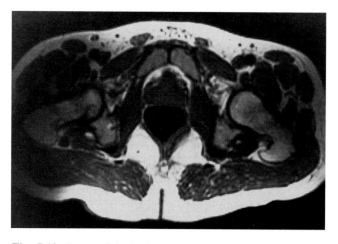

Fig. 5-12. Image of the body at the level of the prostate using a Helmholtz coil. Note improved detail in subcapsular zone.

vorably in the central pelvis for Helmholtz coil examination. Subregions of the abdomen (for instance, the right upper quadrant) can be examined to good advantage with the smaller FOV and high filling factor provided by this design. Cardiac imaging can be accomplished with less wasted coverage of the surrounding lung fields. One manufacturer has designed a movable table with an imbedded Helmholtz pair so that the operator can position the coil around various body regions to maximize filling factor and SNR. For a linear coil this represents the highest performance achievable in a volume configuration (Fig. 5-12).

At this point further improvements in performance can only be achieved by developing a two (quadrature) or more channel system. As we will see in the next section, this design is more complex but is well worth the extra effort.

Quadrature body coils

Quadrature designs are important because from them one can obtain an improvement of 40% over single-channel designs with a modest increase in acquisition system complexity. The idea of quadrature detection has been a part of phase-sensitive MRI receivers for many years;

however, it was not applied to RF coil design until recently. The key to the process is to obtain two orthogonal channels containing the same signal information but independent noise contributions. Orthogonal channels are streams of radio signal information separated by 90 degrees of phase angle (phase-shifted by 90 degrees). Here is another important basic principle: Electrical signals 90 degrees out of phase from each other are independent; as long as they remain out of phase, they do not affect each other in any way. How do we cause the signals to become separated in phase? Electrical components in the coil and the transmitter/receiver circuits can be selected to produce any necessary phase delay. This is no problem for design engineers. For the user, it is enough just to understand the importance of phase combination and to know that quadrature designs inherit the advantages of the underlying physical principles.

When two receiver channels detect the same signal information from the two orthogonal outputs of a quadrature coil, the signal from the two outputs is phase shifted again, intentionally, to reverse the 90-degree separation produced by the coils. The modified signals then are added together to double the net received signal amplitude. It is important to note that the noise does not double along with the signal. Because the noise is random, it only adds as the square root of 2. The net result is an improvement in SNR by the root of 2, or 40%. Why is this true?

Useful signals have nonrandom order, which is discernible over time. In all real systems, signal always coexists with noise. The job of the engineer is to maximize the contrast between the signal elements and the background. SNR is a measure of the success of the circuit in doing just that. The order of a signal distinguishes it from the randomness of background noise, providing that the amplitude of the signal is sufficient to allow detection above the noise threshold. Multiple copies of the same signal (for instance, the output of two receivers, say S1 and S2, tuned to the same radio station) when added combine arithmetically so that averaging can be used to enhance the "quality" (or conspicuity) of the received information. In other words, the information content of the two views of the signal is correlated. On the other hand, random noise is uncorrelated. The same two radio receivers would detect a background hiss of white noise simultaneously (N1 and N2) with the desired signal from the station. However, the noise being random would add only in absolute value terms (the noise detected by two separate receivers would be depicted in an unpredictable way, rather than being arithmetically additive). Therefore, noise adds as the square root of the product of the two contributing noise amplitudes. Thus, the effective signal to noise ratio (SNReff) of a system that combines (finds the product of) two views of the same signal is:

$$SNReff = \frac{S1 + S2}{\sqrt{N1 \times N2}} \times S0$$

where signal component S1 and noise component N1 arise from one view of the signal S0 and components S2 and N2 arise from the second view of the same signal. If S1 = S2 = 1 and the noise values N0, N1, and N2 are uncorrelated then $\sqrt{N1 \times N2} = N0$ and:

$$SNReff = \frac{2 \times S0}{\sqrt{2 \times N0}}$$

and

$$\frac{SNReff}{SNR0} = \sqrt{(2)}$$ 5-5

This relationship holds true whether signals plus uncorrelated noise are combined from simultaneous or sequential acquisitions. However, **the greater the correlation of the background noise, the lower the ratio of effective SNR to individual sample SNRs (ratio approaches 1 to 1).** The quadrature coil follows the discussion above because it uses in effect two independent receiver coils.

The introduction of quadrature to the RF probe design has been pioneered by Hoult.[27] He showed that a volume coil could be designed that would effectively orthogonalize the signals from the body so that two RF channels were 90 degrees out of phase (Fig. 5-13).

It was then necessary to develop a means of both splitting and combining these signals so that the RF transmitter could effectively drive the system while providing a path for the RF receiver. The evolution of this technology has been greatly enhanced by Hoult's early work, and many state-of-the-art MRI scanners today are designed with head and body coils operating in quadrature for maximum performance. In fact, those interested in abdominal imaging should demand that the MR system they purchase have a quadrature body coil. This equipment is virtually assured in recent MR scanners—but is a caveat for those considering reconditioned older models.

The previously discussed bird cage coil lends itself very well to quadrature implementation. The currents in each of the coil rungs have a sinusoidal distribution, which results in a homogeneous RF field within the volume of the coil. Although this design is somewhat more difficult to construct, it offers a nearly ideal platform for implementing quadrature. Because each of the elements represents a phase shift, it is a simple matter to choose elements that are 90 degrees out of phase and place drive circuitry at each of these points (Figs. 5-14 and 5-15).

This design then offers the best of two worlds, high homogeneity and high SNR due to the advantage of quadrature drive. Another advantage of the quadrature drive is

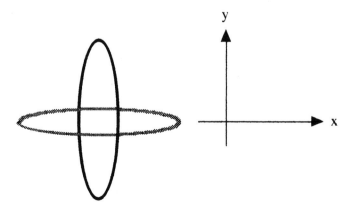

Fig. 5-13. The quadrature coil may be conceptualized as two loops of wire orthogonal to each other. The intent is to produce and receive information from two independent noise sources (the coils are decoupled).

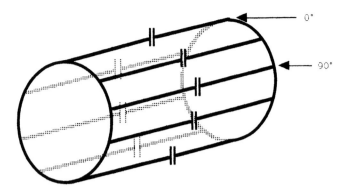

Fig. 5-14. The quadrature bird cage is a particular implementation of the quadrature coil. It is more difficult to visualize the orthogonal elements than in the simple case of two perpendicular loops; however, each element has a particular phase from 0 to 360 degress. This allows the designer to chose the appropriate phases for quadrature operation (0 and 90 degrees).

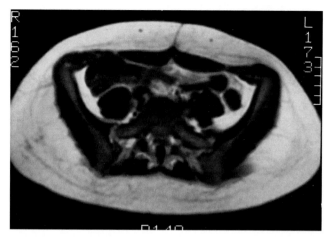

Fig. 5-15. Image of the upper pelvis using a quadrature body coil for improved SNR. Note the improved RF homogeneity in this image as compared to Fig. 5-10.

that it also reduces the required RF power required to tip the spins into the xy plane. This 50% reduction in power reduces the specific absorption rate (SAR) and thus the risk of patient heating due to RF energy absorption.[6]

Coil diameter and length

One further note concerning volume coils for the body is that the coil length and diameter have somewhat different effects on overall coil performance. The typical body coil is about 55 cm in diameter and 60 to 80 cm long. These large coils are obviously designed to accommodate the largest patients; however, they are far from ideal for those patients who have smaller diameters and are shorter. A simple analysis of the sensitivity of a volume coil as a function of length and diameter shows[24] that one can gain more from making the coil shorter than by decreasing its diameter (Fig. 5-16).

Therefore, one could envision smaller body coils for particular applications that could significantly improve the SNR. The only tradeoff is that shorter coils have less homogeneity, so there is a lower limit to improving SNR by coil shortening. This sort of approach would be particularly useful in the pediatric population where typical head coils are too small and the whole body coil is much too large. Such a design emphasizes the importance of optimizing the B1 field strength over the region of interest. If a large volume of pediatric MRI examinations is anticipated, it would be wise to consider purchase of a down-sized coil for abdominal imaging. If the manufacturer does not offer such a configuration, third-party sources should be investigated.

LOCALIZED COILS
Surface coils

Volume coils can be optimized by making their diameter and length appropriate to the size of the body part (i.e.,

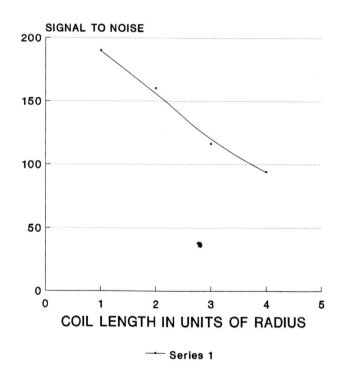

Fig. 5-16. The length effects the performance of a volume coil. In this case the length is shown to be a significant determinant of SNR for a given sample size. These data were collected from clinical volume coils (knee, head, and body).

head coils are smaller than body coils). However, in an effort to fully maximize SNR for regions close to the surface of the body, it is often more productive to abandon the classic volume coil in favor of a much smaller "surface" coil. Such surface coils were introduced by Ackerman et al[1] to improve the SNR from weak nuclei used in spectros-

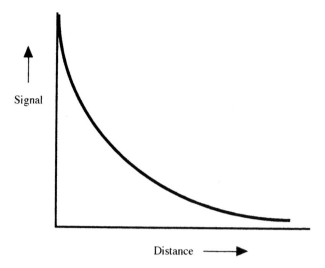

Fig. 5-17. Plot of surface coil sensitivity on axis.

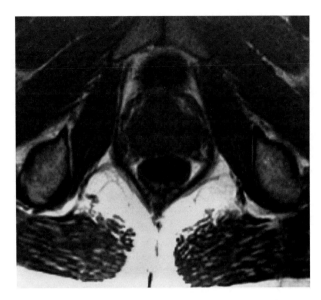

Fig. 5-18. Image of the prostate showing the intensity variation with depth. Note the high intensity of perirectal fat (posterior) as opposed to perivesical fat (anterior).

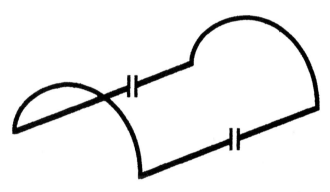

Fig. 5-19. The so-called "half-saddle" coil geometry has been useful in studies requiring open access. The field plot of this design yields modest homogeneity and performance comparable to a surface coil.

copy. It soon became evident, however, that they had broad application to human whole body proton MRI. Early designs included spine imaging,[25] neck imaging,[9] and other body parts. These coils had very poor RF homogeneity when compared to the preceding volume coils; however, they provided significant improvements in SNR. Current surface coil designs can improve the depiction of small regions of the abdomen. It is not always necessary to see the entire abdomen for a study. If only the kidneys or the left lobe of the liver are of interest, for instance, then a spine surface coil may be used. For a small superficial abdominal soft tissue mass, a small diameter coil (such as an orbit coil) may be useful. Coils should be judged by their construction and performance, not necessarily by the name that is on the box (Figs. 5-17 and 5-18).

The rapid fall-off in surface coil sensitivity limits their use to regions no more than 6 to 8 cm from the surface. Beyond this depth the simple surface coil is no more sensitive than the standard whole body coil.

The major difference between the surface coils used for NMR spectroscopy and whole body MRI was that the former were used to transmit and receive signals, whereas the MRI systems took advantage of the large whole body volume coil for excitation. The use of the surface coil for "receive only" application gave much more homogeneous images because the RF excitation process was controlled by the large homogeneous volume coil. The combination of homogeneous excitation and inhomogeneous reception was an acceptable compromise given the large increase in SNR that became available.

Curvilinear surface coils

During the development of the first commercial MRI system, engineers at Technicare realized that the SNR advantage of the surface coil could be combined with the homogeneous field of the volume coil by designing a curvi-

linear surface coil.[10] These coils were very successful in imaging the head and whole body with a single receive only curvilinear surface coil or "half saddle" (Fig. 5-19). Other applications of this design were soon developed for imaging the cervical spine.[3]

These coils were used on over 100 systems from low fields (0.15 T) to intermediate field (0.6 T) whole body systems. However, the desire for higher SNR has led to further refinements on the simple linear surface coil design.

Quadrature surface coils

The advantages of quadrature coils were restricted to volume coil designs until the late 1980s. Then in 1986 Arakawa proposed taking the half saddle design popularized by Technicare and splitting it into two coils with a 90-degree phase shift between them.[3] This approach allowed the

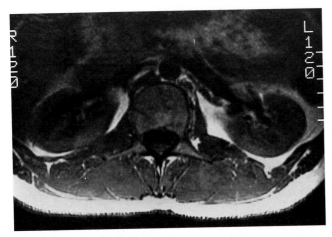

Fig. 5-20. Image of the kidneys demonstrating the high SNR and large FOV in the transverse dimension admitting both kidneys to the FOV.

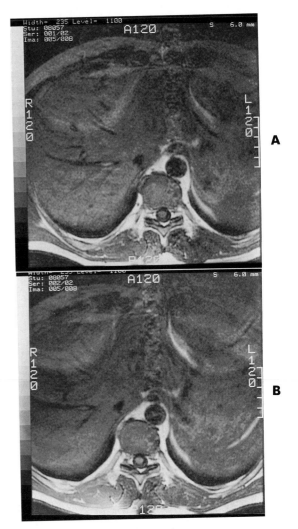

Fig. 5-21. Two images identically obtained except that the experimental two element array used was configured as a generalized quadrature surface coil fixed combined at 45 degrees in **A** and 125 degrees in **B.** Note that **A** has greater depth penetration (increased intensity of ventral subcutaneous fat) but more noise. **B** has a smoother appearance due to lower noise in the mid and posterior upper abdomen, but displays less signal from the anterior structures. These characteristics are produced by signal addition, which varies with position, and noise correlation, which is a global effect. With this array, it is possible to select by remote control either increased depth of penetration or increased near-field SNR—in effect, combining two different coil functions into one unit.

SNR to be increased by up to 40% in a quasisurface coil. This design was quickly applied to imaging the torso with good results. Later, Hyde et al[20] also introduced a quadrature surface coil using three "loop gap resonators" in a flat configuration. They also claimed improvements of up to 40% in the quadrature region of the coil set. An example of what can be achieved is given in Fig. 5-20. Here the kidneys are clearly visible as well as the spine.

Recently, a further innovation has been the optimized phasing of the signals from two adjacent quadrature coils. This sort of optimization can produce images that emphasize regions close to or far away from the surface coil.[8] The potential clinical applications of this new design concept are readily understandable. An electrically steerable coil pattern could be optimized for highest resolution in an area of interest found on a scout sequence, without moving the patient. Fig. 5-21 demonstrates the difference between combining the signals at two different phase angles.

Coil arrays

Several design groups have attempted to optimize the relationship between coil size and FOV by making arrays of surface coils with some method for selecting the number of coils active at any given time.[11,31] Although these coil arrays provide electronic control over FOV, they suffer the same losses as a single large coil when their outputs are combined (Fig. 5-22). One design has even made the FOV continuously variable[7]; however, this design requires mechanical intervention to change the FOV. As a result, newer designs attempt to combine the advantages of a large FOV with the high performance of a small coil. A large FOV scout image can be obtained with all elements operating. Subsequent images, using the most favorable single element, are directed to the precise area of interest (Fig. 5-23).

Closely related to the quadrature surface coil is the surface coil phased array. These coils were first introduced by Roemer et al[26] and promise to provide a number of new and interesting possibilities. The basic concept is to construct a series of coils that have little mutual coupling. Under these conditions the noise contribution of each coil is nearly independent. Each coil is then treated separately by

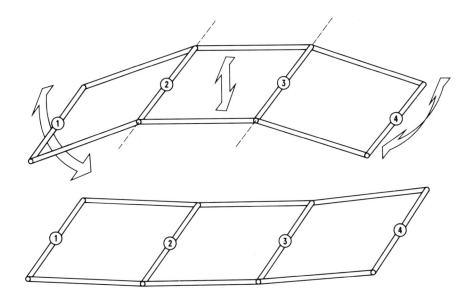

Fig. 5-22. The coil array shown above has been refered to as a "ladder" coil because of its geometry. It is in fact a coil array with switchable`elements. It yields a larger FOV than a single surface coil. Unfortunately, its performance decreases with the selection of a larger FOV because the coils are not noise independent.

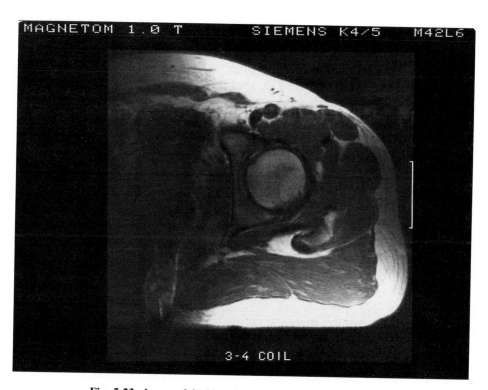

Fig. 5-23. Image of the hip joint using the lateral elements of the ladder coil. Once a large FOV survey scan has been accomplished using all of the elements of the array, small areas can be examined with the appropriate individual coil elements. This array could be used in this way to examine the soft tissue extension of a pelvic mass, or to follow an abscess pointing toward the hip from a retroperitoneal source.

having its own receiver channel. Only when the data are in the computer is the information recombined to form an image. The advantage of a surface coil phased array is that it enables one to obtain the SNR of a small surface coil over an arbitrarily large region of interest. The most immediate application of this technology has been in the area of the spine. However, coil arrays are now being constructed to surround the torso providing high quality images of the body (Fig. 5-24). Examinations of the pelvis, retroperitoneum, kidneys, and omentum could use the wide FOV of

Figs. 5-24. These coil arrays are referred to as "phased" arrays because each coil is noise independent and the outputs are put back into proper phase after acquisition. This design allows an extended FOV with no loss in SNR over a single small surface coil. **A** is a simplified schematic drawing of a three element array; **B** is a drawing of a two element array, including details of the electronic components that are essential to its function.

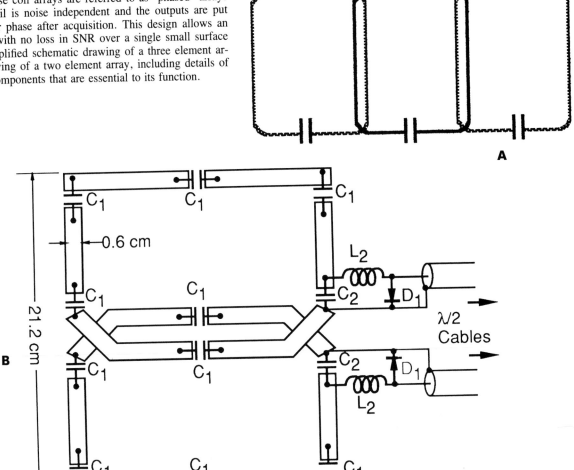

these arrays and the improved SNR at moderate depth (Fig. 5-25). The coils may find powerful applications in combination with fat suppression imaging techniques (Figs. 5-26 and 5-27).

There are, of course, limits to the number of coils one can have in an array, but they are not set by the theory. The cost and marginal benefit of building very large arrays are not very attractive; consequently, arrays will probably be limited to four to six elements for the near future.

Flexible coil designs

Some designers have attempted to give the operator maximum variation in coil shape by going to flexible coils. These coils may be made using transmission lines[4] or a braided or fluid material.[12,22] In any case, these are generally simply linear surface coils with rather poor performance. They do allow the operator to promptly change the configuration to suit the occasion. However, the result is a nonoptimized coil design that does not provide the SNR of quadrature surface and volume coils.

Catheter coils

Highly specific coil design efforts have been focused on small organs such as the prostate. Because the prostate occupies only a small volume, a small diameter coil would be optimal. However, its depth beneath the skin places it out of range of very small surface coils. A coil of nearly optimal dimensions can be placed adjacent to the prostate by insertion into the rectum.[28] The design of insertable coils has been refined so that one manufacturer provides a disposable coil that is connected to a remote tuning box. These coils do provide a high SNR over a limited area near the prostate. However, the small size of the coil (restricted to only 2 to 3 cm for patient comfort) limits the depth penetration to a great extent, and the image quality suffers from very rapid falloff of SNR in the prostate itself (Fig. 5-28).

other things being equal, a better filling factor will yield a better image. With quadrature and multichannel phased coil arrays, there may be a 40% or greater improvement in SNR, but matching the coil geometry to the size of the region of interest is still the most fundamental consideration. RF coil designs are only now becoming widely available to provide the best possible SNR for imaging the kidneys and retroperitoneum, the prostate and other pelvic genitourinary organs, and the detailed anatomy of other subregions of the abdomen.

REFERENCES

1. Ackerman JH, Grove TH, Wong GG, et al: Mapping of metabolites in whole animals by 31P NMR using surface coils, Nature 283: 167-170, 1980.
2. Andrew ER: Nuclear magnetic resonance, London, 1969, Cambridge University Press.
3. Arakawa M, Fehn J, McCarer M: Quadrature surface coils for 0.35T imaging, Annual meeting of the SMRM, Montreal, 1986.
4. Bader R, Zabel H, Lorenz W: Flexible transmission line resonators for high quality MR imaging, Proceedings of Annual Meeting, IEEE, Engineering in Medicine and Biology Society, New York, 1986.
5. Bleaney BI, Bleaney B: Electricity and magnetism, New York, 1985, Oxford University Press.
6. Bottomley PA, Charles HC, Roemer PB, et al: Human in vivo phosphate metabolite imaging with 31P NM, Magn Reson Med 7:319-336, 1988.
7. Duensing GR, Fitzsimmons JR: Continuously variable field of view coil, Magn Reson Med 13:378-384, 1990.
8. Duensing GR, Fitzsimmons JR: Region specific SNR gains by fixed phase non-quadrature combination, Proceedings of the 13th Annual International Conference: IEEE Engineering in Medicine and Biology Society. November 1, 1991, Orlando, Fla.
9. Fitzsimmons JR, Thomas RG, Mancuso A: Proton imaging with surface coils on a 0.15 T resistive system, Magn Reson Med 2:180-185, 1985.
10. Flugen DC: Radio frequency coils for nuclear magentic resonance imaging systems, US Patent #4,649,348, March 10, 1987.
11. Fox T, Nakabayashi K, Segawa T: A linear coil array for spine imaging, Annual Meeting of the SMRM, London, 1990.
12. Fuentas J, Votruba J, Orbach E: A flexible surface coil for general purpose use in high resolution whole body imaging, Annual meeting of the SMRM, London, 1988.
13. Glover GH, Hayes CE, Pelc NJ, et al: Comparison of linear and circular polarization for magnetic resonance imaging, J Magn Reson 64:255-270, 1985.
14. Hayes CE, Edelstein WA, Schenck JF, et al: An efficient, highly homogeneous radiofrequency coil for whole-body NM imaging at 1.5 T, J Magn Reson 63:622-628, 1985.
15. Hinshaw WS: Investigation of samples by NMR Techniques, US Patent 4,468,621, August 28, 1984.
16. Hoult DI: Field, contrast, and sensitivity in imaging. In Cohen JS ed, Magnetic Resonance in Biology, New York, 1980, John Wiley & Sons.
17. Hoult DI, Richards R: The SNR of the NMR receiver, J Magn Reson 24:71-85, 1976.
18. Hoult DI, Lauterbur PC: The sensitivity of the zeugmatographic experiment involving human samples, J Magn Reson 34:425-433, 1979.
19. Hoult DI, Chen CN, Sank VJ: Quadrature detection in the laboratory frame, Magn Reson Med 1: 339-353, 1984.
20. Hyde JS, Jesmanowicz A, Grist TM, et al: Quadrature detection surface coil, Magn Reson Med 4: 179-184, 1987.
21. Loeffler W: Nuclear relaxation and its impact on NMR imaging. In Nuclear magnetic resonance and correlative imaging modalities, New York, 1984, Society of Nuclear Medicine.
22. Malko J, McClees E, Braun I, Davis P: Flexible mercury-filled surface coil for MRI imaging, Am J Neurol Radiol 7:256-247, 1986.
23. Mehdizadeh M, Molyneaux D, Morich M: A quadrature planar surface coil for spine studies, Annual Meeting of the SMRM, San Francisco, 1988.
24. Reiman TH, Heiken JP, Totty WG, Lee JKT: Clinical MR imaging with a Helmholtz-type surface coil, Radiology 169:564-566, 1988.
25. Requart H, Offerman J, Kess H, et al: Surface coil with variable geometry: a new tool for MR imaging of the spine, Radiology 165:574-575, 1987.
26. Roemer PB, Edelstein WA, Souzer SP, et al: Simultaneous multiple surface coil NM imaging, 7th Annual Meeting of the SMRM, San Francisco, 1988.
27. Sank VJ, Chen CN, Hoult DI: A quadrature coil for the adult human head, J Magn Reson 69: 236-242, 1986.
28. Schnall MD, Lenkinski RE, Pollack HM, et al: Prostate: MR imaging with an endorectal surface coil, Radiology 172:570-574, 1989.
29. Sharples T, Lufkin R, Flannigan B, Hanafee W: Dynamic range compression in surface coil MRI, Magn Reson Imag 4:165, 1986.
30. Winkler ML, Ortendahl DA, Mills TC, et al: Characteristics of partial flip angle and gradient reversal MR imaging, Radiology 166:17-26, 1988.
31. Wright SM, Magin RL, Kelton JR: Arrays of mutually coupled local coils for high resolution MR imaging, Annual Meeting of the SMRM, New York, 1987.

Chapter 6

CONTRAST AGENTS

J. Ray Ballinger

Paul Lauterbur's group was the first to demonstrate the feasibility of using paramagnetic contrast agents to improve tissue discrimination in magnetic resonance imaging (MRI).[57] Since then a tremendous amount of work has gone into development of MRI contrast agents for gastrointestinal (GI), intravascular, and hepatobiliary use.

GASTROINTESTINAL

Significant impediments to the acceptance of MR for abdominal imaging include difficulty distinguishing bowel from intraabdominal masses and normal organs, such as the pancreas. Several bowel contrast agents are available or in the developmental stage to solve this problem. They may be classified as either positive agents (appearing bright) or negative agents (appearing dark).

Positive gastrointestinal contrast agents

Positive GI contrast agents can be divided into three categories (1) paramagnetic agents (e.g., gadopentetate dimeglumine), (2) short T1 relaxation agents (e.g., mineral oil), and (3) a combination of these.

Paramagnetic contrast agents. Proposed paramagnetic, positive GI contrast agents include ferric chloride,[128] ferric ammonium citrate,[125,128] manganese chloride,[74] gadolinium oxalate,[90] and gadopentetate dimeglumine (with and without mannitol).[47,54] Paramagnetic materials cause both T1 and T2 shortening. At low concentrations used for bowel opacification, the T1 shortening dominates the signal intensity. This results in high intensity on T1-weighted images (T1WI), T2-weighted images (T2WI), and gradient-echo (GE) images. At high concentrations, T2 shortening causes decreased signal in all but very short echo sequences. This decrease resembles the effect seen with superparamagnetic iron oxide (SPIO) (see Negative Gastrointestinal Contrast Agents). At intermediate concentrations, a mixture of T1 and T2 shortening results in increased signal on T1WI and decreased signal on T2WI.

Ferric ammonium citrate and gadopentetate dimeglumine with mannitol are safe and effective in humans, but both have minor side effects. Ferric iron can cause teeth staining, gastric irritation, nausea, diarrhea, and constipation. Mannitol can cause nausea, vomiting, and diarrhea. Gadopentetate dimeglumine without mannitol is well tolerated but usually fails in opacifying the entire small bowel.[54] It also needs to be buffered when used orally because this chelate is not stable at the low pH found in the stomach.

T1 contrast agents. GI contrast agents with a short T1

Fig. 6-1. Sucrose polyester (SPE) oral contrast in rats. **A,** A coronal section through rats containing peanut oil, control, and SPE. The open arrow shows peanut oil in the stomach at 3 hours postingestion. The curved arrow shows the empty stomach in the control rat with no contrast material. The straight arrow shows SPE in the stomach. **B,** A coronal section of a rat with peanut oil is on the left, and a rat with SPE on the right, at 12 hours postingestion. The curved arrow shows an empty colon in the peanut oil rat. The straight arrow shows contrast agent in the colon of the SPE rat. (From Ballinger R, Margin RL, Webb AG: Magn Reson Med 19:199-202, 1991.)

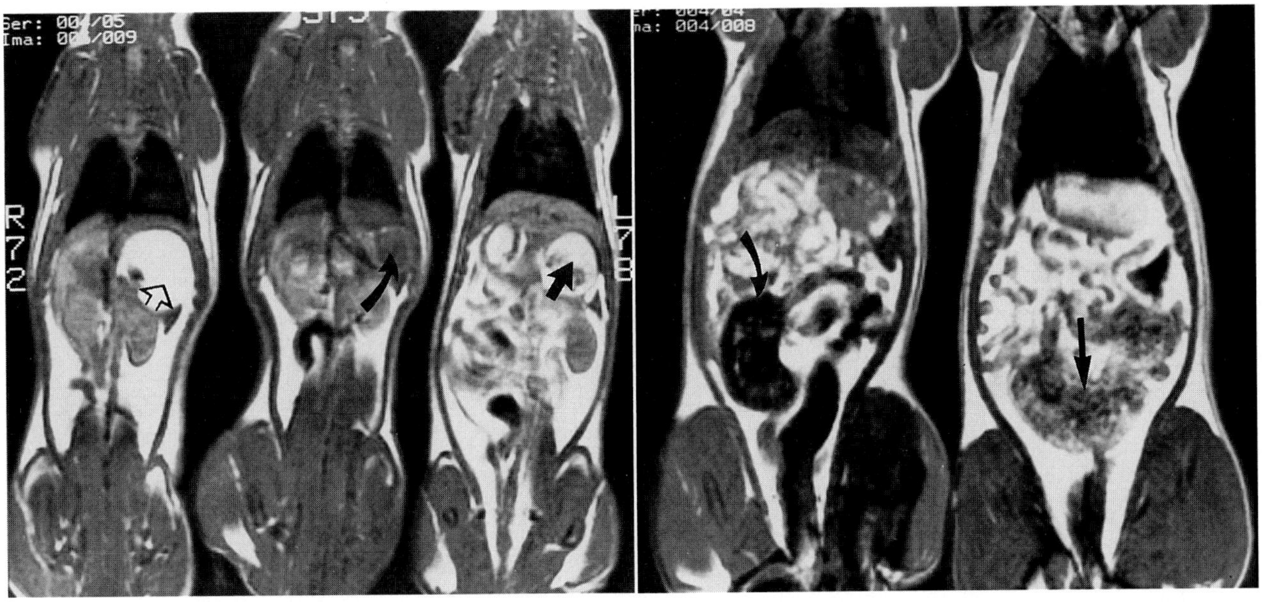

relaxation time include mineral oil,[128] oil emulsions,[60] and sucrose polyester.[5] In these materials, protons contained in $-CH_2-$ groups relax at a faster rate than those in water, resulting in a short T1 time, which produces a bright signal in the bowel on T1-weighted sequences. Of these materials, only oil emulsions have been used successfully in humans. These substances are palatable and produce homogeneous opacification of the stomach and small bowel, but are absorbed in the distal small bowel and fail to fill the colon. This effect is circumvented by using a contrast enema when the colon must be better visualized. A novel approach to retrograde opacification of the colon has been shown in rats with a nonabsorbable fat substitute, sucrose polyester,[5] but no human trials have been conducted (Fig. 6-1).

Combination of agents. Combinations of oil emulsion and paramagnetic substances may be used as bowel contrast agents. In one study, an emulsion containing corn oil and ferric ammonium citrate was used.[63] In two other studies, baby formula with ferrous sulfate was used.[9,31] These are palatable mixtures that distribute uniformly in the bowel; however, signal is lost in the distal small bowel in adults because of absorption of both the oil and the iron (ferrous iron is absorbed three to seven times more than ferric iron[128]). Unlike in adults, the faster transit through the small bowel in infants delivers bright contrast to the colon.[31] The advantage of this combination over oil emulsions alone is the enhancement of signal on T1WI and especially T2WI.

Experimental data show that using a combination of 2% barium sulfate suspension and 0.1% ferric ammonium citrate produces bright signal on T1-weighted, T2-weighted, and gradient-echo (GE) sequences. A homogeneous bright signal is obtained in the stomach and small bowel (Fig. 6-2). Ghosting artifacts are noticeable as with other positive GI contrast agents.[54,125]

Ghosting artifacts from positive contrast agents are projections of bright bowel signal outside the bowel. This phenomenon occurs in the phase-encoded direction, as the result of breathing and peristalsis. This problem is addressed with the use of scopolamine or glucagon to diminish peristalsis.[47] Short, breath-holding sequences,[54] abdominal compression bands, and respiratory gating will also diminish respiratory motion.

Negative gastrointestinal contrast agents

Negative GI contrast materials can be divided into three categories (1) diamagnetic agents, (2) superparamagnetic agents, and (3) perfluorochemicals.

Diamagnetic contrast agents. Two diamagnetic agents have been tested for use as a negative GI contrast agent. The first is a combination of clay minerals found in a popular antidiarrheal medication.*[65] This mixture of kaolin and bentonite is thought to facilitate the relaxation rate of protons in water molecules. The molecules close to the clay have re-

---

*Kaopectate, Upjohn, Kalamazoo, Mich.

Fig. 6-2. Ferric ammonium citrate (FAC)/2% barium sulfate oral contrast. **A,** Axial image through the upper abdomen showing fluid in the stomach of a volunteer *(solid arrow).* **B,** Axial image in a similar position of the same volunteer on a different occasion, after drinking the mixture of FAC/barium. Contrast appears bright within the stomach *(open arrow).*

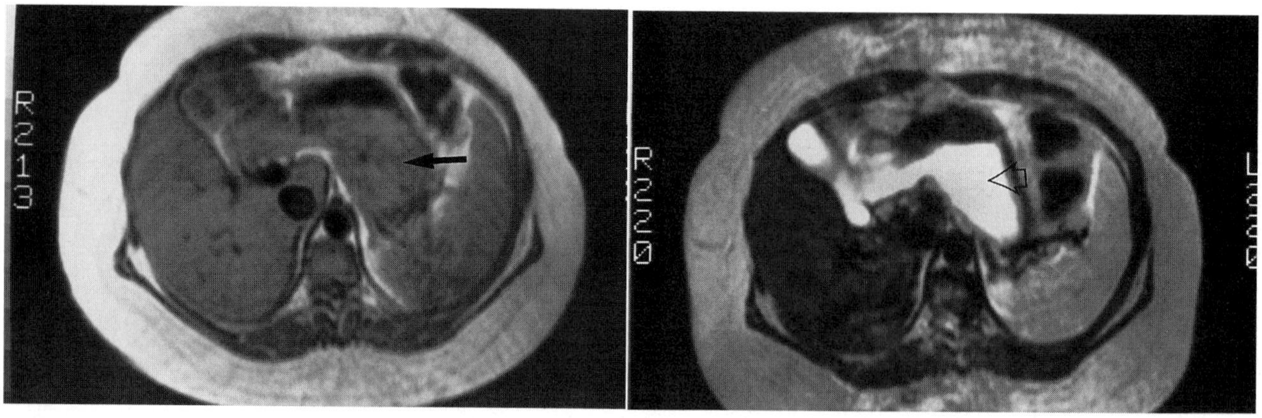

stricted motion, resulting in a shorter correlation time (closer to the Larmor frequency), which produces faster relaxation than the more mobile molecules distant to the clay particles. The water molecules next to the surface of the clay are continually exchanging position with molecules away from the surface, resulting in phase dispersion that also causes loss of signal.[131] When used in volunteers, this mixture causes loss of signal in the stomach and duodenum, resulting in improved visualization of the pancreas. Distribution in the small bowel is reported to be nonuniform.[63]

The second diamagnetic contrast agent causing loss of signal in the bowel is barium sulfate suspension. Barium appears first in the MRI literature as a potential contrast agent in combination with deuterated water (D_2O). The absence of signal results from a lack of protons in the contrast agent. Disadvantages of using D_2O are its high cost and concerns of toxicity.[82] Testing of a conventional barium sulfate suspension (60% w/w) in volunteers and patients gives encouraging results.[61,62,89] In vitro studies at higher concentrations of barium sulfate show that 170% to 220% w/v suspensions give greater loss of signal than the original barium tested.[6] Preliminary results show enhanced loss of signal in the stomach and small bowel when compared to 60% barium sulfate (Fig. 6-3). Marti-Bonmati et al[76] report good results with 250% w/v barium sulfate suspension combined with an anticholinergic drug. The loss of signal from barium sulfate suspensions does not match that seen with SPIO described later. However, barium suspensions and clay suspensions are currently readily available and probably will be much less expensive.

Superparamagnetic contrast agents. Several preparations of superparamagnetic substances are available for use as oral MRI contrast agents. These agents include magnetite albumin microspheres,[127] oral magnetic particles (Ny-

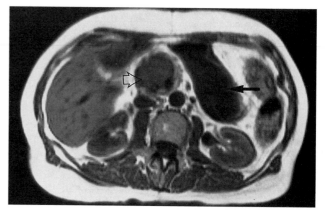

Fig. 6-3. Barium sulfate. Axial image through the upper abdomen showing high density barium in the stomach *(solid arrow)* resulting in loss of signal. The open arrow points to an islet cell tumor in the pancreas.

comed A/S, Oslo, Norway),[66,67,88] and SPIO (AMI-121, Advanced Magnetics, Cambridge, Mass).[40,41] These three contain small iron oxide (Fe_2O_3 and Fe_3O_4) crystals approximately 250 to 350 Å in diameter. The small size of the crystals contributes to their large magnetic moment and their lack of significant residual magnetization after removal from the magnetic field. Therefore, they are superparamagnetic, not ferromagnetic. These crystals are embedded in an inert material, albumin matrix in the first case, and a polymer in the latter two. The particle sizes range from 2 to 5 μm in diameter for the first two contrast agents and 0.2 μm for the third. The inert materials reduce absorption and, therefore, reduce toxicity from the iron. They also help to suspend the particles in solution.

Several clinical trials using the oral magnetic particles[67,88] and the SPIO particles[41] show impressive results

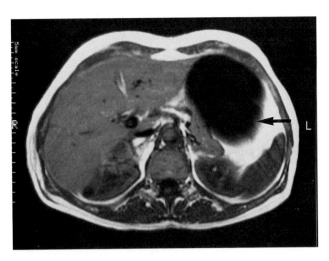

Fig. 6-4. Oral superparamagnetic iron oxide. Axial image through the upper abdomen after ingestion of SPIO, showing loss of signal in the stomach *(arrow)*. Compare with the normal appearance of the stomach in Fig. 6-2, *A*.

(Fig. 6-4). Marked loss of signal in the stomach and small bowel results in excellent visualization of the pancreas, anterior renal margins, and paraaortic regions. Decrease in the phase-encoded artifacts from respiratory and peristaltic motion of the stomach and small bowel is noted.

At certain concentrations and volumes, metallic artifacts are seen in the distal small bowel and colon on delayed imaging. These may be related to settling and concentration of the particles. Optimization of the dose of contrast agent and addition of more suspending agents may overcome this problem. Agents, such as cellulose or polyethylene glycol, may be added to enhance relaxation and thereby allow reduction in the concentration of iron oxide needed. This technique may reduce artifacts.[106]

Perfluorochemicals. Diamagnetic and paramagnetic effects are not the only mechanisms for reducing signal in the bowel. The absence of mobile protons also gives this effect, as with barium sulfate suspended in D_2O, carbon dioxide, and perfluorochemicals.[60,113] CO_2 from effervescent granules is moderately well tolerated by patients, but shows inhomogeneous distribution in the small bowel and requires the use of glucagon to decrease peristalsis.[63]

Perfluorochemicals are organic compounds in which the protons are replaced by fluorine.[77-79] This replacement results in an absence of signal in the bowel. Perfluorooctylbromide (PFOB) ($C_8F_{17}Br$) is the only perfluorochemical that, to date, has been investigated for oral use in humans. Potential advantages are a rapid transit through the small bowel because of its low surface tension, lack of taste or odor, and absence of any known side effects. PFOB is immiscible as are all perfluorochemicals that are in their pure or "neat" state. This effect may be an advantage because PFOB cannot be diluted by bowel contents. However, miscible agents that mix with fluid in the bowel may give more uniform filling of the GI tract.[63] Emulsifying PFOB, which is done for intravascular use of perfluorochemicals, may overcome this potential problem. Perfluorochemicals show promise as future MRI contrast agents.

Positive versus negative gastrointestinal contrast agents

The question of which type of contrast enhancement of the bowel is the best—positive or negative—is still debated. As there is no clear-cut winner of this debate, d'Angincourt[23] suggests that we may want several types of contrast agents to choose from. We may find a positive or negative oral contrast agent better, depending on the specific organ or disease suspected and the pulse sequence used.

Two disadvantages of positive oral contrast agents are ghosting artifacts because of respiratory and peristaltic motion and loss of signal from dilution with secretions and retained fluid in the bowel. One method of reducing ghosting artifacts is to use a drug, such as glucagon or scopolamine, to reduce bowel motion,[47] but this approach increases the invasiveness of the procedure. Other methods include the use of breath-holding pulse sequences, first-order flow compensation, and abdominal compression bands. Further refinements of pulse techniques probably will make breath-holding sequences more popular for abdominal MRI. This will decrease artifacts from both peristalsis and breathing.

Dilution of positive contrast agents by GI secretions occurs in the upper GI tract if the contrast agents are miscible with water. This effect allows for the use of a small dose, but causes loss of signal intensity as the concentration decreases. Immiscible positive agents using oils, especially nonabsorbable oils, do not experience the loss of signal with dilution. However, they probably require a larger volume to replace residual bowel contents.

Another disadvantage of a positive oral contrast agent is the possibility of residual low intensity bowel contents, simulating a mass when surrounded by bright signal. The opposite is also true. A bright mass (such as a lipoma) might be obscured by the contrast agent.

An advantage of positive oral contrast agents is their availability, including ferric ammonium citrate, pediatric formula, and homemade oil emulsions. Positive agents are also inexpensive (except for gadopentetate dimeglumine) and are safe to use.

Disadvantages of negative oral contrast materials include their high cost and lack of general availability (except for CO_2 and barium) and limited evaluations of safety on a large number of patients. The expense may decrease with greater use of these contrast materials and with competition between manufacturers. The two SPIO preparations mentioned in the previous section are undergoing phase II clinical trials and may be approved for use in the future. Metallic artifacts are seen when iron oxide concentrations ideal for spin-echo sequences are used with GE sequences. This is because GE sequences have greater sensitivity to magnetic field inhomogeneity. In addition, some metallic artifacts arise from the colon on delayed (24 hour) imaging with the iron oxide preparations. These artifacts probably could be eliminated as discussed earlier.

Lack of a fat plane between the negative contrast-filled bowel and low signal intensity organs may make it difficult to distinguish normal contours, for example, the plane between the stomach and the pancreas on T2-weighted sequences. The majority of pathology appears bright on T2-weighted sequences and, therefore, is visible.

There are several advantages of negative oral contrast materials. The lack of signal in the bowel removes a source of ghosting artifacts from spin-echo sequences that may be present with positive agents. The loss of signal is fairly independent of concentration of SPIO suspensions on spin-echo sequences so that dilution should not be a problem. The perfluorochemicals are immiscible with water and will not encounter dilution problems.

In conclusion, the most helpful type of oral contrast material for abdominal MRI has yet to be identified. A different agent might be chosen based on the pathology suspected, the degree of suspicion of an abnormal scan, and the pulse sequences used.

INTRAVENOUS CONTRAST AGENTS

Intravenous (IV) contrast agents include the following: chelates of paramagnetic ions, both ionic and nonionic;

particulates, sequestered in the liver, spleen, and lymph nodes; intravascular agents, confined to the blood pool; and tumor-specific agents.

Chelates

Paramagnetic metal ions suitable as MR contrast agents are all potentially toxic when injected intravenously at or near doses needed for clinical imaging. With chelation of these ions, acute toxicity is reduced and the elimination rate is increased, thereby reducing the chance of long-term toxicity. Fig. 6-5 shows the structures of five common ligands to which gadolinium may be chelated. The larger size of the chelate results in a slower tumbling rate and greater T1 relaxation than the ion alone.

Ionics. Chelates of paramagnetic ions with ethylenediaminetetraacetic acid (EDTA) were first used. However, Gd-EDTA was as toxic as $GdCl_2$ when tested in animals.[115] Chelates with higher stability constants have since been used successfully. The stability constant K is defined as:

$$K = [Chelate]/[Gd^{3+}][Ligand]$$

Gadopentetate dimeglumine. Gadopentetate dimeglumine was the first IV MR contrast agent approved for human use. Gadopentetate dimeglumine has a large magnetic moment, exceeded only by dysprosium(III) and holmium(III), explaining its paramagnetic properties at low concentrations.[57] This large magnetic moment is related to its seven unpaired orbital electrons. Gadopentetate dimeglu-

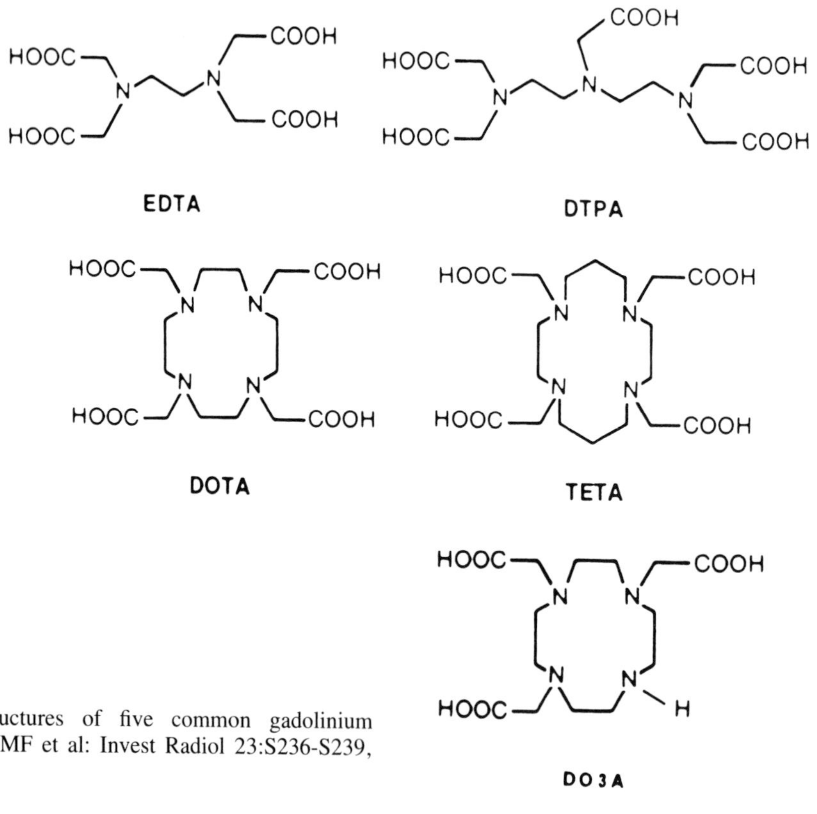

Fig. 6-5. Chemical structures of five common gadolinium ligands. (From Tweedle MF et al: Invest Radiol 23:S236-S239, 1988.)

mine has similar pharmacokinetics as iodinated contrast agents. It is distributed in the intravascular and extracellular fluid spaces, does not cross an intact blood-brain barrier, and is excreted rapidly by glomerular filtration.[83,115]

In the abdomen, IV injection of gadopentetate dimeglumine causes significant enhancement of tumors of the liver,[15,24,43,44,93] bladder,[15] pancreas,[16] ovaries,[16] uterus,[45] and kidneys.[16,99] In the liver, routine spin-echo imaging sequences tend to show a decreased contrast difference between tumor and normal tissue after injection of gadopentetate dimeglumine. This decrease sometimes may result in the tumor becoming isointense to normal liver.[15] This is loss of a problem with bolus injection (over a 15- to 20-second interval) followed by a series of breath-holding, T1-weighted GE images.[24,43,44,93] Doses of contrast used range from 0.1 to 0.2 mmol/kg. Sets of images may be obtained every 60 seconds for 5 minutes, followed by a delay at 10 minutes. Typical low-density malignant lesions appear darkest when compared to the liver at 1 to 2 minutes postinjection, become isointense at 3 to 4 minutes, and then hyperintense at 5+ minutes.[43,93] Hemangiomas show similar findings to those seen on computed tomography (CT) with bolus injection. These findings include precontrast hypointensity and postcontrast peripheral enhancement with central hyperintense fill-in over 5 to 10 minutes.[44]

Gadopentetate dimeglumine is used for physiologic evaluation of the kidney and liver by obtaining multiple rapid images during bolus injection and plotting either signal intensity or relaxation rate versus time curves.[46,83] However, a linear relationship between signal intensity and concentration of contrast does not exist. Signal intensity is a result of competing T1 and T2 relaxation effects, both of which are concentration dependent. In contrast to signal intensity, relaxation rates are linear with respect to concentration over physiologic concentrations. The change in relaxation rate after contrast injection correlates well with creatinine clearance in experimental animals,[46] but takes longer to measure than signal intensity on clinical imagers.

Preliminary data in animals suggest that acute occlusive intestinal ischemia may show measurably less enhancement after contrast injection than normal bowel.[130] Relevant clinical studies have yet to be reported.

Gd-DOTA. Gd-DOTA is the most stable chelate that has been tested as an MR contrast agent.[59] It is also referred to as a cryptelate because of its cyclic structure[51] (Fig. 6-5). The stability constant is 10^{28} versus 10^{22} for gadopentetate dimeglumine. This difference is reflected in the lack of detectable release of free Gd from radiolabeled Gd-DOTA after 150 hours in serum, compared to a 10% to 20% dissociation of gadopentetate dimeglumine.[70] Gd-DOTA has a safety ratio approximately 85% greater than gadopentetate dimeglumine.[1] Elevation of serum iron and bilirubin levels is seen with gadopentetate dimeglumine

but not with Gd-DOTA.[59] The pharmacokinetic properties of Gd-DOTA are essentially the same as gadopentetate dimeglumine in animals and human volunteers.[51,59] In abdominal MRI, the potential of Gd-DOTA is demonstrated in the detection of liver lesions with bolus injection and rapid breath-holding imaging.[75] Gd-DOTA shows definite promise as an MRI contrast agent.

Nonionics. The development of nonionic contrast agents for MRI has paralleled that for iodinated contrast materials. Ionic chelates are also hyperosmolar and some of their side effects may be attributed to this property.

Gadodiamide. Gadodiamide is a nonionic complex with two-fifths the osmolality of gadopentetate dimeglumine.[37] It has a median lethal dose of 34 mmol/kg, resulting in a safety ratio of two to three times that of Gd-DOTA, and three to four times that of gadopentetate dimeglumine. No abnormal serum bilirubin levels occur. However, elevated serum iron levels have been reported, with an incidence of 8.2% in one study of 73 patients.[37] The efficacy of this contrast is shown in at least 439 patients in multicenter clinical trials.[10,105]

Gd-HP-DO3A. Gd-HP-DO3A is a low-osmolar, nonionic complex containing a 12-member ring similar to Gd-DOTA, with one less carboxyl group (Fig. 6-5). It has a similar distribution, safety ratio, and pharmacokinetic profile to Gd-DOTA in animals, except that its elimination half-life is approximately 28% longer.[108] Clinical studies involving 449 patients show efficacy of this agent as a MRI contrast agent with no significant clinical or serologic side effects.[17,91] The signal intensity from Gd-HP-DO3A is equal to that of gadopentetate dimeglumine at similar doses. Initial clinical trials show no adverse effects at doses up to 0.3 mmol/kg, which may be an advantage over gadopentetate dimeglumine in some cases.[92] Both of these nonionic paramagnetic agents show promise of MRI contrast agents.

Safety. Initially, the high soft tissue contrast of MRI was thought to eliminate the need for contrast agents, making MRI a totally noninvasive diagnostic procedure. Since then, contrast agents have become useful in analogous situations to that of CT, such as IV use to help characterize and define abnormalities and oral use to distinguish bowel from intraabdominal masses.

The most commonly reported reactions associated with the injection of gadopenetate dimeglumine are headache (6.5%), injection site coldness (3.6%), injection site pain or burning (2.5%), and nausea (1.9%).[33]

The safety factor or ratio (ratio of the LD_{50} to the imaging dose) may be used to assess the relative acute toxicity of contrast agents. In rats, the safety ratio for $GdCl_3$ is about 5:1 ([0.5 mmol/kg]/[0.1 mmol/kg]). Radiolabeled $GdCl_3$ concentrates in the liver and spleen with a remarkable 98% of the IV dose remaining after 1 week in rats. This delay increases the likelihood of chronic toxicity, including interference with blood formation and coagulation.[11] Chelation of Gd to DTPA increases the safety ratio to approximately 100:1, which is clinically acceptable.[115] Gadopentetate dimeglumine has an excretion half-life of about 20 minutes in rats and 90 minutes in humans with less than 0.3% remaining after 1 week in rats.[8,115]

Gadopentetate dimeglumine usually has no effect on blood chemistries and hematologic studies except transient elevation of serum iron and bilirubin levels.[33,80,104] These elevations peak at 4 to 6 hours postinjection and return to baseline values in 24 to 48 hours. The mechanism of these elevations is uncertain but may be related to mild hemolysis. Hemoglobin breaks down into heme, which is then metabolized to bilirubin and iron. Elevation of intraerythrocyte enzymes, present with large-scale hemolysis, is not seen with gadopentetate dimeglumine, suggesting the insignificance of the hemolysis.[80] The possibility of significant risk to patients with preexisting chronic hemolytic anemias is raised, although there are no reports of such problems.[33] A 10% to 11% increase in the activated partial thromboplastin time and thrombin time occurs in vitro with inhibition of platelet aggregation. The platelet aggregation inhibition is less than that seen with iodinated ionic contrast material,[20] and no bleeding problems have been reported clinically.

Deoxygenated sickle erythrocytes align perpendicular to a magnetic field on in vitro studies, raising the possibility of occlusive complications in patients with sickle cell anemia.[8] No clinical studies of this potential problem are available.

Transient and mild drop in blood pressure is reported in both animals and humans. In dogs, Sullivan et al[103] use the standard 0.1 mmol/kg dose and a 0.5 mmol/kg dose injected over either 10 seconds or 1 minute. A significant but transient drop in mean arterial pressure (20 mmHg) is only noted at the higher dose and with rapid injection. The pressure returns to normal within 1 minute and no other hemodynamic changes occur. They conclude that rapid administration of gadopentetate dimeglumine at a dose of 0.1 mmol/kg should be well tolerated by patients and will be helpful with rapid imaging techniques.[103] A study of 1068 patients reports hypotension in 0.3% of the subjects. Other symptoms, such as syncope, probably are associated with hypotension in 0.8%.[33] Most of these symptoms occur 25 to 85 minutes after the injection.

Reports of several episodes of severe anaphylactoid reactions after IV injection of gadopentetate dimeglumine are published.[48,69,116] The frequency of these reactions is about 1 in 100,000 doses.[49] Potential risk factors may include a history of asthma and significant reaction to previously administered iodinated contrast material. It is suggested that the threshold for injecting gadopentetate dimeglumine be raised in those patients, based on an individual risk/benefit ratio. Weiss states: "If performed, such exams should be done in a hospital setting with close medical supervision."[116] Prophylactic pharmacotherapy with antihistamines and corticosteriods, such as Greenberger's protocol, is suggested for high-risk patients before contrast injections.[38,39] A good review of treatment of contrast reactions by Cohan et al[19] colleagues is recommended for those involved in administering gadopentetate dimeglumine.

Particulates

Although CT is currently the imaging gold standard for detection of liver metastasis, it fails to diagnose approximately 27% of colorectal liver metastases discovered at surgery.[30] Unenhanced MRI is no more accurate than CT. Interest in surgical resection of hepatic metastasis is increasingly making a higher rate of detection and improved anatomic localization desirable. The use of gadopentetate dimeglumine with routine imaging sequences of the liver is unsatisfactory (see the previous section, Chelates). Particulate contrast agents targeted to the reticuloendothelial system (RES) of the liver and spleen achieve the goals of improved detection and localization. This result is analogous to the use of ^{99m}Tc-sulfur colloid in nuclear liver scans.

Gadolinium oxide is a prototype particulate contrast agent.[13] This material accumulates in the liver and spleen of rabbits in Kupffer cells and in sinusoidal vascular spaces and effectively increases T1 and T2 relaxation as desired. The safety ratio (LD_{50}/imaging dose) is only about 7:1, raising concerns of acute and chronic toxicity; therefore, it is precluded from clinical use.

Superparamagnetic iron oxide. As with its use as an oral contrast agent, SPIO causes marked shortening of the T2 relaxation time, resulting in a loss of signal in the liver and spleen with all commonly used pulse sequences. The most common form of iron oxide used is magnetite, which is a mixture of Fe_2O_3 and FeO. A mixture using Fe_3O_4 instead of FeO may also be used.

Three mechanisms are thought to be involved the relaxation enhancement of SPIO. Two are a result of random diffusion (brownian motion) of water protons through local magnetic field gradients, caused by the large magnetic moment of the iron oxide particles. In one of these two mechanisms, a frequency component of the fluctuation in the magnetic field matches the proton resonant frequency, facilitating both T1 and T2 relaxation. In the other mechanism, the random fluctuation in the magnetic field gradients experienced by the various water molecules results in irreversible dephasing of the protons. This T2* relaxation effect increases the loss of signal.[72] The third mechanism is a chemical shift effect on static protons experiencing different local magnetic field strengths, causing line broadening and loss of signal. This last effect can be reversed with spin-echo but not with gradient-echo sequences.[73]

Hepatosplenic imaging. Two major cell types can be targeted for hepatic imaging. Hepatocytes make up about 78% of the liver by volume and Kupffer cells of the RES about 2% by volume.[55] Originally, particulate contrast agents were targeted for the RES but recently developed ultrasmall particles bind to a specific receptor site on the hepatocyte cell membrane.

Reticuloendothelial system. In one of the first reports, magnetite particles, 15 to 25 nm in diameter, are incorporated into serum albumin microspheres (1000 to 5000 nm in diameter) and injected intravenously into animals. Accumulation in the RES of the liver and spleen produces the desired loss of signal in normal liver without affecting the signal from implanted tumors, resulting in marked improvement of the contrast-to-noise ratio (CNR) and thus improved detection. The toxicity ratio is estimated at greater than 20:1.[128]

The use of polymer-coated SPIO particles in animals is found in a report from 1987.[95] These magnetite particles, 100 to 200 nm in diameter, are coated with a hydrophilic polymer yielding an outside diameter of 500 to 1000 nm.[94]

Studies in rats suggest that this material is efficacious in improving detection of metastases in the liver and spleen and in distinguishing lymphomatous from hyperplastic splenomegaly.[95,117,119] However, this material is unsuccessful in detecting diffuse hepatic lymphoma in the rat.[118] In 15 patients, an increased number of hepatic lesions are detected with its use.[102] An increase in detection of splenic lesions is seen in 18 patients with biopsy proven hepatic or other organ metastases (Fig. 6-6).[120]

Pouliquen et al[84] report a test of polymer-coated magnetite "nanoparticles" that are about 49 nm in diameter, with a 3800 nm diameter polymer coat. They obtain results in rats with chemical-induced hepatocarcinoma similar to those with previous SPIO preparations, but at one-third to one-tenth the dose.[84] They feel this improvement is related to two factors: (1) the porosity of the polymer microcapsule, which allows water molecules to diffuse closer to the nanoparticle; and (2) the strong inverse de-

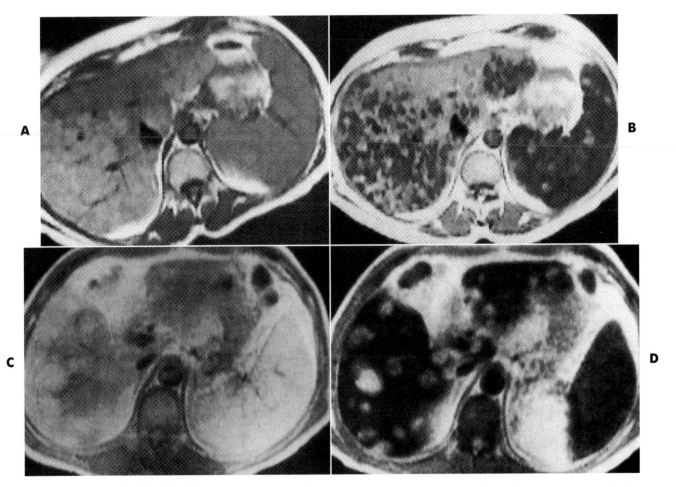

Fig. 6-6. Liver and splenic metastases. **A,** Nonenhanced MR image (TR/TE: 500/28) showing subtle liver lesion but none in the spleen. **B,** Contrast enhanced with superparamagnetic iron oxide (TR/TE: 500/28) showing obvious liver lesions as well as multiple splenic lesions. **C,** Nonenhanced MR image (TR/TE:500/28) showing multiple liver lesions but no splenic abnormalities. **D,** Contrast enhanced image showing obvious liver lesions and replacement of one half of the spleen by a metastasis. (From Weissleder R et al: Radiology 169:399-403, 1988.)

pendence of the relaxation rate of protons on the diameter of the superparamagnetic particle, i.e., faster relaxation with smaller contrast particles.[53]

Kawamura et al[50] use dextran-coated particles with a core diameter of 6.5 nm and mean total diameter of 100 nm in a rat model of hepatocellular carcinoma. They also demonstrate efficacy at low doses (10 μmol/kg).

In rats, Fahlvik et al[29] have tested magnetic starch microspheres, which are produced by precipitating iron oxide in a starch solution. The total particle size ranges from 100 to 500 nm and have a safety ratio of at least 200 in rodents.

Using SPIO particles of mean diameter of 80 nm, Elizondo et al[26] have seen signal intensity changes in the liver corresponding to cirrhosis and regenerating nodules in an animal model (dose 20 μmol/kg). This group also addresses the following problems that can arise with detecting small lesions in the liver using SPIO: (1) small lesions may be indistinguishable from the flow void in small blood vessels seen in cross-section, (2) aortic pulsation artifacts are more noticeable, and (3) the 1-hour delay between injection and imaging makes it impractical to decide at the last minute to give contrast.[42] Their solution is to obtain images within the first 12 minutes of injection while a significant amount of contrast remains in the blood pool. This eliminates signal in small vessels and sometimes eliminates the need for delayed imaging at 1 hour. They also suggest including a fat suppression technique to decrease motion artifacts from subcutaneous and epicardial fat.

Hepatocyte receptors. The development of ultrasmall paramagnetic iron oxide (USPIO) particles that can enter the interstitium allows development of materials that incorporate these particles, which can be targeted to specific cell membrane receptors. Asialoglycoprotein receptors occur in great numbers on the cell membrane of hepatocytes (up to 500,000 per cell).[124] USPIO coated with arabinogalactan (AG-USPIO) has affinity for these receptors because of the galactose termination to the polysaccharide, arabinogalactan. This material binds to receptors on the cell membrane and subsequently undergoes endocytosis and accumulates inside lysosomes where it is degraded.[85] This material is efficacious in detecting hepatic neoplasms in rats at one-half the dose of iron needed for SPIO, targeted to the RES.[85] Differentiation between normal liver and acute and chronic hepatitis or cirrhosis is achieved in rats based on differences in signal intensity.[86]

Lymph node imaging. Two clinical problems common to CT and MRI are (1) distinguishing unenlarged metastatic lymph nodes from normal lymph nodes and (2) differentiating enlarged metastatic nodes from benign hyperplastic nodes. Differentiation of metastases from fibrosis, lipomatosis, and cysts is possible on resected lymph nodes in a 4.7 T magnet using voxels of size $0.1 \times 0.1 \times 1.0$ mm[107]; however, gradient strength and switch capabilities are not adequate in clinical imagers to obtain the necessary

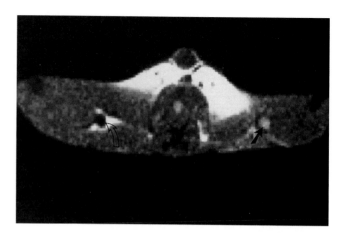

Fig. 6-7. MRI of a rat with a metastatic lymph node (adenocarcinoma) using ultrasmall superparamagnetic iron oxide as a lymph node contrast agent. This is a transverse image of the rat in a "frog-leg" position showing the perineal region and both popliteal areas. The right popliteal node is normal and appears black because of the uptake of USPIO. The left popliteal node contains metastasis and, therefore, appears relatively bright because of lack of USPIO uptake. (From Weissleder R et al: Radiology 175:494-498, 1990.)

spacial resolution. This inadequacy of clinical imagers is circumvented by the use of USPIO.

USPIO particles with a mean diameter of 80 nm may be injected into the interstitium of the foot pad of rats. After a suitable delay, marked loss of signal of normal lymph nodes is seen. Metastatic nodes show less uptake, resulting in less decrease in signal, which allows differentiation of normal-sized, metastatic nodes from uninvolved, normal nodes.[121] From experience with conventional lymphangiography, this route of injection is unlikely to opacify all of the abdominal lymph nodes.

USPIO particles with a median diameter less than 10 nm will localize in lymph nodes after an IV injection.[122,123] This material does not undergo uptake by the RES as rapidly as do larger particles, resulting in a longer plasma half-life in rats (81 versus 6 minutes). This factor plus the small size allow transcapillary passage either into the interstitium and then to the lymph nodes or directly into the lymph nodes. In the rat model, IV injection of USPIO allows differentiation of normal from metastatic nodes despite their size, based on signal characteristics described in the preceding paragraph (Fig. 6-7). MR microscopy of excised lymph nodes, performed at 9.4 T, demonstrates an association between USPIO and macrophages in the medullary sinuses.[58]

Liposomes. A liposome is a spherical vesicle consisting of one or more bilayer phospholipid membranes or lamella (Fig. 6-8). Liposomes for hepatic imaging range in size from about 20 to 400 nm. Reasons to use liposomes as a carrier for paramagnetic contrast materials include (1) to change the interaction between water molecules and the

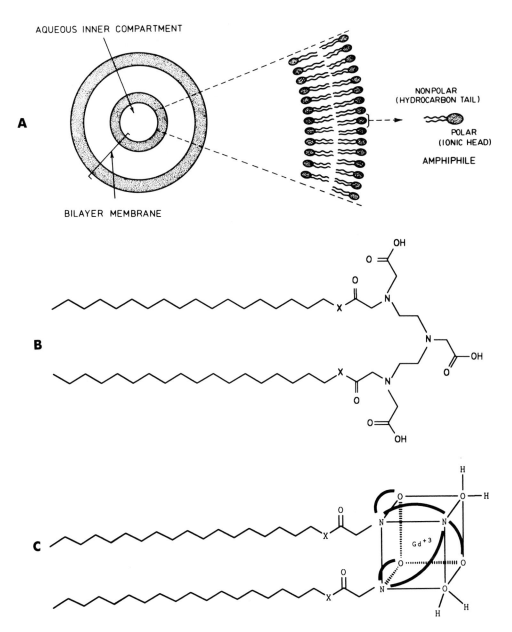

Fig. 6-8. A, Diagram of a liposome illustrating the arrangement of the bilayer lipid membrane. **B** and **C,** Proposed structure of the amphipathic gadolinium complex that is incorporated into the membranes of liposomes. (**A** from Kabalka G, et al: Radiology 163:255-258, 1987.) (**B** from Kabalka GW, et al: Magn Reson Med 19[2]:406-415, 1991.)

contrast agent, (2) to change the rate of removal of the contrast agent from the blood pool, and (3) to target specific organ systems, e.g., liver, spleen, and bone marrow.[71] Paramagnetic materials can be incorporated into either the aqueous inner chamber[4,71,109] or the bilayer membrane.[3,36,98] Encapsulation of SPIO particles into liposomes (ferrosomes) has been reported.[111,126]

Inner chamber encapsulated. Both gadopentetate dimeglumine and $MnCl_2$ can be encapsulated into the aqueous inner chamber of liposomes. $MnCl_2$ may be used in its ionic form to enhance the liver,[74] but acute cardiovascular toxicity is a concern. In addition, $MnCl_2$ is taken up by both normal liver and implanted malignancies in rats. When $MnCl_2$ is encapsulated inside liposomes, its peak concentration in the liver is three times its ionic form, suggesting the affinity of liposomes to Kupffer cells of the liver (Fig. 6-9). This greater affinity of liposomes for the liver and evidence that they are not taken up by cardiac

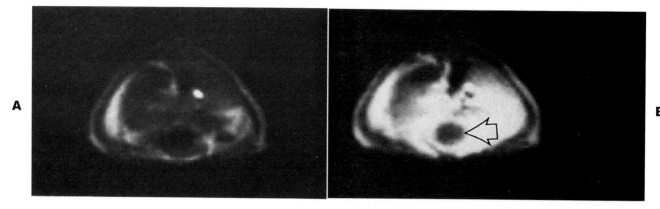

Fig. 6-9. Images of two rats with tumors implanted in the center of the frontal lobe of the liver (TR/TE:100/20; slice thickness = 5 mm.) **A,** The control rat that received no contrast material. **B,** The treated rat that received an injection of MnCl$_2$ (40 μmole/kg) encapsulated in liposomes, acquired 30 minutes postinjection. (From Niesman MR et al: Invest Radiol 25:545-551, 1990.)

tissue suggest reduced toxicity potential.[4] The safety ratio in mice is approximately 10:1. By using the manganese lipophilic chelate, Mn-DTPASA, the safety ratio can be increased to about 100:1, comparable to that for gadopentetate dimeglumine current doses.[98] Liposomes are taken up only by the Kupffer cells. Once in the Kupffer cells, Mn^{+2} ion is slowly released and diffuses into adjacent hepatocytes, resulting in enhancement of normal liver but not malignancies.

Liposomes encapsulating gadopentetate dimeglumine produces sustained signal in small vessels for up to 2 hours in rats, suggesting its use as a perfusion agent. They are also taken up by the RES in the liver and spleen, producing effective enhancement in rats.[109] Safety concerns have not been addressed adequately, particularly because it is unknown if intracellular gadopentetate dimeglumine dissociates into ionic Gd^{+3} more rapidly than extracellular gadopentetate dimeglumine. Subacute toxicity studies in rats indicate splenomegaly, anemia, and decrease in lymphocyte counts at doses 10 to 30 times that needed for imaging when administered intravenously daily for 30 days.[110] In this same study, gadopentetate dimeglumine (with similar doses) results in cardiomegaly and serologic evidence of hepatic dysfunction. Liposomes without contrast produce only mild splenomegaly.

Bilayer membrane incorporated. Three paramagnetic materials can be incorporated into the bilayer lipid membrane of liposomes: gadolinium,[53,98] manganese,[98] and stable nitroxide-free radicals.[3,36]

Nitroxides have been attached to phosphatidylcholine, a common constituent of liposome lamellae.[36] They may also be attached to derivatives of the fatty acid, stearic acid, as may be the DTPA chelates of Mn^{+2} and Gd^{+3}. This effect results in a lipophilic side chain that allows incorporation into the liposome membrane. Membrane incorporation of paramagnetic agents allows greater stability

of the contrast agent when incubated in human plasma.[98] As mentioned earlier, this effect improves the safety ratio of manganese in the form of Mn-DTPASA to about 100:1. Gadopentetate dimeglumine stearic acid (SA) can be administered in a three to six times lower dose than the usual 0.1 mmol/kg of gadopentetate dimeglumine, however, the 61-hour half-life[98] of gadopentetate dimeglumine stearic acid (SA) in the rat liver is considerably longer than the 20-minute elimination half-life[115] of gadopentetate dimeglumine in the rat. The half-life of gadolinium in ionic form is extremely long, with only 2% excreted by 7 days. This characteristic raises the concern that a significant and possibly toxic amount of Gd^{+3} ions may dissociate from DTPASA, resulting in intracellular release within the liver. With the shorter 10-hour elimination half-life of manganese and its physiologic need as a trace element, the liposomes incorporating Mn-DTPASA may have significant potential as contrast agents.

INTRAVASCULAR (BLOOD POOL) CONTRAST AGENTS

Intravascular contrast agents (IVCA) normally remain confined to the intravascular space, whereas gadopentetate dimeglumine disperses throughout the extracellular fluid space. This difference is a result of a molecular weight of approximately 70,000 and greater of IVCA, compared to a molecular weight of 590 for gadopentetate dimeglumine.[25] IVCA have several advantages. They can assess perfusion in areas of ischemia and provide information about capillary permeability in areas of reperfusion. They can show the extent of tumor neovascularity and associated permeability changes. Finally, they are useful in studies requiring prolonged imaging.[114] Three types of IVCA are described here: (1) gadopentetate dimeglumine–labeled albumin, (2) gadopentetate dimeglumine–labeled dextran, and (3) chromium-labeled red blood cells (RBC).

Gadopentetate dimeglumine–labeled albumin

Gadopentetate dimeglumine is covalently bonded to albumin in ratios from 16:1 to 31:1, providing excellent enhancement of liver, spleen, myocardium, brain, and slow-moving blood of rats and rabbits.[96] The albumin has a molecular weight of about 92,000 and a biologic half-life of 88 minutes.[97] The dose of gadopentetate dimeglumine required when bound to albumin is 0.062 mmol/kg compared to usual doses of the chelate alone of 0.1 to 0.2 mmol/kg. No adverse reactions are reported, but in vivo retention of the gadolinium for several weeks in liver and bone raises concerns of long-term toxicity.[114]

Gadopentetate dimeglumine–labeled dextran

Dextran is a polysaccharide consisting of a polymer of glucose molecules. It has a high level of safety and is broken down more rapidly than albumin. The ideal range of molecular weights is 75,000 to 100,000. Approximately 15 gadopentetate dimeglumine molecules are attached to each dextran molecule with an easily hydrolyzable bond. It is hoped that this will reduce the long-term in vivo retention seen with gadopentetate dimeglumine-labeled albumin. The trade-off is a shorter biologic half-life of 43 minutes. In a rat model, satisfactory enhancement of liver, spleen, kidneys, myocardium, and brain is seen for up to 1 hour. The dose of dextran gadopentetate dimeglumine in these studies was 0.01 to 0.05 mmol/kg.[32,114] Elimination and toxicity studies are underway.

Chromium-labeled red blood cells

The use of ^{51}Cr-labeled RBCs in nuclear medicine suggested use of paramagnetic Cr(III)-labeled RBCs as an intravascular contrast agent for MRI.[25] In dogs, significant enhancement of the liver and spleen is noted with minimal enhancement of the kidneys. Ten percent of the blood volume is replaced with labeled RBCs in these studies, corresponding to about one unit in humans. The survival half-life of labeled cells is 4.7 days, compared to 16.6 days for unlabeled cells. The possibility of free Cr^{+3} contributing to the relaxation rates of the liver and spleen is raised. Short-term toxicity appears to be low, but further studies are necessary.

TUMOR-SPECIFIC AGENTS

Tumor-specific agents are pharmaceuticals targeted to tumors, either specifically or nonspecifically. Monoclonal antibodies are targeted to specific tumors, such as adenocarcinoma of the colon. Metalloporphyrins exhibit affinity for many tumor types, including carcinoma, sarcoma, neuroblastoma, melanoma, and lymphoma.[81]

Monoclonal antibodies

Monoclonal antibodies (McAb) are used successfully in nuclear medicine for localization of tumors, but an initial attempt at extending this use to MRI with paramagnetic (Gd^{3+})-labeled antibodies was unsuccessful because of the estimated 800-fold lesser sensitivity of MRI.[2] This problem can be addressed by (1) increasing the number of paramagnetic ions attached to the McAb, (2) attaching several paramagnetic ions to a macromolecule that in turn is attached to a McAb, (3) using more antibodies or those with an affinity to many antigenic sites per cell or both, and (4) using a superparamagnetic particle attached to the McAb.[21,87,100]

Curtet et al[22] attached up to 25 gadopentetate dimeglumine molecules to McAb 19-9 and GA 73-3, specific to human colon adenocarcinoma, with only a slight decrease in immunoreactivity. The GA73-3 also recognizes a large number of antigenic sites, 10^6 versus 8×10^4 for McAb 17-A (recognizes human colorectal carcinoma).[21] They are successful in imaging implanted tumors in the flanks of mice. Shreve and Aisen[100] attached an average of 14 gadopentetate dimeglumine chelates to a macromolecule, polylysine, that is linked to a McAb and tested in vitro for relaxation enhancement. The dose of that particular material, extrapolated to human use, is 1000 mg. This amount is too high for a potentially immunogenic agent.

Two studies report the use of very small magnetite particles coated with McAb.[18,87] The magnetite cores are 10 to 20 nm in diameter with a total particle diameter of 20 to 32 nm. The magnetic moment of these superparamagnetic particles is about 1000 times that of comparable paramagnetic particles.[87] This characteristic allows the use of 1 to 10 nmol concentrations of the McAb-coated magnetite particles. Mixed success is obtained in rodents with implanted neuroblastoma[87] and human colon carcinoma.[18]

Metalloporphyrins

The metalloporphyrin most commonly used as a MRI contrast agent is Mn(III)TPPS$_4$ (manganese[III] tetra-[4-sulfanatophenyl] porphyrin) (Fig. 6-10) because of its low toxicity (compared to Fe[III]TPPS$_4$ for example).[52] The fluorescent and tumor localizing characteristics of porphyrin derivatives are exploited in phototherapy of tumors.[52] A safety ratio of about 6:1 is estimated in mice.[81] This material appears to work the best with tumors that are isointense to surrounding structures on T1-weighted sequences, i.e., ". . . when delineation of the tumor/normal margin is poor."[14]

Nitroxides

Nitroxide-stable free radicals or nitroxyl spin labels, as they may be called, are chemically stable organic compounds that have an unpaired electron that results in paramagnetic properties. They generally consist of a six-member ring piperidine derivative or a five-member ring pyrrolidine derivative (Fig. 6-11). The unpaired electron is protected from chemical reaction by delocalizing between the oxygen and nitrogen atoms and by the stearic hinderance of four surrounding methyl groups.[11,68] The pharmacoki-

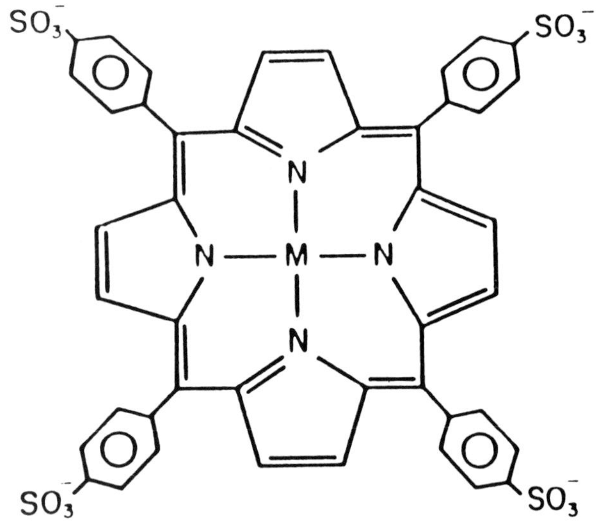

Fig. 6-10. Structure of the metalloporphyrin, TPPS$_4$. M = Manganese (III). (From Fiel RJ et al: Magn Reson Imaging 5:149-156, 1987.)

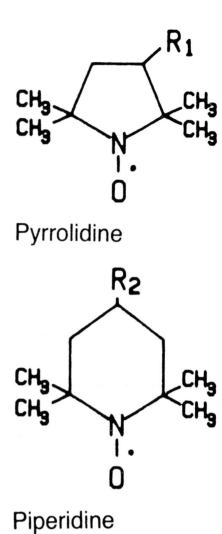

Pyrrolidine

Piperidine

Fig. 6-11. Two common nitroxide stable-free radicals. The unpaired electron *(dot)* is protected from chemical reaction by the stearic hinderance of the four methyl groups and by the delocalization of the electron between the oxygen and nitrogen atoms. (From Eriksson UG et al: J Pharm Sci 77[2]:97-103, 1988.)

netics of nitroxides are similar to iodinated contrast agents and gadopentetate dimeglumine. They do not cross an intact blood-brain barrier and undergo glomerular filtration as the dominant route of elimination.[12] Their ease of conjugation to various biomolecules makes them attractive for targeting to various organ systems. Nitroxides are chemically stable and show limited in vivo metabolism. Their relaxation effects in vivo can be eliminated almost immediately by IV injection of sodium ascorbate, a strong reducing agent.[129] This elimination would allow an unenhanced MR study to be performed immediately after a contrast enhancement study, if the contrast study alone were not satisfactory.

The early ionic derivatives of piperidine have a 38 minute half-life in cats[11] and a safety ratio of between 8:1 and 100:1.[28] Nonionic pyrrolidine derivatives are formulated with a longer half-life of 45 to 50 minutes in dogs and an estimated half-life of about 2 hours in humans. The LD$_{50}$ in mice of this nonionic formulation is about 25 mmol/kg, making it twice as safe as earlier ionic piperidinyl preparations.[35] Mutation and toxicity studies show no evidence of genetic or other cellular damage in mammalian cell preparations.

Larger molecular weight nitroxides exhibit increased relaxation rates[68] as do paramagnetic ions attached to macromolecules. This phenomenon occurs when attaching five-membered nitroxide rings to fatty acids. The fatty acids attach to human serum albumin, either in vitro or in vivo, resulting in a significant increase in relaxation rate.[7] Safety studies and clinical trials must be performed before nitroxides will be available for use.

Ferrioxamine

Ferrioxamine methanesulfonate is a paramagnetic contrast agent that has undergone phase I and phase II clinical trials for use as an IV and retrograde contrast agent for the kidneys, ureters, and bladder.[135] It is more stable than gadopentetate dimeglumine, although its relaxivity is somewhat less, as expected from having five unpaired electrons versus seven unpaired electrons for gadopentetate dimeglumine.[133] Eighty percent is excreted by the kidneys and 20% by the liver. Ferrioxamine undergoes renal excretion by glomerular filtration and also by active tubular reabsorption, resulting in a longer plasma half-life than gadopentetate dimeglumine (128 versus 20 minutes in rats).

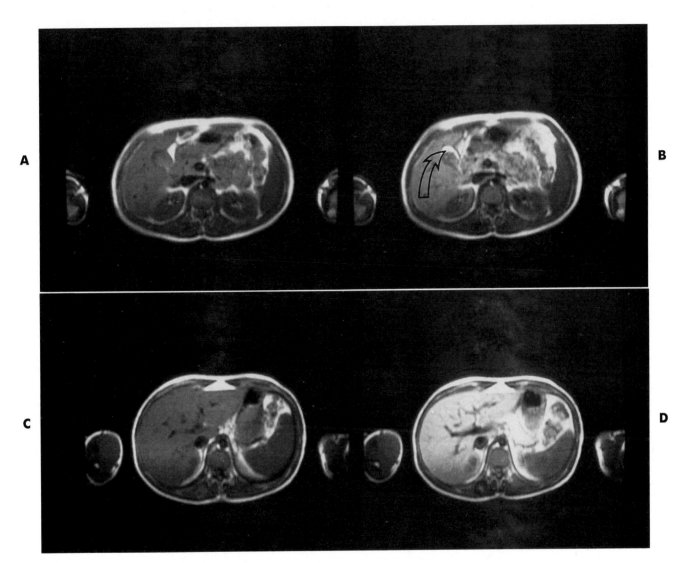

Fig. 6-12. MR images of the liver of human volunteers before and after the injection of Mn-DPDP(TR/TE:150/20). **A,** Before injection through the level of the porta hepatis. **B,** Ten minutes after injection (10 μmole/kg) showing enhancement of the liver. **C,** Before injection in another subject at the level of the gallbladder. **D,** 15 minutes after injection (3 μmol/kg) showing a relative increase in the signal intensity in the gallbladder, indicating accumulation of the agent in the bile. (From Lim KO et al: Radiology 178:79-82, 1991.)

In clinical imaging the long plasma half-life allows enhancement of the kidneys for 60 minutes with little change in intensity. Significant improvement in detectability of lesions in the kidneys is demonstrated over unenhanced controls. Side effects in 24 patients include one case of epigastric distress and one case of transient burning at the injection site. Increase in serum iron levels is expected and was noted in the phase I trial because the iron in the contrast agent is measured by a particular laboratory test. One patient had transient elevation of serum liver enzymes (SGOT/SGPT) at 24 hours postinjection that returned to normal at 8 days.[135]

HEPATOBILIARY CONTRAST AGENTS

Hepatobiliary contrast agents are desirable (1) to detect mass lesions such as metastases within the liver, (2) to evaluate the functional status of the liver in diffuse hepatocellular diseases such as cirrhosis, and (3) to obtain high resolution images of the gallbladder and biliary tree.[57]

Three advantages exist for a hepatobiliary contrast agent over a particulate agent targeted for Kupffer cells. First, there are many more hepatocytes than Kupffer cells (78% versus 2% by volume) in the liver, improving uptake efficiency of contrast material.[55] Second, the biliary ducts are opacified by excreted contrast material, eliminating confusion of normal bile ducts with focal abnormalities, as may occur with particulate agent contrast materials. Third, the contrast agent is rapidly excreted from the body, reducing potential toxicity.[55] In contrast, materials phagocytized by the RES (including Kupffer cells) remain in the body for a long time.

The uptake and excretion of contrast material allow visual assessment of basic hepatocyte function. Biliary opacification allows functional information to be obtained as with radionuclide hepatobiliary studies, but with significantly higher spatial resolution.

Manganese chloride

Manganese chloride ($MnCl_2$) is a prototype hepatobiliary contrast agent.[74] IV and oral administration in animals results in rapid decrease in the T1 relaxation time of liver, spleen, kidneys, heart, and bile, causing a bright signal on T1WI. In its ionic state, Mn^{+2}, it is relatively toxic. In imaging doses of 0.2 mmol/kg, it has caused severe hypotension and ventricular fibrillation in dogs because of its calcium-channel blocking properties.[132] Cerebral damage has resulted from chronic manganese toxicity.[132] It can be used in the form of a chelate with diminished toxicity for hepatobiliary imaging in humans.

Chelates

Chelates used as hepatobiliary contrast agents consist of a paramagnetic ion bound to an organic ligand, forming a complex that shows affinity for hepatocytes.[27] This type of complex is desirable to increase uptake of the con-

trast agent by the hepatocytes and to reduce toxicity of the paramagnetic metal ion. Possible chelates for hepatobiliary imaging include Fe-EHPG and derivatives,[55,56,101] Gd-HIDA,[134] Cr-HIDA,[34] B-19036,[112] and Mn-DPDP.[27,64,136]

The compound Iron(III) ethylenebis-(2-hydroxyphenylglycine) (Fe[EHPG]$^-$) is a structural analog of the radionuclide ^{99m}Tc-iminodiacetate (Tc-IDA) used for hepatobiliary imaging in nuclear medicine.[55] Fe(EHPG)$^-$ is a stable complex over a large pH range, making it likely to be nontoxic. It undergoes both renal and biliary excretion, the latter being approximately 6%, significantly less than for ^{99m}Tc-IDA. This biliary excretion is increased to 47% by substituting a chlorine atom for two hydrogen atoms on the two phenolic rings. This substitution makes the complex more lipophilic, which may improve binding to hepatocyte membrane receptors or cytosolic proteins.[56] Fe-EHPG improves visualization of small and medium-sized, bloodborne liver metastases in mice.[101] No clinical studies with this material have yet been performed.

Chromium diethyl HIDA meglumine (Cr-HIDA) is another analog of a hepatobiliary drug that has been tested in rats and rabbits. Excretion was 45% to 77% after 1 hour. The dose required to give significant increased signal in the liver (0.25 mmol/kg) results in a safety ratio in mice of 6:1, compared to 100:1 for gadopentetate dimeglumine. This low ratio for Cr-HIDA precludes clinical use.[34]

An octadentate chelate of gadolinium-coded B-19036 (Bracco Industria Chimica S.p.A., Milan, Italy) may be used as a hepatobiliary contrast agent. It is a highly stable complex with an LD_{50} in mice comparable to gadopentetate dimeglumine.[112] This agent has yet to be tested in humans.

Manganese(II)-dipyridoxal diphosphate (Mn-DPDP) is a manganese chelate derived from vitamin B_6, pyridoxal-5-phosphate. It is efficacious in detecting small liver metastases in rabbits[136] and has undergone phase I clinical trials which demonstrated its safety and efficacy in enhancing the signal intensity of the liver (Fig. 6-12).[64] It has a safety ratio of 200:1 in rats, which is somewhat better than that for gadopentetate dimeglumine. Unlike Fe-EHPG (and its derivatives) whose uptake by hepatocytes depends on lipophilic attraction to the cell membrane, Mn-DPDP is recognized by a vitamin B_6 transport system in the cell membrane.[27]

REFERENCES

1. Allard M, et al: Experimental study of DOTA-gadolinium: pharmacokinetics and pharmacologic properties, Invest Radiol 23(suppl 1):S271, 1988.
2. Anderson-Berg WT, et al: Nuclear magnetic resonance and gamma camera tumor imaging using gadolinium-labeled monoclonal antibodies, J Nucl Med 27:829-833, 1986.
3. Bacic G, et al: Modulation of water proton relaxation rates by liposomes containing paramagnetic materials, Magn Reson Med 6:445-458, 1988.

4. Bacic G, et al: NMR and ESR study of liposome delivery of Mn^{2+} to murine liver, Magn Reson Med 13:44-61, 1990.

5. Ballinger R, Magin RL, Webb AG: Sucrose polyester: a new oral contrast agent for MRI, Magn Reson Med 19:199-202, 1991.

6. Ballinger R, Ros PR, Rappaport D: Barium sulfate as MR contrast agent: in vitro comparison of ten preparations, Poster presented at the 20th Annual Meeting of the Society of Gastrointestinal Radiologists, LaCosta, Carlsbad, Calif, February 17-21, 1991.

7. Bennett HF, et al: Interaction of nitroxides with plasma and blood: effect on 1/T1 of water protons, Magn Reson Med 14:40-55, 1990.

8. Berlex Laboratories, Inc: Magnevist package insert, Wayne, NJ, 1989.

9. Bisset GS: Evaluation of potential practical oral contrast agents for pediatric magnetic resonance imaging: preliminary observations, Pediatr Radiol 20:61-66, 1989.

10. Brant-Zawadzki MN, et al: Multicenter clinical trial of gadodiamide injection: nonionic MR contrast agent for the central nervous system-brain, Radiology 177(P):159, 1990.

11. Brasch RC, et al: Work in progress: nuclear magnetic resonance study of a paramagnetic nitroxide contrast agent for enhancement of renal structures in experimental animals, Radiology 147:773-779, 1983.

12. Brasch RC, et al: Brain nuclear magnetic resonance imaging enhanced by a paramagnetic nitroxide contrast agent: preliminary report, AJR 141:1019-1023, 1983.

13. Burnett KR, et al: Gadolinium oxide: a prototype agent for contrast-enhanced imaging of the liver and spleen with magnetic resonance, Magn Reson Imaging 3:65-71, 1985.

14. Button TM, Fiel RJ: Isointense model for the evaluation of tumor-specific MRI contrast agents, Magn Reson Imaging 6:275-280, 1988.

15. Carr DH, et al: Gadolinium-DTPA as a contrast agent in MRI: initial clinical experience in 20 patients, AJR 143:215-224, 1984.

16. Carr DH: The use of proton relaxation enhancers in magnetic resonance imaging, Magn Reson Imaging 3:17-25, 1985.

17. Carvlin MJ, et al: Report on clinical trials of Gd-HP-DO3A, a low-osmolar MR imaging contrast medium: results in the head and spine, Radiology 177(P):159, 1990.

18. Cerdan S, et al: Monoclonal antibody-coated magnetite particles as contrast agents in magnetic resonance imaging of tumors, Magn Reson Med 12:151-163, 1989.

19. Cohan RH, Dunnick NR, Bashore TM: Treatment of reactions to radiographic contrast material, AJR 151:263-270, 1988.

20. Corot C, et al: In vitro interactions of gadolinium DOTA meglumine and gadolinium DTPA meglumine on hemostasis, Invest Radiol 23(Suppl 1):S261-S263, 1988.

21. Curtet C, et al: Selective modification of NMR relaxation time in human colorectal carcinoma by using gadolinium diethylenetri-aminepentaacetic acid conjugated with monoclonal antibody 19-9, Proc Natl Acad Sci USA 83:4277-4281, 1986.

22. Curtet C, et al: Gd-25 DTPA-MAb, a potential NMR contrast agent for MRI in the xenografted nude mouse: preliminary studies, Int J Cancer (Suppl 2):126-132, 1988.

23. d'Agincourt L: MR contrast media open new avenues of diagnosis, Diagn Imaging 4:80-90, 1988.

24. Edelman RR, et al: Dynamic MR imaging of the liver with Gd-DTPA: initial clinical results, AJR 153:1213-1219, 1989.

25. Eisenberg AD, et al: MRI enhancement of perfused tissues using chromium labeled red blood cells as an intravascular contrast agent, Invest Radiol 24:742-753, 1989.

26. Elizondo G, et al: Hepatic cirrhosis and hepatitis: MR imaging enhanced with superparamagnetic iron oxide, Radiology 174:797-801, 1990.

27. Elizondo G, et al: Preclinical evaluation of MnDPDP: new paramagnetic hepatobiliary contrast agent for MR imaging, Radiology 178:73-78, 1991.

28. Eriksson UG, et al: Pharmacokinetics in the rat and the dog of a nonionic nitroxide contrast agent for magnetic resonance imaging, J Pharm Sci 77:97-103, 1988.

29. Fahlvik AK, et al: Magnetic starch microspheres, efficacy and elimination: a new organ-specific contrast agent for magnetic resonance imaging, Invest Radiol 25:113-120, 1990.

30. Ferrucci JT: MR imaging of the liver, AJR 147:1103-1116, 1986.

31. Gerscovich EO, et al: The rediscovery of infant feeding formula with magnetic resonance imaging, Pediatr Radiol 20:147-151, 1990.

32. Gibby WA, et al: Biodistribution and magnetic resonance imaging of cross-linked DTPA polysaccharides, Invest Radiol 25:164-172, 1990.

33. Goldstein HA, et al: Safety assessment of gadolinium dimeglumine in U.S. clinical trials, Radiology 174:17-23, 1990.

34. Golman K, et al: A magnetic resonance imaging contrast medium for the liver and bile, Invest Radiol 23(1):S243-S245, 1988.

35. Gordon DG, et al: Pyrroxamide, a nonionic nitroxyl spin label contrast agent for magnetic resonance imaging: mutagenesis and cell survival, Invest Radiol 23:616-620, 1988.

36. Grant CWM, et al: A phospholipid spin label used as a liposome-associated MRI contrast agent, Magn Reson Med 5:371-376, 1987.

37. Greco A, et al: Gadodiamide injection: nonionic gadolinium chelate for MR imaging of the brain and spine: phase II-III clinical trial, Radiology 176:451-456, 1990.

38. Greenberg PA: Contrast media reactions, J Allergy Clin Immunol 74:600-605, 1984.

39. Greenberg PA, Patterson, R, Radin RC: Two pretreatment regimens for high-risk patients receiving radiographic contrast media, J Allergy Clin Immunol 74:540-543, 1984.

40. Hahn PF, et al: Ferrite particles for bowel contrast in MR imaging: design issues and feasibility studies, Radiology 164:37-41, 1987.

41. Hahn PF, et al: First clinical trial of a new superparamagnetic iron oxide for use as an oral gastrointestinal contrast agent in MR imaging, Radiology 175:695-700, 1990.

42. Hahn PF, et al: Clinical application of superparamagnetic iron oxide to MR imaging of tissue perfusion in vascular liver tumors, Radiology 174:361-366, 1990.

43. Hamm B, Wolf KJ, Felix R: Conventional and rapid MR imaging of the liver with Gd-DTPA, Radiology 164:313-320, 1987.

44. Hamm B, Fischer E, Taupitz M: Differentiation of hepatic hemangiomas from metastases by dynamic contrast-enhanced MR imaging, J Comput Assist Tomogr 14:205-216, 1990.

45. Hirano Y, et al: Gd-DTPA enhanced MR imaging in uterine neoplasms with dynamic study, Radiology 177(P):356, 1990.

46. Iaina A, Weininger J, Abrashkin S: Paramagnetic enhanced proton magnetic resonance measurement in rats: correlates with renal function, Magn Reson Imaging 6:131-134, 1988.

47. Kaminsky S, et al: Gadopentetate dimeglumine as a bowel contrast agent: safety and efficacy, Radiology 178:503-508, 1991.

48. Kanal E, Applegate GR, Gillen CP: Review of adverse reactions, including anaphylaxis, in 4,260 intravenous bolus injections, Radiology 177(P):159, 1990.

49. Kanal E, Shellock FG, Talagala L: Safety considerations in MR imaging, Radiology 176:593-606, 1990.

50. Kawamura Y, et al: Use of magnetite particles as a contrast agent for MR imaging of the liver, Radiology 174:357-360, 1990.

51. Knop RH, et al: Gadolinium cryptelates as MR contrast agents, J Comput Assist Tomogr 11:35-42, 1987.

52. Koenig SH, Brown RD, Spiller M: The anomalous relaxivity of $Mn^{3+}(TPPS_4)$, Magn Reson Med 4:252-260, 1987.

53. Koenig SH, Gillis P: Transverse relaxation (1/T2) of solvent protons induced by magnetized spheres and its relevance to contrast enhancement in MRI, Invest Radiol 23(Suppl 1):S224-S228, 1988.

54. Laniado M, et al: MR imaging of the gastrointestinal tract: value of Gd-DTPA, AJR 150:817-821, 1988.

55. Lauffer RB, et al: Iron-EHPG as an hepatobiliary MR contrast agent: initial imaging and biodistribution studies, J Comput Assist Tomogr 9(3):431-438, 1985.

56. Lauffer RB, et al: Hepatobiliary MR contrast agents: 5-substituted iron-EHPG derivatives, Magn Reson Med 4:582-590, 1987.

57. Lauffer RB: Magnetic resonance contrast media: principles and progress, Magn Reson Q 6(2):65-84, 1990.

58. Lee AS, et al: Lymph nodes: microstructural anatomy at MR imaging, Radiology 178:519-522, 1991.

59. Le Mignon MM, et al: Gd-DOTA: pharmacokinetics and tolerability after intravenous injection into healthy volunteers, Invest Radiol 25:933-937, 1990.

60. Li KCP, et al: MRI oral contrast agents: comparative study of five potential agents in humans (abstract). In Book of abstracts, Berkeley, Calif, 1989, Society of Magnetic Resonance in Medicine 1989.

61. Li KCP, et al: Barium sulfate suspension as an oral MRI contrast agent: initial clinical results (abstract). In Book of abstracts: Berkeley, Calif, 1989, Society of Magnetic Resonance in Medicine 1989.

62. Li KCP, et al: Barium sulfate suspension as a negative oral MRI contrast agent: in vitro and human optimization studies, Magn Reson Imaging 9:141-150, 1991.

63. Li KCP, Ho-Tai PCK: The search for the ideal enteric MR contrast agent, Diagn Imaging 3:110-114, 1990.

64. Lim KO, et al: Hepatobiliary MR imaging: first human experience with MnDPDP, Radiology 178:79-82, 1991.

65. Listinsky JJ, Bryant RG: Gastrointestinal contrast agents: a diamagnetic approach, Magn Reson Med 8:285-292, 1988.

66. Lonnemark M, et al: Superparamagnetic particles as an MRI contrast agent for the gastrointestinal tract, Acta Radiol 29(5):599-602, 1988.

67. Lonnemark M, et al: Effect of superparamagnetic particles as oral contrast medium at magnetic resonance imaging: a phase I clinical study, Acta Radiol 30(2):193-196, 1989.

68. Lovin JD, et al: Magnetic field dependence of spin-lattice relaxation enhancement using piperidinyl nitroxyl spin-labels, Magn Reson Imaging 3:73-81, 1985.

69. Lufkin RB: Severe anaphylactoid reaction to Gd-DTPA (letter), Radiology 176:879, 1990.

70. Magerstadt M, et al: Gd(DOTA): an alternative to Gd(DTPA) as a T1,2 relaxation agent for NMR imaging or spectroscopy, Magn Reson Med 3:808-812, 1986.

71. Magin RL, et al: Liposome delivery of NMR contrast agents for improved tissue imaging, Magn Reson Med 3:440-447, 1986.

72. Majumdar S, et al: A quantitative study of relaxation rate enhancement produced by iron oxide particles in polyacrylamide gels and tissue, Magn Reson Med 9:185-202, 1989.

73. Majumdar S, Zoghbi SS, Gore J: The influence of pulse sequence on the relaxation effects of superparamagnetic iron oxide contrast agents, Magn Reson Med 10:289-301, 1989.

74. Mamourian AC, et al: Proton relaxation enhancement in tissue due to ingested manganese chloride: time course and dose response in the rat, Physiol Chem Phys Med NMR 16:123-128, 1984.

75. Marchal G, et al: Gadolinium-DOTA enhanced fast imaging of liver tumors at 1.5 T, J Comput Assist Tomogr 14:217-222, 1990.

76. Marti-Bonmati L, et al: High density barium sulfate as an MRI oral contrast, Magn Reson Imaging 9:259-261, 1991.

77. Mattrey RF, et al: Perfluorochemicals as gastrointestinal contrast agents for MR imaging: preliminary studies in rats and humans, AJR 148:1259-1263, 1987.

78. Mattrey RF, Long DC: Potential role of PFOB in diagnostic imaging, Invest Radiol 23(Suppl 1):S298-S301, 1988.

79. Mattrey RF: Perfluorooctylbromide: a new contrast agent for CT, sonography, and MR imaging, AJR 152:247-252, 1989.

80. Niendorf HP, Seifert W: Serum iron and serum bilirubin after administration of Gd-DTPA-dimeglumine: a pharmacologic study in healthy volunteers, Invest Radiol 23(Suppl 1):S275-S280, 1988.

81. Ogan MD, Revel D, Brasch RC: Metalloporphyrin contrast enhancement of tumors in magnetic resonance imaging: a study of human carcinoma, lymphoma, and fibrosarcoma in mice, Invest Radiol 22:822-828, 1987.

82. Parikh AM, Mezrich RS: Deuterated barium sulphate as an oral MRI contrast agent (abstr). In Book of abstracts: Berkeley, Calif, 1988, Society of Magnetic Resonance in Medicine, 1988.

83. Pettigrew RI, et al: Fast-field-echo MR imaging with Gd-DTPA: physiologic evaluation of the kidney and liver, Radiology 160:561-563, 1986.

84. Pouliquen D, et al: Superparamagnetic iron oxide nanoparticles as a liver MRI contrast agent: contribution of microencapsulation to improved biodistribution, Magn Reson Imaging 7(6):619-627, 1989.

85. Reimer P, et al: Receptor imaging: application to MR imaging of liver cancer, Radiology 177:729-734, 1990.

86. Reimer P, et al: Asialoglycoprotein receptor function in benign liver disease: evaluation with MR imaging, Radiology 178:769-774, 1991.

87. Renshaw PF, et al: Immunospecific NMR contrast agents, Magn Reson Imaging 4:351-357, 1986.

88. Rinck PA, et al: Oral magnetic particles in MR imaging of the abdomen and pelvis, Radiology 178:775-779, 1991.

89. Ros P, et al: Pre- and post-barium MR imaging: normal abdominal/pelvic anatomy (abstract), Radiology 177(P):379, 1990.

90. Runge VM, et al: Work in progress: potential oral and intravenous paramagnetic NMR contrast agents, Radiology 147:789-791, 1983.

91. Runge VM, et al: Clinical safety and efficacy of Gd-HP-DO3A, Radiology 177(P):159, 1990.

92. Runge VM, Gelblum DY, Jacobson S: Gd-HP-DO3A—experimental evaluation in brain and renal MR, Magn Reson Imaging 9:79-87, 1991.

93. Saini S, et al: Dynamic spin-echo MRI of liver cancer using gadolinium-DTPA: animal investigation, AJR 147:357-362, 1986.

94. Saini S, et al: Ferrite particles: a Superparamagnetic MR contrast agent for the reticuloendothelial system, Radiology 162:211-216, 1987.

95. Saini S, et al: Ferrite particles: a Superparamagnetic MR contrast agent for enhanced detection of liver carcinoma, Radiology 162:217-222, 1987.

96. Schmiedl U, et al: Comparison of the contrast-enhancing properties of albumin-(Gd-DTPA) and Gd-DTPA at 2.0 T: an experimental study in rats, AJR 147:1263-1270, 1986.

97. Schmiedl U, et al: Albumin labeled with Gd-DTPA as an intravascular blood pool-enhancing agent for MR imaging: biodistribution and imaging studies, Radiology 162:205-210, 1987.

98. Schwendener RA, et al: A pharmacokinetic and MRI study of unilamellar gadolinium-, manganese-, and iron-DTPA-stearate liposomes as organ-specific contrast agents, Invest Radiol 25:922-932, 1990.

99. Semelka RC, et al: Combined gadolinium-enhanced and fat-saturation MR imaging of renal masses, Radiology 178:803-809, 1991.

100. Shreve P, Aisen AM: Monoclonal antibodies labeled with polymeric paramagnetic ion chelates, Magn Reson Med 3:336-340, 1986.

101. Shtern F, et al: MR imaging of blood-borne liver metastases in mice: contrast enhancement with Fe-EHPG, Radiology 178:83-89, 1991.

102. Stark DD, et al: Superparamagnetic iron oxide: clinical application as a contrast agent for MR imaging of the liver, Radiology 168:297-301, 1988.

103. Sullivan ME, et al: Hemodynamic effects of Gd-DTPA administration via rapid bolus or slow infusion: a study in dogs, Am J Neuroradiol 11:537-540, 1990.

104. Sze G, et al: Multicenter study of gadolinium dimeglumine as an MR contrast agent: evaluation in patients with spinal tumors, Am J Neuroradiol 11:967-974, 1990.

105. Sze G, et al: Multicenter clinical trial of gadodiamide injection: nonionic MR contrast agent for the central nervous system-spine, Radiology 177(P):159, 1990.

106. Tilcock C, Unger E, Fritz T: Novel polymeric contrast agents for improved MR imaging of the GI tract (abstract). In Book of abstracts, Berkeley, Calif, 1990, Society of Magnetic Resonance in Medicine, 1990.

107. Tsyb AF, Slezarev VI: NMR investigations of lymph nodes and lymph in the diagnosis of malignant tumors (abstract), Presented at the Second European Congress of NMR in Medicine and Biology, Berlin, Germany, June 23-26, 1988.

108. Tweedle MF, et al: Comparative chemical structure and pharmacokinetics of MRI contrast agents, Invest Radiol 23(Suppl 1):S236-S239, 1988.

109. Unger E, et al: Gadolinium-DTPA liposomes as a potential MRI contrast agent: work in progress, Invest Radiol 23:928-932, 1988.

110. Unger E, et al: Paramagnetic liposomes: MR imaging and detailed toxicological studies (abstract). In Book of abstracts, Berkeley, Calif, 1990, Society of Magnetic Resonance in Medicine, 1990.

111. Vinitski S, et al: Superparamagnetic ferrosomes in MR imaging of lung parenchyma, pulmonary emboli, liver and Heart (abstract). In Book of abstracts, Berkeley, Calif, 1990, Society of Magnetic Resonance in Medicine, 1990.

112. Vittadini G, et al: B-19036, a potential new hepatobiliary contrast agent for MR proton imaging, Invest Radiol 23(Suppl 1):S246-S248, 1988.

113. Wall SD, et al: Improved imaging of the GI tract and pancreas, MRI Decisions 2(4):27-32, 1988.

114. Wang SC, et al: Evaluation of Gd-DTPA-labeled dextran as an intravascular MR contrast agent: imaging characteristics in normal rat tissues, Radiology 175:483-488, 1990.

115. Weinmann HJ, et al: Characteristics of gadolinium-DTPA complex: a potential NMR contrast agent, AJR 142:619-624, 1984.

116. Weiss KL: Severe anaphylactoid reaction after IV Gd-DTPA, Magn Reson Imaging 8:817-818, 1990.

117. Weissleder R, et al: MR imaging of splenic metastases: ferrite-enhanced detection in rats, AJR 149:723-726, 1987.

118. Weissleder R, et al: Ferrite-enhanced MR imaging of hepatic lymphoma: an experimental study in rats, AJR 149:1161-1165, 1987.

119. Weissleder R, et al: Splenic lymphoma: ferrite-enhanced MR imaging in rats, Radiology 166:423-430, 1988.

120. Weissleder R, et al: Superparamagnetic iron oxide: enhanced detection of focal splenic tumors with MR imaging, Radiology 169:399-403, 1988.

121. Weissleder R, et al: Experimental lymph node metastases: enhanced detection with MR lymphography, Radiology 171:835-839, 1989.

122. Weissleder R, et al: Ultrasmall superparamagnetic iron Oxide: an intravenous contrast agent for assessing lymph nodes with MR imaging, Radiology 175:494-498, 1990.

123. Weissleder R, et al: Ultrasmall superparamagnetic iron oxide: characterization of a new class of contrast agents for MR imaging, Radiology 175:489-493, 1990.

124. Weissleder, et al: MR receptor imaging: ultrasmall iron oxide particles targeted to asialoglycoprotein receptors, AJR 155:1161-1167, 1990.

125. Wesbey GE, et al: Dilute oral iron solutions as gastrointestinal contrast agents for magnetic resonance imaging: initial clinical experience, Magn Reson Imaging 3:57-64, 1985.

126. White DL, et al: Plasma clearance of ferrosomes, a long-lived superparamagnetic MRI contrast agent (abstract). In Book of abstracts. Berkeley, Calif, 1990, Society of Magnetic Resonance in Medicine, 1990.

127. Widder DJ, et al: Magnetite albumin suspension: a superparamagnetic oral MR contrast agent, AJR 149:839-843, 1987.

128. Widder DJ, et al: Magnetite albumin microspheres: a new MR contrast material, AJR 148:399-404, 1987.

129. Wikstrom MG, et al: Ascorbate-induced cancellation of nitroxide contrast media enhancement of MR images, Invest Radiol 24:692-696, 1989.

130. Wilkerson DK, et al: Magnetic resonance imaging of acute occlusive intestinal ischemia, J Vasc Surg 11:567-571, 1990.

131. Woessner DE, Snowden BS, Meyer GH: A tetrahedral model for pulsed nuclear magnetic resonance transverse relaxation: application to the clay-water system, J Colloid Interface Sci 34:43-52, 1970.

132. Wolf GL, Baum L: Cardiovascular toxicity and tissue proton T_1 response to manganese injection in the dog and rabbit, AJR141:193-197, 1983.

133. Wolf GL, et al: Contrast agents for magnetic resonance imaging. In Kressel HY, editor: Magnetic resonance annual 1985, New York, 1985, Raven Press.

134. Wolf GL, Joseph PM, Goldstein EJ: Optimal pulsing sequences for MR contrast agents, AJR 147: 367-371, 1986.

135. Worah D, et al: Ferrioxamine as a magnetic resonance contrast agent: preclinical studies and phase I and II human clinical trials, Invest Radiol 23(Suppl 1):S281-S285, 1988.

136. Young SW, et al: Detection of hepatic malignancies using Mn-DPDP (manganese dipyridoxal diphosphate) hepatobiliary MRI contrast agent, Magn Reson Imaging 8:267-276, 1990.

Chapter 7

MAGNETIC RESONANCE ANGIOGRAPHY

Barry B. Kraus

Magnetic resonance angiography (MRA) is one of the most potentially valuable new applications of magnetic resonance imaging (MRI) in the abdomen. It is currently possible to evaluate the vasculature for a wide range of pathology, including aneurysm, thrombosis, stenosis, and arteriovenous malformation. Techniques are available to track blood flow and to determine both its direction and rate. Proper interpretation of an MR angiogram, however, requires knowledge of its production.

Many factors influence the MRI appearance of flowing blood. Its intensity may be low, intermediate, or high, depending on velocity, position within a multislice volume, and many local effects.

VELOCITY OF BLOOD FLOW

All protons in a volume of stationary tissue receive both a 90- and a 180-degree radiofrequency (RF) pulse in a standard spin-echo (SE) sequence. However, flowing blood contains protons that move. Thus, to the factors that affect signal emission from stationary protons must be added new factors related to flow. Flowing protons, depending on their position relative to the excited slice, may receive only the 90-degree RF pulse, only the 180-degree RF pulse, or both RF pulses. The signal intensity of a volume of flowing blood depends on the relative proportion of these three groups of protons because only those that receive both pulses will emit full-intensity echo signals (Fig. 7-1). Flow rate, slice thickness, and echo time (TE) are the controlling factors. They are related as follows:

$$V = dZ\, /\, (TE/2) \qquad \textbf{7-1}$$

where V represents the velocity of blood flow, dZ represents the slice thickness, and $TE/2$ represents the time between the 90-degree RF pulse and the 180-degree RF pulse.

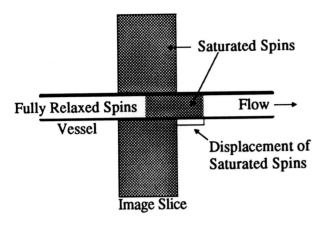

Fig. 7-1. Inflow effect: TOF phenomenon. RF pulses saturate stationary tissue and blood in the selected slice. Fresh blood entering the slice contains unsaturated spins that produce high signal and contrast relative to stationary tissue. (From Haacke EM, Hausmann R, Laub G, et al: MR angiography. In Magnetom SP, editor: Erlangen, Germany, 1990, Siemens Aktiengesellschaft.)

The fraction of protons that receive both RF pulses is:

$$1 - V(TE/2)/dZ \qquad 7\text{-}2$$

For velocities greater than TE/2dZ, signal intensity is zero.[62]

FLOW-VOID PHENOMENA (BLACK BLOOD)
High velocity signal loss

Rapidly flowing blood may not receive both the 90- and the 180-degree RF pulses administered to a given slice. Rapid arterial flow results in a very low intraluminal signal. Conversely, slowly flowing blood often receives both RF pulses. Thus slow venous flow results in high intraluminal signal.[6]

Turbulence

Ideally, flowing blood is either laminar or turbulent. In a straight vessel with smooth sidewalls, steady flow is primarily laminar.[5] Any turbulence in this idealized vessel would occur in the center of the volume, where velocity is greatest. Flow along the walls is slower, owing to drag from the interaction between blood and the walls.[1] The point at which turbulent flow occurs depends on the density, velocity, and viscosity of the blood and the diameter of the vessel. The Reynolds number describes the relationship between these factors:

$$Re = (p \times V \times D)/m \qquad 7\text{-}3$$

where *Re* is the Reynolds number, *p* is density, *V* is velocity, *D* is tube diameter, and *m* is viscosity.[5,7] For Reynolds numbers greater than 2100, turbulent flow occurs.[62]

The Reynolds number is a predictor of turbulent flow only under ideal circumstances—steady flow in a smooth-walled, unbranched vessel. Several factors lead to turbulent flow at lower Reynolds numbers, including pulsatile

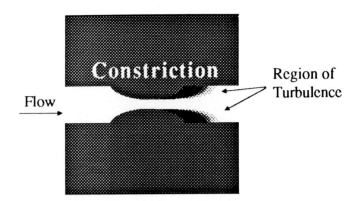

Fig. 7-2. Higher order motion. Turbulent flow contains variations in velocity, but acceleration and other higher order motion results in dephasing, which causes signal loss. Here, turbulence across a stenotic vessel creates enough signal loss to cause overestimation of the length and degree of narrowing.

flow, endothelial irregularities, stenoses, and branching. Large eddy currents (recirculation areas) downstream from sites of partial obstruction may contain smaller areas of relatively laminar flow.[1,7,52] Turbulent flow causes dephasing of blood-pool protons and a reduction in signal intensity. This signal void may be mistaken for an area of stenosis or occlusion (Fig 7-2).

Loss of phase coherence

Variation in flow velocity across the vessel cross-section results in local dephasing of protons. With wider variations in velocity, more rapid loss of phase coherence occurs.[65,67] In addition, steeper magnetic field gradients result in greater dephasing.[65,67] The slice selection gradient (Z) is weaker than either the readout (Y) or phase-encoding (X) gradients. As a result, less dephasing occurs for flow perpendicular to the imaging plane than for flow within the plane. In a multiecho train dephasing occurs on the odd echoes, and rephasing occurs on the even echoes.[9,69]

FLOW ENHANCEMENT PHENOMENA (BRIGHT BLOOD)
Even-echo rephasing

The first echo of a multiecho sequence disperses the phases of protons in flowing blood so that the signal intensity in that volume of blood decreases. If a second even echo occurs at a time t = 2TE (where TE = echo time of the first echo), the spin phases realign, producing bright signal (Fig. 7-3). Even-echo rephasing occurs only with constant velocity flow in a linear gradient.[69] Acceleration or irregular (higher order) motion or similar change in the gradient prevents the effect.

Even-echo rephasing can be used to evaluate thrombosis. If an even echo produces a bright signal, then flow exists within the vessel. If the signal is not enhanced, then the vessel likely contains no flow.

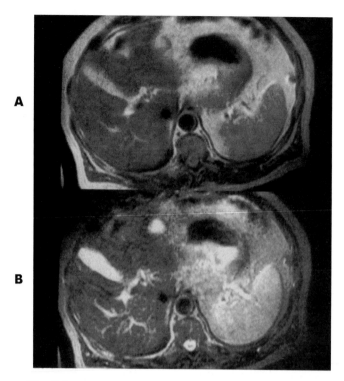

Fig. 7-3. Even-echo rephasing. **A,** Density-weighted transverse image through the gallbladder fossa. Note poor delineation of intrahepatic vessels and blurring of the gallbladder margins. **B,** T2-weighted (even-echo) image at the same slice location. Note the marked improvement in intrahepatic vessel appearance and sharpness of gallbladder margins. Even-echo rephasing results from the realignment of previously dephased spins. (From Spritzer CE: Magn Reson Q 5[3]:205, 1989.)

Diastolic pseudogating

In an ECG-gated SE acquisition, images of many slices are obtained within each cardiac cycle (R-R interval). Each slice is acquired at a different point within the cycle.[12,42] The slices acquired during systole have low intensity blood and those acquired during diastole have higher intensity blood signal due to variations in flow velocity during the cardiac cycle.

Diastolic pseudogating is physiologic gating, which simulates the effect of ECG gating. If the TR interval is set to match the R-R interval, physiologic gating occurs, as long as the heart rate remains regular for most of the scan time. About one-third of the resultant set of images are acquired during systole, and about two-thirds are acquired during diastole. Because most of the images are acquired during diastole, the arteries contain bright blood.

Diastolic pseudogating may occur unexpectedly. High signal within the lumen of an artery could represent thrombosis or tumor but must be differentiated from unintentional pseudogating. This differentiation can be achieved by repeating the acquisition gated to the ECG and triggered so that the image in question is acquired during a different point in the cardiac cycle. If a vascular lesion does exist, then the bright signal remains unchanged.

Flow-related enhancement

The group of magnetized protons subjected to the 90-degree RF pulse becomes partially or fully saturated and is temporarily unable to accept further RF energy. Those protons that do not receive the 90-degree pulse remain in the low energy state and are capable of accepting and emitting a full RF signal. As the latter group of protons flows into the imaged slice, it replaces the former group of saturated protons, thereby increasing the signal within the blood pool. This phenomenon is known as flow-related enhancement (FRE), or entry slice phenomenon (Fig. 7-4).[6]

The blood pool signal within an image thus depends on the proportion of unsaturated to saturated protons. As more unsaturated protons flow into a slice, the intraluminal signal increases. The maximum signal results when blood flows fast enough for unsaturated protons to completely replace saturated protons. This event occurs when the velocity is:

$$V = dz/TR \qquad \textbf{7-4}$$

where V represents velocity, dz represents slice thickness, and TR represents the repetition time. The typical velocity of venous flow is 1 cm/sec.[62] Thus, for typical slice thicknesses of 0.5 to 1 cm and typical T1-weighted images (T1WI) (TR = 0.5 to 1 sec), the ratio of slice thickness to TR (dz/TR) approaches the threshold for FRE.

As unsaturated blood flows deeper into the imaged volume of tissue, it is subjected to successive 90-degree RF pulses as deeper slices are excited. These 90-degree pulses progressively saturate this blood, thereby reducing its potential to emit an echo. Thus, as blood flows deeper into the imaged volume, its signal decreases progressively. The rate at which the signal decreases depends on the rate of flow, the slice thickness, and the TR. For a fixed slice thickness, fast flowing blood can traverse many more slices than slow flowing blood in a given TR. As a result, fast flowing blood will emit high signal on more slices than slower flowing blood.[1] A small imaging volume will contain mostly bright vessels (Fig. 7-5). The first slice of a scan volume contains inflowing vessels, which return high amplitude echoes. These signals weaken progressively as deeper direction of flow is important. Blood in the aorta emits a bright signal in the most superior slice. The signal weakens in more inferior slices until a signal void is present. The inferior vena cava demonstrates high signal in the most inferior slice and a signal void in more superior slices. Because flow in the aorta is faster than flow in the inferior vena cava, more slices of the aorta will be bright.

COMBINATIONS OF FLOW PHENOMENA

Rarely does any one of these flow phenomena occur alone. More commonly, they occur in combinations, making interpretation of the vascular signal complicated.

A

PRIOR TO FIRST 90

FOLLOWING FIRST 90

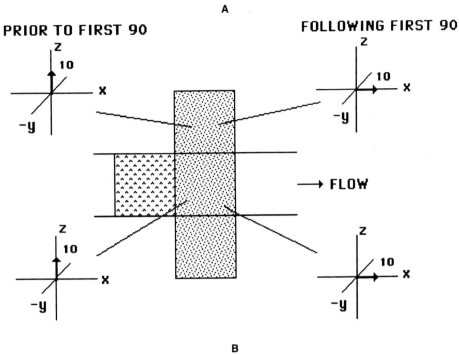

B

PRIOR TO SECOND 90

FOLLOWING SECOND 90

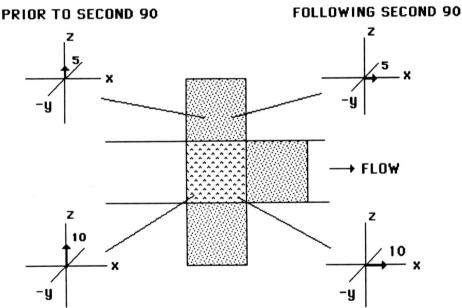

Fig. 7-4. Entry-slice phenomenon. **A,** If flowing blood and stationary tissues have the same proton density, T1, and T2, then there is equal transverse magnetization in both after the first 90-degree RF pulse. This results in equal signal. **B,** Partial regrowth of longitudinal magnetization occurs before the second 90-degree RF pulse for both blood and surrounding tissue. If blood flows rapidly, partially saturated spins become replaced with unsaturated spins in the fresh blood. This effect results in higher signal for rapidly flowing blood than for surrounding tissues. This phenomenon is enhanced with short repetition times and long tissue T1 relaxation times. (From Spritzer CE: Magn Reson Q 5[3]:205, 1989.)

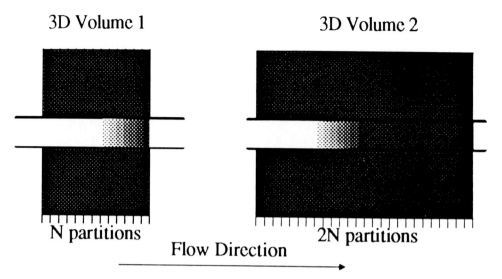

Fig. 7-5. Penetration of intravascular signal in 3-D volumes. With a fixed flow rate and repetition time (TR), the length of a vessel that exhibits bright signal remains fixed. If a small volume (3-D volume 1) is examined, inflow (TOF) effects maintain high vascular signal through nearly the entire slab. If a larger volume (3-D volume 2) is examined, inflow effects become lost due to progressive spin saturation much earlier within the slab. Faster flow yields inflow effects that penetrate deeper into a slab. Here, white represents high signal and black represents lower signal. (From Haacke EM, Hausmann R, Laub G, et al: MR angiography. In Magnetom SP, editor: Erlangen, Germany, 1990, Siemens Aktiengesellschaft.)

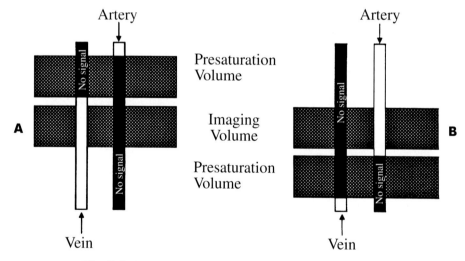

Fig. 7-6. Presaturation pulses: scheme of selective saturation. MR angiography suffers image degradation from vessel overlap on the processed images. Presaturation pulses may be used to eliminate signal from unwanted vessels. **A,** For example, a presaturation pulse placed cephalad in the abdomen will eliminate signal within the aorta and allow for better interpretation of the inferior vena cava. **B,** A presaturation pulse placed caudally in the abdomen will eliminate signal within the inferior vena cava and allow for evaluation of the aorta. Placement of parallel presaturation pulses will eliminate all signal within vessels flowing perpendicular to them. (From Haacke EM, Hausmann R, Laub G, et al: MR angiography. In Magnetom SP, editor: Erlangen, Germany, 1990, Siemens Aktiengesellschaft.)

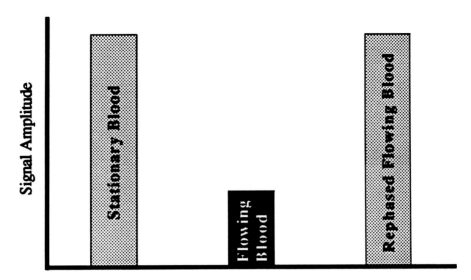

Fig. 7-7. Gradient moment rephasing. Rapidly flowing blood possesses low signal due to dephasing of protons. Gradient moment rephasing corrects for first order dephasing, but can only increase signal to that of stationary blood. (From Haacke EM, Hausmann R, Laub G, et al: MR angiography. In Magnetom SP, editor: Erlangen, Germany, 1990, Siemens Aktiengesellschaft.)

When the flow rate varies, high signal intensity contributions generally have greater influence than low signal intensity contributions on the resultant signal.[62] An occasional brief Valsalva maneuver, during which venous return decreases, may significantly increase signal intensity.[62]

METHODS TO CONTROL FLOW PHENOMENA
Presaturation

Flow-rated enhancement results from inflow of fully magnetized, unsaturated protons. A 90-degree pulse (and spoiler gradient) administered upstream from the imaging volume saturates inflowing protons and prevents FRE.[24] A presaturation pulse superior to a set of transverse images eliminates signal within the abdominal aorta. A presaturation pulse caudal to the imaging volume suppresses the inferior vena cava (Fig. 7-6).

Gradient moment nulling (flow compensation)

Phase dispersion due to magnetic field gradients in stationary tissue can be corrected by applying a gradient of equal magnitude and opposite polarity (the second lobe of a bilobed gradient). However, flowing protons acquire more complex phase dispersion than protons in stationary tissue. Application of a different combination of gradients (a trilobed gradient combination) can compensate for the additional effects of flow on dephasing. This technique is called gradient moment nulling (GMN) or flow compensation (Figs. 7-7 and 7-8).[30,31,57,71,72]

GMN can produce artifacts. It enhances susceptibility artifacts and causes spatial misregistration of intravascular

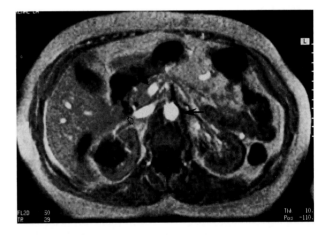

Fig. 7-8. Gradient moment rephasing. Transverse T2*-weighted gradient-echo image, using gradient moment rephasing, through the kidneys displays bright signal in the aorta *(arrow)*, inferior vena cava *(open arrow)*, and portal vein *(arrowhead)*. This signifies that all of these vessels are patent at this level. Also note good delineation of intrahepatic vessels.

signal for vessels flowing obliquely within the plane of imaging. This misregistration artifact results from the presently unavoidable time separation of phase- and frequency-encoding.[43,67,71]

Widely used methods of GMN correct for dephasing due to constant velocity. Higher order effects, such as those due to acceleration, can be corrected only by application of more gradient pulses.[11,30,31] Additional gradient pulses increase scan times to unacceptable clinical levels, allow other modes of dephasing to occur, and further enhance susceptibility effects. Therefore, at present they are not used in routine clinical sequences.

GMN results in high intravascular signal because the protons are rephased at the time of the echo. No enhancement of stationary tissue occurs. Therefore, MRA algorithms frequently use GMN in combination with GE sequences to acquire the data used in image production.

Gradient-echo imaging

Gradient-recalled-echo (GRE) imaging renders vessels as high intensity structures.[62] FRE is the primary cause of increased signal on GRE images acquired in a sequential, two-dimensional (2-D) mode. Images can be acquired within a single breath-hold (less than 15 sec). FRE can occur in each separately acquired slice. In combination with GMN, GRE can provide images with blood signal intensity near its maximum if flow is present.

GRE images can also be obtained as a volume (three-dimensional (3-D) mode from which individual slices are reconstructed. Because blood is imaged repetitively through a greater distance in order to acquire a 3-D data set, phase dispersion time of flight (TOF) nulls the effects of FRE deep within the volume. Scan volume size, flow rate, and depth of penetration of bright blood are related. Phase dispersions result in artifactual loss of signal within large 3-D acquisition volumes. For imaging of rapid flow within small volumes, however, 3-D GRE imaging with GMR can be used successfully.

MRA TECHNIQUES

For MRA to provide diagnostic images of vascular pathology, several conditions must be met. These conditions include maximizing the signal of flowing blood, minimizing the signal of surrounding tissue, providing adequate spatial resolution, and avoiding artifacts that may reduce sensitivity and specificity. GRE sequences and gradient moment rephasing maximize blood signal intensity. Blood signal intensity relative to tissue signal intensity is called *flow contrast*.* Currently, two methods are used clinically to maximize flow contrast. One method exploits TOF effects and the other uses gradient pulses to elicit a phase shift.

Time-of-flight MRA

The TOF method exploits the high intensity of unsaturated inflowing blood to produce angiographic images. Because TOF effects are reduced in deeper sections, the success of the method depends on the rate and direction of flow, the thickness of the slices, and the TE.

The TOF method can be used in two ways: to acquire data for a volume of tissue (3-D acquisition) or to acquire data for contiguous or overlapping slices (2-D acquisition). A volume acquisition excites a slab of tissue, usually 32 or

*References 4, 19, 20, 35, 40, 53-55, 63.

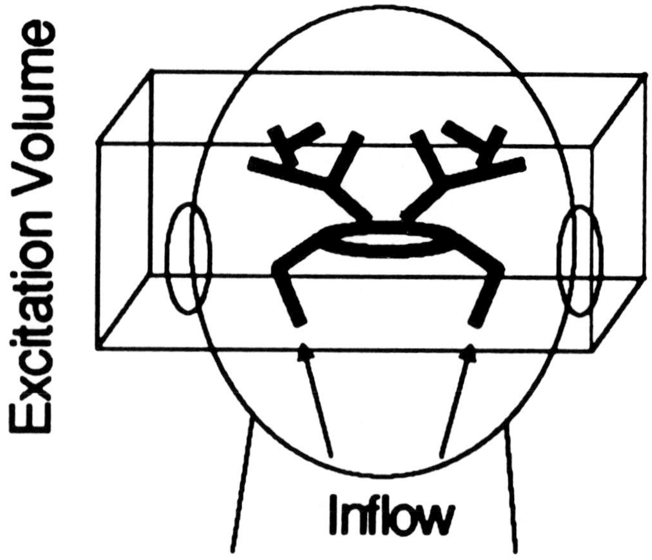

Fig. 7-9. 3-D volume acquisition for MR angiography. The imaging slab generally is of a fixed size (32 to 64 mm). The slab should be positioned so as to maximize the effects of the TOF (inflow) phenomenon. (From Haacke EM, Hausmann R, Laub G, et al: MR angiography. In Magnetom SP, editor: Erlangen, Germany, 1990, Siemens Aktiengesellschaft.)

64 mm thick (Fig. 7-9). Then a phase-encoding gradient in the slice-selection direction produces slices (called partitions in this algorithm).

Effective partition thicknesses of less than 1 mm enable the 3-D TOF method to produce higher resolution MRA than the 2-D TOF method. Volume acquisition also results in a higher signal-to-noise ratio (SNR). A matrix of 256×256 is used; thus, pixel size is changed by varying slice/partition thickness. Generally, 3-D imaging allows for use of shorter TEs, thereby reducing flow-related dephasing. Because this method relies on the TOF effects of inflowing protons, small volumes must be used for 3-D acquisition. Imaging two or more small slabs in a contiguous fashion increases the imaging volume at the expense of examination time. Slower flowing blood may not traverse the entire imaged volume before it becomes saturated. Severe intravascular pathology may cause blood flow to decrease, also enhancing signal loss. In addition to these limitations, volume imaging is sensitive to patient motion, such as that from respiration or peristalsis.[15,47]

3-D TOF imaging is best used in the abdomen and pelvis for examination and characterization of arteries within a localized, small area. Evaluation of veins may be complicated by intravascular signal loss from slower flow. However, evaluation of renal artery stenosis is an ideal application of this method. Splenorenal shunts may be adequately examined with 3-D TOF if flow through them is rapid.

Individual 2-D slices may also be obtained and processed to form the angiogram. Using a GRE technique

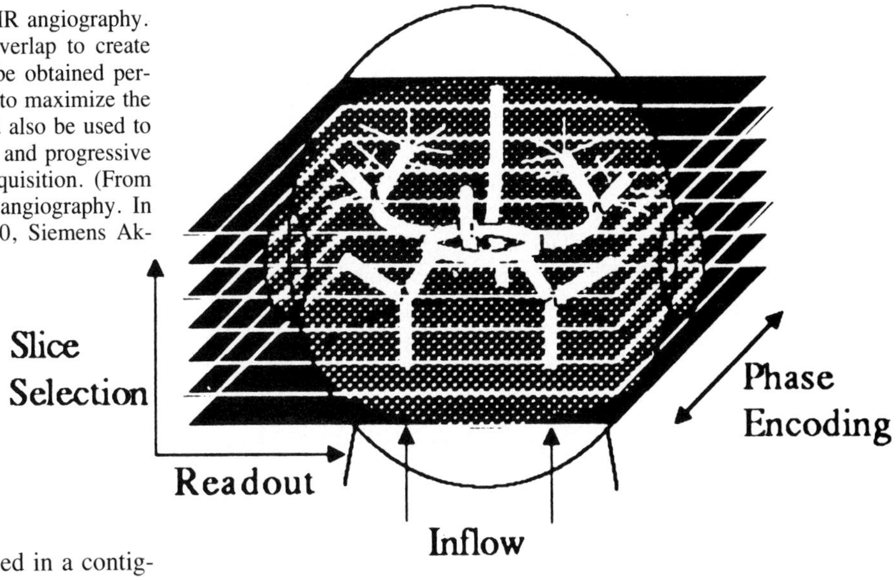

Fig. 7-10. 2-D sequential slice acquisition for MR angiography. Individual 2-D slices are obtained with some overlap to create smooth edges on the angiogram. Slices should be obtained perpendicular to the flow in the vessel(s) of interest to maximize the inflow effect. Gradient moment rephasing should also be used to further enhance vascular signal. Motion artifacts and progressive spin saturation are reduced compared to 3-D acquisition. (From Haacke EM, Hausmann R, Laub G, et al: MR angiography. In Magnetom SP, editor: Erlangen, Germany, 1990, Siemens Aktiengesellschaft.)

with GMN, sequential 2-D slices are obtained in a contiguous or overlapping fashion (Fig. 7-10). Each acquisition is short enough (less than 15 seconds) to be obtained within a single breath-hold. While only a single slice per breath-hold usually is obtained, total examination time may be reduced by obtaining multiple slices if equipment permits.

2-D TOF angiography offers some advantages over 3-D TOF angiography. By using slices of approximately 5 mm, TOF effects are enhanced, even for slower flow in veins or diseased arteries. Thus, signal loss from progressive saturation may be avoided. As a result, 2-D imaging may be used to examine a large volume of tissue (Fig. 7-11). In addition, breath-hold 2-D sequences reduce the motion artifacts that hamper 3-D imaging.

2-D TOF angiography is less advantageous than 3-D imaging with respect to some other factors. It yields lower SNR than 3-D imaging. As a result, slice thicknesses much less than 5 mm will not return enough signal for reliable interpretation. The thicker 2-D slices produce larger pixels and decreased spatial resolution versus 3-D TOF angiography. Longer TEs result in more flow-related dephasing in 2-D TOF imaging than in 3-D TOF imaging.

Several other factors influence the quality of both 2-D and 3-D TOF images, including choice of flip angle and use of intravenous (IV) contrast. With 3-D imaging, a flip angle of approximately 60 degrees produces the best images of vessels in the first few centimeters of the imaging volume; smaller flip angles (e.g., 20 degrees) better enhance the deeper vessels.[20] For 2-D imaging, flip angles of approximately 30 degrees give good flow contrast.[20]

Gadopentetate dimeglumine may improve vascular contrast. Because gadopentetate dimeglumine enhances signal within any tissue in which it accumulates, however, the signal of stationary background tissue could be as high or higher than that of blood. This result could produce a bright artifact. In addition, the shortened T1 may make the use of presaturation ineffective.

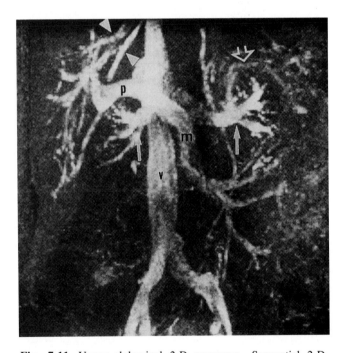

Fig. 7-11. Upper abdominal 2-D venogram. Sequential 2-D venogram of the upper abdomen in a normal subject. Scan variables for each breath-hold acquisition: 72/10/35°/1 (TR/TE/flip angle/NEX), three slices per breath-hold. 5 mm slice thickness with 40 mm interslice gap, 256 × 192 acquisition matrix, and 38 cm FOV. The thickness of the projection image, created from multiple overlapping breath-hold acquisitions, is 120 mm. Presaturation slab *(black stripe across top of image)* above diaphragm eliminates signal from arterial blood flowing into abdomen. Inferior vena cava *(v)* and iliac veins, superior mesenteric vein *(m)* and small branches, renal veins *(solid arrows)*, main protal vein and its intrahepatic branches, and hepatic veins *(arrowheads)* are visualized. Splenic vein *(open arrow)* is not well shown because it is partially outside imaging volume. (From Edelman RR, Mattle HP, Atkinson DJ, et al: Am J Roentgenol 154:937, 1990.)

Phase shift MRA

In contrast to TOF angiography, phase shift angiography exploits differences in phase between flowing blood and stationary tissue. Various methods of phase shift imaging have been developed since its first clinical application in 1982.[50] Some use thin slices (in-plane technique) to acquire and display the data,[51,55] whereas others use larger volumes to display the data angiographically (projective techique).[14,16,18,70] Of these, some detect flow as a loss of phase uniformity from velocity dispersion in a vessel,[70] and others detect flow as a discrete phase shift.[14,16,18]

Several properties are common to all phase shift methods. The velocity component on axis with the magnetic field gradient causes phase shift in transverse magnetization. The induced phase shift is proportional to the velocity of blood flow (Fig. 7-12).[17] Phase incoherence results in loss of signal in areas of turbulent flow. Intravoxel phase dispersion also causes signal loss. As a result, phase-shift angiograms often have worse SNR than TOF angiograms.

Phase contrast angiography. Blood contains protons that flow at different rates: those in the center of the vessel flow fastest and those near the wall flow slowest (Fig. 7-13, *A*). In a uniform magnetic field, the axis of precession of each proton aligns along the direction of the field. If a magnetic field gradient is present, the protons move through a range of field strengths. Moving protons dephase as they travel through the gradient (Fig. 7-13, *B*). However, stationary tissue undergoes no phase shift in a gradient field. This accumulated phase shift is proportional to velocity. Fast-flowing blood appears dark; slow-flowing blood appears bright.

For 3-D angiographic imaging, three sets of encoded data are acquired in orthogonal planes. However, this triple data set alone may not provide adequate blood-tissue contrast. A fourth set of information is obtained using GMN to eliminate phase shifts from first-order effects. A postprocessing algorithm uses flow information from the first three data sets and background information from the fourth data set to create a single data set with phase information in all three planes (Fig. 7-14).

Magnitude contrast angiography. In this method, GMN is used to provide contrast. The range of flow velocities within a vessel creates phase dispersion, which produces a flow void. This intravascular phase incoherence is corrected by GMN, which restores phase coherence and results in a high amplitude signal for flowing blood.

Magnitude contrast angiography uses a subtraction algorithm. Specifically, two sets of images are obtained: one with GMN and one without. Stationary tissue emits similar signal on both. GMN increases only the signal of flowing blood. The images without GMN result in a display of bright flowing blood against a dark background (Fig. 7-15).

Comparison of MRA techniques

Four techniques of MRA have been described. They are 3-D TOF (also called *3-D inflow*), 2-D TOF (also called *2-D inflow*), phase contrast, and magnitude contrast angiography. Their relative performance differs in regard to several parameters (Fig. 7-16). Inflow TOF methods require less imaging time and are less sensitive to turbulence and pulsatile flow than phase methods. However, inflow methods may be complicated by progressive signal loss due to spin saturation. Thus, phase methods are superior for imaging slowly flowing blood. Phase contrast techniques also provide better suppression of background signal than do inflow techniques.

3-D and 2-D techniques have useful different properties that must be understood. In general, 3-D TOF methods

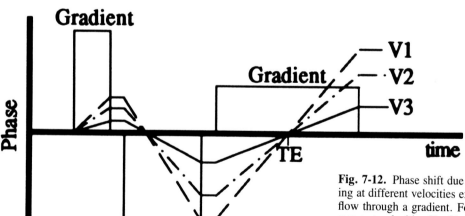

Fig. 7-12. Phase shift due to flow through gradients. Spins moving at different velocities experience different phase shifts as they flow through a gradient. For example, three populations of spins move at velocities V_1, V_2, and V_3. Due to differences in velocity, the protons dephase as they flow through each gradient. In this example, the gradients are arranged so that the spins are rephased at the echo time *(TE)*. (From Haacke EM, Hausmann R, Laub G, et al: MR angiography. In Magnetom SP, editor: Erlangen, Germany, 1990, Siemens Aktiengesellschaft.)

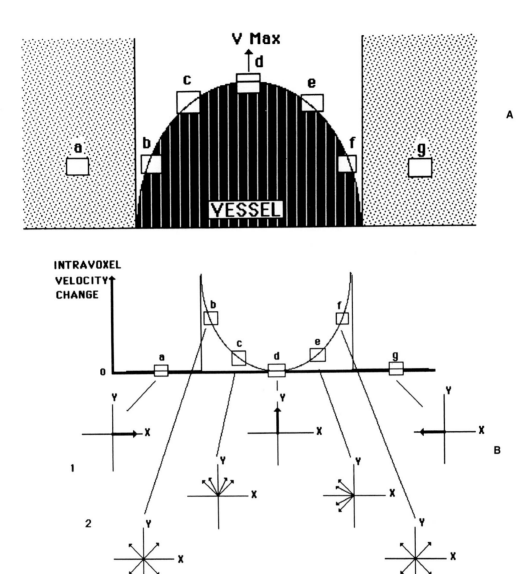

Fig. 7-13. Spin phase phenomena. **A,** Theoretical flow profile of blood moving through stationary tissue. Highest flow rate occurs at the center of the vessel *(d)* and the lowest occurs near the vessel wall *(f)*. **B,** Rate of velocity changes with location. Spins within stationary tissues *(a,g)* and the center of the vessel *(d)* are phase coherent because there is no variation of velocity at those areas. This yields maximum signal. Gradient fields elicit phase shifts among the three areas. Small differences in flow result in some dephasing in the middle third of the vessel *(c,e)*, which reduces signal. Greater changes in flow at the walls causes complete dephasing *(b,f)*, yielding absent signal. (From Spritzer CE: Magn Reson Q 5[3]:205, 1989.)

Fig. 7-14. Reconstruction algorithm for phase contrast MRA. Three sets of flow-encoded data—one of each axis—and one data set with gradient moment rephasing are acquired to create a phase contrast image. The set with gradient moment rephasing is subtracted from each of the other three to yield three new data sets, each containing phase information for a different flow direction. Summation of the resultant three sets yields a phase contrast set with phase (flow) information in all three directions. (From Haacke EM, Hausmann R, Laub G, et al: MR angiography. In Magnetom SP, editor: Erlangen, Germany, 1990, Siemens Aktiengesellschaft.)

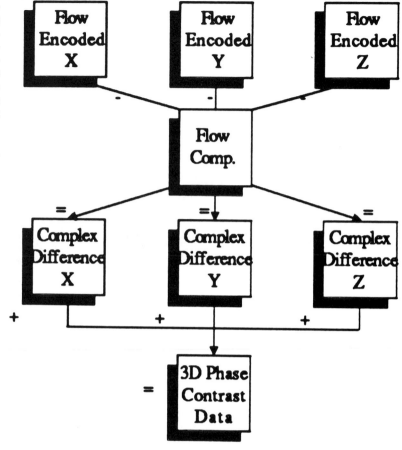

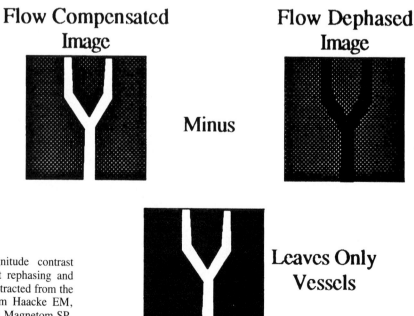

Fig. 7-15. Reconstruction algorithm for magnitude contrast MRA. Two images, one with gradient moment rephasing and one without, are acquired. The latter image is subtracted from the former to leave only signal from vessels. (From Haacke EM, Hausmann R, Laub G, et al: MR angiography. In Magnetom SP, editor: Erlangen, Germany, 1990, Siemens Aktiengesellschaft.)

Summary of Flow Imaging Techniques

	2D Inflow	3D Inflow	Magnitude Contrast (1 Flow Dir.)	Phase Contrast (3 Flow Dir.)
Acquisition Time	Positive	Positive	Moderate	Negative
Spin Saturation	Negative	Negative	Positive	Positive
Turbulence Sensitivity	Moderate	Positive	Negative	Negative
Pulsatile Sensitivity	Moderate	Positive	Negative	Negative
Spatial Resolution	Negative	Positive	Moderate	Positive
Direction Sensitivity	Negative	Positive	Negative	Positive
T1 Sensitivity	Negative	Negative	Positive	Positive
Background Suppression	Moderate	Negative	Positive	Positive

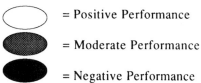

○ = Positive Performance

◍ = Moderate Performance

● = Negative Performance

Fig. 7-16. Summary of flow imaging techniques. In general, phase/magnitude contrast techniques provide better T_1 sensitivity and background suppression than inflow techniques but suffer from longer scan times and increased sensitivity to physiologic motion. 3-D methods have better spatial resolution and direction sensitivity than 2-D methods. (From Haacke EM, Hausmann R, Laub G, et al: MR angiography. In Magnetom SP, editor: Erlangen, Germany, 1990, Siemens Aktiengesellschaft.)

provide superior spatial resolution and direction sensitivity. They are less sensitive to turbulence and pulsatile flow than 2-D methods. However, 3-D methods suffer more from spin saturation artifacts (Fig. 7-17). Thus 3-D imaging is most advantageous for small regions of interest with complex vascular anatomy and fast flow. 2-D imaging excels for large FOVs, large vessels, and slower flow.

It should be apparent that none of the four angiographic techniques is perfectly suited for all vascular imaging. Each has unique advantages and disadvantages, and the parameters discussed here vary in relative importance from case to case. The diagnostician must choose the technique that maximizes contrast and spatial resolution and minimizes artifacts.

MAXIMUM INTENSITY PROJECTION

Maximum intensity projection (MIP) is an algorithm for converting an MRA data set into a format similar to a conventional angiogram. High signal values along a ray through the data set are projected onto a plane (Fig. 7-18). Blood vessels are depicted as bright structures against a dark background. In areas of high background signal intensity, vascular contrast is degraded.

Vessels in a volume of tissue appear to overlap when viewed in a planar projection. To overcome this problem, the MIP is performed in multiple orientations. Each MIP image may be reviewed separately or in a rapid sequence, similar to a cine loop. This gives the radiologist a perspective view. If vessels overlap in one orientation, rotating the image may show them to better advantage. MIP images can be acquired at intervals ranging from 1 to 360 degrees of rotation. Small increments produce a smoother cine loop, but require more postprocessing time. Generally, production of MIP images at 5- to 20-degree intervals is sufficient.

The axis about which the MIP images rotate is chosen

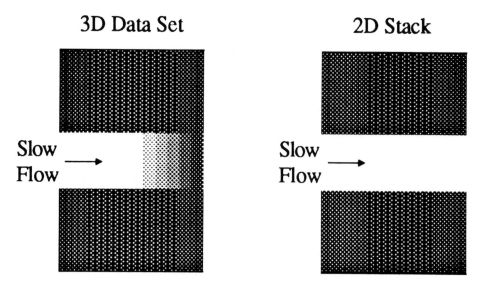

Fig. 7-17. Spin saturation in slow flow. In TOF MRA, slowly flowing blood becomes saturated a short distance within a 3-D slab. Each slice in a 2-D acquisition takes full advantage of the inflow effect. A stack of 2-D slices acquired perpendicular to the plane of flow can cover the course of a vessel over a great distance. (From Haacke EM, Hausmann R, Laub G, et al: MR angiography. In Magnetom SP, editor: Erlangen, Germany, 1990, Siemens Aktiengesellschaft.)

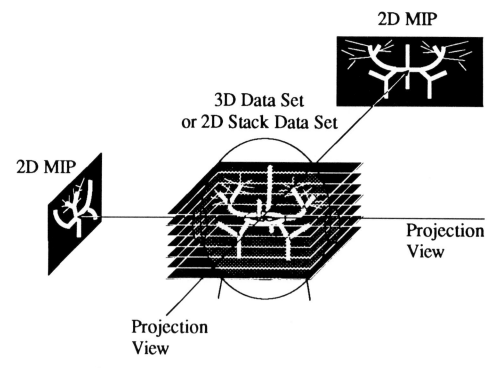

Fig. 7-18. Maximum intensity projection. One view of a 3-D structure may be projected on to a 2-D plane. A ray is projected through the 3-D data set and only those pixels with "maximum signal intensity" are projected on to the final image. One may project successive images at varying angles to yield rotated views. (From Haacke EM, Hausmann R, Laub G, et al: MR angiography. In Magnetom SP, editor: Erlangen, Germany, 1990, Siemens Aktiengesellschaft.)

by the operator. Generally, one of the three standard orthogonal axes (craniocaudal, left-right, or posterior-anterior) is chosen according to the anatomy of the vessels of interest. For example, rotation about the craniocaudal axis demonstrates the aorta and inferior vena cava well. The maximum intensity projection algorithm has some characteristic artifacts. Areas of stationary tissue with high signal intensity (such as ascites and free blood) may cause bright artifacts on the angiogram. Conversely, if the vessel intensity is within approximately 0.5 standard deviation of that of a low intensity background, the vascular signal may appear artifactually to drop out, creating a false-positive diagnosis of stenosis or occlusion on the MIP.[2] Because of laminar flow and partial volume averaging, signal intensity is brighter at the center of a vessel than near its walls. Turbulence or streamlining also produces alterations in intravascular signal intensity, which can cause signal drop out on MIP, particularly at vessel bifurcations and stenoses. Signal dropout could lead to overestimation of the degree of stenosis.

Partial volume averaging within pixels may create a stripe artifact.[2] As a vessel passes obliquely through the plane of imaging, its signal intensity is shared by pixels of adjacent sections. If the adjacent tissue is low intensity, the vessel appears narrowed by partial volume averaging. This effect results in stripes of low intensity across the vessel (Fig. 7-19). The stripes are most apparent when the pixel size is large compared to the vessel diameter.[2] In fact, if the vessel diameter is very small, the vessel may drop out completely from the MIP image.

The intensity of the vessel relative to its background tissue, the topography of the vessel (branched, stenosed), the orientation of the vessel relative to the imaging plane, and the diameter of the vessel relative to pixel size all affect MIP image quality. For example, MIP angiograms of proximal renal artery stenosis are compromised by turbulence from vessel branching and from the stenosis itself. The radiologist must review the individual planar sections and compare them with the processed MIP angiogram to assess accurately the degree of stenosis.

VELOCITY MEASUREMENTS

Blood flow rates may be roughly estimated from intravascular signal intensity. Other techniques exploit phase or presaturation effects for more precise quantitative evaluation of flow.

Phase shift method

Long before MRI came into widespread clinical use, investigators found that the velocity of moving protons could be measured.[34,60,61] The phase shift resulting from movement of protons through a magnetic field gradient is expressed by the following equation:

$$\text{phase shift} = (K)(G)(t_1 - t_0)(V_1 - V_0) \qquad \textbf{7-5}$$

where K represents the gyromagnetic ratio, G is magnitude

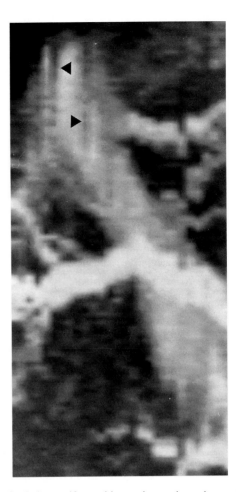

Fig. 7-19. Stripe artifact with maximum intensity projection. Partial volume averaging, which results from flow oblique to the plane of data acquisition, results in stripes of signal loss *(arrowheads)* on certain projections with maximum intensity projection.

of the gradient, t_0 is starting time of the MRI sequence, t_1 is ending time of the sequence, V_0 is the velocity at time t_0, and V_1 is the velocity at time t_1.[8] Because K, G, t_0, and t_1 are known constants for a given imaging sequence, the measured phase shift is directly proportional to the change in flow velocity (Fig. 7-20).

Early recognition of the phase-velocity relationship led investigators to make phase shift imaging the first method of measuring flow velocity with MRI.[50] Several methods for this type of imaging have been proposed. All have in common the use of selective magnetic field gradients. Blood flowing along the axis of a gradient experiences a phase shift proportional to its flow velocity. Blood flowing in any other plane experiences an effect that ranges from partial to none (vessel perpendicular to gradient axis). Vessels with random orientations can be studied by application of three gradients in orthogonal planes (Fig. 7-21).

The phase shift technique may suffer from artifacts.

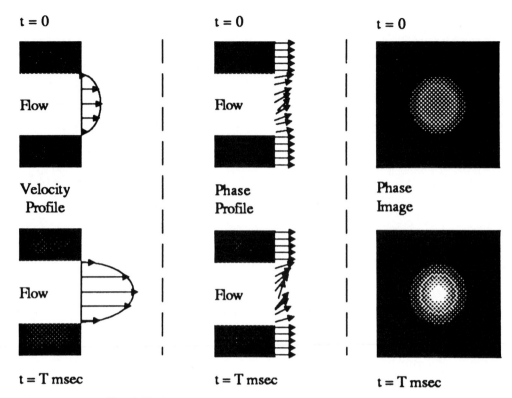

Fig. 7-20. 2-D phase mapping. A slice-selection gradient tags flow. Blood that flows rapidly incurs a greater phase change than more slowly flowing blood. Phase differences at points in the image are displayed as signal differences. In this example, the more rapidly flowing blood, in the bottom row, results in a higher signal on the resultant phase image. (From Haacke EM, Hausmann R, Laub G, et al: MR angiography. In Magnetom SP, editor: Erlangen, Germany, 1990, Siemens Aktiengesellschaft.)

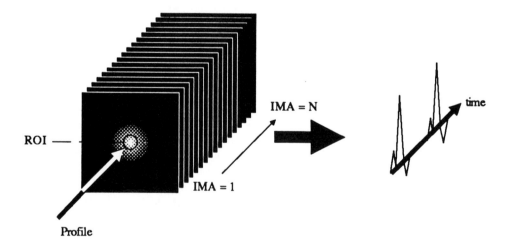

Fig. 7-21. Quantitative analysis of 2-D phase mapping. A series of phase-mapped images may be obtained over time to evaluate flow throughout the cardiac cycle. The operator determines the mean signal amplitude in a region of interest (ROI) on each image. The resultant data generate a curve of flow velocity as a function of time (i.e., during the cardiac cycle). (From Haacke EM, Hausmann R, Laub G, et al: MR angiography. In Magnetom SP, editor: Erlangen, Germany, 1990, Siemens Aktiengesellschaft.)

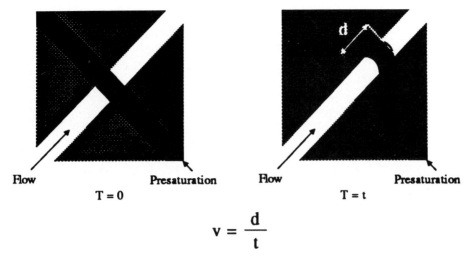

$$v = \frac{d}{t}$$

Fig. 7-22. Bolus tracking. A presaturation slab, placed orthogonal to the vessel of interest, tags the flowing blood within the slab. The blood carries the presaturated spins through the vessel a certain distance between the time *(t)* of tagging and image data acquisition. This time usually ranges from 20 to 50 msec. The distance *(d)* is measured directly from the position of the leading or trailing edge of the bolus in relation to its original location. The velocity *(v)* is then calculated as the distance traveled divided by the acquisition time. (From Haacke EM, Hausmann R, Laub G, et al: MR angiography. In Magnetom SP, editor: Erlangen, Germany, 1990, Siemens Aktiengesellschaft.)

Ghost images produced by pulsatile flow along the phase-encoding direction may be reduced by various interventions. Cardiac gating reduces pulsatile flow artifacts.[8] However, this extends scan time and decreases SNR. Alternatively, a nongated rapid scanning technique may be used.[16,68] In this method, pairs of echoes are acquired as the flow-encoding gradient polarity is reversed. One of each pair is sampled with a positive gradient and one with a negative gradient. Repetition times are approximately 35 msec. Each phase-encoding step spans an integral multiple of cardiac cycles. Even echoes are subtracted from odd echoes and the difference of each pair is averaged.[68] This technique decreases scan time and increases SNR. A combination of cardiac gating with a fast Fourier flow method also allows rapid scan times and high SNR, while suppressing phase ghosts.[37]

Bolus tracking method

Intravascular signal intensity and phase shift measurements both determine flow velocity indirectly. Such methods often suffer from artifacts, although novel variations of the latter method have minimized this problem. Other methods used to determine flow velocity measure directly the distance that blood flows within a given time.[21,27,38,59] All of these tag a bolus of blood in some manner. One method uses an SE technique in which the 90-degree excitation pulse is applied at one location and the 180-degree refocusing pulse is applied at another location.[72] Another method uses selective saturation, in which a plane is selec-

tively excited by an RF pulse and various delay times between excitation and imaging are used to measure the flow of unsaturated spins into the plane.[73] Although these TOF tagging methods are useful, they are hindered by flow artifacts. Another method of tagging, which is similar to TOF tagging, decreases vascular artifacts by allowing concurrent use of GMN. This method is called *bolus tracking* or *bolus tagging*.[21]

Bolus tracking uses a presaturation slice within the volume of interest to tag flowing blood by making it dark on images. GE sequences are then used to follow visually the tagged blood as it flows through the images (Fig. 7-22). The presaturation technique uses a 90-degree RF pulse to tip the protons into the transverse plane. A series of spoiler gradients then disperses the transverse magnetization, so that the presaturated tagged volume of blood emits little or no signal on subsequent GE images.[21] A flip angle of 20 degrees provides the maximum contrast between untagged and tagged blood and also provides good SNR.[21] Lower flip angles produce less signal and higher flip angles reduce contrast.

The GE sequence produces a series of snapshots of flowing tagged blood (Fig. 7-23). Measurement of distance traveled, with knowledge of the time intervals between scans, allows direct calculation of velocity of flow.

This simple bolus tracking method can reliably assess venous flow. However, pulsatile arterial flow may require cardiac gating or rapid GE sequences.

Bolus tracking techniques demonstrate not only the rate

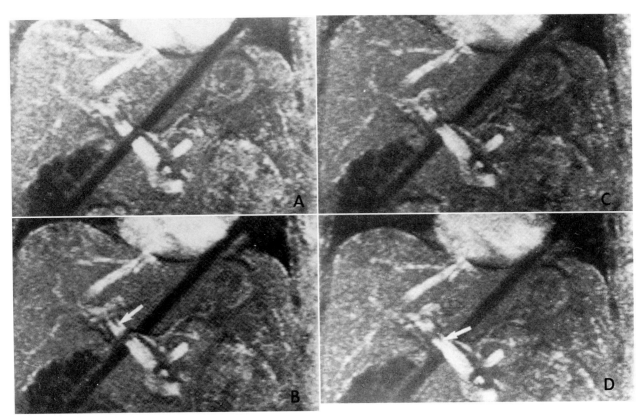

Fig. 7-23. Bolus tracking in normal portal vein. Coronal MRA with bolus tracking. The presaturation slab *(black stripe)* is placed perpendicular to the axis of the main portal vein. Note the hepatopetal flow: **A,** 20.4; **B,** 58.3; **C,** 96.3; and **D,** 134.2 msec after the tagging. Also note the dark stripe *(arrow)*. The significance of this stripe is uncertain, but may represent phase dispersion due to shear flow at divider separating flow into right and left portal veins. (From Edelman RR, Zhao B, Liu C, et al: Am J Roentgenol 153:755, 1989.)

but the character of flow. Plug flow can readily be distinguished from parabolic flow. Flow jet phenomena also may be seen and are helpful to evaluate stenoses. Collateral pathways may be evaluated for flow direction as well as rate.

Comparison of velocity measurement methods

Phase shift methods have one major advantage over bolus tracking methods for velocity measurement. Because information from the same raw data used to form the magnitude image is also used to determine velocity, physiologic measurements require no additional data collection. However, phase shift methods have several disadvantages: (1) The amplitude of a phase shift depends in part on the strength of the magnetic field gradient; imaging parameters must be reset when the gradient is changed; (2) phase shift techniques are sensitive to magnetic field inhomogeneity and to motion; (3) background phase shifts must be eliminated by subtraction processing of multiple sequences; (4) data are not accessible for phase shift analysis on some current MR systems; and (5) phase shift analysis of rapid flow is impeded by signal drop-out and aliasing artifacts.[21]

Bolus tracking techniques have some advantages over

phase shift techniques: (1) Data may be obtained throughout the cardiac cycle, (2) GMN may be used to reduce or eliminate flow artifacts, (3) velocity may be calculated simply from direct measurements, (4) no recalibration of sequence parameters is required as gradient strength changes, (5) flow profiles are readily apparent, and (6) thin sections may be used to reduce volume averaging.[21]

Bolus tracking has one major disadvantage. Because velocity is measured by direct tracking of specific tagged blood sample, the entire length of the vessel along which the blood flows during the sequence must lie completely within the imaging plane. Fortunately, this length need be only a few centimeters, particularly if short duration pulse sequences are used.[21]

CLINICAL APPLICATIONS OF MRA

Although various MRA techniques have been developed to examine both anatomic and physiologic abnormalities, application of these methods to disease in the abdomen has so far been limited. As more MRI sites develop the capability to perform MRA, its use will become routine. This section reviews the current indications for MRA in the abdomen.

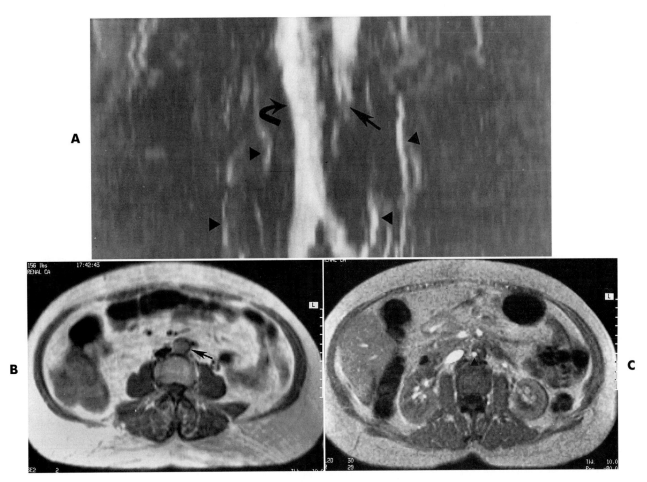

Fig. 7-24. MRA of abdominal aorta. **A,** Sequential axial images using 2-D inflow technique are projected in the coronal plane after processing with maximum intensity projection. The inferior vena cava *(curved arrow)* is patent, but the abdominal aorta is thrombosed, as evidenced by an abrupt end to the high signal *(straight arrow)*. Note the abundant collateral circulation *(arrowheads)*, indicating that occlusion of the aorta was not acute. **B,** Axial T1-weighted spin-echo and **C,** gradient-echo images obtained at the superior edge of the thrombus. The spin-echo image shows fairly uniform high signal in the aorta *(arrow)*, suggesting slow flow or thrombus. The gradient-echo image shows absence of the usual high signal within the vessel, except for a focal area posteromedially *(arrowhead)*, suggesting that some flow is present at this level.

Abdominal aorta

MRA techniques are useful to examine various pathologic conditions of the abdominal aorta. Because the aorta travels a relatively straight course within the abdomen, either coronal or transverse images may be acquired for reconstruction of an MIP angiogram. However, one must limit coronal acquisition to a small FOV because of dephasing effects. The length of the aorta that can be examined in this way depends on the flow velocity. Although coronal acquisition saves time by covering the abdomen with fewer sections, transverse acquisition is generally preferred because of reduced artifacts. TOF MRA is preferred for the abdominal aorta because high flow rate artifacts are more pronounced with phase shift techniques.

Thrombosis. MRA, combined with SE and GRE MRI, can display occlusion or anomalies of the abdominal aorta quite well. Areas of suspected thrombosis on conventional SE scans can be evaluated with MRA to determine their extent (Fig. 7-24).

Aneurysm. Abdominal aortic aneurysms may be evaluated by several techniques, including ultrasound, contrast angiography, and computed tomography (CT). MRI also displays vessel caliber and may also be used. Atherosclerotic stenoses or thromboses often complicate aortic aneurysms, and it is necessary to exclude their presence whenever an aneurysm is seen. Although all of these imaging techniques have some success depicting these complications, MRA may provide more information.

Conventional SE MRI can assess the size of the aneurysm and the presence of plaques or clots, but provides

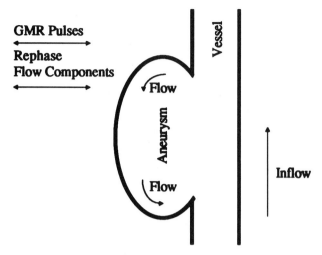

Fig. 7-25. Flow physics of aneurysms. Aneurysms create areas of turbulence and slow flow. Gradient moment rephasing will correct for phase dispersion due to flow through gradients. It will not correct for higher order causes of dephasing, such as acceleration and jerk. This results in loss of signal and underestimation of the size of the aneurysm. (From Haacke EM, Hausmann R, Laub G, et al: MR angiography. In Magnetom SP, editor: Erlangen, Germany, 1990, Siemens Aktiengesellschaft.)

limited information about its effects on flow. However, MRA may reveal aneurysm size, the presence and extent of plaques or clots, and any adverse changes in blood flow.

Flow across the area of dilation is often turbulent. The presence of mural disease may increase this effect (Fig. 7-25). As a result, spinning protons within flowing blood dephase, creating signal loss. This effect may be seen on MRAs of the aorta as sites of absent or, more commonly, reduced signal. Plaque or thrombus will narrow the expected widened luminal signal.

Dephasing effects complicate interpretation. Signal loss due to turbulent flow occurs most prominently near the vessel walls. This effect causes artifactual narrowing of the aortic caliber, leading to the overdiagnosis of mural disease. To avoid this pitfall, compare the angiogram with conventional SE images. Mural disease tends to be asymmetric. Therefore, circumferential narrowing frequently is artifact, whereas asymmetric narrowing is more likely plaque or thrombus.

Dissection. Similar to aortic aneurysm, dissection of the abdominal aorta may be evaluated with various modalities, including MRI and MRA.[13,48,65,75] Conventional angiography depicts vascular anatomy well but carries with it significant morbidity. Ultrasound can evaluate both structure and flow, but portions of the aorta may be hidden by bowel gas artifact. SE MRI and MRA can assess both the anatomy of the dissection and the presence or absence of flow in both lumina (Fig. 7-26).

SE images of the suspected abnormality first are obtained in the transverse and the coronal planes. Coronal images help to define the craniocaudal extent of the dissection and often show whether the dissection extends into any major branches arising from the abdominal aorta. Axial images best reveal the intimal flap and the two lumina.

SE images may distinguish between the true and false lumina based on differences in flow. However, if flow in the false lumen is extremely fast, SE images may not distinguish the false from the true lumen (both may exhibit a signal void). Conversely, if flow in the false lumen is very slow, the high signal that results may be difficult to distinguish from thrombosis. MRA, especially cineangiography, can be quite helpful in these cases. GE images are acquired in the transverse plane for reconstruction into a coronal angiogram. Differences in dephasing due to flow become more pronounced. Subtle variations in flow velocity between the true and false lumina may become apparent, especially if phase shift methods are used.[13] Phase shift methods may also help to distinguish slow flow from thrombus.

Cine loop display of MRA makes differences in flow even more apparent. To produce a cine display, GE images are gated at 40 to 50 msec increments during the cardiac cycle. The resultant images depict pulsatile flow when played back in a cine loop. Because of time constraints, only one or two slices may be obtained at a time (scan time of about 5 to 10 minutes). Therefore, the coronal plane must be used to view the full length of the affected aorta.

Atherosclerotic disease. Conventional angiography, CT, and ultrasonography are usually imaging modalities typically used to diagnose atherosclerotic disease within the abdominal aorta. Signs of atherosclerosis also are detectable by MRI and MRA. In general, atherosclerotic plaques appear dark on GE images and can easily be seen against the bright background of flowing blood. In one study using conventional angiography for comparison, MRA correctly graded the pathology in 88% of patients.[41] However, further study comparing MRA to ultrasound and contrast-enhanced CT is needed to determine the appropriate role of each in the noninvasive evaluation of atherosclerosis.

Flow measurements. Bolus tracking may be used to evaluate flow within the abdominal aorta. The technique is described in an earlier section of this chapter. MRI measurements correlate well with those obtained by ultrasound.[46,48] Flow parameters with good correlation include the pulsatile change of flow velocity, the peak flow velocity, and the velocity integral.[48]

Portal vein

MRA has made noninvasive imaging of the portal vein and its main branches practical (Fig. 7-27). In three different studies the portal vein was visualized in 83% to 100%

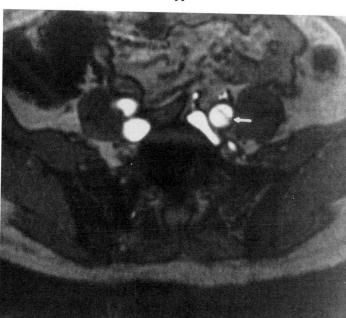

A

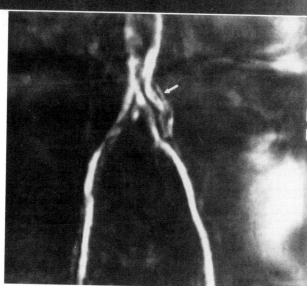

B

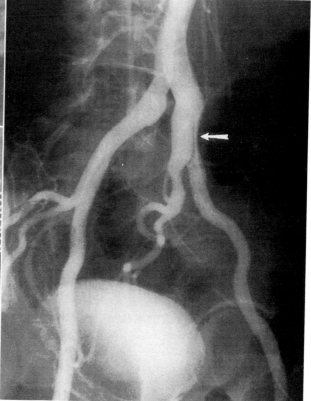

C

Fig. 7-26. Dissection. **A,** Axial gradient-echo image just distal to the aortic bifurcation reveals a dissection, as evidenced by the intimal flap *(arrow)*. High signal in both lumina indicates that both contain flowing blood. **B,** Coronal MRA reveals the extent of the dissection, with the intimal flap again seen *(arrow)*. The internal and external iliac arteries are not seen because they project posterior to the imaging volume. The MRA correlates well with **C,** the intravenous contrast angiogram. (From Spritzer CE, et al: Magn Reson Q 5[3]:205-227, 1989.)

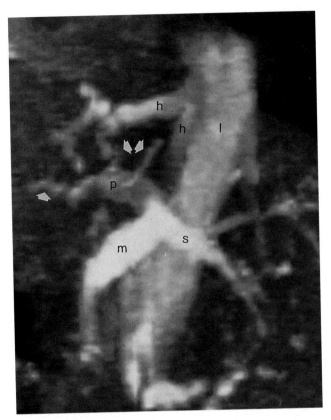

Fig. 7-27. Portal MR angiogram. Coronal MR of the portal venous system was obtained using the 2-D inflow technique. Sequential slices were rotated from the sagittal plane to a plane nearly perpendicular to the plane of the portal vein to maximize inflow effects. Note the splenic *(s)*, superior mesenteric *(m)*, portal *(p)*, and hepatic *(h)* veins; the inferior vena cava *(i)*; and the branches of the portal vein *(arrowheads)*. In this normal individual, aortic and hepatic arterial flow was eliminated by placing a presaturation slab superior to the imaging volume and over the diaphragm.

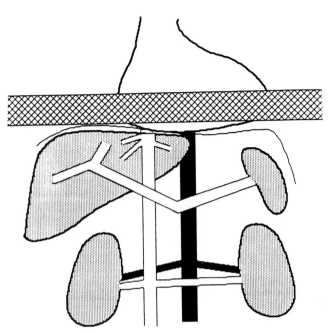

Fig. 7-28. Scheme for placement of presaturation slab in portal vein imaging. Assessment of the portal vein system suffers on maximum intensity projection from vessel overlap. Placement of a presaturation slab over the diaphragm eliminates arterial flow downstream. Thus, the vein can be seen without overlap from the hepatic artery. (From Edelman RR, Wentz KU, Mattle HP, et al: Radiology 172:351, 1989.)

of subjects.[23,39,66] MRA can be used to evaluate anatomic variations, thrombosis, cavernous transformation, collateral vessels, portal hypertension, and reversal of flow.

Thrombosis and cavernous transformation. The portal vein originates at the confluence of the splenic and superior mesenteric veins, courses obliquely to the liver hilus, and divides into left and right branches. SE imaging can be used to evaluate thrombosis and the main portal vein and the development of collateral vessels.[26,56] However, the radiologist may not appreciate the extent of collateral flow on single-plane images. MRA provides additional information; it may be better than contrast angiography for evaluating the extent of collaterals.[66] Because slow flow may be present, the best technique for portal vein MRA is 2-D TOF imaging. Transaxial GE sections are reconstructed into a 3-D data set, which is viewed as a 2-D coronal MIP image. This technique usually is sufficient to demonstrate the main portal vein and any collaterals.

However, the MIP algorithm may cause troublesome overlap of vessels on the 2-D coronal image, which may interfere with interpretation. The MIP image can be rotated to avoid overlap of veins with the hepatic artery. Alternatively, overlapping can be overcome by the use of presaturation. A 90-degree presaturation pulse placed judiciously over the descending aorta (outside the area of interest) will saturate arterial protons and create a signal void downstream. Placement of the pulse over the aorta at the level of the diaphragm usually yields adequate presaturation (Fig. 7-28). Because the hepatic artery arises from the aorta, its signal also will be suppressed. Therefore, it will not interfere with the final MIP image of the portal venous anatomy.

Several studies have shown that MRA and SE MRI can effectively demonstrate thrombosis of the portal vein. Williams et al[74] diagnosed two out of three cases of portal vein obstruction with SE alone. Torres et al[64] demonstrated correctly two of two angiographically proven positive cases of portal vein thrombosis and 39 of 40 angiographically proven negative cases. This study also revealed that for the evaluation of portosystemic shunts (splenorenal, mesoatrial, and mesocaval), MR agreed with angiography on the presence or absence of shunt flow in 41 of 42 cases. The sole false-negative result occurred because the site of the shunt was not included in the FOV of

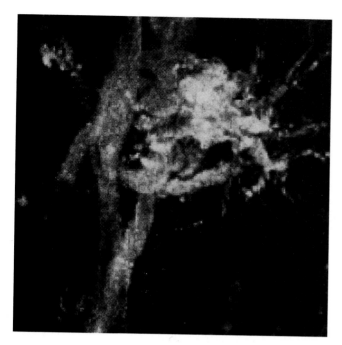

Fig. 7-29. Cirrhosis and portal hypertension. Sequential 2-D MRA of the upper abdomen, projected in the coronal plane, was acquired in a patient with liver cirrhosis. The angiogram shows massive gastric varices. The aorta and portal venous system overlap because no presaturation slab was placed. (From Edelman RR, Mattle HP, Atkinson DJ, et al: Am J Roentgenol 154:937, 1990.)

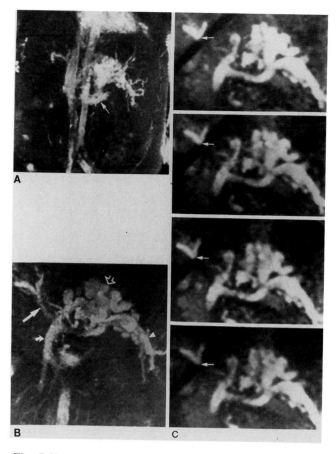

Fig. 7-30. Cirrhosis and portal hypertension. This patient was suspected to have portal vein thrombosis by duplex ultrasound. **A,** A coronal MRA reveals massive collaterals and splenorenal shunting. Note the enlarged left renal vein *(arrow).* **B,** Another coronal MRA was created from the same data as for **A,** but slices containing the upper abdominal portions of the aorta and inferior vena cava were excluded from postprocessing, eliminating overlap of the portal vein with these vessels. The MRA reveals a patent portal vein *(straight solid arrow)* and massive collaterals *(open arrow).* Note the superior mesenteric vein *(curved arrow)* and splenic vein *(arrowhead).* **C,** A series of images from a dynamic bolus tracking sequence reveals that flow in the portal vein moves away from the liver *(reversed flow).* The presaturation slab *(black stripe)* was positioned just proximal to the junction of the right and left portal veins. Four time points are shown, the earliest at the top and the latest at the bottom. (From Edelman RR, et al: Am J Roentgenol 153:755, 1989.)

the MRI. A more recent study has demonstrated portal vein thrombosis in a patient using MRA only.[23] More clinical investigation is needed to assess the sensitivity and specificity of MRA, alone or in combination with SE imaging, for the detection of portal vein thrombosis.

Portal hypertension and flow reversal. Radiographic evidence of portal hypertension includes abnormalities in hepatic size and configuration, splenomegaly, ascites, and presence of collateral flow (including gastric and esophageal varices and a recanalized paraumbilical vein). These signs allow for a presumptive diagnosis. MRA can provide additional evidence by direct visualization of collaterals and by determination of the rate and direction of flow.

Both TOF and phase shift techniques may be used to produce the angiogram. In addition, either 2-D or 3-D acquisition may be used. The operator should place a presaturation pulse over the aorta at the level of the diaphragm to eliminate signal from the hepatic artery.

Several signs of portal hypertension may be detected by MRA (Figs. 7-29 through 7-31). Reversal of flow is a frequent sign of increased portal vein pressure. Edelman et al[23] used the bolus tracking technique to evaluate flow. Peak flow velocities and direction of flow as determined by MR were found to correlate well with duplex sonography.

Liver transplantation

The patient with liver failure must meet several criteria to be considered a candidate for transplantation. One of the most important requirements is a patent portal vein or a large collateral to which donor vessels may be anastomosed. Generally, absence of a sufficient portal inflow vessel precludes transplantation. Thus, radiographic evaluation of the portal system is an essential component of pretransplantation assessment.

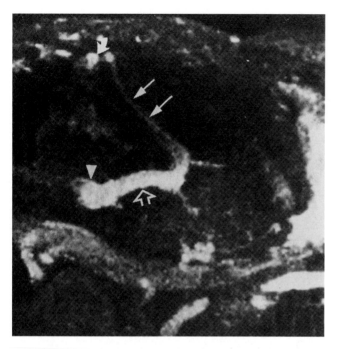

Fig. 7-31. Cirrhosis and portal hypertension. Sagittal MRA reveals a patent umbilical vein *(solid arrows)* originating from the left portal vein *(open arrow)* and extending to the abdominal wall. Abdominal wall venous collaterals are also seen *(curved arrow)*. Only a small part of the main portal vein, seen end-on *(arrowhead)*, projected onto the angiogram due to the limited FOV. (From Edelman RR, et al: Am J Roentgenol 153:755, 1989.)

In the past, sonography and dynamic CT have been used preoperatively to evaluate portal vein patency. However, recent data suggest that MRA can provide high sensitivity and specificity (Fig. 7-32). Finn et al[25] evaluated 30 patients who were about to undergo liver transplantation. Angiography and bolus tracking were used. MRA demonstrated portal vein patency in 96% (26 of 27 patients) and portal vein thrombosis in 100% (three of three patients). MRA accurately determined reversed flow in one patient (Fig. 7-33). Duplex ultrasound demonstrated patency in 96% (24 of 25 patients), agreeing with MRA as to the direction of flow in all cases, and thrombosis in 66% (two of three patients). Ultrasound provided indeterminate results in two patients. MRA correctly determined patency in one portal vein and occlusion in the other (confirmed at surgery). In addition, MRA revealed the extent of collateral vessels, whereas ultrasound tended to underestimate their size and number. The results of this study suggest that MRA is as accurate as duplex ultrasound and may be more useful for preoperative evaluation of the portal vein and collateral vessels (Fig. 7-34).

Renal vessels

Renal artery stenosis. Of all types of intraabdominal vascular pathology, renal artery stenosis has to date been the one most frequently studied by MRA. Early investigation revealed that the renal arteries could be seen. However, it was conceded that inferior spatial resolution and the possibility of flow artifacts made MRA less desirable

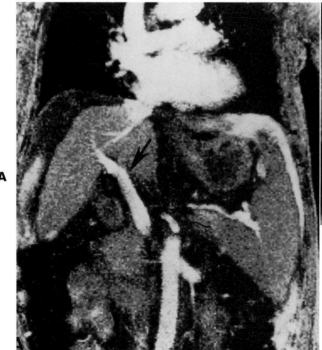

A

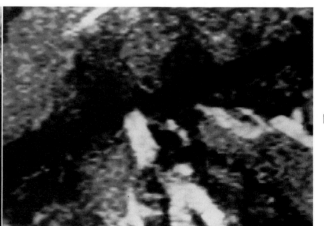

B

Fig. 7-32. Normal portal vein in liver transplant. **A,** Coronal projection image shows a normal main portal vein *(straight arrow)*. Note the ascites, some of which is of high signal intensity. The left renal vein and part of the celiac trunk are also seen. **B,** A bolus tracking sequence shows hepatopetal movement of the trailing edge, confirming antegrade flow. (From Finn JP, Edelman RR, Jenkins RL, et al: Radiology 179:265, 1991.)

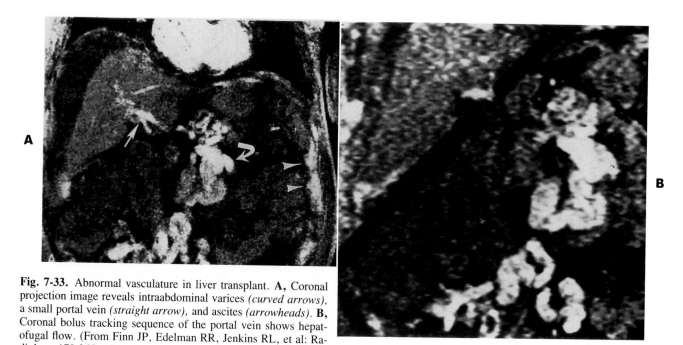

Fig. 7-33. Abnormal vasculature in liver transplant. **A,** Coronal projection image reveals intraabdominal varices *(curved arrows),* a small portal vein *(straight arrow),* and ascites *(arrowheads).* **B,** Coronal bolus tracking sequence of the portal vein shows hepatofugal flow. (From Finn JP, Edelman RR, Jenkins RL, et al: Radiology 179:265, 1991.)

than conventional angiography.[22] At that time, MRA was considered an adjunct to conventional angiography. More recent studies have demonstrated that MRA may become a screening procedure for renal artery stenosis. Because of the relatively high velocity renal flow rate, either 2-D sequential overlapping slices or a 3-D volume may be used.

In general, evaluation of the renal arteries requires presaturation of the renal veins to avoid overlap on MIP images. This technique may be accomplished by administering presaturation pulses to the volume containing each kidney (Fig. 7-35). Injudicious use of these pulses could either fail to saturate the venous flow or could saturate the distal renal artery near the renal hilus.

Both TOF and phase shift methods have been used to generate renal arteriograms. One study using the TOF method yielded a sensitivity of 100% and specificity of 92% for detecting a stenosis of 50% or greater.[41] MRA overgraded the degree of stenosis in 4 of 55 renal arteries. The number of renal arteries was correctly assessed in every case. Evaluation with the 3-D phase shift method yielded detection rates in normal volunteers of 91% and 100% for the right and left arteries, respectively. Another evaluation of 18 patients by MRA showed 89% sensitivity and 100% specificity for occluded or stenosed arteries.[66]

These recent studies show that MRA has high sensitivity and specificity for detection of proximal and mid-portion renal artery stenosis. However, the distal renal artery is much more difficult to interpret at present. Progressive spin saturation can cause loss of intravascular signal in the distal part of the artery. Also, physiologic movement is more pronounced distally, creating blur artifact.[41,45] Thus,

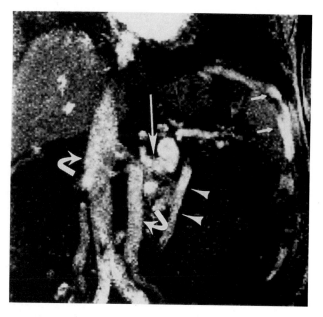

Fig. 7-34. Collateral vasculature in liver transplant. Coronal projection image shows enlarged gonadal veins *(arrowheads),* retroperitoneal varices *(long straight arrow),* and ascites *(short straight arrows).* The aorta and inferior vena cava *(curved arrows)* can also be seen. (From Finn JP, Edelman RR, Jenkins RL, et al: Radiology 179:265, 1991.)

MRA may currently be used to assess most cases of renal artery stenosis. However, the unusual case of isolated distal atherosclerotic stenosis could be missed. In addition, the MRA examination might also yield false-negative results for distal lesions of fibromuscular dysplasia.

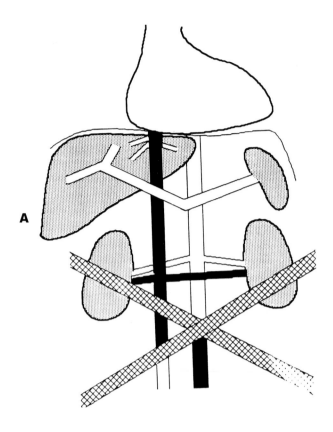

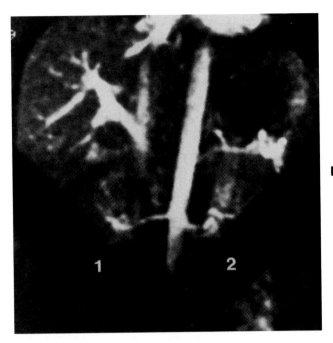

Fig. 7-35. Renal artery MRA: placement of presaturation slabs. Evaluation of the renal arteries may be hampered by overlap from the inferior vena cava and renal veins. **A,** Placement of criss-crossing presaturation slabs will eliminate flow in the inferior vena cava and renal veins. **B,** Nulling venous flow allows for more clear visualization of the renal arteries. (From Edelman RR, Wentz KU, Mattle HP, et al: Radiology 172:351, 1989.)

Each angiographic method has its individual technical drawbacks. 3-D TOF methods are sensitive to variations in contrast between the renal arteries and the surrounding tissue. Placement of the imaging volume so that the arteries lie within the upper half of the slab will yield better contrast than if the arteries lie within the lower half, owing to the effects of progressive spin saturation.[45]

Phase shift methods often suffer from spin dephasing due to intravoxel velocity gradients or higher order motion. In the renal arteries, these effects may be responsible for the signal drop often seen at the inferior convexity.[66] This cause of signal loss can be minimized by shortening the TE.

Renal vein. Investigators realized early that MRI could be used to evaluate the patency of renal veins. One study correctly identified thrombus in 12 of 12 renal veins and slow flow in five of five renal veins.[39] MRA often provides little additional morphologic information, but may supply valuable flow data. Renal vein flow differences in patients with unilateral renal artery stenosis can be evaluated. Edelman et al[20] demonstrated reduction in renal vein blood flow on the side of the arterial stenosis in five patients. These measurements can be used to confirm the significance of an arterial stenosis.

Arteriovenous malformations. With CT, renal arteriovenous malformations (AVM) may be distinguished from neoplasms by their degree of contrast enhancement, feeding and draining vessels, and mural calcifications.[44] Because of the vascularity of these lesions, SE MRI and MRA can display their anatomy well. Unless an AVM is thrombosed, flowing blood within it will appear bright on MRA (Fig. 7-36). The size and location of feeding vessels may be seen to good advantage.

Inferior vena cava

Various congenital anomalies of the inferior vena cava (IVC) can be assessed with MRA, but they are relatively uncommon entities. More often, MRA is used to evaluate the extent of intraluminal thrombus (Fig. 7-37). Tumor thrombus from renal cell carcinoma is a common cause of IVC thrombosis. The cranial extent of thrombosis is of critical importance to the surgeon. Extension into the right atrium necessitates cardiopulmonary bypass for complete removal of the thrombus. MRA, in combination with standard SE imaging, can be used as the initial examination. SE images give excellent anatomic detail of the primary tumor site and can accurately stage the disease. MRA provides valuable information about extension into the venous system. Should intraatrial extension be suspected, an electrocardiogram-gated cineangiogram is indicated. This tech-

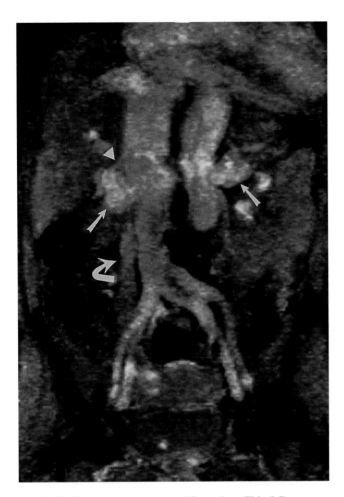

Fig. 7-36. Renal arteriovenous malformation. This 2-D sequential TOF MRA projected in the coronal plane demonstrates large arteriovenous malformations (AVMs) in both kidneys *(straight arrows)*. The draining vessel for the right AVM *(arrowhead)* may be seen entering the inferior vena cava, which is greatly enlarged due to increased flow. The aorta is thrombosed 1 to 2 cm below the level of the AVMs. Also note the prominent collateral vessels *(curved arrow)*. Additional collateral vessels, present on axial imaging, are not seen because they lie outside of the FOV.

nique can demonstrate intracardiac thrombus in spite of motion that precludes conventional SE imaging.

WORK IN PROGRESS

MRA is being tested to assess pathology affecting various other intraabdominal vessels. Investigation of vascular shunts by MRA has begun.[10] Blood flow to organ transplants has been demonstrated (Fig. 7-38); however, significant barriers remain. For example, evaluation of smaller vessels, such as the mesenteric arteries, may be unreliable because of limited spatial resolution. The same may hold true for evaluation of the intrahepatic vessels and the internal iliacs. However, under favorable conditions, MRA can successfully display smaller vessels (Figs. 7-39 and 7-40). Assessment of the splenic vein is difficult because of its

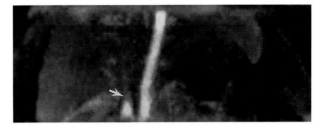

Fig. 7-37. Inferior vena cava thrombosis. This patient suffered from a renal cell carcinoma, which invaded the renal vein and inferior vena cava. The coronal TOF MRA demonstrates lack of signal within the cava from the level of entry of the right renal vein superiorly *(arrow)*, which is due to tumor thrombus occluding the suprarenal inferior vena cava.

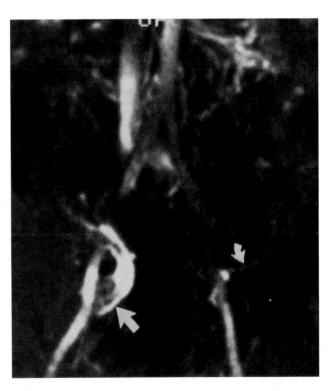

Fig. 7-38. Evaluation of transplant vascularity. Coronal projection MRA in a patient with renal and pancreatic transplants. The vascular supply to the kidney *(straight arrow)* and the pancreas *(curved arrow)* is well demonstrated. (From Edelman RR, Wentz KU, Mattle HP, et al: Radiology 172:351, 1989.)

tortuosity (which may cause turbulence and artifactual signal loss). Anecdotal reports of MRI of puerperal ovarian vein thrombosis raise the possibility of using MRA for this condition.[49,58] Additional applications will be discovered as clinical experience with abdominal MRA increases.

Fig. 7-39. Appearance of gonadal vein. Coronal MRA demonstrates a normal left gonadal vein *(arrow)*. The superior end of the vein cannot be seen because it lies outside of the field of view. (From Edelman RR, Wentz KU, Mattle HP, et al: Radiology 172:351, 1989.)

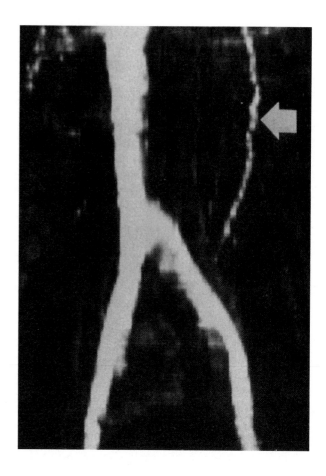

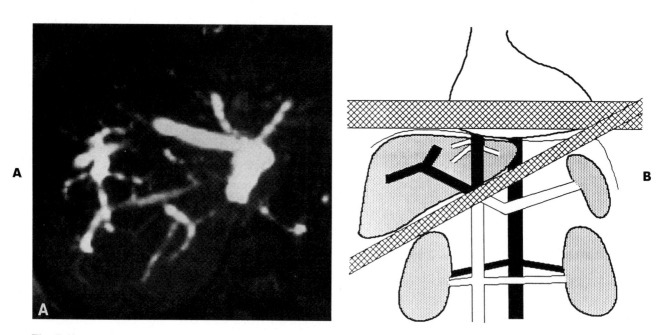

Fig. 7-40. Hepatic venography. **A,** Axially projected MRA reveals the confluence of the middle and left hepatic veins with the inferior vena cava. Usually, overlap of the portal venous branches obscure the hepatic veins. The operator may exclude the caudal portion of the image data to eliminate the portal veins. **B,** Alternatively, one may apply presaturation slabs—one over the diaphragm to eliminate hepatic arterial flow and one orthogonal to the portal vein to eliminate portal venous flow. (From Edelman RR, Wentz KU, Mattle HP, et al: Radiology 172:351, 1989.)

SUMMARY

MRA techniques can provide valuable information in many cases of abdominal vascular pathology. The two methods of MRA, TOF and phase shift, offer relative advantages and disadvantages. Both 2-D sequential and 3-D volume acquisitions are possible for either method. No one of these is ideal for all cases. Choice of the appropriate technique depends on several factors: the flow rate within the vessels of interest, the length of the vessel to be evaluated, the imaging coil types available, patient compliance (i.e., with breath-holding), and scan time. All of these factors affect image quality and patient throughput.

Flow imaging techniques have only recently become clinically practical. Velocity measurement is possible by phase shift and bolus tracking methods. Bolus tracking techniques probably will become the most useful method, but further evaluation is necessary.

Until recently, examination of intraabdominal vessels was limited to conventional angiography, duplex ultrasound, CT, and occasionally radionuclide scans. These modalities currently remain the examinations of choice in many instances, but MRI and MRA have become increasingly valuable. MRA is less invasive than conventional angiography, but is currently limited by worse spatial resolution and variability in vascular contrast. MRA offers wide FOV and is less dependent on patient habitus than is duplex ultrasound. Like ultrasound, it yields both anatomic and flow data. MRA currently offers less spatial resolution than CT but can image vessels in several planes, often with superior contrast, and offers angiographic images not obtainable by CT. As investigation continues, new angiographic methods will no doubt surface, as will new applications of MRA to the evaluation of intraabdominal vascular disease.

REFERENCES

1. Alvarez O, Hyman RA: Even echo MR rephasing in the diagnosis of giant intracranial aneurysm, J Comput Assist Tomogr 10(4):699-701, 1986.
2. Anderson CM, Salouer O, Tsuruda JS, et al: Artifacts in maximum-intensity-projection display of MR angiograms, Am J Roentgenol 154:623-629, 1990.
3. Atlas SW, Mark AS, Fram EK, et al: Vascular intracranial lesions: applications of gradient-echo imaging, Radiology 169:455-461, 1988.
4. Axel L, Morton D: MR flow imaging by velocity-compensated/uncompensated difference images, J Comput Assist Tomogr 11(1):31-34, 1987.
5. Bird RB, Stewart WE, Lightfoot EN: Transport phenomena, New York, 1960, John Wiley & Sons.
6. Bradley WG, Waluch V: Blood flow: magnetic resonance imaging, Radiology 154:443-450, 1985.
7. Bradley WG, Waluch V, Lai KS, et al: The appearance of rapidly flowing blood on magnetic resonance images, Am J Roentgenol 143:1167-1174, 1984.
8. Bryant DJ, Payne JA, Firmin DN, et al: Measurement of flow with NMR imaging using a gradient pulse and phase difference technique, J Comput Assist Tomogr 8(4):588-593, 1984.
9. Carr HY, Purcell EM: Effects of diffusion on free precession in nuclear magnetic resonance experiments, Phys Rev 94:630-638, 1954.
10. Chezmar JL, Bernardino ME: Mesoatrial shunt for the treatment of Budd-Chiari syndrome: radiologic evaluation in eight patients, Am J Roentgenol 149:707-710, 1987.
11. Constantinesco A, Mallet J, Boumartin A, et al: Spatial or flow velocity phase encoding gradients in NMR imaging, Magn Reson Imaging 2:335, 1984.
12. Crooks LE, Baker B, Chang H, et al: Magnetic resonance imaging strategies for heart studies, Radiology 153:459, 1984.
13. Dinsmore RE, Wedeen VJ, Miller SW, et al: MRI of dissection of the aorta: recognition of the intimal tear and differential flow velocities, Am J Roentgenol 146:1286-1288, 1986.
14. Dumoulin CL, Hart HR: Magnetic resonance angiography, Radiology 161:717-720, 1986.
15. Dumoulin CL, Cline HE, Souza SP, et al: Three-dimensional time-of-flight magnetic resonance angiography using spin saturation, Magn Reson Med 11:35-46, 1989.
16. Dumoulin CL, Souza SP, Hart HR: Rapid scan magnetic resonance angiography, Magn Reson Med 5:238, 1987.
17. Dumoulin CL, Souza SP, Walker MF, et al: Three-dimensional phase contrast angiography, Magn Reson Med 9:139-149, 1989.
18. Dumoulin CL, Souza SP, Walker MF, et al: Time-resolved magnetic resonance angiography, Magn Reson Med 6:275-286, 1988.
19. Edelman RR, Chien D, Atkinson DJ, et al: Fast time-of-flight MR angiography with improved background suppression, Radiology 179:867-870, 1991.
20. Edelman RR, Mattle HP, Atkinson DJ, et al: MR angiography, Am J Roentgenol 154:937-946, 1990.
21. Edelman RR, Mattle HP, Kleefield J, et al: Quantification of blood flow with dynamic MR imaging and presaturation bolus tracking, Radiology 171:551-556, 1989.
22. Edelman RR, Wentz KU, Mattle HP, et al: Projection arteriography and venography: initial clinical results with MR, Radiology 172:351-357, 1989.
23. Edelman RR, Zhao B, Liu C, et al: MR angiography and dynamic flow evaluation of the portal venous system, Am J Roentgenol 153:755-760, 1989.
24. Felmlee J, Ehman R: Spatial presaturation: a method for suppressing flow artifacts and improving depiction of vascular anatomy in MR imaging, Radiology 164:559-564, 1987.
25. Finn JP, Edelmann RR, Jenkins RL, et al: Liver transplantation: MR angiography with surgical validation, Radiology 179:265-269, 1991.
26. Fisher MR, Wall SD, Hricak H, et al: Hepatic vascular anatomy on magnetic resonance imaging, Am J Roentgenol 144:739-746, 1985.
27. Foo TK, Perman WH, Poon CS, et al: Projection flow imaging by bolus tracking using stimulated echoes, Magn Reson Med 9:203-218, 1989.
28. Frahm J, Haase A, Matthaei D, et al: FLASH MR imaging: from images to movies. Presented at the 71st Annual Meeting of the Radiological Society of North America, Chicago, November 17-22, 1985.
29. Gullberg GT, Wehrli FW, Shimakawa A, et al: MR vascular imaging with a fast gradient refocusing pulse sequence and reformatted images from transaxial sections, Radiology 165:241-246, 1987.
30. Haacke EM, Lenz GW: Improving image quality in the presence of motion by using rephasing gradients, Am J Roentgenol 148:1251, 1987.
31. Haacke EM, Hausmann R, Laub G, et al: MR angiography. In Magnetom SP, editor: 1990, Erlangen, FRG, Siemens Aktiengesellschaft.
32. Haase A, Frahm J, Matthei D, et al: FLASH imaging: rapid NMR imaging using low flip angle pulses, J Magn Reson 67:217-225, 1986.
33. Haase A, Frahm J, Matthei D, et al: Rapid images and NMR movies. Proceedings of the Fourth Annual Meeting of the Society of Magnetic Resonance in Medicine, London, August 19, 1985.
34. Hahn et al: Detection of sea-water motion by nuclear precession, J Geophys Res 65:776, 1960.

35. Hale JD, Valk PE, Watts JC, et al: MR imaging of blood vessels using three-dimensional reconstruction: methodology, Radiology 157:727-733, 1985.

36. Hendrick RE, Kneeland JB, Stark DD: Maximizing signal-to-noise and contrast-to-noise ratios in FLASH imaging, Magn Reson Imaging 5:117-127, 1987.

37. Henning J, Muri M, Brunner D, et al: Quantitative flow measurement with the fast fourier flow technique, Radiology 166:237-240, 1988.

38. Henning J, Muri M, Friedburg H, et al: MR imaging of flow using the steady state selective saturation method, J Comput Assist Tomogr 11(5):872-877, 1987.

39. Hricak H, Amparo E, Fisher MR, et al: Abdominal venous system: assessment using MR, Radiology 156:415-422, 1985.

40. Keller PJ, Drayer BP, Fram EK, et al: MR angiography with two-dimensional acquisition and three-dimensional display, Radiology 173:527-532, 1989.

41. Kim D, Edelman RR, Kent KC, et al: Abdominal aorta and renal artery stenosis: evaluation with MR angiography, Radiology 174:727-731, 1990.

42. Lanzer P, Botvinick EH, Schiller EB, et al: Cardiac imaging using gated magnetic resonance, Radiology 150:121, 1984.

43. Larson TC III, Kelly WM, Ehman RL, et al: Spatial misregistration of vascular flow during MR imaging: theory and clinical significance in the CNS, Am J Neuroradiol, 155:1117, 1990.

44. Lee, Sagel: Computed tomography of the abdomen with MRI correlation, New York, 1989, Raven Press.

45. Lewin JS, Laub G, Hausmann R: Three-dimensional time-of-flight MR angiography: applications in the abdomen and thorax, Radiology 179:261-264, 1991.

46. Maier SE, Meier D, Boesiger P, et al: Human abdominal aorta: comparative measurements of blood flow with MR imaging and multigated doppler US, Radiology 171:487-492, 1989.

47. Marchal G, Bosmans H., Van Fraeyenhoven L, et al: Intracranial vascular lesions: optimization and clinical evaluation of three-dimensional time-of-flight MR angiography, Radiology 175:443-448, 1990.

48. Matsuda T, Shimizu K, Sakurai T, et al: Measurement of aortic blood flow with MR imaging: comparative study with doppler US, Radiology 162:857-861, 1987.

49. Mintz MC, Levy DW, Axel L, et al: Puerperal ovarian vein thrombosis: MR diagnosis, Am J Roentgenol 149:1273-1274, 1987.

50. Moran PR: A flow velocity zeugmatographic interlace for NMR imaging in humans, Magn Reson Imaging 1:197-203, 1982.

51. Moran PR, Moran RA, Karstaedt N: Verification and evaluation of internal flow and motion, Radiology 54:433-441, 1985.

52. Motomiya M, Karino T: Flow patterns in the human carotid artery bifurcation, Stroke 15:50-56, 1984.

53. Nishimura DG, Macovski A, Jackson JI, et al: Magnetic resonance angiography by selective inversion recovery using a compact gradient echo sequence, Magn Reson Med 8:96-103, 1988.

54. Nishimura DG, Macovski A, Pauly JM: Considerations of magnetic resonance angiography by selective inversion recovery, Magn Reson Med 7:472-484, 1988.

55. O'Donnell M: NMR blood flow imaging using multiecho, phase contrast sequences, Med Phys 12:59-64, 1985.

56. Ohtomo K, Itai Y, Furui S, et al: MR imaging of portal vein thrombus in hepatocellular carcinoma, J Comput Assist Tomogr 9(2):328-329, 1985.

57. Prorok RJ: Signa applications guide, vol II, Milwaukee, 1989, GE Medical Systems.

58. Savader SJ, Otero RR, Savader BL: Puerperal ovarian vein thrombosis: evaluation with CT, US, and MR imaging, Radiology 167:637-639, 1988.

59. Shimizu K, Matsuda T, Sakurai T, et al: Visualization of moving fluid: quantitative analysis of blood flow velocity using MR imaging, Radiology 159:195-199, 1986.

60. Singer et al: Nuclear magnetic resonance blood flow measurements in the human brain, Science 221:654-656, 1983.

61. Singer JR: NMR diffusion and flow measurement and an introduction to spin phase graphing, J Phys (E) 11:281-291, 1978.

62. Stark DD, Bradley WG: Magnetic resonance imaging, St Louis, 1988, Mosby–Year Book.

63. Tasciyan TA, Lee JN, Riederer SJ, et al: Fast limited flip angle MR subtraction angiography, Magn Reson Med 8:261-274, 1988.

64. Torres WE, Gaylord GM, Whitmire L, et al: The correlation between MR and angiography in portal hypertension, Am J Roentgenol 148:1109-1112, 1987.

65. Valk PE, Hale JD, Kaufman L et al: MR imaging of the aorta with three-dimensional vessel reconstruction: validation by angiography, Radiology 157:721-725, 1985.

66. Vock P, Terrier F, Wegmuller H, et al: Magnetic resonance angiography of abdominal vessels: early experience using the three-dimensional phase-contrast technique, Br J Radiol 64:10-16, 1991.

67. Von Schulthess GK, Higgins CB: Blood flow imaging with MR: spin-phase phenomena, Radiology 157:687-695, 1985.

68. Walker MF, Souza SP, Dumoulin CL: Quantitative flow measurement in phase contrast MR angiography, J Comput Assist Tomogr 12(2):304-313, 1988.

69. Waluch V, Bradley WG: NMR even echo rephasing in slow laminar flow, J Comput Assist Tomogr 8:594-598, 1984.

70. Wedeen VJ, Meuli RA, Edelman RR, et al: Projective imaging of pulsatile flow with magnetic resonance imaging, Science 230:946-948, 1985.

71. Wehrli FW: Fast-scan magnetic resonance: principles and applications, Magn Reson Q 6(3):165-236, 1990.

72. Wehrli FW, Shimakawa A, Gullberg GT, et al: Time-of-flight MR flow imaging: selective saturation recovery with gradient refocusing, Radiology 160:781-785, 1986.

73. Wehrli FW, Shimakawa A, MacFall JR, et al: MR imaging of venous and arterial flow by a selective saturation-recovery spin echo (SSRSE) method, J Comput Assist Tomogr 9(3):537-545, 1985.

74. Willimas DM, Cho KJ, Aisen AM, et al: Portal hypertension evaluated by MR imaging, Radiology 157:703-706, 1985.

75. Yamada T, Tada S, Harada J: Aortic dissection without intimal rupture: diagnosis with MR imaging and CT, Radiology 168:347-352, 1988.

Part II

UPPER ABDOMEN

Chapter 8

OVERVIEW OF ABDOMINAL MAGNETIC RESONANCE IMAGING

Pablo R. Ros
Luis H. Ros Mendoza

This chapter presents an overview of the applications of magnetic resonance imaging (MRI) in the upper abdomen (liver, spleen, pancreas, kidneys, mesentery, and retroperitoneum). The major indications and contraindications, both absolute and relative, are outlined. The major advantages and disadvantages of MRI are compared with other imaging techniques (computed tomography [CT], ultrasound [US], and angiography). The chapter is a general introduction to subsequent chapters that present individual organs and regions in detail, with emphasis on specific indications for MRI.

INDICATIONS
General indications

Since the early publications on the clinical applications of MRI in 1982 and 1983, it has been obvious that MRI would eventually play an important role in the evaluation of abdominal diseases. At first, however, the indications for MRI in the upper abdomen were more limited than in other areas of the body, due primarily to the challenges of respiratory and cardiac motion and to the lack of adequate intravascular and gastrointestinal (GI) contrast agents in the early years of MRI.

Because CT clearly depicts the gross anatomy and pathology of the upper abdominal organs, the role of MRI has depended on its capability to depict biochemical changes resulting from pathologic abnormalities at a molecular level, which cannot be obtained with CT.[1]

The intrinsic stengths of MRI, well known in other organ systems (central nervous system, musculoskeletal system, etc.), must be exploited fully to complement or supplant other imaging modalities, particularly CT.

In the current climate of regulation and cost containment in health care, it is of paramount importance to know when to use MRI or CT, as duplication of similar information by multiple modalities is not justified. The increased sensitivity of MRI, based on its superb contrast resolution, goes beyond morphology (demonstrable by CT at lower cost) and allows more specific characterization of certain pathologic processes in the abdomen.

The general characteristics of MRI that make it a useful modality in the upper abdomen are listed here and summarized in the box on p. 166:

1. Superb sensitivity to minimal physical differences between tissues and fluid collections.
2. Exquisite contrast resolution.
3. Flexible capability to modify the imaging technique to enhance certain specific differences. A wide range of pulse sequences and techniques is available for tailored application to particular situations.
4. Multiplanar capability to fit the pathologic process or organ to be studied. This implies not only to the three orthogonal planes (axial, sagittal, and coronal), but also off-axial and oblique planes that depict organs such as the uterus or pancreas to better advantage.
5. Intrinsic sensitivity to blood flow, allowing evaluation of vessels without administration of contrast material.
6. Lack of ionizing radiation and apparent absence of significant biologic risk.
7. Availability of a gamut of different contrast agents, both for intravascular and GI use, that may be chosen according to the particular area to be studied (similar to different radionuclides in nuclear medicine).

The general properties making MRI a useful modality in the upper abdomen and applying to general indications for abdominal MRI are listed here and summarized in the box below:

1. The high contrast resolution of MRI makes it the ideal technique to evaluate patients in whom the quality of ultrasound and/or CT scans is suboptimal for whatever cause (multiple abdominal clips for CT, obesity for ultrasound, etc.).
2. The superb sensitivity of MRI, based on high contrast resolution, justifies its use in cases where CT and/or ultrasound are negative or equivocal, particularly when there are bonified clinical symptoms or laboratory results that indicate the presence of an abnormality.
3. In those cases in which a significant allergy to iodine is known, it is logical to use an imaging technique that provides diagnostic information without the risk of a severe allergic reaction. This is of particular interest in patients who, due to the nature of their illness, must be followed with serial scans (such as those having abdominal malignancies). To prevent allergic contrast reactions, MRI should be encouraged versus CT for follow-up studies.
4. Due to lack of ionizing radiation and no biologic risks, the use of MRI is preferable to CT for patients whose exposure to ionizing radiation should be minimized or nil (infants, pregnancy, and in general women of childbearing age).

Specific indications

Specific indications are divided into two groups. The first is the group of specific indications that apply to the entire abdomen. The second is the group of organ-specific indications, presented in table form.

The specific indications for MRI that apply to the entire upper abdomen (see box below) as follows.

Detection and characterization of focal masses in different organs. A typical example is the evaluation of focal liver lesions, where MRI has been proven to be helpful in distinguishing nonsurgical benign lesions (hemangioma and cyst) from primary and secondary malignant neoplasms. MRI has been considered the most successful imaging technique for the evaluation of focal liver lesions.[2,3] In this textbook, we dedicate particular attention to MRI of the liver, as this organ is considered the major target for the application of abdominal MRI.

Characterization of fluid collections. MRI is highly specific, as well as sensitive, for determining the presence of fat and/or blood in fluid collections. It is a useful technique to characterize abdominal fluid collections as hemorrhagic or fatty versus serous. This is important in the evaluation of pancreatic pseudocysts, lymphangiomas, complex renal cysts, etc.

Origin of large abdominal masses. The multiplanar capability of MRI is helpful in determining the origin of large intraabdominal masses, both intraperitoneal and retroperitoneal. Likewise, MRI is helpful in detecting invasion of adjacent organs, as a second plane (coronal or sagittal) can supplement transverse images to clarify possible questions.

Vascular pathology. Because MRI does not require injection of contrast material to identify major abdominal vessels, and because it can also be obtained in multiple planes, it is considered the modality of choice to evaluate the patency of large abdominal vessels, as well as vascular pathology in the retroperitoneum.[5-7]

Detection of neuroendocrine neoplasms (islet cell tumors, pheochromocytoma). For the diagnosis of primary neuroendocrine neoplasms in the abdomen (pheochromocytoma and islet cell tumors), MRI is the favored diagnostic imaging technique. The appearance of neuroendocrine tumors is characteristic, with marked hyperintensity in T2-weighted images (T2WI) due to the high contents of neuroendocrine secretions within the cells. An added advantage of MRI is the avoidance of intravenous contrast material that could result in undesired reactions. This commonly encountered potential complication of abdominal CT is obviated by MRI.

In addition to these indications for MRI survey of the upper abdomen, other specific indications are grouped in the accompanying boxes, according to the major upper abdominal organs: pancreas/spleen, mesentery/retroperitoneum/abdominal vessels, and kidney/adrenal. (Chapters 9 to 17 cover these applications of MRI in detail.)

Specific indications: pancreas/spleen

Pancreas

1. Islet cell tumors
2. Peripancreatic effusions and pseudocysts (detection of hemorrhage)
3. Cystic neoplasms
4. Unusual neoplasms
   - Solid and papillary epithelial neoplasms

Spleen

1. Focal lesions
   - Hematoma
   - Hemangioma
   - Candidiasis
   - Infarcts
2. Diffuse lesions
   - Gaucher disease
   - Sickle cell disease
   - Lymphoma
3. Splenomegaly

Specific indications: liver

Focal lesions

1. Hemangioma
2. Metastasis (particularly if hypovascular)
3. Primary hepatic neoplasms
   - Hepatocellular carcinoma
   - Fibrolamellar carcinoma
   - Hepatoblastoma
   - Focal nodular hyperplasia
   - Hepatocellular adenoma
4. Focal fatty change
5. Focal sclerosing cholangitis
6. Hemorrhagic lesions/fluid collections
7. Abscess

Diffuse lesions

1. Iron deposition disease
2. Cirrhosis
3. Diffuse fatty change

Liver transplant

Specific indications: mesentery/retroperitoneum/ abdominal vessels

Mesentery

- Characterization of fluid collection/cystic masses
- Demonstration of mesenteric origin in large abdominal masses
- Abscesses

Retroperitoneum

- Extraadrenal pheochromocytoma
- Adenopathy
- Primary retroperitoneal tumors
- Abscess
- Hemorrhage
- Fibrosis
- Psoas muscle abnormalities

Abdominal vessels

- Congenital anomalies
- Aortic aneurysm/dissection
- Postoperative aorta
- Venous thrombosis
- Tumor thrombi (i.e., from RCC)

Specific indications: kidney/adrenal

Kidney

- Mass characterization/staging
- Angiomyolipoma
- Renal transplant
- Vascular invasion in RCC
- Iron deposition in renal cortex (sickle cell disease)

Adrenal

- Pheochromocytoma
- Myelolipoma
- Adenoma versus metastasis

Contraindications

Absolute

- Cardiac pacemaker
- Ferromagnetic intracranial clips
- Cochlear implants
- Neurostimulators
- Some IVC filters

Relative

- Claustrophobia
- Unstable patients
- Severely ill patients
- Patient on ventilators/monitors
- Pregnancy

LIVER

The liver is the most common target organ for MRI in the upper abdomen. The success of MRI in differentiating some benign, nonsurgical processes, such as hemangioma and cysts, from primary and secondary malignancy is well known. This ability has been heralded by some authors as the major contribution of MRI to the study of the liver. For some radiologists, MRI is preferred over CT to diagnose focal liver diseases.[2,3] The specific indications for MRI in the evaluation of focal liver disease are as follows:

1. Solitary focal lesion before resection
2. Known metastatic disease in patients who are candidates for segmental resection
3. Normal CT in patients with bonified clinical suspicion for liver metastases or primary liver tumors (i.e., hepatocellular carcinoma in chronic cirrhotics)
4. Survey for recurrent postpartial hepatectomy, particularly in patients with multiple surgical clips

CONTRAINDICATIONS

In general, abdominal MRI is contraindicated clinically when the MRI study could be dangerous because of potential interactions between either the static magnetic field, the pulsed gradient fields, or the radiofrequency field and the patient.[8] Contraindications are classified as either absolute or relative.

Absolute contraindications

Absolute, as well as relative, contraindications are summarized in the box at top right.

Patients with cardiac pacemakers constitute an absolute contraindication for MRI as the exposure to magnetic fields with rapid changes in gradients may induce currents in the pacemaker leads that may produce untoward effects.[9] It has been proven that the magnetic relays contained within pacemakers are susceptible to magnetic fields of less than 5 gauss.[9]

Leads left behind after removal of a pacemaker do not constitute an absolute contraindication for MRI, although it is not possible to completely rule out induction of currents in them.[10,11]

It is also general knowledge that patients with intracranial ferromagnetic clips, particularly after aneurysm repair, cannot be examined under any circumstances with MRI. In these cases, displacement or torsion of the intracranial clip as a response to the external magnetic field could provoke rupture of an intracranial vessel.[10,11]

On the other hand, conventional vascular clips, as well as intracranial aneurysm clips made out of titanium or some stainless steel alloys, are not ferromagnetic, and therefore, are compatible with MRI.[13,14]

The overwhelming majority of surgical clips, as well as sutures, do not constitute a contraindication to MRI.

Prosthetic cardiac valves are not a contraindication except in the older models, such as Starr-Edwards, although in many cases cardiac valves produce local artifacts.[15]

Regarding inferior vena cava filters, the majority of them are not ferromagnetic (Greenfield) and, therefore, are not a contraindication for abdominal MRI; however, some bird nest filters may be ferromagnetic. Therefore, one should check with the manufacturer for MRI compatibility in cases where a bird nest filter is identified.[16]

In patients with large orthopedic devices such as hip or knee prostheses or Harrington rods, abdominal MRI can be performed. However, in patients with Harrington rods in the thoracolumbar spine, the degree of distortion of the magnetic field could be sufficient to produce significant local degradation of the image.

In patients with cochlear implants as well as neurostimulators, MRI cannot be performed because these devices constitute an absolute contraindication. Likewise, patients with ferromagnetic ocular implants are also not candidates for MRI.

In general, in patients with metallic foreign bodies that contain either iron (metal workers, carpenters) or shrapnel fragments (of unknown composition) more particular precautions have to be exercised. If a metallic foreign body is in or near a critical location, such as the ocular globe, MRI may not be indicated because the risks may outweigh the benefits. These patients should go through a rigorous pre-MRI screening process. In general, it is accepted that plain radiographs of the skull, or in some cases, CT limited to the orbit, may be needed to rule out the presence of a metallic foreign body in the eye.[6,14]

Ultimately, if there is a question regarding the compatibility of a particular surgical or medical device, it may be necessary to obtain an identical prosthesis, implant, or other device and place it at the entrance of the gantry to determine whether it is displaced or otherwise affected by the magnetic field.

Relative contraindications

Relative contraindications are summarized in the box on p. 168.

Up to 10% of patients scheduled for an MRI examination have claustrophobia and may require sedation. In some cases, despite sedation, a patient may refuse to be examined due to severe claustrophobia.

Other possible relative contraindications are unstable medical conditions and the requirement for continuous monitoring. The majority of conventional devices for monitoring of vital signs are not designed to be compatible with MRI. However, some MRI-compatible systems on the market, such as pulse oximeters and others, allow adequate monitoring of unstable patients.[17]

Severely ill patients also represent another relative contraindication, as a relatively long examination (particularly in abdominal MRI) may not be tolerated.

Pregnancy does not constitute a contraindication for MRI, as there are no proven biologic effects to the fetus. However, ultrasonography is considered the preferred method for evaluation. If alternative methods, such as ultrasound, do not provide the needed information, MRI is preferable to CT or other radiologic studies using ionizing radiation.[18,19]

GENERAL PRECAUTIONS

Patients should be gowned so that ferromagnetic objects that may be in the patient's clothes are not introduced into the magnetic field (coins, belt buckles, keys, etc.). Dentures, hairpins, shoes (often having ferromagnetic nails in the heel or sole), and other metallic objects should also be removed.

Regarding technical personnel, magnetic field safety precautions should also be observed routinely. Metallic objects such as pens, scissors, and badges, should be removed. Pregnant medical personnel are advised to remain beyond the 10 gauss line and to avoid exposure to time-variable radiofrequency magnetic fields or time-variable magnetic field gradients. It is preferable for pregnant technologists and/or physicians not to enter the imaging room for positioning or monitoring purposes.[9]

ADVANTAGES
General advantages

The major advantage of MRI versus other imaging techniques is its superb contrast resolution that allows definition of abnormal versus normal tissues. The contrast resolution of MRI is based on the fact that several physical parameters play a role to produce an MRI. Therefore, if one of these physical parameters is altered in an abnormal tissue, a change in signal characteristics results. Tissue contrast can be intensified by the appropriate selection of pulsing sequences. This marked contrast resolution is the basis for the high sensitivity of MRI, as well as for its capacity to specifically characterize certain processes.

MRI vs CT

Unlike CT, which uses x-rays, MRI does not use ionizing radiation and, therefore, avoids a major class of biologic risks. As is well known, MRIs can be obtained directly in any orientation without the need of image reformatting. Therefore, MRI can provide identical resolution in any possible spatial planes superior to reformatted images produced by conventional CT.[20] Vascular structures can be identified by MRI without need of contrast material unlike in CT.

An additional advantage of MRI is the lack of beam-hardening artifacts (which are troublesome in CT, due to metallic clips or residual barium and/or air). Therefore, MR scans do not require the same degree of patient preparation as needed in CT. Because in abdominal MRI there is no routine administration of intravenous contrast material (and, when intravenous contrast is needed, gadolinium does not have the same risk of nausea and vomiting as iodine), prolonged fasting is not indicated before MRI of the abdomen, as it often is in iodine-enhanced CT. In pediatric patients, an added advantage is that MRI is less dependent on the presence of fat planes when compared to CT of abdominal structures.

MRI vs ultrasound

Regarding ultrasound, the advantages of MRI can be summarized as follows:

1. MRI is not operator-dependent.
2. MRI is easily reproducible.
3. There are no artifacts secondary to air or bone.
4. MRI allows a "global vision" of the entire abdomen, of particular interest in large lesions.
5. MRI is not as limited as ultrasound in the examination of obese and postsurgical patients.

MRI vs angiography

The advantages of MRI regarding angiography are primarily its noninvasiveness due to the lack of ionizing radiation, and its avoidance of iodinated contrast material. For abdominal vessels, the multiplanar capability of MRI is particularly appealing, as pathologic processes in major

Advantages of MRI

1. Excellent organ visualization without need of contrast material
2. Multiplanar imaging
3. No ionizing radiation
4. Vascular visualization in a noninvasive manner
5. High sensitivity
6. Biochemical information—tissue characterization
7. Spectroscopy
8. Lack of artifacts caused by bone or air

Table 8-1. CT versus MRI: technical aspects

	CT	MRI
Radiation	W	B
Equipment cost	B	W
Space/installation	B	W
Running costs	B	W
Speed of examination	B	W
Uncooperative patient	B	W
Screening	B	W

B, Better; W, Worse.
Modified from Steiner RE: Am J Roentgenol, 145:883-893, 1985.

abdominal vessels can be identified without the need to move the patient between sequences.

MRI combines some of the major advantages of the principle imaging techniques, such as the following:

1. Multiplanar capabilities of ultrasound
2. Spatial and contrast resolution of CT
3. Vascular visualization of angiography

The major advantages of MRI as compared with other techniques are summarized in box above.

DISADVANTAGES
General disadvantages

Abdominal MRI is in continuous evolution. The major disadvantages that have limited the complete development of MRI in the abdomen are disappearing. Due to the rapid technologic change in abdominal MRI, it is difficult to establish meaningful comparison with other more established techniques.

In the upper abdomen, two major drawbacks have not allowed a full development of MRI:

1. Lack of adequate GI contrast
2. Motion artifacts secondary to physiologic motion (breathing, intestinal peristalsis, diaphragmatic excursion and heartbeat). All these motions produce marked degradation of the upper abdominal images, when compared with other areas of the body.[21]

MRI vs CT

When compared to CT, MRI has inferior spatial resolution, lack of established protocols and techniques, and lack of universally accepted oral contrast agents.

Regarding intravenous contrast, gadolinium-DTPA has not been as successful in the abdomen as it has been in other areas, primarily due to the long examination times in the abdomen. However, iodine vascular enhancement has been a consistent success in widespread clinical use in conventional abdominal CT protocols.

Because the examination times are more prolonged in abdominal MRI than in CT, patient cooperation is of paramount importance. Therefore, image degradation occurs in

Table 8-2. Abdominal CT versus abdominal MRI: imaging/clinical aspects

	CT	MRI
Contrast resolution	W	B
Spatial resolution	B	W
Sensitivity	W	B
Specificity	B	W
Multiple sequences	W	B
Contrast media	B	W
Contrast reactions	W	B
Dynamic studies	B	W
Bone, metal artifacts	W	B
Calcification	B	W

B, Better; W, Worse.
Modified from Steiner RE: Am J Roentgenol, 145:883-893, 1985.

patients that cannot cooperate completely for an extended time for MRI as compared to CT.

In addition, in some situations the sensitivity and specificity of MRI is intrinsically less than those of CT, for example the detection of calcifications. Another factor that must be considered when comparing MRI to CT is that MRI requires more attention to detail in the protocol and better clinical knowledge so that studies can be designed specifically. Because there are many more variables in MRI than in CT, the physician must devote more time and the need for monitoring of the study is greater.

Tables 8-1 and 8-2 summarize a comparison between MRI and CT regarding clinical aspects, image quality, and clinical applications.

MRI vs ultrasound

When MRI is compared with ultrasound, the major disadvantages of MRI are its long examination time and its high cost.

Another advantage of ultrasound is its portability. Ultrasound examinations can be performed at bedside in the intensive care units, operating room, and emergency room. Ultrasound also provides ease of access for biopsies and drainages.

MRI vs angiography

When compared with angiography, MRI is limited in the evaluation of small vessels. Conventional angiography routinely provides a dynamic display of arterial capillary and venous phases. MRA lags in this capability, but is improving rapidly. Another major pitfall of MRI is the presence of flow phenomena, that are much more complex to interpret than findings in conventional angiography.

REFERENCES

1. Becker RL, Norfray JF, Teitelbaum GP, et al: MR imaging in patients with intracranial aneurysm clips, Am J Neuroradiol 9:891-897, 1988.
2. Edelman RR, Kim D, Wentz KU, et al: Projection arteriography and venography of the body with MR imaging (abstract), Radiology 173(P):320, 1989.
3. Ferrucci JT: MR imaging of the liver, Am J Roentgenol 147:1103-1116, 1986.
4. Hotas S, Olsson M, Romner B, et al: Comparison of MR imaging and CT in patients with intracranial aneurysm clips, Am J Neuroradiol 9:891-897, 1988.
5. Hricak H, Demas BE, Williams RO, et al: Magnetic resonance imaging in the diagnosis and staging of renal and perirenal neoplasms, Radiology 154:709-715, 1985.
6. Kanal E, Shellock FG, Talagala L: Safety considerations in MR imaging, Radiology 176:593-606, 1990.
7. LaRoy LL, Cormier PJ, Matalon TAS, et al: Imaging of abdominal aortic aneurysms, Am J Roentgenol 152:785-792, 1989.
8. Laakman RW, Kaufman B, Hau JS, et al: MRI in patients with metallic implants, Radiology 157:777-714, 1985.
9. Mitchell DG, Burk DL Jr, Vinitski S, et al: The biophysical basis of tissue contrast in extracranial MR imaging, Am J Roentgenol 149:831-837, 1987.
10. Paulicek W, Geisenger M, Castle L, et al: Effects of nuclear magnetic resonance on patients with cardiac pacemakers, Radiology 147:149-153, 1983.
11. Randall PA, Kohman LJ, Scalzetti EM, et al: MR imaging of prosthetic cardiac valves in vitro and in vivo, Am J Cardiol 62:973-976, 1988.
12. Shellock FG: Monitoring during MRI: an evaluation of the effect of high-field MRI on various patient monitors, Med Electron 100:93-97, 1986.
13. Shellock FG: Biological effects of MRI, Diagn Imag 9:96-101, 1987.
14. Shellock FG: MR imaging of metallic implants and materials: a compilation of literature, Am J Roentgenol 151:811-184, 1988.
15. Shellock FG, Crves JV: Potential adverse effects and safety considerations, MRI Decis 2:25-30, 1988.
16. Stark DD, Felder RC, Wittenberg J, et al: Magnetic resonance imaging of cavernous hemangioma of the liver: tissue specific characterization, Am J Roentgenol 145:213-222, 1985.
17. Steiner RE: Magnetic resonance imaging: its impact on diagnostic radiology, Am J Roentgenol 145:883-893, 1985.
18. Teitelbaum GP, Bradley WG, Klein BD: MR imaging artifacts, ferromagnetism, and magnetic torque of intravascular filters, stents and coils, Radiology 166:657-664, 1988.
19. Yuasa Y, et al: MR angiography in pelvic and abdominal venous occlusion, Magn Reson Imaging 8:54, 1990.

Chapter 9

ANATOMY OF THE UPPER ABDOMEN

Christophoros Stoupis
Eugenio Erquiaga

Liver
Spleen
Pancreas
Adrenal glands
Kidneys
Gastrointestinal (GI) tract
Blood vessels
Abdominal wall

Magnetic resonance imaging (MRI) provides anatomic detail that is comparable to or better than other imaging modalities. Although computed tomography (CT) is considered the gold standard for abdominal imaging by most authors, MRI provides important diagnostic information in multiple planes and allows characterization of lesions based on signal characteristics in various pulse sequences. Although it is well known that T1 spin-echo (SE) sequences are useful for anatomic details and that T2-weighted images (WI) are useful in the detection of pathologic lesions, other sequences are useful as well, for both normal anatomy and abnormal conditions.[11] This chapter illustrates the normal appearance of the solid and nonsolid organs of the upper abdomen and demonstrates how to approach them in a practical way.

LIVER

The liver occupies the upper right portion of the abdomen and is the largest abdominal organ. Due to its relaxation time, liver on MRI has a homogeneous signal intensity between muscle and fat on both T1WI and T2WI.[5] In comparison with other organs, on T1WI liver has an inter-

mediate signal intensity similar to that of the pancreas or almost similar to the signal intensity of the renal cortex (Fig. 9-1); on T2WI liver intensity decreases. Fat supression imaging reveals the liver as a slightly hyperintense organ. The vascular anatomy of the liver is clearly delineated by MRI without injection of contrast agent.[6,7] MRI can serve as a noninvasive guide to hepatic surgical anat-

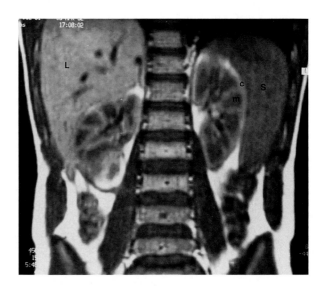

Fig. 9-1. Coronal T1WI of the abdomen in a young person. The liver *(L)* intensity is almost identical to that of the renal cortex *(c)*. The spleen *(S)* is hypointense to the liver. Note the superb cortico *(c)*-medullary *(m)* differentiation in the kidneys. Note also the position of the kidneys and their relationship to the liver and spleen.

172

omy. Refinements in surgical techniques permit extensive resection in liver tumors; and in the preoperative assessment of potential candidates for hepatic resection, a precise definition of the tumor extension is necessary.[1]

The multiplanar approach allows better definition of segmental liver anatomy and, therefore, more accurate localization of liver lesions. The hepatic veins separate the liver into the following segments: The left hepatic vein separates segment 2 from segment 3; the middle hepatic vein separates segment 4 from segments 8 (superior) and 5 (inferior); the right hepatic vein separates segments 8 and

5 from segments 7 (superior) and 6 (inferior).[1] The main right portal vein separates segment 8 from segment 5. Segment 6 is the part of the liver closest to the right kidney. Segment 4 (quadrate lobe) is separated from segments 2 and 3 by the falciform ligament. Segment 1 (caudate lobe) is bordered anteriorly by the left portal vein, posteriorly by the inferior vena cava (IVC) and laterally by the ligamentum venosum. The caudate lobe has one or more hepatic veins, which drain directly to the IVC independent of the three major hepatic veins (Fig. 9-2, A).

Axial MRI demonstrate these major vascular structures

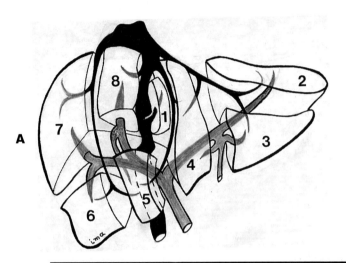

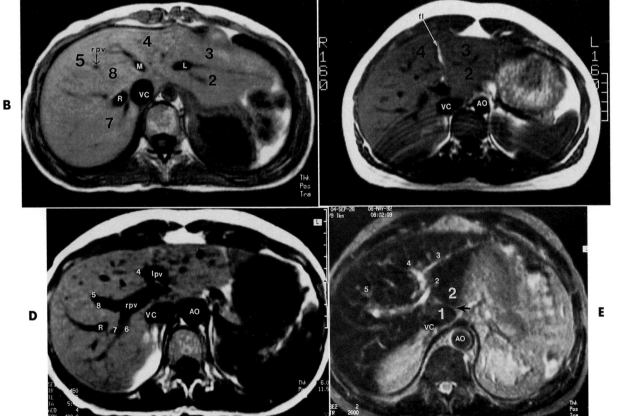

Fig. 9-2. Segmental anatomy of the liver in MRI. **A,** Hepatic segments with their hepatic and portal vein branches. The numbers represent the segments (redrawn according to Bismuth[1]). Note the direct venous drainage of the caudate lobe into the inferior vena cava. **B,** Separation of the liver segments by the hepatic veins in axial T1WI. *R,* right, *M,* middle and *L,* left hepatic veins; *rpv,* right portal vein; *VC,* vena cava; *AO,* aorta. The numbers represent the segments. **C,** The falciform ligament *(fl)* is hyperintense in T1WI due to its fat content and separates the quadrate lobe (4) from segments 2 and 3. **D,** Portal branches to the segments in T1WI. *rpv,* right portal vein; *lpv,* left portal vein; *R,* right hepatic vein. The small numbers represent the portal branches to the liver segments (*vc,* vena cava; *AO,* aorta). **E,** T2WI reveals hyperintense portal branches (flow compensation technique). Big numbers represent the segments; small numbers are the portal branches to the liver segments. The ligamentum venosum *(arrow)* separates the caudate lobe (1) from segment 2.

Fig. 9-3. Sagittal T1WI through the liver. The middle hepatic vein *(m)* is shown draining into the inferior vena cava *(VC)*. The right renal artery *(arrow rra)* is also demonstrated in this plane.

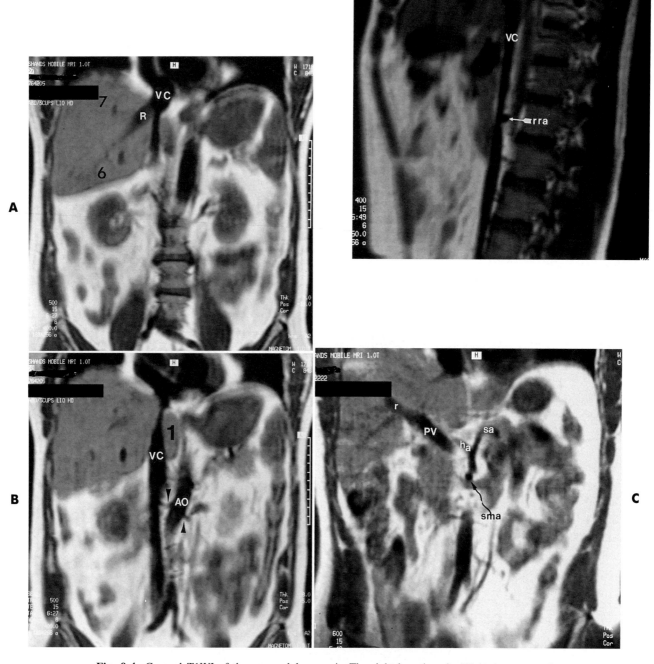

Fig. 9-4. Coronal T1WI of the upper abdomen. **A,** The right hepatic vein *(R)* is demonstrated draining into the vena cava *(CV)*. Segment 7 (superior) and 6 (inferior) are also shown. **B,** The caudate lobe *(1)* is also demonstrated in coronal plane (compare with Fig. 9-2, *A*). The renal arteries *(arrowheads)* are shown arising from the aorta *(AO)*. **C,** A section anterior to the vena cava reveals the main portal vein (PV) and its right branch *(r)*. The celiac axis also is demonstrated *(ha,* hepatic artery; *sa,* splenic artery). The arrow shows the proximal segment of the superior mesenteric artery *(sma)*.

most consistently (Fig. 9-2, *B* to *E*). Sagittal sections often show the middle hepatic vein draining into the IVC (Fig. 9-3). Coronal images demonstrate the right hepatic vein and the main portal vein with its major branches (Fig. 9-4).

The relationship of the liver to the adjacent viscera and to the thoracic cavity and diaphragm is well demonstrated in the sagittal and coronal planes. The common hepatic duct is often visible as a low-intensity, rounded structure in the liver hilus anterior to the portal vein and lateral to the hepatic artery. The intrahepatic bile ducts are usually not visible if not dilated. The gallbladder, an important landmark for liver anatomy, demonstrates different signal intensities depending upon chemical composition and concentration of bile. Usually bile in the gallbladder is hypointense in T1WI, but can be hyperintense on both

T1WI- and T2WI (Fig. 9-5) if it is filled with concentrated bile. Fluid level formation within is not uncommon. (See Chapter 11 for further discussion of biliary MRI.)

SPLEEN

The spleen is located intraperitoneally in the left upper quadrant. It normally has a smooth surface. Because of its large fractional blood content, the spleen has long T1 and T2 relaxation times[5] and produces a signal intensity isointense or hypointense to the liver in T1WI (see Fig. 9-1) and hyperintense to the liver in T2WI (with an intensity similar to that of the renal cortex) (Fig. 9-6).

The intensity of the spleen can be used as a comparative reference for metastatic liver cancer, as the signal intensities of normal splenic parenchyma and hepatic metastases are similar. The splenic artery sometimes can be seen as it

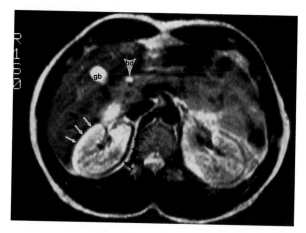

Fig. 9-5. Axial T2WI through the liver. The gallbladder *(gb)* and the common bile duct *(bd)* are seen as hyperintense structures. Note the usual chemical shift artifact in the kidneys in this sequence *(black and white arrows)*.

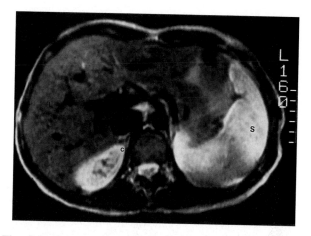

Fig. 9-6. Signal intensities of the spleen *(S)* and liver *(L)* in T2WI. The spleen is hyperintense to the liver, and its signal intensity is similar to that of the renal cortex *(c)*. The pancreas *(P)* is isointense to the liver.

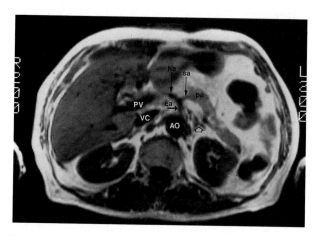

Fig. 9-7. Axial T1WI at the level of celiac axis *(ca)*. The hepatic artery *(ha)* and the splenic artery *(sa)* are seen arising from the celiac axis. The open arrow shows the left adrenal gland. *AO*, aorta; *VC*, inferior vena cava; *PV*, portal vein; *pa*, pancreas.

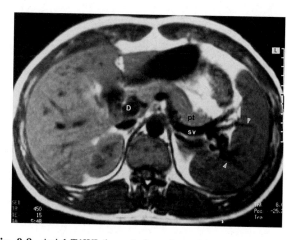

Fig. 9-8. Axial T1WI through the spleen. The splenic vein *(sv)* is seen dorsal to the pancreatic tail *(pt)*. The branches of the splenic vein are partially seen beyond the hilus *(white arrowheads)*. *D*, duodenum.

arises from the celiac axis (Fig. 9-7). The splenic vein is well imaged in spin-echo sequences as a signal void dorsal to the pancreatic body and tail. The vessels in the splenic hilus are also readily visible. However, the branches of the splenic vein can be visualized only partially beyond the hilus (Fig. 9-8).

The protocol for MR spleen examination is similar to that for the liver. Estimation of splenic size is facilitated in the coronal and sagittal planes. The relationship of the spleen to the left hemidiaphragm and to the intraperitoneal and retroperitoneal organs is also demonstrated well with multiplanar imaging. Accessory spleens sometimes can be seen; the advantage of the MRI in these cases is not only the multiplanar approach to these structures (e.g., evaluation of patients with malignant diseases) but in tissue characterization and differentiation, especially when using hepatosplenic contrast agents (such as superparamagnetic iron oxide). (See Chapter 13 for further discussion of splenic MRI.)

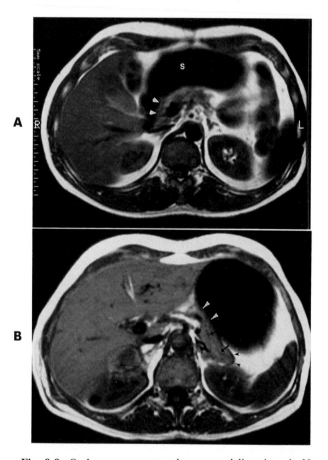

Fig. 9-9. Oral contrast agent and pancreas delineation. **A,** Negative contrast agent in the stomach *(S)* and duodenum demarcates the pancreatic head *(arrowheads)* and body. **B,** Oral contrast agent in the stomach demarcates the pancreatic body *(white arrowheads)*. Retroperitoneal fat is helpful to delineate the tail *(black arrowheads)*. The pancreatic duct is visible as a thin hypointense structure in T1WI *(arrows)*.

PANCREAS

Imaging of the pancreas has always been difficult and remains so with MRI. The pancreas is located in the retroperitoneum (anterior pararenal space) oriented with its long axis transverse to the midline and oblique to the axial plane. The normal pancreas has a homogeneous signal intensity similar to that of the liver (Fig. 9-6).[10] The splenic vein delimits the gland dorsally in the majority of individuals. The anterior margin of the pancreas is often difficult to distinguish from the adjacent gastric body and fundus. The pancreatic head is not easily delineated from the adjacent descending duodenum.

The use of enteric contrast agents, with negative or positive signal, has greatly improved delineation of the pancreas (Fig. 9-9).[3,12] On T1WI the pancreas can be well delineated when some peripancreatic retroperitoneal fat is present (as in CT). The pancreatic duct is seen as a linear structure without signal on T1WI and with high or low signal on T2WI. Recently, special MRI techniques, such as fat suppression sequences, have improved the demonstration of normal anatomy of the gland (Fig. 9-10).

Because of the orientation of the pancreas, serial axial sections are necessary to demonstrate the entire gland. Oblique planes are useful in pancreas imaging. Echo-planar imaging[9] and rapid-acquisition spin-echo techniques overcome motion artifacts and pulsation artifacts from midline vessels, which can obscure the pancreas on conventional spin-echo images.

ADRENAL GLANDS

The adrenal glands vary in configuration and may not be visible if they are thin and the perinephric fat is sparse.

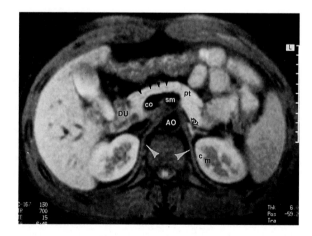

Fig. 9-10. Fat suppression technique and pancreas. The pancreas is hyperintense on this sequence; the pancreatic duct *(black arrowheads)* is visible as a hypointense structure. *Du,* duodenum; *pt,* pancreatic tail; *co,* confluence of superior mesenteric vein and splenic vein; *sm,* superior mesenteric artery; *AO,* aorta. Note the cortico *(c)*-medullary *(m)* differentiation of the kidneys and the appearance of the left adrenal *(open arrow-a)*. The white arrowheads show the diaphragmatic crura.

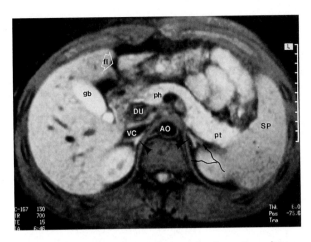

Fig. 9-11. Fat suppression technique in the retroperitoneum. Liver is hyperintense to the spleen *(SP)* and has the intensity of the pancreas. Due to fat suppression, stuctures with fat content are markedly hypointense, such as falciform ligament *(open arrow-fl)* and retroperitoneal fat. The adrenals *(black arrowheads)* are well demonstrated as intense structures. Compare the thickness of the limbs to that of the crus *(curled arrows).* *AO,* aorta; *VC,* vena cava; *DU,* duodenum; *ph,* pancreatic head; *pt,* pancreatic tail; *gb,* gallbladder.

The width of the limbs of the glands usually ranges from 2 to 4 mm. As a general rule, the thickness of the normal gland should be equal or less than the thickness of the ipsilateral crus of the hemidiaphragm. A landmark for the left adrenal gland is the splenic vein. The right adrenal gland is positioned cephalad to the upper pole of the right kidney.

The adrenals have low signal intensity on both T1WI (see Fig. 9-7) and T2WI. Using fat suppression technique, the glands can be visualized easily (Fig. 9-11). Adrenal MRI is usually performed in the axial plane. However, the coronal (see Fig. 9-14, *A*) and sagittal planes are ideal for imaging and localization of adrenal or suprarenal masses. Signal differences between the normal adrenal cortex and the medulla cannot be demonstrated with current imaging systems.

KIDNEYS

The kidneys are located in the perirenal space between the anterior renal fascia (Gerota's fascia) and the posterior renal fascia (Zuckerkandl's fascia). The left kidney usually is located 1 to 2 cm cephalad to the right.

The kidneys are well visualized on MRI.[8] The renal cortex has shorter T1 and T2 relaxation times than the renal medulla, allowing the differentiation of these two structures. On T1WI the renal cortex has less intense signal than the surrounding perinephric fat. The renal medulla, with a longer T1 relaxation time, is darker than the cortex. As a result, there is excellent corticomedullary differentiation on T1WI (see Fig. 9-1).

Renal sinus fat has a high signal on T1WI. On T2WI, the renal cortex continues to have higher signal than the medulla, although the difference is not as pronounced as on T1WI (see Fig. 9-6). The renal vessels can be easily demonstrated in MRI (as low intensity tubular structures on T1WI and high intensity structures on flow-compensated, gradient-echo sequences) (Fig. 9-12). On T1WI the renal pelvis and the ureter are hypointense (Fig. 9-13). Urine is hypointense on T1WI but becomes hyperintense on heavily T2WI. The renal fascial compartments are often outlined by adjacent fat, and Gerota's fascia can be visualized as a low-intensity line (Fig. 9-14). The coronal plane is useful in renal MRI to demonstrate the renal axis (see Fig. 9-1). Sagittal images can improve the demonstration of the renal pelvis and the proximal ureter and can display the relationship of the right kidney and the liver to better advantage than the other planes.

GASTROINTESTINAL (GI) TRACT

One of the greatest obstacles in abdominal MRI is the delineation of normal bowel. Contracted or fluid-filled bowel has signal characteristics indistinguishable from soft tissue. As a result, normal nondistended bowel is confused easily with abnormal masses. The problem can be overcome with the use of GI contrast (see Fig. 9-9). The coronal plane is useful to demonstrate the entire colon (Fig. 9-15). The sagittal plane is best for the rectosigmoid colon, as it demonstrates the relationship of the colon to other pelvic structures.

BLOOD VESSELS

With MRI the abdominal vasculature can be distinguished from other structures without contrast agent injections. In heavily T2WI, slow-flowing blood may generate signal. The celiac axis can be demonstrated easily in axial plane and is frequently well demonstrated in the coronal plane (Fig. 9-16 and see Figs. 9-4, *C* and 9-7). The splenic vein and the renal veins, with their relationship to the aorta and the superior mesenteric artery, can be nicely demonstrated in the axial (Fig. 9-12, *C* and *D*) and sagittal (Fig. 9-17) planes. MRI can depict small vascular structures that may appear isodense to lymph nodes and are poorly differentiated in suboptimal enhanced CTs. Various gradient-echo imaging techniques can be used to demonstrate flow and thus vessel patency, both in slices (see Fig. 9-12, *D*) and en bloc two- or three-dimensional MR angiography (Fig. 9-18). MRI can also demonstrate normal variants such as retroaortic left renal vein and azygos continuation.

ABDOMINAL WALL

Abdominal muscles are less intense than the liver on both T1WI and T2WI. They are usually clearly delineated by surrounding fat on T1WI. The ribs and the sternum are easily identified in upper abdominal MRI by the high intensity of bone marrow (Fig. 9-19). The vertebral bodies, *Text continues on p. 182.*

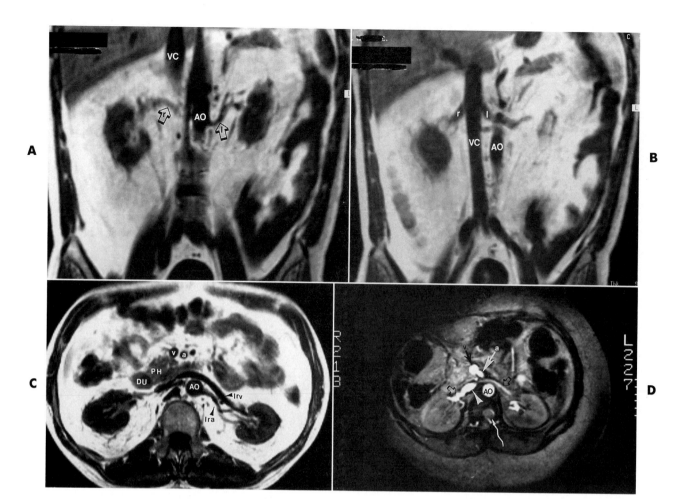

Fig. 9-12. Renal vessels in T1 and T2 sequences. **A,** Coronal T1WI through the aorta *(AO)* reveals the right *(r)* and left *(l)* renal arteries *(open arrows)*. *VC,* vena cava. **B,** Coronal plane through the inferior vena cava *(VC)* demonstrates the right *(r)* and left *(l)* renal veins draining into the vena cava. *AO,* aorta. **C,** Axial T1WI at the level of the renal hilus reveals the renal vessels as hypointense structures. *AO,* aorta; *lrv,* left renal vein; *lra,* left renal artery; *v,* superior mesenteric vein; *a,* superior mesenteric artery; *PH,* pancreatic head; *DU,* duodenum. **D,** Gradient-echo imaging in axial plane at the level of renal hilus. The vessels are hyperintense. The renal veins *(open arrows)* are shown draining into the inferior vena cava *(white arrowhead)*. The superior mesenteric artery *(a-white arrow)* and vein *(v-black arrow)* are also demonstrated. Note the typical artifact *(curled white arrow)* produced by the pulsations of the aorta *(AO)*.

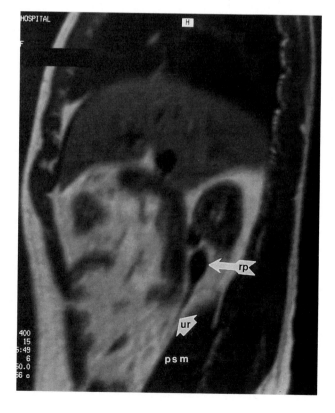

Fig. 9-13. Sagittal T1WI of the right kidney. The renal pelvis *(rp)* and the ureter *(ur)* are hypointense. Note the relationship of the right kidney to the liver and the course of the ureter in front of the psoas muscle *(psm)*.

Fig. 9-14. Gerota's fascia. **A,** Coronal T1WI through the kidneys showing the proximal ureter *(open arrow)* and Gerota's fascia *(arrows)* on the left. Note that the crus of the left hemidiaphragm extends down to the level of the renal hilum *(arrowheads)*. The curved arrow shows the normal right adrenal *(psm, psoas muscle)*. **B,** Sagittal T1WI through the right kidney demonstrates Gerota's fascia as a thin hypointense line *(arrows)*.

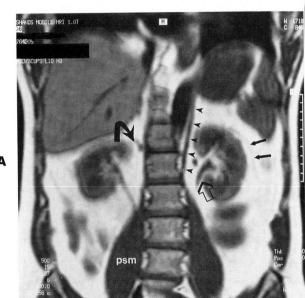

A

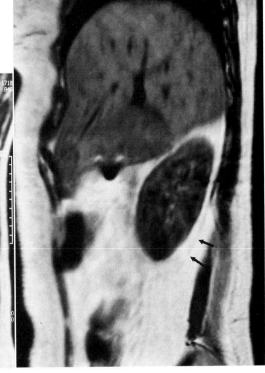

B

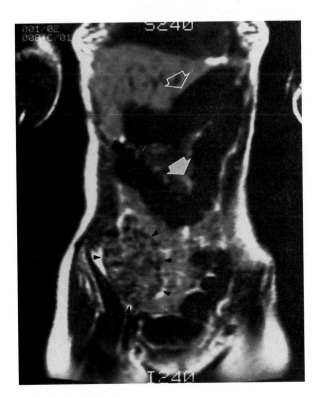

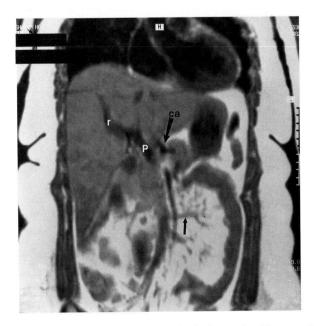

Fig. 9-15. GI MRI contrast and bowel delineation. Negative oral MR contrast delineates the stomach *(open white arrow)* and the transverse colon *(closed white arrow)* on this coronal T1WI. Nonopacified bowel can mimick intraabdominal mass *(arrowheads)*.

Fig. 9-16. Coronal T1WI and abdominal vessels. The portal vein *(p)* and its right main branch *(r)* are clearly demonstrated. A left colic vein *(arrow)* receiving branches from the splenic flexure and the descending colon is also seen. The celiac axis *(ca)* branching into hepatic and splenic arteries can be identified in the center of the image.

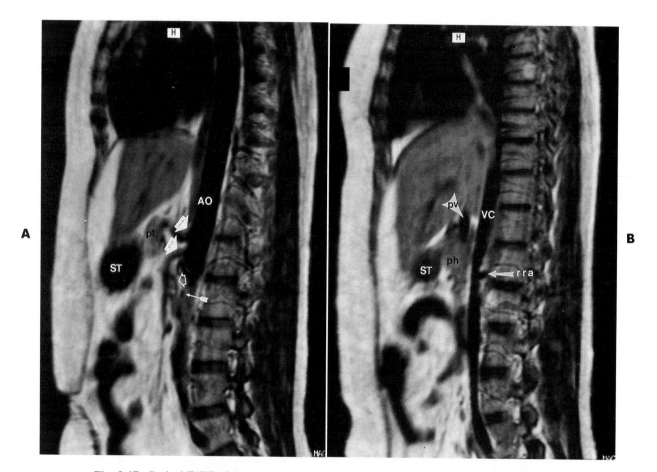

Fig. 9-17. Sagittal T1WI of the descending aorta *(AO)* and the inferior vena cava *(VC)*. **A,** Section through the aorta shows the origins of the celiac axis *(white arrow 1)* and superior mesenteric artery *(white arrow 2)*. The pancreatic tail *(pt)* is seen posterior to the stomach *(ST)*. The duodenum *(open white arrow)* and left renal vein *(small white arrow)* course between the superior mesenteric artery and aorta. **B,** Section through the inferior vena cava. The pancreatic head *(ph)* is between the portal vein *(pv-white arrowhead)* and stomach *(ST)*. *(rra,* right renal artery).

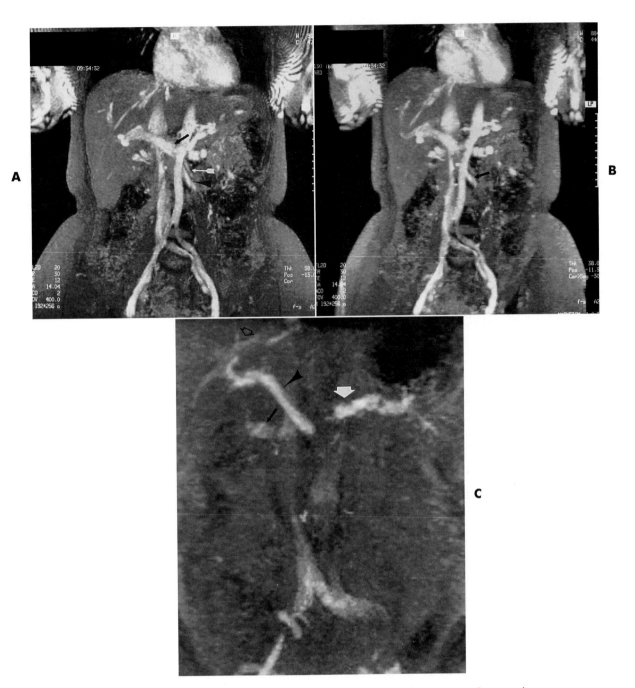

Fig. 9-18. MR angiography of the abdomen. **A,** Both arterial flow and venous flow are shown. The left renal artery *(white arrow)* and the superior mesenteric artery *(arrowhead)* are seen arising from the aorta. The splenic vein *(arrow)* enters the portal vein. Note volume averaging with the aorta. **B,** A left posterior oblique view of the same study better demonstrates the origin of the superior mesenteric artery *(arrow)*. **C,** MR angiogram to evaluate venous flow. A spatial presaturation zone was placed above the diaphragm to eliminate signal from high velocity arterial flow. This image demonstrates flow in the inferior vena cava, hepatic veins *(open black arrow)*, right renal vein *(arrow)*, portal vein *(arrowhead)*, and splenic vein *(white arrow)*. Minimal residual signal is present in the aorta.

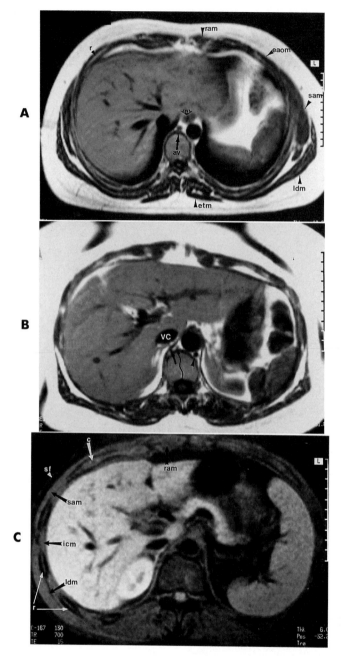

although not of major interest in body imaging, can some-times be used as landmarks for the intraabdominal organs.

REFERENCES

1. Bismuth H: Surgical anatomy and anatomical surgery of the liver, World J Surg 6:3-9, 1982.
2. Bradley WG: Flow phenomena. In Stark DD, Bradley WG, editors: Magnetic resonance imaging, 1988, Mosby–Year Book.
3. Burton SS, Ros PR, Otto PM, et al: Barium MR imaging of the pancreas: initial experience (abstract), Radiology 173(P):517, 1989.
4. Davis PL, Hricak H, Bradley WG: Magnetic resonance imaging of the adrenal glands, Radiol Clin North Am 22:891, 1984.
5. Ehman RL, Kjos BO, Hricak H, et al: Relative intensity of abdominal organs in MR images, J Comput Assist Tomogr 9:315, 1985.
6. Fisher MR, Wall SD, Hricak H, et al: Hepatic vascular anatomy on magnetic resonance imaging, Am J Roentgenol 144: 739-746, 1985.
7. Gazelle GS, Haaga JR: Hepatic neoplasms: surgically relevant segmental anatomy and imaging techniques, Am J Roentgenol 158: 1015-1018.
8. LiPuma JP: Magnetic resonance imaging of the kidney, Radiol Clin North Am 22:925, 1984.
9. Reimer P, Saini S, Hahn PF, et al: Techniques for high-resolution echo-planar imaging of the pancreas, Radiology 182:175-179, 1992.
10. Stark DD: Biliary system, pancreas, spleen and alimentary tract. In Stark DD, Bradley WG, editors: Magnetic resonance imaging, 1988, Mosby–Year Book.
11. Stark DD: Magnetic resonance imaging of the upper abdomen: technical advances. In Taveras JM, Ferrucci JT, editors: Radiology diagnosis—imaging—intervention, Philadelphia, 1987, Lippincott.
12. Weinreb JC, Maravilla KR, Redman HC, et al: Improved MR imaging of the upper abdomen with glucagon and gas, J Comput Assist Tomogr 8:835, 1984.

Fig. 9-19. Abdominal wall. **A,** Axial T1WI through the liver. The esophagus *(open arrow-e)* and the azygos vein *(arrow-av)* are shown. The rectus abdominis muscle *(ram),* the external abdominal oblique muscle *(eaom),* the serratus anterior muscle *(sam),* the latissimus dorsi muscle *(ldm),* and the erector trunci muscles *(etm)* are well demonstrated. The ribs *(r)* are recognized from their high intensity signal. **B,** In this axial T1WI the azygos vein *(arrow),* the hemiazygos vein *(arrowhead)* and the thoracic duct *(curled arrow)* are demonstrated *(VC,* vena cava). **C,** Fat suppression technique and the abdominal wall. Note that musculature and ribs *(r)* are hypointense, and cartilage *(c)* is more intense than ribs. Subcutaneous fat *(sf)* is markedly hypointense *(ldm,* latissimus dorsi muscle; *icm,* intercostal muscle; *sam,* serratus anterior muscle; *ram,* rectus abdominis muscle).

Chapter 10

LIVER

Liver imaging techniques
Hemangioma
Benign tumors and tumorlike conditions
Malignant liver tumors
Hepatic metastasis
Focal infectious processes
Vascular diseases
Diffuse diseases

Section one
Liver imaging techniques

Christophoros Stoupis
Pablo R. Ros

Motion reduction
Spin-echo imaging
Gradient-echo imaging
Inversion recovery
Phase contrast
Future directions

The magnetic resonance imaging (MRI) technique for the liver is similar to the one in other areas of the abdomen. However, because of special characteristics in this large, solid organ located immediately below the diaphragm and heart, selection of an ideal imaging technique is still controversial.

Although MRI of the liver is used primarily to detect focal liver lesions, especially tumors, a unique scheme for imaging techniques cannot be given, as, in an ideal liver MRI study, not only do masses have to be differentiated from normal liver but also portal vein and hepatic veins have to be visualized, lesions seen by other imaging techniques have to be characterized, and motion control has to be considered (see accompanying box). It is obvious that if an ideal MRI study has to achieve all the goals described in the accompanying box, compromises must be made to obtain an optimal study within a reasonable time. The best techniques are those that produce great anatomic resolu-

tion, offering sufficient contrast and signal-to-noise ratio (SNR).

The major factors needed to produce a good MRI scan of the liver are (1) the T1 and T2 relaxation time differences between normal liver and lesion, (2) the parameters used for pulsing sequences, and (3) imaging artifacts. Only selection of pulsing sequences can be controlled. The relaxation differences between normal and abnormal tissue depend on the particular lesion to be studied, and the presence of image artifacts depends on patient cooperation. Nevertheless, in each system, and depending on the particular field strength and software produced by different manufacturers, an array of motion-reducing techniques is currently available, which can be used to decrease some of the motion artifacts that has plagued abdominal MRI.

It is also important to spend time to optimize pulsing sequences that can improve image contrast. In addition, it is advisable to have several slightly different protocols that consider the major goal of the particular study and the overall patient's condition (i.e., ascites, dyspnea, dysrhythmia, encephalopathy, etc.). Modifications of the technique should be considered if the objective of the study is to detect potential lesions (i.e., staging of oncologic patients), characterize a lesion detected by other imaging techniques (i.e., hemangioma versus other focal lesions), or visualize vessels (e.g., thrombosis of hepatic veins or portal vein).

This section reviews the major techniques available to study the liver by MRI by major pulsing sequences. However, it is likely that in a particular patient a combination

---

Goals for ideal liver imaging technique

- Maximization of lesion detection
- Characterization of detected lesions
- Vessel patency (hepatic veins, portal vein)
- Differentiation between vessel and lesion
- Motion reduction

of pulsing sequences (e.g., spin-echo plus gradient-echo, spin-echo plus fat suppression) would be performed.

MOTION REDUCTION

Motion can be reduced in several ways when performing MRI of the liver (see accompanying box). All of these techniques have advantages and disadvantages.

Increasing the number of excitations is one of the earlier "tricks" used to produce better images (Fig. 10-1). However, this method increases the length of the examination, and the longer pulsing sequence (T2-weighted images [T2WI]) is likely to result in voluntary motion of the patient, which will end produce poor quality images.

Respiratory ordered phase-encoding (ROPE) is used routinely in some software programs. ROPE decreases "ghosting" but increases blurring, which also may counteract the effectiveness of this motion-reduction technique.

The use of saturation pulses, initially designed to reduce vascular artifacts (Fig. 10-2), has proved effective and relatively easy and inexpensive (regarding time penalty) to reduce motion in the abdomen. Superior and infe-

---

Motion reduction techniques

- Increase number of excitations (NEX)
- Respiratory ordered phase-encoding (ROPE)
- Saturation pulses
- Flow compensation (gradient moment nulling)
- Fat suppression

---

rior saturation planes are used routinely to reduce vascular artifacts, but an anterior saturation plane will also reduce the "ghosting" produced by the fat in the anterior abdominal wall. This technique is used routinely by many centers. Saturation pulses are primarily used in T2WI where motion is more marked and also where elimination of few images invested in the saturation pulses is not as essential as in T1-weighted images (T1WI), where the number of images produced is inherently small.

Flow compensation, or gradient moment nulling (GMN), another technique developed to reduce vascular

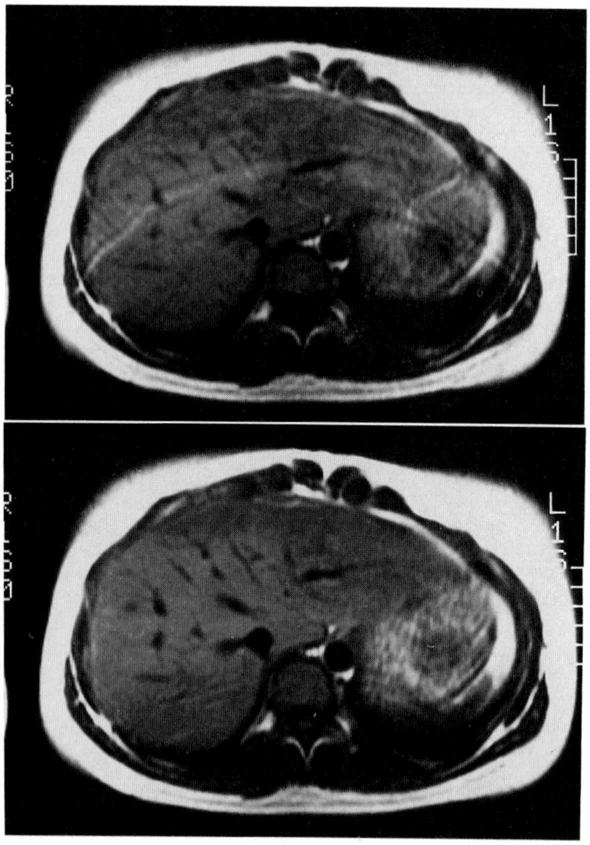

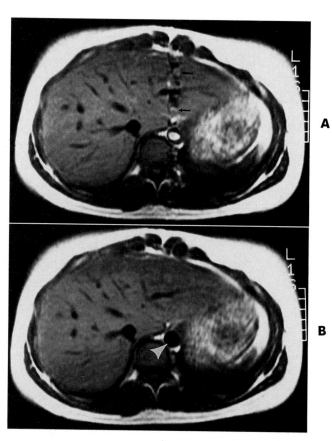

Fig. 10-1. Effect of varying number of excitations (NEX) on image quality. **A,** Axial T1WI of the liver (TR 300 msec/TE 20 msec) performed with 2 NEX. **B,** Image at the same level performed with 4 NEX (other image parameters unchanged) demonstrates overall better image quality when compared with **A.** Note superior delineation of the hepatic vessels and lack of artifacts.

Fig. 10-2. Use of saturation pulses on vascular artifacts. **A,** Axial T1WI (TR 300 msec/TE 20 msec/4 NEX) without saturation pulse shows typical aortic ghosting artifact on the left lobe of the liver *(arrows).* **B,** With the additional superior saturation pulse (other image parameters unchanged) aortic ghosting is suppressed. The aorta is now black *(white arrowhead).*

artifacts, has had unexpected success in reducing motion in the abdomen. Flow compensation renders vessels "bright" while reducing motion artifacts (Fig. 10-3). Its application to the liver has been slightly more controversial than in other abdominal areas, as all liver vessels become "bright" and somewhat more difficult to distinguish from small focal lesions. With experience, however, it is easy to learn the normal distribution of hepatic vessels and the use of flow compensation, and its benefit in reducing motion takes precedence over potential confusion between vessel and lesion, which can be solved with T1WI and/or gradient-echo images.

Finally, fat saturation decreases "ghosting" because it renders fat "dark" and thus less susceptible to respiratory motion (Fig. 10-4). Cardiac gating is not used routinely to evaluate the liver. To reduce motion, simple "tricks" can be used such as placing a restraining band in the upper abdomen, using an anteroposterior direction for phase-encoding.

SPIN-ECHO IMAGING

Conventional spin-echo imaging remains the basic staple for the study of the liver, as well as the rest of the body. Ideally, the best contrast is obtained in T1WI when the repetition time (TR) chosen is less than the T1-relaxation time of the lesion. The majority of T1-relaxation times in liver lesions ranges between 250 and 500 msec. The fact that the T1-relaxation time of lesions varies with the magnetic field strength should be considered, but this range includes the majority of lesion relaxation times at the available magnetic fields.

Choice of echo time (TE) is also important and, in general, the shortest possible TE (ideally less than 20 msec) should be obtained to minimize contribution from T2 in image and to reduce motion artifacts.[5] An additional advantage of using short TE is the increased number of sections with the same TR.

Generally, in T1WI, liver lesions appear hypointense relative to normal liver. Because vascular structures also appear hypointense to flow void, it sometimes may be difficult to distinguish small hepatic lesions from vessels.

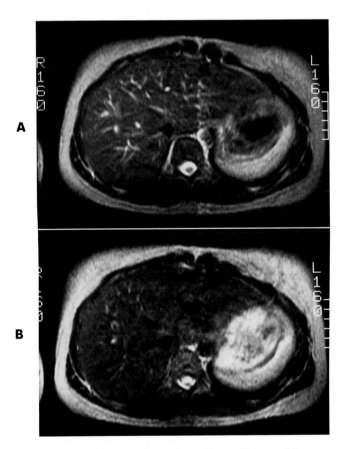

Fig. 10-3. Reduction of vascular artifacts with use of flow compensation. **A,** T2WI (TR 1800 msec/TE 90 msec) with flow compensation technique. The hepatic vessels appear bright. At this level, hepatic vein branches appear longitudinal and portal branches are small, round, bright, and difficult to differentiate from lesions. **B,** Same image parameters without flow compensation technique. The vessels are isointense or hypointense. However, the overall image quality is inferior when compared to **A** due to motion artifacts.

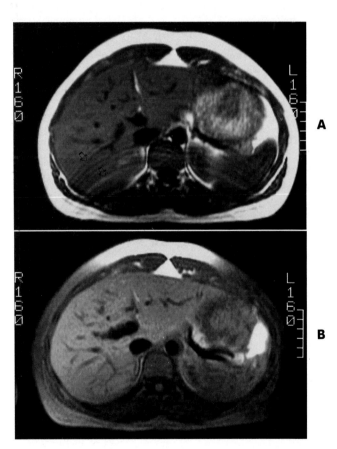

Fig. 10-4. Fat saturation technique. **A,** Spin-echo T1WI (TR 300 msec/TE 20 msec/4 NEX). Typical ghosting artifacts from subcutaneous fat *(open arrows)* due to motion. **B,** Fat saturation technique (other parameters unchanged) produces marked decrease of these artifacts because the signal intensity of fat is markedly reduced.

SE T2WIs are obtained with long TR and TE. With this technique the majority of focal liver lesions are hyperintense due to the increase of free water within them. In T2WI, vascular structures remain hypointense due to flow void and may be distinguished from small hepatic lesions in comparison with T1WI. If flow compensation (or GMN) is used in T2WI, however, vessels will be hyperintense as lesions, and gradient-echo imaging techniques

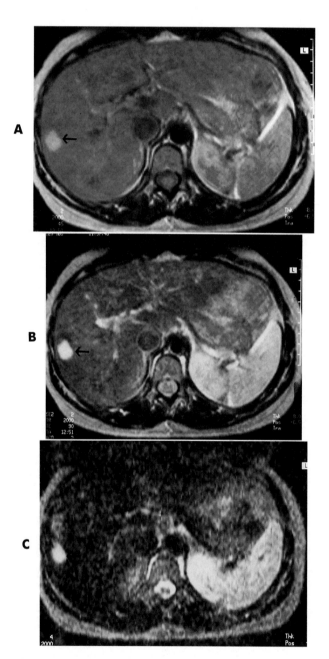

Fig. 10-5. Multiple echo T2 spin-echo technique used to characterize a solitary lesion as benign (hemangioma). **A,** TR 2000 msec/TE 45 msec. **B,** TR 2000 msec/TE 90 msec. **C,** TR 2000 msec/TE 180 msec. Typical appearance of hemangioma *(arrows)* with "light bulb" sign. With increased TE the intensity of the hemangioma increases proportionally.

have to be used to differentiate between vessels and small focal abnormalities. The usual TR used is long—between 2000 and 2500 msec, which produce a large amount of artifacts and poor SNR. Nevertheless, the benefits of being able to confirm lesions with this technique and to characterize some of these lesions as hemangiomas make the use of spin-echo T2WI an essential component of liver MRI.

As stated earlier, because T2WI is an excellent tool for tissue characterization between hemangioma and malignant tumors, a different technique will be used when the major goal of a study is to characterize a lesion detected by another imaging technique. In these cases, a multiple echo (ME) pulse sequence will be used with increasing TE times with at least three steps (i.e., 45, 90, 120, 180) to allow discrimination between malignant lesions and hemangioma (Fig. 10-5). It is well known that on heavily T2WI with a TE of 120 to 180 msec, hemangioma will increase its intensity, whereas metastases will not. In addition, the "blooming" of hemangiomas at these very high TEs will "erase" inhomogeneities due to fibrosis seen in lower TEs. SNR also increases between malignancy and liver, improving the conspicuity of lesions when the TE increases from 60 to 120 msec.[11]

In general, for both T1 and T2 spin-echo images, a maximum thickness of 10 mm is recommended, with a 2 mm gap between slices. If there is a low index of suspicion for liver abnormalities, some centers perform 15 mm sections with a 2 mm gap.

GRADIENT-ECHO IMAGING

The main use of gradient-echo imaging in the liver is delineation of vessels and determination of their patency.[4] The use of a low FLIP angle (less than 30 degrees) is recommended for better image quality because "ghosting" occurs with larger FLIP angles.[14] Although the major advantage of gradient-echo imaging is its short time of acquisition, which allows combination with suspended respiration for true motion-free images of the abdomen, severe drawbacks have not allowed the widespread use of gradient echo as the sole technique for the liver.[3,15] Some of the disadvantages of gradient-echo imaging are its poor tissue contrast and high sensitivity to field inhomogeneities. With poor tissue contrast, in comparison with spin-echo imaging, gradient-echo imaging is not useful for either lesion detection or characterization.

Because of its speed, gradient-echo imaging has been used in combination with the intravenous administration of gadopentetate dimeglumine, as perfusion of tumors (in particular, to differentiate hemangioma from other hepatic neoplasms) can be followed in a timely manner with gradient-echo images.

The acronyms for gradient-echo pulsing sequences vary, depending on the manufacturer, and terms such as GRASS, FLASH, and FISP have been used, making gradient-echo terminology somewhat confusing. The most

Table 10-1. Gradient-echo sequences

Manufacturer's acronym	Name	Main feature
FLASH (Siemens)	Fast low angle shot	Prototype for GRE sequences
GRASS (GE)	Gradient recalled acquisition in the steady state	Free induction decay of steady-state signal sample
FISP (Siemens)	Fast imaging with steady-state processing	Similar to GRASS
CE-FAST (Picker)	Contrast-enhanced fast scan	Steady-state GE sampled (not FID)
MP-GR (GE)	Multiplanar GRASS	Combination of GRASS + multiecho + multiplanar
SP-GR	Spoiled GRASS	T1 contrast predominance
		T2 contrast eliminated

Key: GRE = gradient echo
     FID = free induction decay
Modified from Tanabe J: Introduction to fast MRI, Appl Radiol No. 20 (March 1992), 13-17.

common gradient-echo pulsing sequences and its variants are listed in Table 10-1.[13]

INVERSION RECOVERY

Inversion recovery techniques are primarily T1 techniques, and the contrast depends on the inversion time (TI).[1] The choice of TI is related to the T1 relaxation time of the tissue of interest. Therefore, because nonvascular liver metastases have a T1 of approximately 500 msec, a standard inversion recovery technique that has been successful at demonstrating liver metastases at 1.5 T, will have a TI of 500 to 600 msec.[8] To maximize contrast between lesions and normal liver, it is possible to find a particular TI so that the normal liver signal is suppressed, thereby enhancing the appearance of lesions.[7]

Although standard TI techniques have been practically abandoned, as they are lengthy and produce images of poorer quality than spin-echo sequences, a modification of inversion recovery technique, the so-called short inversion time recovery (STIR) has been useful for liver MRI. STIR sequences provide high contrast images of the liver with relatively little motion degradation.[1,2]

Using STIR, the signal from fat can be reduced to zero, and soft tissue lesions that have an increased T2 will not be confused with fat. Lesions appear hyperintense, as the effect of T1 and T2 relaxation times on soft tissue contrast is additive. STIR is a promising sequence for liver imaging because a significant but opposite degree of T1 and T2 contrast is present between lesions and normal liver, and therefore most lesions are enhanced with this "opposing" imaging technique.

PHASE CONTRAST

Conventional pulsing sequences are based on in-phase imaging. However, opposed-phase imaging techniques for both SE and inversion recovery have been name phase-contrast imaging. Phase-contrast techniques differ from conventional techniques only by decreasing the signal intensity from tissues containing both water and fat.[12] For instance, fatty liver appears hyperintense in phase-contrast images because it contains both fat and water. Spleen and focal malignancies, however, do not remain hyperintense in phase-contrast images, unlike in conventional T2WI, because they do not contain a mixture of fat and water.

T1-weighted opposed-phase images are not suggested for liver malignancies because the intensity of both the normal and malignant liver decreases. However, phase-contrast techniques may be used in T1 to exclude fatty liver.

In patients with fatty liver, T1-weighted opposed-phase images demonstrate marked improvement in SNR for liver metastases and can be valuable for screening in patients with fatty liver and malignancy.[12]

It is apparent that as the majority of metastases are devoid of fat (with the exception of liposarcoma), metastases appear hyperintense in comparison with fatty liver when opposed-phase T2WI is used with greater sensitivity than in-phase or conventional T2WI.[10]

FUTURE DIRECTIONS

It is obvious that high-speed MRI, ultrafast MRI, rapid acquisitions spin echo (RASE), and fast spin-echo techniques will change the face of MRI of the abdomen, and in particular, of the liver. Echo-planar imaging, Instascan, GRASS (a gradient SE hybridization sequence), and others will be available for general use in the future. As with the initial experience with gradient echo, these techniques will have to face the well-established conventional spin-echo techniques.[6,9] (See Chapter 2 for a description of some of these high-speed MRI sequences.) The major advantage of fast scanning is reduction in motion; however, contrast-to-noise ratio (CNR) and SNR is at best comparable to that of standard T1WI and T2WI.

It is apparent that in the future, with developments occurring in magnetic resonance angiography (MRA), the ideal evaluation of the liver may consist of fast MR scanning for the study of the liver parenchyma, as well as MRA for the study of the portal and hepatic vascular systems. A time frame for these two techniques is comparable to that for current computed tomography (CT) and has similar spatial and contrast resolution. This technique may become the ideal preoperative work-up, with conventional spin echo and CT scan performed when questions arise after completion of fast MRI and MRA of the liver.

REFERENCES

 1. Bydder GM, Young IR: MR imaging: clinical use of the inversion recovery sequence, J Comput Assist Tomogr 9(4):659-675, 1985.
 2. Bydder GM, Steiner RE, Blumgart LH, et al: MR imaging of the liver using short T1 inversion recovery sequences, J Comput Assist Tomogr 9(6):1084-1089, 1985.
 3. Edelman RR, Hahn PF, Buxton R, et al: Rapid MR imaging with suspended respiration: clinical application in the liver, Radiology 161:125-131, 1986.
 4. Gehl H, Bohndorf K, Klose K-C, et al: Two-dimensional MR angiography in the evaluation of abdominal veins with gradient refocused sequences, J Comput Assist Tomogr 14(4):619-624, 1990.
 5. Mitchell DG, Vinitski S, Soponaro S, et al: Liver and pancreas: improved spin-echo T1 contrast by shorter echo time and fat suppression at 1.5 T, Radiology 178:67-71, 1991.
 6. Mitchell DG: Rapid-acquisition spin-echo MR imaging of the liver: a critical view, Radiology 179:609-614, 1991.
 7. Paling MR, Abbitt PL, Mugler JP, et al: Liver metastases: optimization of MR imaging pulse sequences at 1.0 T, Radiology 167:695-699, 1988.
 8. Reinig JW, Dwyer AJ, Miller DL, et al: Liver metastases: detection with MR imaging at 0.5 and 1.5 T, Radiology 170:149-153, 1989.
 9. Riederer SJ: High-speed MR assists in abdominal diagnoses, Diagn Imaging 149-167, 1991.
10. Rummeny E, Saini S, Stack DD, et al: Detection of hepatic metastases with MR imaging: spin-echo vs phase-contrast pulse sequences at 0.6 T, Am J Roentgenol 153:1207-1211, 1989.
11. Stark DD, Wittenberg D, Edelman RR, et al: Detection of hepatic metastases by magnetic resonance: analysis of pulse sequence performance, Radiology 159:365-370, 1986.
12. Stark DD, Wittenberg J, Middleton MS, et al: Liver metastases: detection by phase-contrast MR imaging, Radiology 158:327-332, 1986.
13. Tanabe J: Introduction to fast MRI, Appl Radiol 13(5), March 1992, 13-17.
14. Teitelbaum GP, Ortega HV, Vinitski S, et al: Optimization of gradient-echo imaging parameters for intracaval filters and trapped thromboemboli, Radiology 174:1013-1019, 1990.
15. Winkler ML, Thoeni RF, Luh N, et al: Hepatic neoplasia: breathhold MR imaging, Radiology 170:801-806, 1989.

Section two
Hemangioma

Pablo R. Ros

Technique
Typical hemangioma
Atypical hemangioma
Hemagioma vs other focal masses
Comparison of MRI with other imaging techniques
Current role of MRI in work-up of hemangioma

Hemangioma is one of the most successfully studied lesions with MRI in the liver. The work-up of hepatic hemangiomas constitutes one of the major applications of MRI in the upper abdomen. From early reports it has been well known that hemangioma has the potential of being characterized with MRI due to both its unusual high intensity in T2WI and some morphologic criteria.[19] Hemangioma and metastases are the most common indications for MRI of the liver. Due to their incidence and clinical importance, each is covered in a separate section in this chapter.

This section on hemangioma includes technique considerations, features of both typical and atypical hemangiomas, key differential points between hemangioma and other focal masses by MRI, a comparison of MRI with other imaging techniques, and the current role of MRI in the work-up of hemangiomas.

TECHNIQUE

The technique for studying hemangioma of the liver has evolved since 1985, along with the evolution of MRI itself. From the basic spin-echo techniques, the evolution has included the application of gradient-echo and liver contrasts.

Since 1985, it has been known that the unique property of hemangioma in MRI has been its high SNR in heavily weighted T2WI.[19] Therefore, the units in 1985 used spin-echo technique with TR of 2000 msec and TE of 120 msec with contiguous 1.5 cm thick sections, 128 × 256 matrix and 4 NEX.[19] This initial technique has proved successful and is still performed as the main staple to diagnose hemangioma of the liver, with high yield in both sensitivity and specificity with state-of-the-art equipment[6] (Fig. 10-6). T1WI are also routinely performed, although the information provided (hypointensity compared to normal liver) is nonspecific and similar to many other focal lesions of the liver. In addition, T1WI are inferior to T2WI in the detection of small hemangiomas because in T1WI small hemangiomas have a similar appearance to hepatic vessels.[18]

Gradient-echo sequences have been used to diagnose hemangioma. Like T1WI, gradient-echo technique is sig-

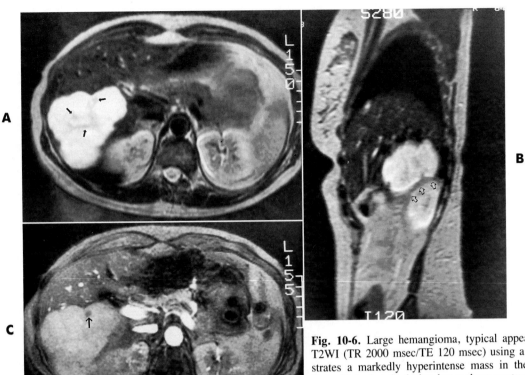

Fig. 10-6. Large hemangioma, typical appearance. **A,** Heavily T2WI (TR 2000 msec/TE 120 msec) using a 1.5 T unit demonstrates a markedly hyperintense mass in the right lobe of the liver. Note that the lesion has a sharp contour, is lobulated, and although it extends to the surface of the liver, does not produce an abnormality of contour. Note also that within the hemangioma there are hypointense areas, corresponding to fibrosis *(arrows)*. **B,** Sagittal T2WI confirms the lack of deformity of the contour of the liver. The renal-hepatic margin *(open arrows)* is undisturbed by the presence of the large hemangioma. **C,** Gradient echo fails to demonstrate flow within hemangioma. Note that the areas of fibrosis are seen with slightly lower intensity than the hemangioma *(arrow)*, but no vessels are seen within the hemangioma, as the flow through the tumor is very slow and without arteriovenous shunting.

nificantly inferior to spin-echo T2WI because of its reduced CNR (due to shorter acquisition time) and incomplete suppression of motion artifacts. However, certain gradient-echo images, with their property of single slice breath-hold capability, have been used to complement findings obtained with spin-echo T2 values to diagnose hemangioma.[16]

Tumor-to-liver signal ratio between hemangioma and primary hepatocellular carcinoma (HCC) seems to benefit not only from measurements in T2WI, but also from measurements obtained with gradient-echo (FLASH) images. As stated earlier, the major advantage of FLASH techniques to spin-echo T2WI is its speed with the capability of breath-hold images. As demonstrated by Ohtomo,[16] FLASH technique is helpful to distinguish small hemangiomas (smaller than 2 cm) from malignancy.

With state-of-the-art equipment, attempts have been made to establish the optimal spin-echo T2WI technique to provide the highest sensitivity and specificity for hemangioma. Choi et al[5] has tested a T2-weighted pulsing sequence of TR 2000 msec and variable TEs increasing from 60 to 180 msec (60, 90, 120, 150, and 180 msec). In a series of 38 hemangiomas analyzed with a 2 T superconducting magnet, the technique with highest sensitivity to detect hemangioma was TR 2000 msec/TE 60 msec.[5]

However, the best technique for characterization was TR 2000 msec/TE 180 msec, but no statistical difference was noted between TR 2000 msec/TE 180 msec and TR 2000 msec/TE 150 msec. Therefore, use of a TR of 2000 msec with TE of 60 and 150 msec is recommended. A technique composed of a 128 × 256 matrix, slice thickness of 8 mm, intersection gap of 2 mm, and 2 NEX was used.

The application of gadopentetate dimeglumine has also been used to increase the specificity of MRI for the study of hemangiomas. As routinely demonstrated in angiography, dynamic CT, and red blood cell scintigraphic studies, one of the hallmarks of hemangiomas is a very prolonged and delayed enhancement due to its unique lack of intratumoral shunting. The advent of gradient-echo images has made it possible to harvest this property of hemangioma by performing dynamic-gradient-echo image postintravenous injection of gadopentetate dimeglumine to differentiate hemangioma from other focal liver masses, primarily malignancies.[21] Gradient-echo (FLASH) images are obtained without contrast injection, selecting the section that best demonstrates the abnormality. At that level, repeated FLASH images are performed after administering a bolus injection of gadopentetate dimeglumine (.05 mmol/kg). After the first minute, images are performed at a rate of two images per minute for the first 5 minutes, followed by one image per minute for 10 minutes.

Another technique has been to perform both spin-echo T2WI and gradient-echo T1WI before contrast administration, followed by gradient-echo T1WI post-gadopentetate dimeglumine administration (Fig. 10-7). A typical gradient-echo T1WI of TR 315 msec/TE 14 msec and FLIP angle of 90 degrees has been described with a total duration of 10.2 sec data acquisition.[8] In this particular series where 14 hemangiomas were studied with dynamic MRI with gadopentetate dimeglumine and compared with 15

metastases, images were obtained at 30-second intervals in the first 5 minutes and at 60-second intervals between 5 and 10 minutes. Delayed postcontrast studies were performed at 11 minutes and 60 minutes. However, late postcontrast images at 60 minutes did not yield any diagnostic information.

The typical appearance of hemangiomas is that of peripheral contrast enhancement with subsequent hyperintense fill-in. In delayed postcontrast examination at 11 minutes, hemangiomas present a high and usually homogeneous intensity with contrast between tumor and liver. It appears that the use of gadopentetate dimeglumine may be helpful to further characterize hemangiomas and decrease the overlap between hemangioma and some hypervascular metastases, as will be discussed later.

In summary, hemangioma of the liver should be studied

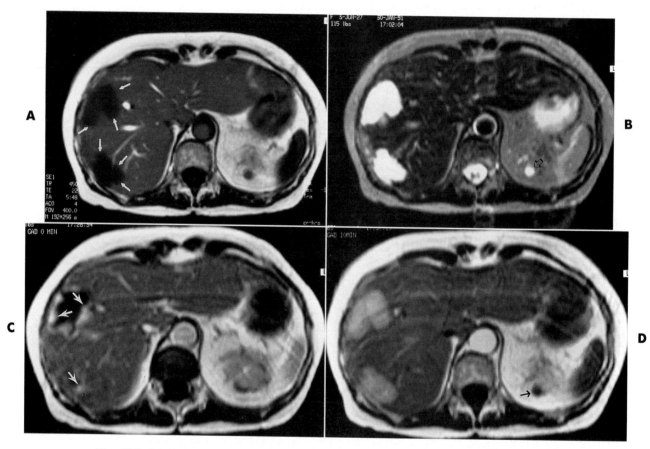

Fig. 10-7. Multiple hemangiomata before and after gadopentetate dimeglumine injection (1.0 T unit). **A,** Spin-echo (TR 450 msec/TE 22 msec) demonstrates two markedly hypointense well-defined areas in the right lobe *(white arrows).* This is the typical appearance on T1WI of hemangioma. **B,** T2WI (TR 2500 msec/TE 180 msec) demonstrates the "light bulb" sign of hemangioma with both tumors being homogeneous and markedly hyperintense. Note some of the typical morphologic findings of hemangiomas such as sharp contour, lobulated edges, and lack of deformity of the liver. Incidentally noted is a cyst in the upper pole of the left kidney *(open arrow).* **C,** T1WI obtained immediately after injection of gadopentetate dimeglumine demonstrates peripheral enhancement in the margin of both tumors *(white arrows),* similar to that seen typically in hemangioma in iodine-enhanced CT. **D,** Delayed MRI 10 minutes postcontrast injection demonstrates complete filling of the two hemangiomas with persistence of the gadopentetate dimeglumine within the tumor. Note that there is no enhancement in the left kidney cyst *(arrow).*

not only with T1WI but also with T2WI with extended TE. A T2 pulsing sequence that includes at least 3 TE values (i.e., 40, 80, and 120 msec or 45, 90, and 180 msec) is imperative. Likewise, the possibility of injection of gadopentetate dimeglumine should be considered. A dynamic MRI study is recommended, particularly when it is necessary to differentiate hemangioma from hypervascular metastases.

TYPICAL HEMANGIOMA

Typically, a hemangioma is a markedly hyperintense focal lesion in T2WI and markedly hypointense in T1WI. This appearance is caused by the hemangioma's multiple vascular channels, which are filled with red blood cells. There is minimal fibrous stroma; therefore, hemangiomas behave like a primarily blood-filled mass, with blood slowly flowing through the vascular channels. Thus, hemangiomas act like cystic masses as the blood is slowly moving and not capable of producing flow void. On the other hand, the blood is not extravasated and does not behave like a hematoma or other blood collections.

Hemangiomas have been defined as spherical or ovoid, with smooth and well-defined margins and with a homogeneous appearance on T2WI.[11,19] With this basic criteria, in one of the initial papers describing hemangioma, Stark et al[19] found that 25 of 30 hemangiomas complied with the preceding criteria, yielding a 19% sensitivity, 92% specificity, and 90% accuracy for hemangioma when compared with other tumors. Typically, hemangiomas measure 1 to 3 cm and, therefore, both specificity and accuracy are required, as in general, hemangiomas are small lesions.[11]

If one considers the definition of hemangioma by MRI as a homogeneous, well-marginated hypointense lesion in T2WI, it has been well known since 1987 that hemangiomas may be difficult to distinguish from cysts, and that hemangiomas may be heterogeneous.[4,17] Cysts are focal lesions, which are also well defined and markedly hyperintense in T2WI and hypointense in T1WI. Clinically, however, it is not important to distinguish hemangiomas from cysts, as both lesions are benign and nonsurgical. In addition, if MRI is the initial imaging study performed and there is a need to distinguish between hemangioma and cyst, ultrasound can perform this function.

It is well known that hemangiomas are heterogeneous lesions when examined pathologically. On cut section, there are almost always areas of fibrosis and/or necrosis. Cystic change, thrombosis, and hemorrhage within the tumor may also be present. Therefore, the criterion of heterogeneity cannot be applied to rule out hemangioma if a lesion is seen with areas of either lower intensity (fibrosis) or higher intensity (cystic change on necrosis).

Other morphologic criteria are important in distinguishing hemangioma from other lesions. Hemangiomas, although not encapsulated, have an extremely well-defined margin with the normal liver. The margin is frequently lobulated with a geographic pattern. Frequently, hemangiomas, particularly when large, extend to the surface of the liver, but deformity of the normal liver contour is not seen except in cases of pedunculated hemangiomas.[9,14]

Several attempts have been made to add quantitative criteria to the preceding qualitative criteria of hyperintense signal and morphology. Signal intensity measurements have been proposed to differentiate hemangioma from metastases.[1,13,14,18] Due to significant overlap, however, qualitative criteria have been more accurate than quantitative ones.

Morphologic patterns have also been applied to describe hemangiomas, the "light bulb" pattern being typical.[20]

The most serious attempt to establish a quantitative criterion to differentiate hemangioma from other lesions was attempted by Lombardo, et al.[14] After reviewing 15 hemangiomas and measuring lesion/liver signal intensity ratio, CNRs and T2-relaxation time on long TR/TE spin-echo sequences, there was statistical significant data on the T2 measurements to distinguish hemangioma from other lesions, primarily metastases. A T2 value of 88 msec was determined to be the cut off quantitatively, with hemangiomas measuring higher than 88 msec. However, the authors recognized that despite both quantitative and qualitative analyses, there is overlap between hemangiomas and some hypervascular metastases.

ATYPICAL HEMANGIOMA

Hemangiomas can be atypical in size, as well as other MRI findings. Although the majority of hemangiomas are smaller than 3 cm, they may be much larger; when they are larger than 10 cm, they are called *giant* and appear different in MRI from typical hemangiomas. In a review of 10 giant hemangiomas, Choi, et al[5] noted that in T2WI giant hemangiomas are always heterogeneous. The mean size of the tumors was 10.8 cm, and in all cases a cleftlike lower intensity area was seen in both T1WI and T2WI. On T2WI, a large portion of giant hemangiomas have high intensity. Low-intensity areas seen within hemangiomas correlate to lower-density areas seen on dynamic bolus CT, corresponding to central areas of fibrosis. Therefore, it is important to be familiar with the appearance of giant hemangiomas in MRI, as their heterogeneity may be confused with malignant tumors. Necrotic metastatic tumors and HCC should be included in the differential diagnosis of giant hemangiomas, as these two tumors may appear, primarily by CT, as large, heterogeneous masses.

T2WI may be extremely helpful in differentiating the hypodense areas seen in CT as areas of fibrosis (hypointense and suggestive of hemangioma) versus areas of necrosis (hyperintense and suggestive of necrotic tumor, such as HCC or metastases).

Other atypical appearances of hemangiomas have to be considered. If a patient has underlying iron deposition disease (hemochromatosis), the baseline intensity of the liver is lower than normal; therefore, metastases may appear very hyperintense when compared with the surrounding liver. This appearance is similar to that of hemangioma in normal liver. Such a case of confusion of metastases with hemangioma in a patient with hemochromatosis has been described.[15] Likewise, inhomogeneity in hemangiomas, not with areas of hypointensity but with areas of hyperintensity, has also been described in large hemangiomas with cystic change, corresponding to zones of liquefactive necrosis.[9]

HEMANGIOMA VS OTHER FOCAL MASSES

As the ability to study hemangioma of the liver by MRI has advanced, efforts have been made to distinguish hemangioma and other common nonsurgical lesions (cysts) from malignant focal lesions, such as metastases and HCC. This differentiation is particularly important as hemangioma is currently considered the most common benign tumor of the liver, with reported incidence as high as 20%.[12]

In addition, although hemangiomas are considered congenital, they present primarily in postmenopausal women (female/male is 5:1). Therefore, the age of presentation of hemangioma usually coincides with that of metastases and HCC. Although there is a different geographic distribution for metastases (commonly seen in Europe and the United States) and HCC (more commonly seen in Asia), hemangioma has no geographic distribution pattern. Several studies have been performed comparing the imaging diagnosis of hemangioma with other common lesions in the liver, primarily metastases and HCC.

In comparing hemangioma with metastases, several authors report similar findings, which can be summarized as follows.[4,8,13,14,18,20]

1. MRI has excellent sensitivity and specificity for hemangioma based primarily on qualitative and morphologic criteria, but it is difficult to differentiate between some hypervascular metastases and hemangioma.

However, this difficulty is in practical terms not important, because as discussed in the metastases subsection of this chapter, it is uncommon for primarily hypervascular tumors to present as liver metastasis. Nevertheless, as both metastases and hemangiomas are prevalent, it may be important when planning resection to know which lesions detected by MRI correspond to metastases and which to hemangiomas.

2. Some morphologic criteria have been used to differentiate metastases from hemangioma, and signs described for metastases such as "halo" and "target" do not occur with hemangiomas. Conversely, the classic "light bulb" sign of hemangioma has been described to have a 10% overlap with malignancy, primarily hypervascular metastases.[20]

At first assessment, it may appear that differentiating between hemangioma and hypervascular metastases would be difficult when only signal criteria are applied. In both cases, the same underlying abnormality (presence of large amounts of blood flowing through a mass) is present. In many cases, however, the use of intravenous gadopentetate dimeglumine with dynamic MRI effectively distinguishes these lesions.[8,13]

Using gadopentetate dimeglumine, researchers in the University of Berlin compared 14 hemangiomas with 15 metastases.[8] Marked homogeneous hyperintensity was present in the postcontrast examination of hemangiomas, whereas metastases were inhomogeneous and hypointense. In this series, a combination of dynamic MRI with delayed postcontrast T1WI was a useful method to diagnosing hepatic hemangiomas and to distinguish them from metastases, even when they were hypervascular.

In Asia efforts have been made to distinguish hemangioma from HCC. The use of highly T2WI is sufficient to differentiate between hemangioma and HCC.[6] Gadopentetate dimeglumine and gradient-echo dynamic MRI has also yielded excellent results.[21] Hemangiomas appeared as low-intensity masses before gadopentetate dimeglumine was administered, with a peak enhancement more than 2 minutes after injection in the majority of cases (72%). There was marked delayed enhancement in all cases of hemangioma. In cases of HCC, peak enhancement after gadopentetate dimeglumine was less than 2 minutes, and there was no delayed enhancement in any of the cases.

It is apparent that to differentiate hypervascular metastases or HCC from hemangioma, the use of gadopentetate dimeglumine in dynamic MRI may be extremely helpful (Fig. 10-8).

COMPARISON OF MRI WITH OTHER IMAGING TECHNIQUES

The "acid test" of MRI in the abdomen and, in particular, in the liver is its comparison with CT. Since Stark et al published their first report in 1985, MRI has been accepted as more sensitive than CT in the discovery of typical hemangiomas (smaller than 3 cm).[19] In fact MRI has not only better sensitivity but also better specificity than CT in identifying hemangiomas. Because hemangiomas are frequently less than 2 cm, no respiratory "misses," typical in small tumors studied by CT, occur in MRI. In addition, when compared with dynamic CT, MRI is a more simple technique without technical variations (i.e., injection rate, timing of delayed sections, selection of the "single level" for dynamic CT, etc.).

It is now well recognized that dynamic-bolus incremental technique in CT is not specific for hemangioma, with significant overlap in the appearance of hemangioma and malignant neoplasm. Peripheral contrast enhancement occurs in up to 54.5% of enhancing hepatic neoplasms studied with dynamic CT.[7]

Despite the fact that CT may be highly accurate when findings are positive, it does not consistently yield characteristic enhancement patterns; therefore, its clinical use is

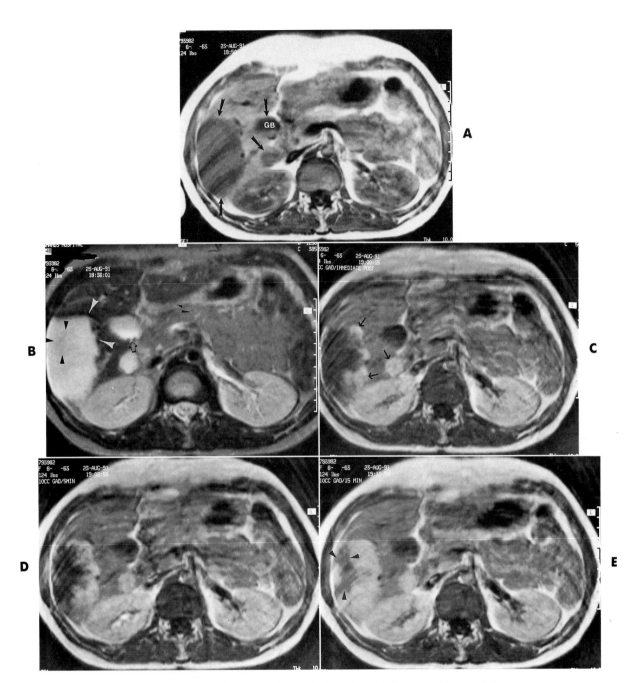

Fig. 10-8. Multiple hemangiomas. **A,** Spin-echo T1WI (TR 450 msec/TE 15 msec) demonstrates three hypointense areas in the liver *(arrows)*. One of these *(GB)* corresponds to the gallbladder, whereas the other two are hemangiomas. **B,** In T2WI (TR 2000 msec/TE 90 msec) these three areas become markedly hyperintense. Feeding vessels are seen in the periphery of the largest hemangioma *(white arrowheads)* with no signal due to flow void. Note fibrotic strands *(black arrowheads)*. Two small gallstones are seen in the gallbladder *(open arrow)*. **C,** Spin-echo T1WI (TR 250 msec/TE 22 msec) performed immediately after administration of 10 ml of gadopentetate dimeglumine demonstrates peripheral enhancement in the hemangiomas *(arrows)*; the gallbladder does not enhance. **D,** In the 5-minute delayed view there is further enhancement in a centripetal manner seen in the larger hemangioma. **E,** In the 15-minute delayed view there is persistence of gadopentetate dimeglumine in both hemangiomas, although areas of fibrosis do not enhance *(arrowheads)*.

reduced, especially because other imaging techniques (i.e., RBC-^{99m}TC or MRI) are more accurate.

When studied by ultrasound, hemangiomas are typically hyperechoic and well delimited and may have faint acoustic enhancement.[3] However, the degree of echogenicity may be variable and the tumor may contain hypoechoic, hyperechoic, and anechoic areas.[4] Therefore, although ultrasound is a sensitive method to discover hemangioma, it is not specific enough to characterize it particularly, when compared with other imaging modalities.

Angiography is a highly specific imaging modality to characterize hemangioma with its typical "cotton wool" sign. There is also typical persistence of contrast well beyond the venous phase in pools without arteriovenous shunting.

Technetium-99m-labeled red blood cell studies, particularly if performed with single proton emission computed tomography (SPECT) technique, has proved to be a highly specific and sensitive method to confirm a hepatic lesion as a hemangioma.[1] The classic finding of early defect with filling of it in delay scans is virtually diagnostic of this lesion.

SPECT has been compared with MRI in a series where 69 suspected hemangiomas were studied with CT, ultrasound, MRI, and SPECT with technetium-99m labeled red blood cells.[1] SPECT provided a sensitivity of 78% and an accuracy of 80%, whereas qualitative analysis of signal intensity on T2WI produce a sensitivity of 91% and an accuracy of 90%. The authors recommend the performance of SPECT to diagnose hemangioma, primarily because of its lower cost.[1] MRI is reserved for lesions smaller than 2 cm or lesions larger than 2 cm that are adjacent to the heart of major hepatic vessels.

CURRENT ROLE OF MRI IN WORK-UP OF HEMANGIOMA

Several schemes have been proposed in the diagnosis and characterization of hepatic hemangioma.[1,4] These schemes are based on a work-up that includes at least two imaging techniques and may or may not include the use of fine needle aspiration biopsy. In addition, combination studies such as a fusion technique between MRI and technetium-99m-labeled red blood cell SPECT images has also been proposed.[2] However, there are many opinions regarding the "ideal work-up" for questionable hepatic hemangiomas.

Imaging techniques in the diagnosis of hemangioma can be divided into highly specific tests including (1) MRI, (2) technetium-99m-labeled red blood cells, and (3) angiography. The less specific imaging techniques are ultrasound and dynamic CT.

It seems logical to consider in the work-up of a hemangioma the clinical situation where hemangioma needs to be confirmed. The current approach is to consider the potential hemangioma. If a patient is asymptomatic, has normal liver function, and no known malignancy, it is likely that a well-marginated echogenic hepatic mass by ultrasound or a peripherally enhancing mass by CT is a hemangioma. In these cases, follow-up with ultrasound in a few months may suffice to confirm the suspected diagnosis of hemangioma.

However, if a patient is symptomatic and has abnormal liver function or known malignancy, it is also likely that an echogenic liver "nodule" or a peripherally enhancing mass in CT may not be a hemangioma. Therefore, other studies must be performed to confirm or rule out this lesion. Both SPECT with red blood cells tagged with technetium-99m or MRI with a hemangioma protocol (with potential use of intravascular paramagnetic contrast) have superb specificity, which is greater than 90%. Either of these tests is advisable according to clinical availability and expertise.

If findings are questionable in one or two of the tests and/or there is a need to close the "10% gap" left by MRI or tagged red blood cell studies, two options are available—aspiration biopsy or angiography. Although it is clear that core biopsies have been performed in hemangiomas without significant complications, this procedure should not be encouraged when there is strong clinical and/or imaging suspicion of hemangioma.

The role of aspiration biopsy is controversial. Although some authors propose it, the material obtained (red blood cells and endothelial cells) is not specific for a definitive diagnosis.[4] In atypical cases, angiography is as accurate as aspiration biopsy to confirm the diagnosis of hemangioma.

In summary, MRI is one of the choice techniques to diagnose hemangioma because of its noninvasiveness, ease of performance with simplicity of technique, and ability to study of the entire liver without respiration misregistrations. MRI is considered superior to all other imaging modalities, particularly when supplemented with gadopentetate dimeglumine.

REFERENCES

1. Birnbaum BA, Weinreb JC, Megibow AJ, et al: Definitive diagnosis of hepatic hemangiomas: MR imaging versus Tc-99m-labeled red blood cell SPECT, Radiology 176:95-101, 1990.
2. Birnbaum BA, Noz ME, Chapnick J, et al: Hepatic hemangiomas: diagnosis with fusion of MR, CT, and Tc-99m-labeled red blood cell SPECT images, Radiology 181:469-474, 1991.
3. Bree RL, Schwab RE, Neiman HL: Solitary echogenic spot in the liver: is it diagnostic of a hemangioma?, Am J Roentgenol 140:41-45, 1983.
4. Bree RL, Schwab RE, Glazer GM, et al: The varied appearances of hepatic cavernous hemangiomas with sonography, computed tomography, magnetic resonance imaging and scintigraphy, Radiographics 7:1153-1175, 1987.
5. Choi BI, Han MC, Park JH, et al: Giant cavernous hemangioma of the liver: CT and MR imaging in 10 cases, Am J Roentgenol 152:1221-1226, 1989.
6. Choi BI, Han MC, Kim CW, et al: Small hepatocellular carcinoma versus small cavernous hemangioma: differentiation with MR imaging at 2.0 T, Radiology 176:103-106, 1990.

7. Freeny PC, Marks WM: Hepatic hemangioma: dynamic bolus CT, Am J Roentgenol 147:711-719, 1986.

8. Hamm B, Fischer E, Taupitz M: Differentiation of hepatic hemangiomas from metastases by dynamic contrast-enhanced MR imaging, J Comput Assist Tomogr 14:205-216, 1990.

9. Itai Y, et al: Atypical cavernous hemangioma of the liver, Radiat Med 6:135-140, 1988.

10. Itai Y, Ohtomo K, Furui S, et al: Noninvasive diagnosis of small cavernous hemangioma of the liver: advantage of MRI, Am J Roentgenol 145:1195-1199, 1985.

11. Itoh K: Differentiation between small hepatic hemangiomas and metastases on MR images: importance of size-specific quantitative criteria, Am J Roentgenol 155:61-65, 1990.

12. Karhunen PJ: Benign hepatic tumors and tumor-like conditions in men, J Clin Pathol 139:183-188, 1986.

13. Li KC, Glazer GM, Quint LE, et al: Distinction of hepatic cavernous hemangioma from hepatic metastases with MR imaging, Radiology 169:409-415, 1988.

14. Lombardo DM, Baker ME, Spritzer CE, et al: Hepatic hemangiomas vs metastases: MR differentiation at 1.5 T, Am J Roentgenol 155:55-59, 1990.

15. Mirowitz S, Heiken JP, Lee JKT: Potential MR pitfall in relying on lesion/liver intensity ratio in presence of hepatic hemochromatosis, J Comput Assist Tomogr 12:323-324, 1988.

16. Ohtomo K, Itai Y, Yoshida H, et al: MR differentiation of hepatocellular carcinoma from cavernous hemangioma: complementary roles of FLASH and T2 values, Am J Roentgenol 152:505-507, 1989.

17. Ros PR, Lubbers PR, Olmstead WW, et al: Hemangioma of the liver: heterogeneous appearance on T2-weighted images, Am J Roentgenol 149:1167-1170, 1987.

18. Rummeny E, Weissleder R, Stark DD, et al: Primary liver tumors: diagnosis by MR imaging, Am J Roentgenol 152:63-72, 1989.

19. Stark DD, Felder RC, Wittenberg J, et al: Magnetic resonance imaging of cavernous hemangioma of the liver: tissue-specific characterization, Am J Roentgenol 145:213-222, 1985.

20. Wittenberg J, Stark DD, Forman BH, et al: Differentiation of hepatic metastases from hepatic hemangiomas and cysts by using MR imaging, Am J Roentgenol 151:79-84, 1988.

21. Yoshida H, Itai Y, Ohtomo K, et al: Small hepatocellular carcinoma and cavernous hemangioma: differentiation with dynamic FLASH MR imaging with Gd-DTPA, Radiology 171:339-342, 1989.

Section three
Benign tumors and tumorlike conditions

Pablo R. Ros

Focal nodular hyperplasia
Hepatocellular adenoma
Lipoma
Cystadenoma/cystadenocarcinoma
Pediatric tumors
    Infantile hemangioendothelioma
    Mesenchymal hamartoma
Miscellaneous benign tumors
    Nodular regenerative hyperplasia
    Cysts
    Adenomatous hyperplastic nodules

This section describes benign tumors of the liver in both pediatric and adult patients. Most of the section is dedicated to focal nodular hyperplasia (FNH) and hepatocellular adenoma (HCA), the two most common tumors in the adult after hemangioma. Sections on pediatric tumors, lipoma, and miscellaneous tumors are included.

Each tumor is discussed by reviewing the underlying pathologic findings followed by the typical features in magnetic resonance imaging (MRI) and concluding with the comparison of MRI findings to other imaging modalities.

FOCAL NODULAR HYPERPLASIA

Other than hemangioma, the evaluation of FNH by MRI is more common than any other benign tumor of the liver. FNH is defined microscopically as a tumorlike condition characterized by a central fibrous scar with surrounding nodules of hyperplastic hepatocytes that contain bile ductules.[6] The gross appearance of FNH is unusual when compared to other benign and malignant tumors. FNH is a predominantly homogeneous tumor, except for its scar, due to its excellent vascularity. This characteristic results in a lack of areas of necrosis or hemorrhage, which are present in the majority of both benign and malignant liver neoplasms.

The majority of FNHs are solitary (95%) and smaller than 5 cm. Pathogenetically, FNH is believed to be a hyperplastic response to an underlying spiderlike arterial malformation.[30] An arteriovenous malformation would be the nidus of the FNH and will be present within the scar as a collection of vessels and bile ductules that are seen surrounded by collagenous tissue. Therefore, the central scar of FNH is different than areas of fibrosis seen in other neoplasms such as hemangioma, HCC, or metastases.

FNH is seen predominantly in women from the third to fifth decades of life and usually is discovered (75% of cases) as an incidental finding. FNHs are almost always

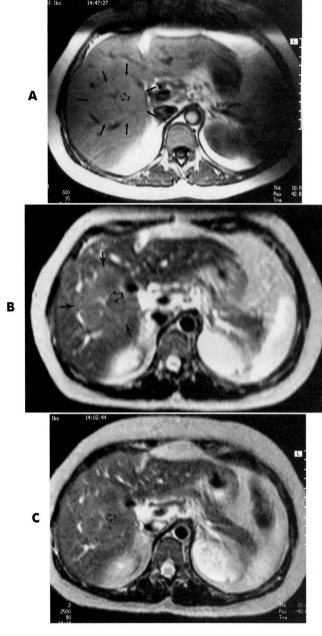

Fig. 10-9. Typical appearance of FNH. **A,** Spin-echo T1WI (TR 300 msec/TE 15 msec) demonstrates an isointense lesion in the right lobe of the liver *(arrows)*. The lesion is identified primarily due to the presence of a central scar *(open arrow)*, as well as displacement of the normal hepatic vessels. **B,** T2WI spin-echo (TR 2500 msec/TE 90 msec) demonstrates the lesion hyperintense to the rest of the liver *(arrows)*. Note that the central scar becomes hyperintense indicating its hypervascular nature *(open arrow)*. Normal vessels seen in the periphery have normal flow. **C,** Follow-up image performed seven months after study displayed in A and B, demonstrates no change in size, shape, or signal intensity in the FNH. Again, the spiculated central scar is seen hyperintense *(open arrow)*. Radiologic stability is typical in FNH.

solitary (90% of cases), and its incidence is much smaller than hemangioma (involving up to 3% of adult women) and typically occurs as a solitary lesion.[13] It may be associated with hemangioma, and it has been linked to oral contraceptive use.

The majority of the 77 cases of FNH with MRI correlation that have been reported belong to only two large series (35 cases in one and 25 in the other).[2,16,17,23,25-28] The remaining publications are primarily based on case reports or on small series of two to three cases.

From the early report by Butch et al[2] in 1986, it was clear that MRI could distinguish among FNH, metastases, HCC, and hemangioma and thus could be useful in diagnosis. It is particularly important to make this diagnose because FNH does not require surgery and has never resulted in complications or death. In fact, the only mortality and morbidity associated with this tumorlike lesion is secondary to surgical resection.

The initial description in 1986 of FNH, based on a single case, was that of an isointense tumor in T1WI that became slightly hyperintense with the rest of the liver in T2WI and that had a central area, corresponding to the central scar of FNH, which was hypointense in T1WI and became hyperintense in T2WI (Fig. 10-9).

Other descriptions[17,27] made it possible to establish a fairly consistent MRI appearance of FNH, which was based on the following triad:

1. Isointensity of the tumor on T1WI and T2WI
2. Presence of a central scar, which is hyperintense in T2WI
3. Homogeneous signal intensity, except for the presence of a scar

It must be noted, however, that atypical cases have been described in which the appearance of the tumor was markedly hypointense compared to the normal liver in T1WI or in which the scar was isointense in T2WI.[23]

A large series of 35 cases by Korobkin, et al, et al[13] demonstrated that only 20% of FNHs were isointense in both T1WI and T2WI and that there was variable appearance ranging from isointense (60%), to hypointense (34%), to even hyperintense (6%) in T1WI. On T2WI, 66% of FNHs were hyperintense, and 34% were isointense. Central scar was present in 49% of the FNHs, in all cases being hypointense in T1WI and hyperintense on T2WI. Fifty percent of the lesions were of homogeneous intensity, except for the presence of a central scar. However, of the preceding triad of MRI characteristics, central scar was present in only 9% of all cases.

This large series illustrates the variable appearance of FNH on MRI. Although the classic triad described initially was present in a minority of patients, some of the key features of FNH, such as its relative similar intensity to a normal liver in either T1WI or T2WI, may be sufficient to differentiate FNH from liver metastases, especially because metastases are almost never isointense with the liver in either T1WI or T2WI. In addition, the behavior of the scar, which is frequently hyperintense in T2WI, may be of help to distinguish FNH from other lesions that also have central areas of fibrosis.

The issue of central scars in primary liver tumors have been reviewed by Rummeny et al.[26] FNH has a hypervascular scar with multiple vascular channels that have blood flow within them. Therefore, it appears by MRI similar to a hemangioma with long T1-and T2-relaxation times. Like hemangiomas, the central scar will appear in spin-echo images as hypointense in T1WI, as well as hyperintense in T2WI. However, it is hard to distinguish hypervascular scars in FNH and adenoma from inflammatory scars,

which are characterized by the presence of edema and which may be present in both HCC and giant hemangiomas (Fig. 10-10). Therefore, the scar itself cannot be used solely to distinguish FNH from other tumors, especially those that require resection, such as HCC.

The use of gadopentetate dimeglumine in FNH has been described in one case using conventional spin-echo techniques.[29] In that particular case, there was marked hyperintensity after injection of gadopentetate dimeglumine, indicating the vascularity of the tumor, as well as the presence of radiating septa that could be seen in images obtained 6 minutes after gadopentetate dimeglumine injection. Radiating septa were seen as low signal intensity structures that separated the nodular lobules of high signal intensity, corresponding to areas of cellular hyperplasia.

Occasionally, as FNH may be isointense in both T1WI and T2WI, the presence of a mass can be distinguished only by displacement of vessels or by the presence of the central scar.[2,26] Use of gradient echo images is helpful in assessing FNH, supplementing findings seen by spin-echo images. By gradient echo, high signal intensity indicating flow can be seen within the central scar (see Fig. 10-11), a phenomenon not present in other masses with scars.

A recent review including 25 FNHs describes the use of fast imaging (turboFLASH images) after the administration of gadolinium tetraazacyclododecanetetraacetic acid (DOTA).[16] The use of turboFLASH, a gradient-echo sequence, was coupled with the injection of gadolinium-DOTA to ascertain the capabilities of combining a fast dynamic motion-free technique and an intravenous contrast.

TurboFLASH without contrast administration demonstrated good T1 contrast in FNH when compared to the liver. FNH always appeared hypointense, as it had already been reported in cases where heavily T1WI were obtained.[2,23] After bolus injection of gadolinium-DOTA, lesions appeared hyperintense with marked high signal intensity in the arterial phase, indicating the vascular nature of FNH. Enhancement of the scar was seen after injection of contrast at approximately 40 to 80 seconds.

The use of advanced fast imaging coupled with administration of intravenous contrast allows the obtention of images that demonstrate the vascularity of tumors, and, as with angiography, the patterns of enhancement of hepatic neoplasms may be of help to further characterize focal lesions. Although the patterns described in the paper by Mathieu et al[16] are suggestive of FNH, similar findings can be seen in other tumors that have central areas of fibrosis, as well as a hypervascular nature such as HCC.

There is little experience with the use of SPIO particles in the study of FNH. Because FNH is known to have Kupffer cells as well as an excellent vascular supply, however, preliminary experience suggests that FNH uptakes SPIO particles in a similar proportion as the normal liver. Therefore, the use of intravenous SPIO may be of help to further distinguish tumors such as FNH or adenoma that

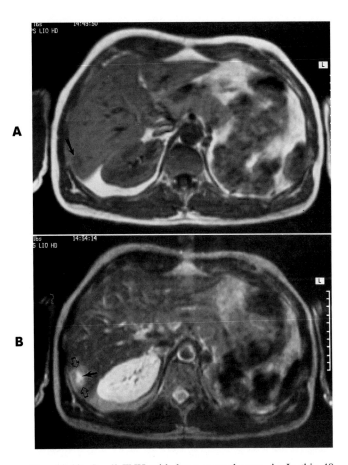

Fig. 10-10. Small FNH with large central scar. **A,** In this 48-year-old man with prior left nephrectomy due to renal cell carcinoma, a small hypointense lesion in T1WI (TR 450 msec/TE 15 msec) is seen in the right lobe *(arrow),* which has a central area that is isointense with normal liver. **B,** Heavily T2WI demonstrates that the periphery of this lesion is slightly hyperintense compared to the normal liver parenchyma *(open arrows).* However, the central portion is markedly hyperintense (TR 2200 msec/TE 80 msec) *(arrow).* This lesion was resected and proved to be an FNH with a large central scar. If the central scar is proportionally large in comparison with the entire tumor, the scar of FNH may be mistaken for necrosis, and the overall appearance be confused with metastases or other tumors that may have areas of necrosis.

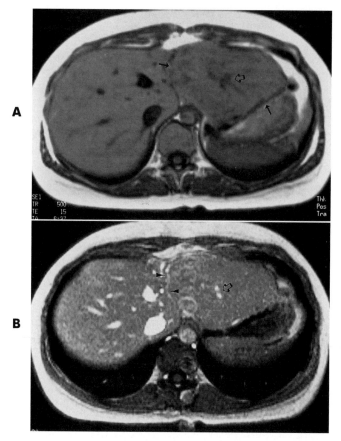

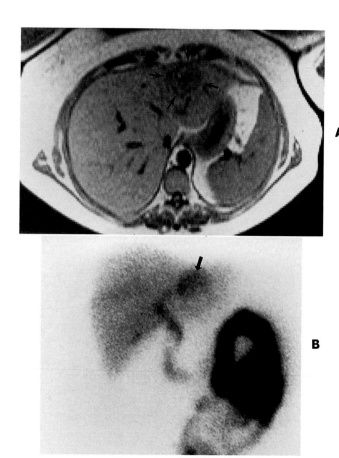

Fig. 10-11. FNH findings with gradient-echo imaging. **A,** In this 26-year-old woman, a large mass *(solid arrows)* is seen replacing the left lobe of the liver (lobar FNH) (TR 500 msec/TE 15 msec). The low signal in the center of the lesion *(open arrow)* corresponds to the typical scar. **B,** Gradient-echo image (TR 80 msec/TE 70 msec, FLIP angle 80 degrees) demonstrates flow within the scar *(open arrow)* indicating the presence of flowing vessels within it, one of the hallmarks of FNH. Note displaced vessels in the periphery of the tumor *(arrowheads).*

Fig. 10-12. Hypointense FNH at 0.35 T. **A,** Axial T1WI spin-echo image (SE 500/30) in a 0.35 T unit demonstrates a slightly hypointense lesion *(arrows)* in the left lobe of the liver. **B,** Corresponding iminodiacetic acid (IDA) derivative scintigram demonstrates uptake in the lesion *(arrow).* Uptake with excretion of biliary contrast is also a typical finding in FNH.

contain Kupffer cells from all other primary or metastatic liver lesions that do not contain Kupffer cells.

The decision whether to use other imaging techniques in the diagnosis of FNH, when compared to MRI, has to consider that sulfur colloid scintigraphy is a helpful technique to prove the presence of Kupffer cells, as well as good vascularity, a hallmark of FNH. Using biliary scintigraphy with IDA (iminodiacetic acid) derivatives, there is usually uptake in FNH followed by excretion of the radionuclide by the tumor (Fig. 10-12). By ultrasound and CT, FNH appears as primarily a homogeneous mass, except for the presence of the central scar that appears hypodense and hyperechoic. However, identification of a central scar by CT is less frequent than in MRI, particularly when injection of intravascular contrasts such as gadopentetate dimeglumine is performed.

Although the MRI characteristics of FNH are not as specific as those of hemangioma, MRI may play a signifi-

cant role in characterizing this benign nonsurgical tumor-like lesion of the liver. The presence of a homogeneous, isointense tumor, either in T1WI or T2WI (or slightly hypointense in T1WI and hyperintense in T2WI to the normal liver), is suggestive of FNH. Furthermore, if the mass has a central hyperintense scar in T2WI and there is marked enhancement of the tumor-post gadolinium administration, it may be possible to characterize FNH.

HEPATOCELLULAR ADENOMA

The few reports describing MRI of hepatocellular adenoma (HCA) are limited to either single case reports or a description of a few adenomas in larger series dealing with primary liver tumors.[8,18,19,26] The paucity of reports of adenoma reflects the fact that HCA is an unusual neoplasm, with an incidence approximately half that of FNH.

HCA is defined pathologically as composed of hepatocytes arranged in courts that occasionally form bile.[6] The tumor lacks portal tracts, hepatic veins, and biliary canaliculi, although it is known to have Kupffer cells.[9,14] Hepatocytes rich in fat and glycogen are frequently present. It is encouraged to use the prefix "hepatocellular," as there are other adenomas within the liver, primarily in the biliary tree (biliary adenomas or papillomas).

Grossly, HCA is a large tumor (8 to 10 cm in diameter at discovery) with pedunculation seen in 10% of cases, frequently encapsulated, and with multiple large vessels running through the capsule. On cut-section, HCA are inhomogeneous with frequently large areas of hemorrhage or infarction. Internal hemorrhage is one of the hallmarks of adenoma. Rupture of an adenoma with subsequent peritoneum is one of the reasons why HCA is a surgical lesion. Occasionally, adenomas are homogeneous without areas of hemorrhage or infarction and with possible central scars and blood vessels seen throughout the tumor.

The majority of adenomas are seen in women of childbearing age who are using oral contraceptives. The cause-effect relationship between oral contraceptives and HCA has been proven, with an overall incidence of 4 adenomas for every 100,000 users.[5] The majority of adenomas are single, although multiple adenomas can occur.

The MRI appearance of HCA is not well established. To date, only eight cases have been reported, and a variety of appearances have been described.[8,18,19,25]

The reports of Moss et al[19] (two cases) and Rummeny et al[26,27] (four cases) performed with superconducting magnets of 0.35 T and 0.6 T, respectively, demonstrated that the tumor was hyperintense in T2WI, and isointense or slightly hyperintense to normal liver in T1WI. The slight hyperintensity in T1WI that has been attributed to fatty change, which is frequent in adenomas, makes it impossible to differentiate it from HCC (Fig. 10-13).

A single case report by Nokes et al[20] demonstrated that HCA can also be isointense with normal liver in both T1WI and T2WI, thereby making it impossible to differentiate it from FNH[20]. In this case, however, there was no evidence of a central scar, which is typically seen in FNH.

A recent report by Gabata et al[8] provides another different appearance from the one reported for HCA. Their single case described a heterogeneous tumor, primarily with hyperintensity in T1WI, similar to the appearance seen in HCC and in adenomatous hyperplasia of the liver. However, fatty change was noted. The somewhat surprising finding is the hypointense appearance of this HCA in T2WI. The relative hypointensity of HCA has also been seen in adenomatous hyperplasia (a precancerous lesion to HCC seen in chronic cirrhotic livers). That the adenoma was hypointense in T2WI suggests that HCA may be distinguished from HCC, which is always hyperintense. In this case, an area that appears hypointense compared to the tumor was noted in T1WI and hyperintense compared to tumor in T2WI due to the presence of central hemorrhage. A thin rim of hypointensity was noted in both T1WI and

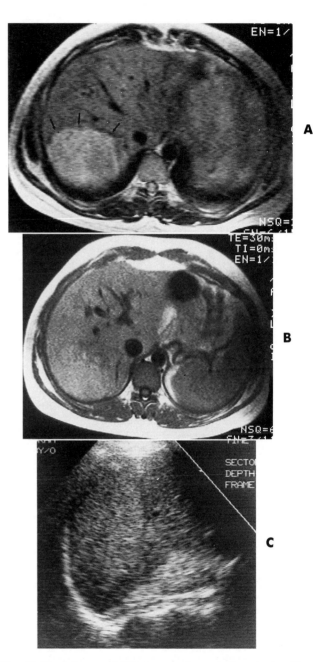

Fig. 10-13. Adenoma: MRI-ultrasound correlation. **A,** In this 27-year-old pregnant woman, a large lesion is seen in right lobe of the liver in this T2-weighted spin-echo image (TR 2000 msec/TE 60 msec) at 0.35 T. Note that the lesion is well-defined *(arrows)*, and it is predominantly hyperintense, although there are some inhomogeneous areas. **B,** T1WI (TR 500 msec/TE 30 msec) demonstrates slight hyperintensity of this lesion compared to normal liver, as well as displacement of normal hepatic vessels. **C,** Ultrasound scan performed in the operating room, before resection, demonstrates the hyperechoic nature of this lesion. Fatty change was noted within the hepatocytes pathologically.

T2WI and corresponded pathologically to the capsule, which is frequently seen in adenomas.

We have studied five adenomas by MRI and have noted some of the features described here. Adenomas are frequently inhomogeneous tumors that have in T1WI areas that are hyperintense compared to normal liver, likely due to the presence of fatty change. However, in T2WI the tumors are either hyperintense to normal liver or hypointense, depending on their internal contents (Fig. 10-14). It is essential to understand that adenomas are large tumors that frequently undergo areas of internal hemorrhage; therefore, multiple areas corresponding to hemorrhages in different stages may be present at the same in an adenoma. Thus, due to blood by-products, the appearance of adenomas by MRI, particularly in T2WI, may vary greatly from case to case.

It is also important to remember that adenomas are usually seen in noncirrhotic livers, and frequently encapsulated. Capsules will be seen as a hypointense rim surrounding the tumor.

Not infrequently, patients seek medical attention due to acute abdominal pain secondary to massive internal hemorrhage (Fig. 10-15). We have encountered one case that was classified pathologically as "burned out adenoma," which appeared as a markedly hypointense lesion in T1WI and markedly hyperintense in T2WI, mimicking the appearance of an abscess. Rings of hemosiderin were noted by MRI, indicating the hemorrhagic nature of the tumor. Therefore, in a differential diagnosis of a cystic lesion by MRI, adenoma should be considered as well as abscess and other cystic tumors.

In the work-up of adenomas, MRI may play a role, albeit less important than with hemangioma or even FNH. There are no characteristic signs in adenoma, and further study is needed of larger series of adenomas to better understand its appearance by MRI (Fig. 10-16). Its potential hyperintensity on T1WI overlaps with HCC. Its heterogeneity in both T1WI and T2WI is also nonspecific. The use of contrast material has not been reported in adenoma. In our experience, with the use of SPIO there was no uptake in a large adenoma, corresponding with the findings seen with the use of sulfur colloid, where 80% of adenomas demonstrated no uptake. This characteristic is due not to the lack of Kupffer cells, but to the presence of poor vascularity and inability of the sulfur colloid or SPIO particles to be delivered to the Kupffer cells present in adenomas.

LIPOMA

Hepatic lipomas are extremely rare and are asymptomatic. These tumors as well as hepatic angiomyolipomas may occur in patients with tuberous sclerosis; however, solitary liver lipomas may be present without associated lesions.[25]

Only one case of an intrahepatic lipoma has been published.[15] In this case, the MRI appearance was characteris-

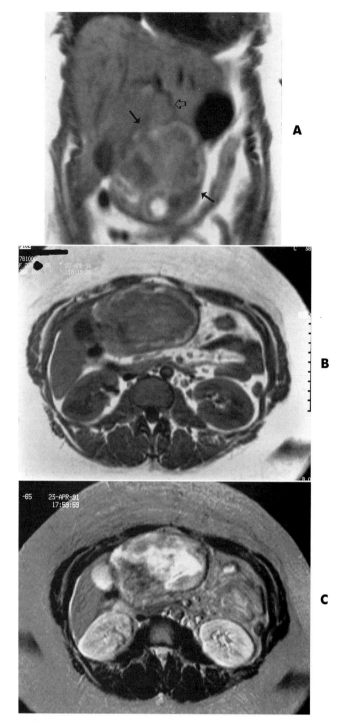

Fig. 10-14. Typical appearance of adenoma at 1 T. **A,** Coronal T1-weighted spin-echo (TE 400 msec/TE 15 msec) demonstrates a large heterogeneous lesion arising from the inferior edge of the liver *(arrows).* Note areas of hyperintensity, corresponding to fresh hemorrhage, as well as darker areas corresponding to older hemorrhage. Note also a large feeding vessel *(open arrow).* **B,** Axial T1WI (TR 500 msec/TE 15 msec) through the center of the pedunculated mass demonstrates the heterogeneous nature of the tumor, as well as its overall hyperintensity compared to the normal. **C,** Spin-echo T2WI (TR 2000 msec/TE 90 msec) demonstrates heterogeneity, as well as markedly hyperintense areas, corresponding to necrosis, and hypointense areas, corresponding to old hemorrhage.

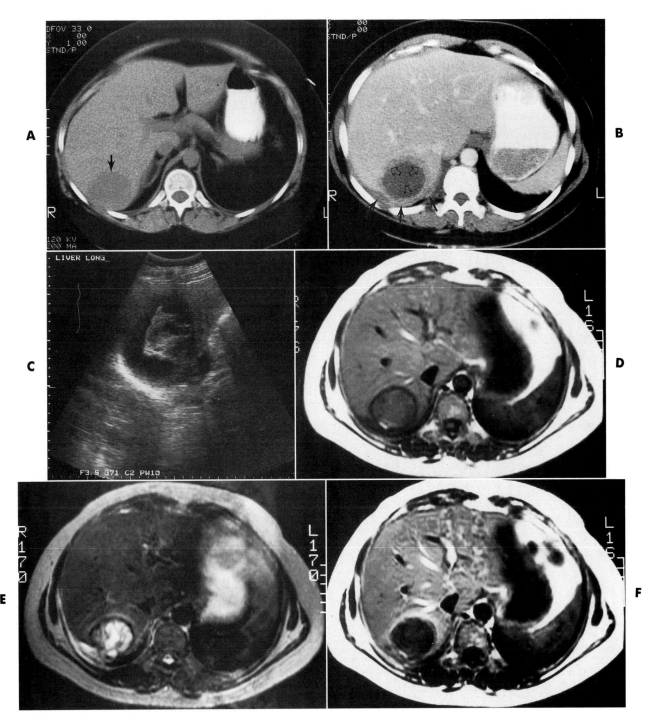

Fig. 10-15. "Burned out" adenoma mimicking metastases: CT-MR correlation. **A,** Nonenhanced CT section demonstrates an ill-defined lesion of the right lobe of the liver *(arrow)* in this young woman that was felt to correspond to an abscess. **B,** After enhancement there appears to be a peripheral rim *(open arrows)* of higher density than the water-density center. Note extension into the surface of the liver *(arrows).* **C,** Correlative ultrasound demonstrates a slight amount of debris in a predominantly cystic lesion. Ultrasound and CT findings suggest the presence of an abscess. **D and E,** T1WI and T2WI demonstrate the complex nature of the mass, as well as its extension into the subcapsular liver. Note a hypointense rim in both T1WI and T2WI. **F,** Postgadolinium injection. There is evidence of an area of rim enhancement, corresponding to viable tumor. At pathology, a "burned out" or completely hemorrhagic adenoma was found with rupture into the subcapsular space of the liver.

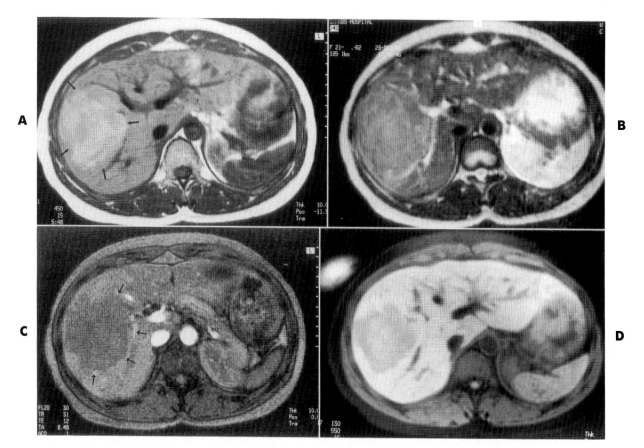

Fig. 10-16. Adenoma, usual appearance (spin-echo, gradient-echo, and fat suppression techniques.) **A,** T1WI (spin-echo TR 450 msec/TR 15 msec) demonstrates a well-delimited, slightly hyperintense and inhomogeneous mass of the right lobe of the liver *(arrows)*. **B,** T2WI (TR 2000 msec/TE 90 msec) demonstrates that the lesion is hyperintense compared to the normal liver parenchyma. There are some isointense areas within the tumor. **C,** Gradient-echo image (TR 31 msec/TE 12 msec/FLIP angle 30 degrees) demonstrates that no large vessels are seen within the tumor, unlike in FNH. However, vessels are seen in the periphery of the tumor *(arrows)* frequently noted in adenomas. **D,** Fat suppression technique (TR 550 msec/TE 15 msec) demonstrates that the lesion is hypointense compared to the normal liver, suggesting fat content.

tic of a lipoma, as seen in other areas of the body (Fig. 10-17). The tumor appeared homogeneous and well demarcated, with the same signal intensity as retroperitoneal fat in all pulsing sequences used. The lesion/fat ratio was always 1, indicating the unquestionable fatty nature of the tumor.

This tumor was also studied with CT, which also produced the characteristic appearance of a lipoma. In cases where a tumor appears in the liver with fat characteristics by MRI, CT may be used to confirm its diagnosis.

CYSTADENOMA/CYSTADENOCARCINOMA

Cystadenoma is a rare neoplasm of the liver, which is currently considered as a spectrum of disease, including both cystadenoma and cystadenocarcinoma. Cystadenocarcinoma is an obviously malignant tumor, whereas cystadenoma is considered a tumor of malignant potential. Trans-

formation of a cystadenoma into cystadenocarcinoma is a recognized complication; therefore, a cystadenoma-cystadenocarcinoma sequence has been established,[11] similar to the concept well known with ovarian tumors, as well as with mucinous cystic tumors of the pancreas.

Although the CT and ultrasound appearance of cystadenoma of the liver is well known, the MRI appearance is limited to a case report.[4,12,22] In this case the MRI findings are primarily compared to CT and ultrasound findings.

In our experience with cystadenoma, MRI was helpful not only to display the internal structure of the tumor, but also to be able to recognize that the tumor recurred at the site of excision and that the recurrence was not accumulation of fluid or bile (biloma). The appearance by MRI is that of a multiseptated tumor with diverse signal intensities within the locules, both in T1WI and T2WI.

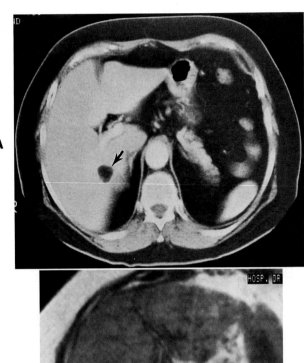

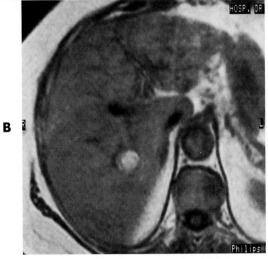

Fig. 10-17. Lipoma of the liver: CT and MRI correlation. **A,** Enhanced CT of the abdomen demonstrates a homogeneous low-density lesion *(arrow)* in the posterior segment of the right lobe. **B,** T1WI (TR 500 msec/TE 30 msec) at the same level demonstrates a hyperintense localized lesion, corresponding with the findings in CT and of the same signal intensity of subcutaneous fat. (From Marti-Bonmati L, Menoz F, Vizcaino I, et al: Gastrointest Radiol 14:155-157, 1989.)

CT and ultrasound are able to demonstrate multiple septations and therefore, the multiloculated nature of cystadenomas; however, they are not able to demonstrate the variable nature of the different locules. MRI allows the demonstration of differences in fluid concentration, which in T1WI is isointense or hypointense material with the presence of fluid-fluid levels. In T2WI, the mass is primarily hyperintense, indicating the fluid contents. Different levels of intensity correspond to the different concentrations of proteinaceous material, as well as bile and blood residue within the different loculi. A capsule can be distinguished in both T1WI and T2WI as a low signal rim (Fig. 10-18).

A major differential diagnosis with cystadenoma/cystadenocarcinoma should include complicated abscesses, as well as echinococcal cysts. In the pediatric age group, mesenchymal hamartomas and embryonal sarcomas should also be included in the differential diagnosis.

In summary, although the experience is limited in the use of MRI for cystadenoma/cystadenocarcinoma of the liver, the high sensitivity of MRI to determine the nature of fluid collections may be helpful to distinguish that a multiseptated cystic mass may be of neoplastic origin (i.e., cystadenoma/cystadenocarcinoma) if the intensity in different locules varies, corresponding to different concentrations of proteinaceous material and/or debris (bloody/bilious). On the other hand, postsurgical seromas or bilomas tend to be multiloculated with locules of similar intensity, which is particularly important because cystadenomas tend to recur.

PEDIATRIC TUMORS

The major pediatric benign tumors are infantile hemangioendothelioma and mesenchymal hamartoma.

Infantile hemangioendothelioma

Infantile hemangioendothelioma (IHE) is a vascular tumor derived from endothelial cells forming vascular channels. Usually IHEs are multiple and diffuse, being uncommonly solitary.[10]

Microscopically and grossly, IHEs are similar to hemangiomas; they can fibrose and eventually calcify. A major difference with hemangiomas is that IHEs have arteriovenous shunting that may produce hemodynamic consequences and ultimately cardiac failure. IHE will involute spontaneously. Cutaneous hemangiomas are commonly concurrent in patients with IHE (40%).

The knowledge of the MRI appearance of IHE is limited to scant reports.[21] In these few cases, IHE appears inhomogeneous in both T1WI and T2WI due to its hemorrhagic, necrotic, and fibrotic areas. On T2WI, the nodules of IHE display varying degrees of hyperintensity, reflecting its vascular nature, therefore, having a similar appearance of hemangioma by MRI (Fig. 10-19).

MRI allows a noninvasive method to confirm the vascular nature of infantile hemangioendotheliomas that may be on occasion extraordinarily large. Since typically IHE presents in the first 6 months of life, it is preferable to confirm the diagnosis by MRI than to perform angiography.

Mesenchymal hamartoma

Mesenchymal hamartoma of the liver is another benign cystic lesion that occurs in children, but is considered developmental in origin and, therefore, not a "true" neoplasm. Grossly, mesenchymal hamartoma is a large predominantly cystic mass averaging at discovery 12 to 15 cm.[10] On cut-section, mesenchymal hamartoma are either

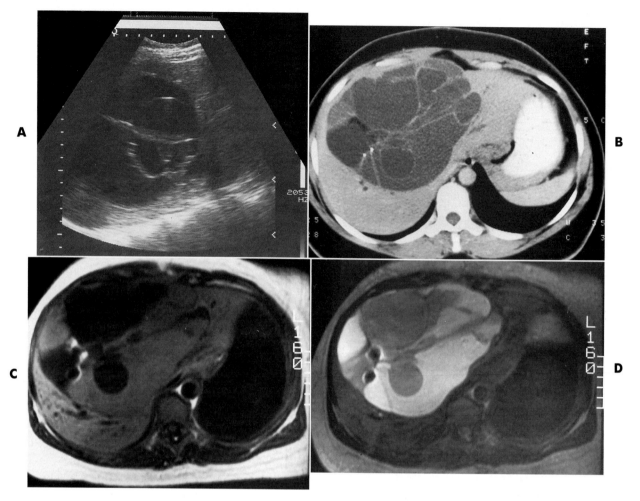

Fig. 10-18. Cystadenoma of the liver: ultrasound, CT, and MRI appearance. **A,** Ultrasound demonstrates a multiloculated mass in the liver. Note that there is no appreciable difference in echogenicity in the fluid seen in different locules. **B,** Corresponding CT demonstrates a multiseptated lesion. Minimal differences in density are seen in between certain locules. Clips are seen, corresponding to prior surgery. (This is recurrent tumor.) **C,** T1WI at 1.5 T (TR 500 msec/TE 20 msec) demonstrates multiple locules, which have different signal intensity. The signal varies from markedly hypointense to isointense with the liver. **D,** T2WI (TR 2200 msec/TE 80 msec) demonstrates the variable intensity of the multiple locules of this cystadenoma. A mass with locules seen with multiple densities suggests a neoplasm and not a seroma or biloma. Note surgical clips with metallic artifact. Pathologic analyses of the fluid contents of this cystadenoma revealed hemorrhagic, as well as bilious contents of various proportions in different locules in this cystadenoma. Incidentally noted, in both **C** and **D** is barium seen within the stomach.

of mesenchymal predominance (solid appearance) or cystic predominance (multiloculated cystic appearance).

The appearance of mesenchymal hamartoma on MRI varies, depending on stromal or cystic predominance. If there is a stromal predominance due to increased fibrosis, intensity in T1WI will be lower than that of normal liver. Conversely, if there is cystic predominance, the appearance would be similar to that of other cystic masses with hypointense appearance and marked hyperintensity in T2WI. Multiple septations are seen in both T1WI and

T2WI transversing the tumor, indicating that the mass is not a simple cyst. The intensity of the different locules may vary, indicating different concentrations of proteinaceous material and/or debris (Fig. 10-20). Thus the appearance of mesenchymal hamartoma of the liver is similar to that of cystadenoma of the liver, but the age of presentation is so different (mesenchymal hamartoma seen in the first 2 years of life with peak incidence at 18 months; cystadenomas in women in the sixth or seventh decade of life) that there is usually no need to differentiate between these two tumors.

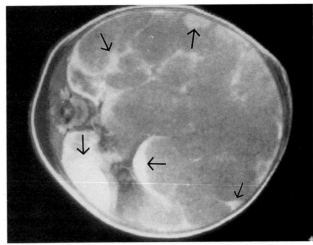

Fig. 10-19. Infantile hemangioendothelioma. T1WI demonstrates a massive infantile hemangioendothelioma in this child. Due to the massive size of the tumor, the patient had to be scanned in or on the left lateral decubitus. Note the multiple nodules of infantile hemangioendothelioma, as well as some internal hemorrhage *(arrows)*.

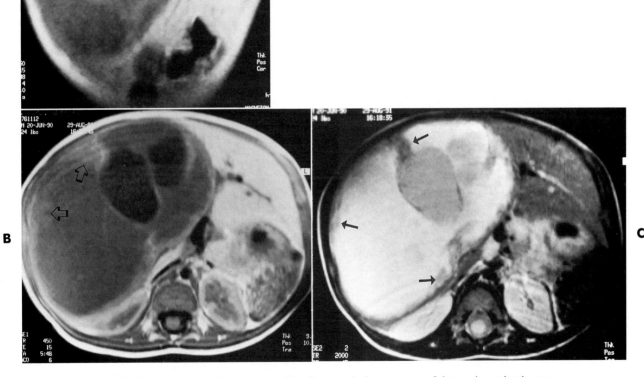

Fig. 10-20. Mesenchymal hamartoma of the liver: typical appearance of the cystic predominance. **A,** Coronal T1WI (TR 450 msec/TE 15 msec) demonstrates a large mass occupying the right lobe of the liver and displacing the left lobe. Note that the intensity of the different locules of this predominantly cystic mesenchymal hamartoma varies. **B,** Axial T1WI demonstrates some solid components *(open arrows),* as well as a predominantly cystic mesenchymal hamartoma of the liver. Note the variable signal intensity in different locules of mesenchymal hamartoma. **C,** T2WI (TR 2000 msec/TE 45 msec) demonstrates the mural nodules in the periphery of the mesenchymal hamartoma *(arrows),* as well as the multiple locules seen within the tumor. A multicystic mass, in a child of 1 to 2 years of age without history of trauma and with different signal intensities in different locules suggest mesenchymal hamartoma.

MISCELLANEOUS BENIGN TUMORS
Nodular regenerative hyperplasia

Nodular regenerative hyperplasia (NRH) is defined as diffuse nodularity of the liver produced by many regenerative nodules, which are associated with fibrosis.[7] NRH is grossly characterized by the presence of bulging nodules, which appear discrete on cut-surface, resembling diffuse involvement with metastatic carcinoma. These nodules are composed microscopically of cells resembling normal hepatocytes, and there is no evidence of fibrosis. NRH is associated with a variety of systemic diseases, as well as multiple drugs that have in common their hepatotoxicity.[7]

Only one case report of NRH studied by MRI has been published.[23] In this case, a large nodule of NRH, which appeared angiographically as multiple hypervascular lesions and ultrasonographically as multiple well-delimited hyperechoic lesions, had a normal appearance by CT and MRI.

The spectrum of radiologic findings seen in NRH vary from a normal-appearing liver with associated portal hypertension to multiple masses that have a nonspecific appearance by ultrasound, CT, and angiography.

With a single case reported, it appears that nodules of NRH may not be seen by MRI; therefore, its role in the diagnosis of this rare entity may be one of exclusion.

Cysts

True cyst of the liver or bile duct cyst is defined by the presence of epithelial lining in the inner surface of the cyst. Simple hepatic (bile duct) cyst is defined as a single (less than 10) unilocular cyst. The wall is composed of a thin layer of fibrous tissue if the adjacent liver is normal. If more than 10 cysts are seen, adult polycystic kidney-liver disease should be considered (Fig. 10-21).

The incidence of simple hepatic cyst has been reported to be as high as 14% in autopsy series; it is more common in women than in men.[6] The MRI appearance of simple cyst is that of an extremely hyperintense lesion in T2WI, which becomes homogeneously hypointense in T1WI. It is impossible in some cases to differentiate a cyst from a typical hemangioma in MRI. Small cysts are also difficult to differentiate from small vessels.

Adenomatous hyperplastic nodules

Adenomatous hyperplastic nodule (AHN) is the preferred term for a lesion that appears in the chronically cirrhotic liver. These lesions should not be confused with small liver cancers. AHN also has been referred to as adenomatoid hyperplasia, adenomatous hyperplasia, macroregenerative nodule, and nodular hyperplasia.[17]

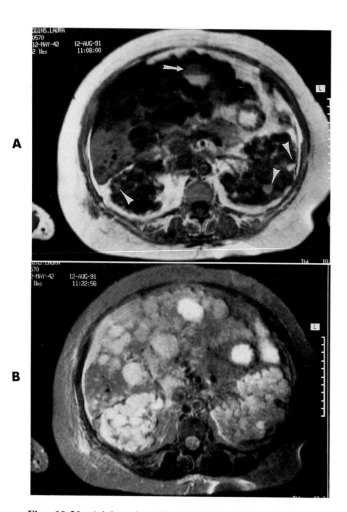

Fig. 10-21. Adult polycystic kidney-liver disease. **A,** T1WI demonstrates multiple lesions in the liver and the kidneys with low signal intensity. Some lesions are hyperintense due to secondary internal hemorrhage *(arrowheads)*. Fluid-fluid level is found in one hemorrhagic liver cyst *(arrow)*. **B,** T2WI reveals the cysts as hyperintense areas.

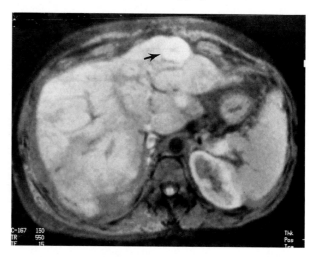

Fig. 10-22. Adenomatous hyperplastic nodule. Fat suppression T1WI (TR 150 msec/TE 15 msec) of this young patient with long-standing hepatic cirrhosis demonstrates at least one hyperintense nodule *(arrow)*. This corresponds to a nodule of adenomatous hyperplasia (macroregenerative nodule). Adenomatous hyperplastic nodules are typically multiple and appear hyperintense in T1WI and T2WI, as well as in fat suppression technique images.

Table 10-2. Hyperplastic hepatocellular conditions

	FNH	HCA	NRH	Multiple HCA	AHN
Number of lesions	1	1	Many	Many	Many or few
Size	1-6 cm	4-12 cm	>1.5 cm	2-9 cm	1-6 cm
Key feature	Pseudoductules	Neohepatocytes	Small nodules No fibrosis	Normal cords	Portal tracts
Prior liver disease	None	None	None	None	Cirrhosis

FNH, Focal nodular hyperplasia
HCA, Hepatocellular adenoma
NRH, Nodular regenerative hyperplasia
AHN, Adenomatous hyperplastic nodule or macroregenerative nodules

AHN is a nodular lesion significantly larger than other regenerative nodules of the cirrhotic liver and, therefore, has also been called macroregenerative nodule. AHN has no true capsule but has portal areas and bile ducts. It is considered a precancerous lesion in the cirrhotic liver, and its differentiation from HCC may be important in order to plan resection and/or liver transplantation in chronic cirrhotic patients (Fig. 10-22).

Although further detail in the discussion of AHN is included in section four of this chapter, it is important to mention it here because AHN should not be confused with other hyperplastic hepatocellular conditions (Table 10-2).

Multiple hepatocellular adenomas is defined as the presence of multiple adenomas (more than four by definition), which are usually present in both lobes. Very few cases have been reported.[3]

There are other benign tumors of the liver that have not been described by MRI. These tumors include lymphangiomatosis, leiomyoma, fibroma (fibrous mesothelioma), adrenal rest tumors, and pancreatic heterotopias.

REFERENCES

1. Boechat MI, Kangarloo H, Ortega J, et al: Primary liver tumors in children: comparison of CT and MR imaging, Radiology 169:727-732, 1988.
2. Butch RJ, Stark DD, Malt RA: MR imaging of hepatic focal nodular hyperplasia, J Comput Assist Tomogr 10:874-877, 1986.
3. Chen KT, Bocian JJ: Multiple hepatic adenomas, Arch Pathol Lab Med 107:274-275, 1983.
4. Choi BI, Lim JH, Han MC, et al: Biliary cystadenoma and cyst-adenocarcinoma: CT and sonographic findings, Radiology 171:57, 1989.
5. Christopherson WM, Mays ET, Barrows G: A clinicopathologic study of steroid-related tumors, Am J Surg Pathol 1:31-41, 1977.
6. Craig GR, Peters RL, Edmonson HA: Tumors of the liver and intrahepatic bile ducts. Atlas of tumor pathology, 2nd series, Washington, DC, 1989, Armed Forces Institute of Pathology.
7. Dachman AH, Ros PR, Goodman ZD, et al: Nodular regenerative hyperplasia of the liver: clinical and radiologic observations, Am J Roentgenol 148:717-722, 1987.
8. Gabata T, Matsui O, Kadoya M, et al: MR imaging of hepatic adenoma, Am J Roentgenol 155:1009-1011, 1990.
9. Goodman ZD, et al: Kupffer cells in hepatocellular adenomas, Am J Surg Pathol 11:191-196, 1987.
10. Ishak KG, Rabin L: Benign tumors of the liver, Med Clin North Am 59:995-1013, 1975.
11. Ishak KG, et al: Biliary cystadenoma and cyst-adenocarcinoma, Cancer 38:322-338, 1977.
12. Reference deleted in proof.
13. Korobkin M, Stephens DH, Lee JKT, et al: Biliary cystadenoma and cystadenocarcinoma: CT and sonographic findings. Am J Roentgenol 153:507-511, 1989.
14. Lubbers PR, Ros PR, Goodman ZD, et al: Accumulation of technetium-99m sulfur colloid by hepatocellular adenoma: scintigraphic-pathologic correlation, Am J Roentgenol 148:1105-1108, 1987.
15. Marti-Bonmati L, Menor F, Vizcaino J, et al: Lipoma of the liver: US, CT and MRI appearance, Gastrointest Radiol 14:155-157, 1989.
16. Mathieu D, Rahmouni A, Anglade MC, et al: Focal nodular hyperplasia of the liver: assessment with contrast-enhanced turboFLASH MR imaging, Radiology 180:25-30, 1991.
17. Matsui O, Kadoya M, Kameyama T, et al: Adenomatous hyperplastic nodules in the cirrhotic liver: differentiation from hepatocellular carcinoma with MRI, Radiology 173:123-126, 1989.
18. Mattison GR, Glazer GM, Quint LE, et al: MR imaging of hepatic focal nodular hyperplasia: characterization and distinction from primary malignant hepatic tumors, Am J Roentgenol 148:711-715, 1987.
19. Moss AA, Goldberg HJ, Stark DD, et al: Hepatic tumors: magnetic resonance and CT appearance, Radiology 150:141-147, 1984.
20. Nokes SR, Baker ME, Spritzer CE, et al: Hepatic adenoma: MR appearance mimicking focal nodular hyperplasia, J Comput Assist Tomogr 12:885-887, 1988.
21. O'Neil J, Ros PR: Knowing hepatic pathology aids MRI of liver tumors, Diagn Imaging Dec:58-67, 1989.
22. Palacios E, Shannon M, Solomon C, et al: Biliary cystadenoma: ultrasound, CT and MRI. Gastrointest Radiol 15:313-316, 1990.
23. Patriarche C, et al: Ultrasonography, angiography, computed tomography and magnetic resonance in nodular regenerative hyperplasia of the liver: report of a pseudotumoral case, Radiat Med 6:111-114, 1988.
24. Rahman ME, Li KCP, Ros PR: Hepatic focal nodular hyperplasia: new MR findings, Mag Reson Med 7:1-2, 1989.
25. Roberts JL, Fishman EK, Hartman DS, et al: Lipomatous tumors of the liver: evaluation with CT and US, Radiology 158:613-617, 1986.
26. Rummeny E, Weissleder R, Sironi S, et al: Central scars in primary

liver tumors: MR features, specificity, and pathologic correlation, Radiology 171:323-326, 1989.

27. Rummeny E, Weissleder R, Stark DD, et al: Primary liver tumors: diagnosis by MR imaging, Am J Roentgenol 152:63-72, 1989.
28. Schiebler ML, Kressel HY, Saul SH, et al: MR imaging of focal nodular hyperplasia of the liver, J Comput Assist Tomogr 11:651-654, 1987.
29. Tham R, et al: Focal nodular hyperplasia of the liver: features on Gd-DTPA-enhanced MR, Am J Roentgenol 153:884-885, 1989.
30. Wanless IR, Mawdsley C, Adams R: Pathogenesis of focal nodular hyperplasia, Hepatology 5:1194-1200, 1985.

Section four
Malignant liver tumors

Pablo R. Ros

Hepatocellular carcinoma
Fibrolamellar carcinoma
Intrahepatic cholangiocarcinoma
Angiosarcoma
Hepatoblastoma
Undifferentiated embryonal sarcoma
Other primary malignancies

Some of the major advantages of magnetic MRI in the liver have been recognized since early reports of particular importance for the study of hepatic malignancies.[16] In particular, MRI's ability to evaluate vessels, its superb display of location of tumors based on its multiplanar capabilities, the minor artifact production due to clips, compared to CT, and its ability to delineate the internal structure of masses have been pertinent in malignant tumors.

If one considers that all malignant tumors are surgical and that hepatic resections are performed according to vascular territories, it is obvious that MRI plays a choice role in the preoperative evaluation of malignant neoplasms. If in addition, one considers that hepatocellular malignancies frequently have a tendency to grow into vessels (angioinvasion—typical of hepatocellular carcinoma) or encase vessels (intrahepatic cholangiocarcinoma), the role of MRI is further enhanced. Furthermore, because MRI is able to display the liver in sagittal, coronal, and axial planes, location of tumors in relation to essential surgical anatomic structures such as the cava or porta is of interest for the practicing surgeon.

Although MRI has offered a potentially ideal method for preoperative evaluation of malignant tumors, its practical application has lagged behind CT due to some important drawbacks. Because there is tremendous overlap in signal intensity between tumors, no consistent differences are discovered; and, therefore, preoperative characterization of a mass as malignant is not possible. Only hemangioma and at a certain point focal nodular hyperplasia (FNH) may have a characteristic MRI appearance. Therefore,

from adenoma to metastases, as well as many other malignant tumors, the appearance is nonspecific.

Furthermore, there has been controversy in establishing the best pulsing sequence, magnetic field strength, and overall technique to better detect hepatic lesions. There are no significant differences in detecting focal lesions due to magnetic field strengths.[28] When 100 lesions were studied comparing 0.5 T and 1.5 T, both magnetic field strengths were equivalent, although T1-weighted spin-echo sequence at 1.5 T was significantly inferior to other sequences. T2-weighted sequences were optimal for detection of liver lesions in both magnetic field strengths. At 0.5 T, inversion recovery T1WI were also excellent.[28]

This section presents the primary malignant liver tumors by pathologic diagnosis. Knowing the underlying pathology is helpful to better understand the MRI appearance of these different tumors.[22] In addition, with the advent of MRI contrast agents, such as superparamagnetic iron oxide (SPIO) which is taken up by reticuloendothelial cells, it is becoming more important to understand the pathology of lesions. Because in general, all hepatic malignancies contain no Kupffer cells, there will be no uptake of SPIO particles and hepatic malignancies, both primary or metastatic, will have higher signal intensity in T2WI or gradient-echo images compared to the normal liver. This increases the detectability of hepatic lesions, primarily malignancies.[8]

HEPATOCELLULAR CARCINOMA

Hepatocellular carcinoma (HCC) is the most common primary hepatic malignancy and one of the most common visceral malignancies worldwide.[3] It is important to realize that HCC has a dual geographic distribution, not only in incidence but in clinical presentation. HCC is rare in the Western Hemisphere (low incidence areas) and has a relatively high frequency in sub-Saharian Africa and Asia (high incidence areas). Even in the United States, the incidence of HCC ranges from 0.9 per 100,000 in New York women to 30.9 per 100,000 in San Francisco men of Chinese origin.[3] Worldwide, the highest incidence reported of HCC is in Japan with a rate as high as 4.8%.[17] Therefore, this bimodal distribution translates to a relative paucity of MRI descriptions from the Western Hemisphere compared to the large amount of MRI reports coming from Japanese authors.[5,11,12]

Microscopically, HCC has several patterns. In general, HCC is composed of malignant hepatocytes that attempt to differentiate themselves into normal liver, mimicking hepatocyte growth, but unable to form normal hepatic acini. HCC cells are difficult to distinguish from normal hepatocytes and hepatocellular adenoma cells. Malignant hepatocytes may even produce bile. There are microscopic variations with HCC containing fat, tumoral secretions (large amounts of watery material), fibrosis, and rarely even

---

Hepatocellular carcinoma: MRI-pathologic correlation

MRI

- Hypointense (T1W1)
- Isointense (T1W1)
- Hyperintense (T1W1)
- Heterogeneous Hyperintense (T2W1)
- Hypointense peripheral rim
- High signal in vessels

Pathology

- Fibrosis
- Pseudoacinar (water secretion)
- Fatty change
- Internal necrosis/hemorrhage
- Fibrous capsule
- Tumor thrombi (vascular invasion)

---

amorphous calcification. This variable microscopic composition gives rise to different appearances by MRI (box above).

Grossly, there also are several patterns of growth. HCC is called single or massive when there is a solitary large mass. Nodular or multifocal HCC, the second most common pattern, is characterized by multiple separated nodules, mimicking the appearance of metastases. The least common pattern of diffuse or cirrhotomimetic HCC is composed of multiple small foci of tumor distributed throughout the liver, mimicking nodules of cirrhosis.

HCC may be encapsulated when it is completely surrounded by a fibrous capsule, which is detectable by MRI. Encapsulated HCC has better prognosis due to greater resectability.[7,24] Vascular growth of HCC in intrahepatic (portal hepatic vein branches) and perihepatic vessels (inferior vena cava and porta) is common.[29]

Japanese authors have become interested in describing HCC by MRI because of the need to diagnose HCC as early as possible.[5,11] Early reports have shown that HCC can take many different appearances by MRI, ranging from diffuse to nodular and massive, and is microscopically diverse. These differences yield variable success rates in detection.[20,21] Differentiation between metastases and HCC is not possible, but MRI can detect invasion by HCC of the portal vein and other vessels, obviating the need for angiography to assess vascular invasion of these tumors.[19]

MRI is able to detect with greater contrast than CT small foci of tumor. The rate of detection of HCC varies with its size: greater than 95% if the tumor is larger than 2 cm and less than 35% for tumors smaller than 2 cm. The capsule that may be present in HCC (20% to 30% in Western patients and higher in Japanese patients) is demonstrated twice as often by MRI than by CT.

In T1WI four patterns of intensity have been described: (1) low, (2) iso, (3) high, and (4) mixed. These patterns correspond to the presence of watery secretions, fibrosis, and fatty change within malignant hepatocytes. In spin-echo T2WI, almost all HCCs appear with high intensity (Fig. 10-23).

MRI is superior to CT in the depiction of pseudocap-

sules, intratumoral septa, satellite or regenerating nodules, and presence of tumor thrombi.

In a large series of Western patients, HCC was best detected with T2 pulsing sequences with a higher tumor-liver T2 difference (34%) than T1 tumor-liver difference (21%).[26] Some of the expected findings in HCC were present, such as fatty degeneration (47%), tumor capsule (23%), and vascular invasion (28%). Peritumoral edema was noted in 28% of patients. Thus except in a percentage of cases where MRI was able to depict a tumor capsule (45% in Japanese patients versus 28% in Western patients), the appearance for HCC was similar in both Asian and Western populations.

MRI has also been used to try to differentiate small HCCs from regenerating nodules of cirrhosis by both American and Japanese researchers.[10,13,15,18] Differentiating between HCC and adenomatous hyperplastic nodules (AHN) or regenerating nodules is extremely important because in chronic cirrhosis a major complication is the development of HCC. However, large regenerating nodules or AHN are also common in patients with cirrhotic livers. Regenerating nodules are frequently small (0.5 to 1.5 cm) and are not detected by other imaging modalities, particularly CT. With spin-echo T2WI and particularly with gradient-echo sequences, regenerating nodules and AHN appear with low intensity. On the other hand, HCC appears as areas of hyperintensity in T2WI. In T1WI, AHN are frequently hyperintense.

The reason that AHN (regenerating nodules) have low intensity in gradient-echo and T2WI is not known. Some authors consider that this low intensity is due to high levels of hemosiderin.[18] However, the low intensity may be due to the presence of broad fibrous septa. It is also possible to recognize the development of HCC within large AHN or regenerative nodules, which has been described as the "nodule within nodule" sign.[15] On MRI, the nodule within nodule consists of a markedly low intensity, large nodule in gradient-echo images with internal foci that are isointense to the liver. These foci correspond to HCC that has developed in large AHN.

Occasionally, HCC may be confused with FNH, as both exhibit a central area of hyperintensity in T2-

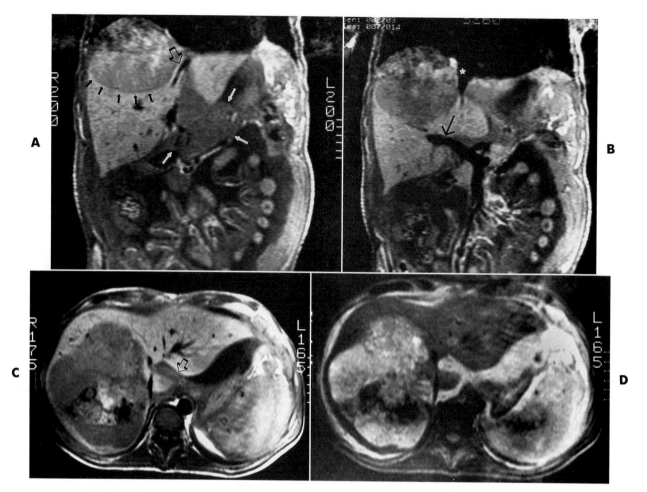

Fig. 10-23. Hepatocellular carcinoma (HCC): MRI appearance. **A,** In this patient with chronic cirrhosis and ascites, there is a large HCC in the dome of the liver *(arrows)* seen as a hypointense mass in this coronal T1WI (TR 600 msec/TE 20 msec). A hepatic vein *(open arrow)* is displaced, but not invaded. There is extrahepatic extension of the tumor through the gastrohepatic ligament *(white arrows)*. Note ascites with floating bowel loops. **B,** A section slightly more anterior demonstrates patency of the portal vein *(arrow)*, as well as extension of the tumor to the level of the inferior vena cava *(*)*. **C,** Axial T1WI (TR 500 msec/TE 20 msec) shows the heterogeneous nature of this HCC. Areas of hemorrhage, as well as fibrosis, are seen within the tumor. However, the overall intensity of the HCC is less than the one of the normal liver. Again, ascites, gastrohepatic ligament extension *(open arrow)*, and extension of the tumor to the inferior vena cava can be identified. **D,** Correlative T2WI (TR 2000 msec/TE 80 msec) demonstrates the overall hyperintensity of HCC compared with the uninvolved liver. Note ascites seen as a thin bright intensity rim surrounding the liver.

weighted spin-echo sequences. This area will correspond to the scar in FNH and to necrosis in HCC. If a central hyperintense region has a stellate appearance, however, it may be difficult to distinguish FNH from HCC.[32]

MRI is well suited to evaluate possible invasion of hepatic and perihepatic vascular structures noninvasively, using not only spin-echo techniques but also MR angiography.[19]

Dynamic MRI with gadopentetate dimeglumine and gradient-echo images has been used to differentiate small HCC from hemangioma.[33] HCC appears as a hyperintense mass before contrast enhancement, and the peak enhance-

ment occurs earlier than in hemangioma (an average of 10 seconds after injection). In HCC, there is no delineated enhancement, as with hemangioma. Gadopentetate dimeglumine is also capable of demonstrating the presence of a capsule surrounding HCC with higher sensitivity than without intravascular enhancement.

The use of SPIO in the diagnosis of HCC has been successful in preliminary reports. After intravenous administration of SPIO, small nodules of HCC may be accurately depicted with greater sensitivity than with unenhanced MRI[6] (Figs. 10-24 and 10-25).

In summary, MRI depicts HCC as either hypointense,

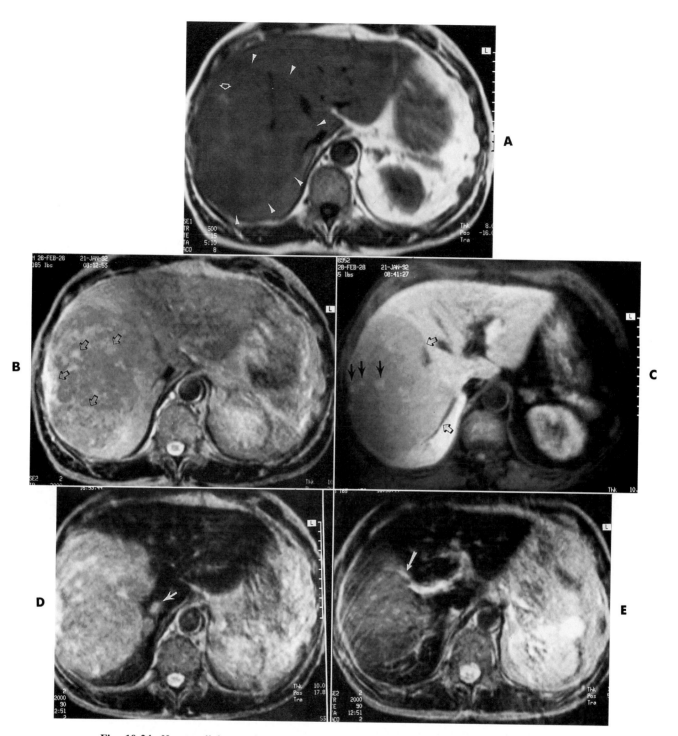

Fig. 10-24. Hepatocellular carcinoma (HCC): Before and after SPIO administration. **A,** T1WI
(TR 300 msec/TE 15 msec) in this 64-year-old man demonstrates a subtle decrease in intensity in
the right lobe of the liver *(arrows)*. This corresponds to a large mass. There is distortion of the
normal liver vascularity within the tumor. There is also ill-defined areas of increased intensity
secondary to hemorrhage *(open arrow)*. The tumor is seen to extend to the area of the inverior
vena cava without invading it. **B,** T2WI (TR 2000 msec/TE 90 msec) demonstrates mild irregularity in the right lobe, as well as heterogeneity of the signal. Figures **A** and **B** demonstrate that
hepatocellular carcinoma may be almost isointense with normal liver in T1WI and T2WI. However, the heterogeneity typical of the tumor with some areas of marked hyperintensity, corresponding to hemorrhagic and/or liquefactive necrosis, can be seen *(open arrows)*. **C,** Fat suppression image demonstrates that the tumor is hypointense compared to the normal parenchyma, suggesting fatty content within the HCC. This may also explain the appearance in T1WI and T2WI.
Note the small areas of hemorrhage and/or necrosis *(black arrows)*. Note how the tumor is seen
displacing hepatic veins *(open arrows)*. **D,** T2WI postintravenous administration of SPIO demonstrates improvement in tumor visualization due to decreased signal in the normal liver. A satellite
or daughter tumor can be seen *(arrow)*. **E,** Section lower than **D** demonstrates invasion of the
right portal branch *(arrow)*.

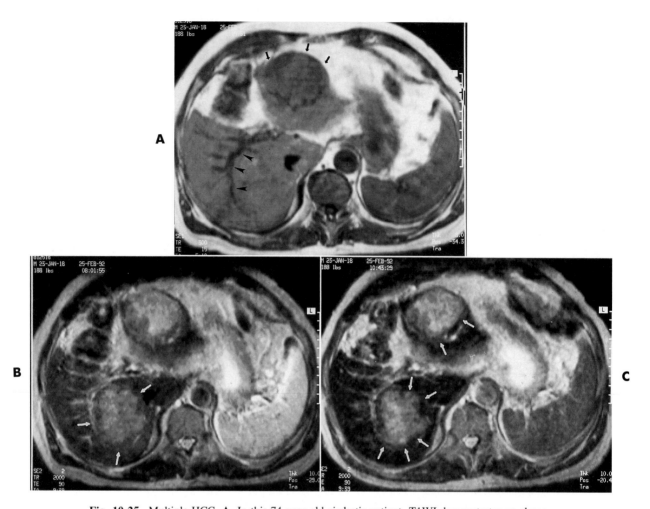

Fig. 10-25. Multiple HCC. **A,** In this 74-year-old cirrhotic patient, T1WI demonstrates an abnormality of the contour of the liver *(arrows),* as well as displacement of the right portal branch *(arrow heads).* However, it is difficult to distinguish definite masses. The cava is not patent (TR 300 msec/TE 15 msec). **B,** T2WI (TR 2000 msec/TE 90 msec) demonstrates a slightly hyperintense mass in the left lobe of the liver, which is responsible for its unusual contour. A second mass is seen in the posterior segment of the right lobe *(arrows),* which is slightly hyperintense than the normal liver. **A** and **B** demonstrate an example of HCC that is isointense in T1 and slightly hyperintense in T2. **C,** T2WI (TR 2000 msec/TE 90 msec) post-SPIO intravenously administered demonstrates decrease in the signal intensity of the normal liver, producing better visualization of the two large foci of HCC *(arrows).*

isointense, or hyperintense in appearance in T1WI. This variable appearance by MRI is secondary to microscopic forms of HCC, including cellular, pseudoacinar, and fatty changes.

HCC appears frequently as a heterogeneous mass with a hyperintense appearance in T2WI. A hyperintense peripheral rim, corresponding to fibrous capsule can be seen up to 45% of cases (high incidence areas in Asia), or 28% of cases (low incidence areas in United States). MRI is an excellent method to depict vascular invasion with tumor thrombi within perihepatic vessels, appearing as high signal intensity in both T1WI and T2WI within vessels.

FIBROLAMELLAR CARCINOMA

Fibrolamellar carcinoma (FLC) is a hepatocellular neoplasm that should not be confused with the usual or typical HCC. Although both tumors are composed of neoplastic hepatocytes, in FLC the hepatocytes are separated by lamellar fibrous strands.[3] Recently, FLC has been recognized as a completely independent biologic entity from the usual HCC.[2]

FLC occurs in adolescents and adults less than 40 years old in a normal liver without underlying cirrhosis. It is associated with a much longer average survival rate than in other types of HCC (45 to 60 months versus 6 months) and a high likelihood of cure if surgically resected.

> **Fibrolamellar carcinoma: MRI-pathologic correlation**
>
> | *MRI* | *Pathology* |
> |---|---|
> | • Hypointense (T1W1) | • Hepatocellular neoplasm |
> | • Hyperintense (T2W1) | |
> | • Hypointense scar (T2W1) | • Lamellar fibrosis |

> **Intrahepatic cholangiocarcinoma: MRI-pathologic correlation**
>
> | *MRI* | *Pathology* |
> |---|---|
> | • Homogeneous Hypointense (T1W1) Hyperintense (T2W1) | • No necrosis/ hemorrhage |
> | • Large fibrotic areas | • Hypointense areas (T2W1) |
> | • Vascular encasement (caliber reduction of vessels without tumor thrombosis) | • Vascular encasement |
> | • Centripetal enhancement (post-gadolinium-DTPA) | |

Microscopically, satellite nodules are often present. The gross appearance of FLC is similar to that of FNH, as both have a central scar and multiple fibrous septa. FLC is a homogeneous tumor compared with typical HCC; hemorrhage and necrosis are rare.

Although few cases of FLC have been published, it is apparent that MRI provides key diagnostic information.[14,30] In 1987, Mattison, et al[14] described two cases at 0.35 T where FLC appears as an isointense tumor in T1WI compared to normal liver, which becomes slightly hyperintense in T2WI. However, the scar is hypointense in both T1WI and T2WI. In 1988, Titelbaum, et al[30] described two additional cases at 1.5 T. That the central scar is never of high signal intensity when compared to the rest of the lesion or the liver in T2WI indicates that the scar is composed of collagenous, cellular fibrosis, as opposed to FNH where the scar is frequently hyperintense in T2WI because it contains multiple vessels.

Thus, MRI plays an important role in differentiating FLC from FNH. This ability is important because both entities are present in noncirrhotic livers of patients who are frequently in the fifth decades or life or younger. In general, other imaging modalities have not been able to differentiate between both tumors.[31]

In addition, although FLC is a tumor composed of malignant hepatocytes, the levels of alpha-fetoprotein are normal. Thus, MRI is the only noninvasive diagnostic test that may be helpful to differentiate FNH from FLC. The hyperintensity (typical of FNH) or hypointensity (typical of FLC) of the central scar in a T2WI becomes an important sign to differentiate these two tumors (see box).

INTRAHEPATIC CHOLANGIOCARCINOMA

Intrahepatic cholangiocarcinoma (I-CAC) is a malignant neoplasm arising from the epithelium of the intrahepatic bile ducts. These neoplasms are characterized grossly as large, firm masses with large amounts of whitish fibrous tissue and rarely small areas of necrosis or hemorrhage. Clinically, I-CAC is the second most common primary hepatic malignancy in the adult, usually seen in the seventh decade of life and with slight male predominance.[3]

Although there is one report on extrahepatic cholangiocarcinoma,[4] the MRI appearance of I-CAC is limited to two published cases.[9,22] In both, the appearance is strikingly identical. I-CAC appears as a large, central mass with irregular borders seen as hypointense in T1WI and hyperintense in T2WI. The mass is heterogeneous with large areas that are hypointense in T2WI, corresponding to large central areas of fibrosis. The periphery of I-CAC is more hyperintense in T2WI.

In the report by Hamrick-Turner et al,[9] progressive, concentric enhancement is seen after intravenous administration of gadopentetate dimeglumine. This centripetal enhancement spares central areas, reflecting the presence of central fibrosis and viable peripheral tumor.

Another feature of I-CAC is encasement of large vessels such as the inferior vena cava or hepatic veins by the tumor without thrombosis or invasion, which would be suggestive of HCC. Gradient-echo images demonstrate the feature of vascular encasement without tumor thrombus in I-CAC (Fig. 10-26).

In summary, the finding of a large tumor that has hypointense appearance in T1WI and hyperintense appearance in T2WI, except for large central areas of scar, is the most common appearance of I-CAC. Other features are the centripetal enhancement after intravenous injection of gadopentetate dimeglumine (Fig. 10-27), except in the hypointense areas corresponding to scar, and encasement of large hepatic vessels (see box).

ANGIOSARCOMA

Angiosarcoma of the liver is a malignant neoplasm derived from endothelial cells. It occurs primarily in adults as a result of occupational exposure to polyvinyl chloride, or PVC, and thorium dioxide (Thorotrast).[3]

Microscopically, angiosarcomas are composed of multiple vascular channels of variable size lined with malignant endothelial cells. Exposure to Thorotrast can result in particles being found within the malignant endothelial cells. Grossly, the majority of angiosarcomas are multiple, with areas of internal hemorrhage. Angiosarcoma is a rare neoplasm (30 times less common than HCC) that is seen more

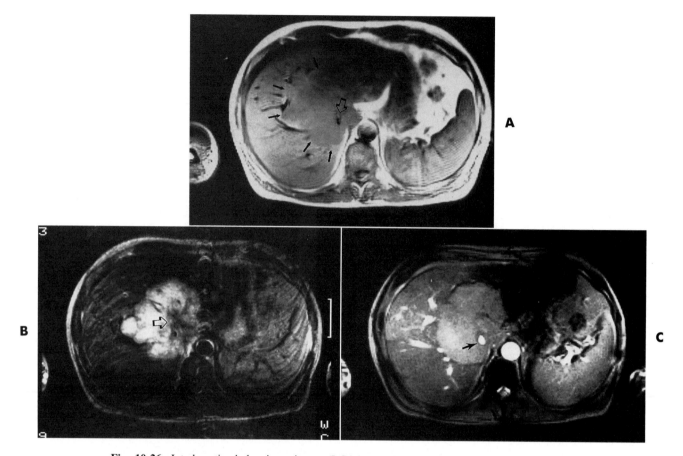

Fig. 10-26. Intrahepatic cholangiocarcinoma (I-CAC) at 1.5 T. **A,** T1WI (TR 550 msec/TE 22 msec) shows lobulated hypointense homogeneous mass *(arrows)*. Note encasement of inferior vena cava *(open arrow)*. **B,** T2WI (TR 2500 msec/TE 80 msec) demonstrates the hyperintense nature of the tumor, primarily in the periphery. A large central area of low density, corresponding to scar, frequent in intrahepatic cholangiocarcinoma is noted *(open arrow)*. **C,** Gradient-echo image (TR 50 msec/TE 18 msec/FLIP angle 30 degrees) shows the mass hyperintense relative to normal liver. In this sequence designed to enhance vascular structures, the encasement of inferior vena cava is well demonstrated *(arrow)*.

frequently in the seventh decade of life and in men.

No cases of angiosarcoma have been reported by MRI. In our experience angiosarcomas appear as a hypointense mass on T1WI that becomes hyperintense in T2WI. Rim enhancement can be noted after injection of gadopentetate dimeglumine, and persistence of gadopentetate dimeglumine can be seen in delayed images, mimicking the appearance of hemangioma (Fig. 10-28). This appearance has been reported angiographically and in dynamic-enhanced CT. Because the underlying pathology of angiosarcoma and hemangioma is similar, with multiple vascular channels, this persistence is not surprising.[27]

Thorotrast-induced angiosarcoma is easy to recognize by CT because of the distinctive pattern of Thorotrast and its circumferential displacement by the nodules of angiosarcoma. Thorotrast is not distinguishable by MRI.[23]

In summary, the MRI findings of angiosarcoma have not been published. However, because Thorotrast is not detected by MRI the appearance of angiosarcoma is that of a nonspecific hepatic mass. Persistence of gadopentetate dimeglumine, as well as centripetal filling as seen in hemangioma, may prove to be a helpful feature. Additional experience is needed to ascertain the value of MRI for angiosarcoma of the liver.

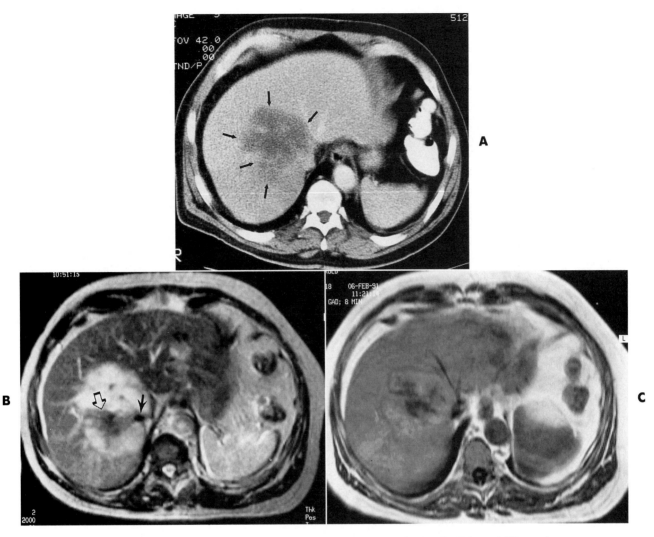

Fig. 10-27. I-CAC: CT and gadopentetate dimeglumine-enhanced MRI. **A,** Enhanced CT scan in this 72-year-old man demonstrates a 10 cm central, homogeneous mass in the liver *(arrows)*. The tumor has markedly low density primarily because of its relative hypovascularity secondary to its fibrous nature. **B,** T2WI (TR 2000 msec/TE 90 msec) shows the mass to be hyperintense relative to liver within a regular area of hypointensity, corresponding to scar *(arrow)*. Note how the inferior vena cava *(curved arrow)* is encased. **C,** T1WI (TR 302 msec/TE 15 msec) MR image obtained 10 minutes after intravenous administration of gadopentetate dimeglumine shows progressive, concentric, peripheral enhancement of the I-CAC. Note persistence of a central area of hypointensity, as well as a hypointense rim surrounding the periphery of the mass.

HEPATOBLASTOMA

Hepatoblastoma, the most common primary hepatic neoplasm in childhood, is composed of malignant hepatocytes, which often contain mesenchymal elements. Although this tumor is described in the pediatric chapter of this textbook, we include a brief description here to compare it with other malignant hepatic neoplasms.

Hepatoblastoma can be classified as either epithelial or mixed (epithelial-mesenchymal).[3] This histologic classification not only has prognostic implications (epithelial type with better prognosis than mixed), but also helps explain the variable gross appearance of this tumor. Epithelial hepatoblastomas are homogeneous, whereas mixed hepatoblastomas are more often heterogeneous, as they contain osteoid tissue, cartilage, and frequently large calcifications, fibroid bands, and larger areas of necrosis and hemorrhage.

Hepatoblastoma appears on MRI as a hyperintense tumor in T2WI, which becomes hypointense in T1WI. However, particularly in T2WI, MRI demonstrates the internal septations usual in this tumor as hypointense bands, corresponding to fibrosis (Fig. 10-29). MRI is able to demon-

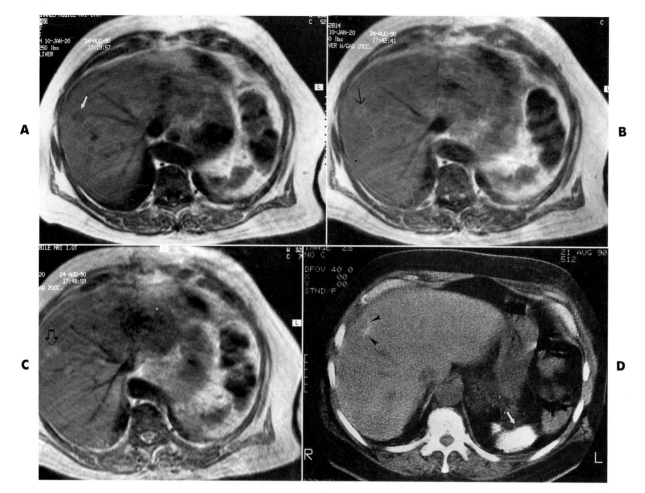

Fig. 10-28. Angiosarcoma: MR-CT correlation. **A,** Axial T1-weighted spin-echo (TR 500 msec/TE 15 msec) at 1.0 T demonstrates a hypointense area in the liver *(white arrow).* **B,** T1WI (TR 500 msec/TE 15 msec) obtained immediately after gadopentetate dimeglumine injection demonstrates peripheral enhancement of the nodule *(arrow).* **C,** Delayed T1WI (6 minutes after gadopentetate dimeglumine injection) demonstrates filling in of the nodular of angiosarcoma with persistence of the enhancement *(open arrow).* **D,** Correlative enhanced CT of the abdomen demonstrates deposits of Thorotrast in the liver *(arrowheads),* as well as marked Thorotrast deposition in the spleen *(white arrow).* Although Thorotrast is exquisitely well seen by CT, it is not detectable by MRI.

strate these fibrotic bands and the nodular architecture of hepatoblastoma with more detail than other techniques, particularly CT.[1,22]

MRI also demonstrates the presence of vessel invasion. Hepatoblastoma, like HCC, has a tendency to invade vessels with tumor thrombi in perihepatic or intrahepatic vessels (hepatic veins, intrahepatic cava, portal vein), which can be easily recognized by MRI.

When compared with CT, MRI is particularly valuable

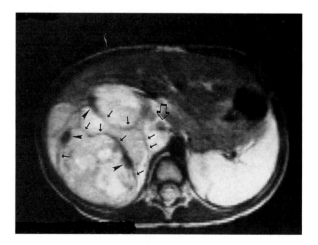

Fig. 10-29. Hepatoblastoma. T2WI (TR 2000 msec/TE 60 msec) at 0.35 T demonstrates a large mixed type hepatoblastoma. Note fibrous bands *(arrow),* as well as large vessels *(arrowhead)* seen within the tumor. There is displacement of the inferior vena cava by the tumor *(open arrow)* without obstruction.

in assessing both the preoperative extension of hepatoblastoma and potential tumor recurrence after surgery.

UNDIFFERENTIATED EMBRYONAL SARCOMA

Undifferentiated embryonal sarcoma (UES) is a malignant tumor occurring primarily in older children (and teenagers) 6 to 15 years of age.[25]

Grossly, UES is a large, usually solitary mass frequently of cystic nature due to a large degree of necrosis and internal hemorrhage. Cystic tumors are seen more frequently than solid ones.

No cases of UES studied with MRI have been published. In our experience, UES appears as a large mass with marked hyperintensity in T2WI and hypointensity in

T1WI, as is usually seen in large cystic masses. T2WI depicts the internal nature of these cystic tumors, displaying internal debris and septations.

OTHER PRIMARY MALIGNANCIES

Other primary malignancies may involve the liver. Lymphoma, both primary and secondary, is discussed in section eight (diffuse diseases) of this chapter. However, other malignant neoplasms such as malignant fibrous histiocytoma, intrahepatic leiomyosarcoma, and other sarcomas have been described. The appearance by MRI is that of a nonspecific mass that appears hypointense in T1WI and hyperintense T2WI (Fig. 10-30). MRI is helpful to identify tumor extension into vessels.

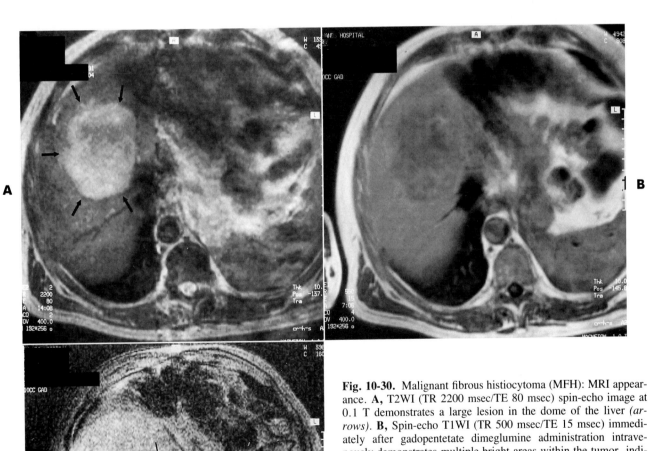

Fig. 10-30. Malignant fibrous histiocytoma (MFH): MRI appearance. **A,** T2WI (TR 2200 msec/TE 80 msec) spin-echo image at 0.1 T demonstrates a large lesion in the dome of the liver (arrows). **B,** Spin-echo T1WI (TR 500 msec/TE 15 msec) immediately after gadopentetate dimeglumine administration intravenously demonstrates multiple bright areas within the tumor, indicating the hypervascular nature of MFH. **C,** T2-weighted gradient-echo image (TR 31 msec/TE 12 msec/FLIP angle 15 degrees) demonstrates that the tumor is seen abutting the inferior vena cava (arrow). However, the tumor is barely distinguishable when compared with T1- or T2-weighted spin-echo images. A thin rim of hypointensity is seen due to chemical-shift artifact, corresponding to the margin of the tumor (arrow).

REFERENCES

1. Boechat MI, Kangarloo H, Ortega J, et al: Primary liver tumors in children: comparison of CT and MR imaging, Radiology 169:727-732, 1988.
2. Craig JR, Peters RL, Edmondson HA: Fibrolamellar carcinoma of the liver, Cancer 46:372-379, 1980.
3. Craig JR, Peters RL, Edmondson HA: Tumors of the liver and intrahepatic bile ducts, second series, Fascicle 26. In Hartmann WH, ed: Atlas of Tumor Pathology, Washington, DC, 1989, Armed Forces Institute of Pathology.
4. Dooms GC, Kerlan RK Jr, Hricak H, et al: Cholangiocarcinoma: imaging by MR, Radiology 159:89-94, 1986.
5. Ebara M, et al: Diagnosis of small hepatocellular carcinoma: correlation of MR imaging and tumor histologic studies, Radiology 159:371-377, 1986.
6. Ferrucci JT, Stark DD: Iron oxide-enhanced MR imaging of the liver and spleen: review of the first five years, Am J Roentgenol 155:943-950, 1990.
7. Freeney PC, Baron RL, Teefey SA: Hepatocellular carcinoma: reduced frequency of typical findings with dynamic contrast-enhanced CT in a non-Asian population, Radiology 182:143-148, 1992.
8. Fretz CJ, Elizondo G, Weissleder R, et al: Superparamagnetic iron oxide-enhanced MR imaging: pulse sequence optimization for detection of liver cancer, Radiology 172:393-397, 1989.
9. Hamrick-Turner J, Abbitt PL, Ros PR: Intrahepatic cholangiocarcinoma: MR appearance, Am J Roentgenol 158:77-79, 1992.
10. Itai Y, Ohnishi S, Ohtomo K, et al: Regenerating nodules of liver cirrhosis: MR imaging, Radiology 165:419-423, 1987.
11. Itoh K, Nishimura K, Togashi K, et al: Hepatocellular carcinoma: MR imaging, Radiology 164:21-25, 1987.
12. Kitagawa K, Matsui O, Kadoya M, et al: Hepatocellular carcinomas with excessive copper accumulation: CT and MR findings, Radiology 180:623-628, 1991.
13. Matsui O, Kadoya M, Kameyama T, et al: Adenomatous hyperplastic nodules in the cirrhotic liver: differentiation from hepatocellular carcinoma with MR imaging, Radiology 173:123-126, 1989.
14. Mattison GR, Glazer GM, Quint LE, et al: MR imaging of hepatic focal nodular hyperplasia: characterization and distinction from primary malignant hepatic tumors, AJR 148:711-715, 1987.
15. Mitchell DG, Rubin R, Siegelman ES, et al: Hepatocellular carcinoma within siderotic regenerative nodules: appearance as a nodule within a nodule on MR images, Radiology 178:101-103, 1991.
16. Moss AA, Goldberg HJ, Stark DD, et al: Hepatic tumors: magnetic resonance and CT appearance, Radiology 150:141-147, 1984.
17. Nakashima T, et al: Pathology of HCC in Japan: 232 consecutive cases autopsied in ten years, Cancer 51:863-877, 1983.
18. Ohtomo K, Itai Y, Yoshida H, et al: Regenerating nodules of liver cirrhosis: MR imaging with pathologic correlation, Am J Roentgenol 154:505-507, 1990.
19. Ohtomo K, Itai Y, Furui S, et al: MR imaging of portal vein thrombus in hepatocellular carcinoma, J Comput Assist Tomogr 9(2):328-329, 1985.
20. Ohtomo K, Itai Y, Furui S, et al: Hepatic tumors: differentiation by transverse relaxation time (T2) of magnetic resonance imaging, Radiology 155:421-423, 1985.
21. Ohtomo K, et al: Magnetic resonance imaging (MRI) of primary liver cancer - MRI-pathologic correlation, Radiat Med 3(1):38-41, 1985.
22. O'Neil J, Ros PR: Knowing hepatic pathology aids MRI of liver tumors, Diagn Imaging 58-67, 1989.
23. Ros PR: Focal liver masses other than metastases, ACR Categor Course Gastrointest Radiol 159-169, 1991.
24. Ros PR: Encapsulated hepatocellular carcinoma: radiologic findings and pathologic correlation, Gastrointest Radiol 15:233-237, 1990.
25. Ros PR, Olmstead WW, Dachman AH, et al: Undifferentiated (embryonal) sarcoma of the liver: radiologic-pathologic correlation, Radiology 160:141-145, 1986.
26. Rummeny E, Weissleder R, Stark DD, et al: Primary liver tumors: diagnosis by MR imaging, Am J Roentgenol 152:63-72, 1989.
27. Silverman PM, Rau PC, Korobkin M, et al: CT appearance of induced angiosarcoma of the liver, J Comput Assist Tomogr 7:655-658, 1983.
28. Steinberg HV, Alarcon JJ, Bernardino ME: Focal hepatic lesions: comparative MR imaging at 0.5 and 1.5 T, Radiology 174:153-156, 1990.
29. Subramanyam BR, Balthazar EJ, Hilton S, et al: Hepatocellular carcinoma with venous invasion: sonographic-angiographic correlation, Radiology 150:793-796, 1984.
30. Titelbaum DS, Hatabu H, Schiebler ML, et al: Fibrolamellar hepatocellular carcinoma: MR appearance, J Comput Assist Tomogr 12(4):588-591, 1988.
31. Titelbaum DS, Burke DR, Meranze SG, et al: Fibrolamellar hepatocellular carcinoma: pitfalls in nonoperative diagnosis, Radiology 167:25-30, 1988.
32. Wilbur AC, Gyi B: Hepatocellular carcinoma: MR appearance mimicking focal nodular hyperplasia, Am J Roentgenol 149:721-722, 1987.
33. Yoshida H, Ohtomo K, Kokubo T, et al: Small hepatocellular carcinoma and cavernous hemangioma: differentiation with dynamic FLASH MR imaging with Gd-DTPA, Radiology 171:339-342, 1989.

Section five
Hepatic metastasis

Christophoros Stoupis
Pablo R. Ros

Diagnostic challenges
Classification
Technical principles
MRI apperance
Differential diagnosis
Contrast agents
Summary

Metastases are the most common malignancy in the noncirrhotic liver. They are surpassed in incidence only by hemangioma, focal fatty change, and cysts as focal lesions in the noncirrhotic liver. It is important to emphasize that metastases are uncommon in the cirrhotic liver, where hepatocellular carcinoma (HCC) is more frequent. Large pathology series have demonstrated that in the noncirrhotic liver, metastases are approximately 30 times more common than any other malignancies. However, in the cirrhotic liver, HCC is approximately nine times more frequent than metastatic disease.[18] Therefore, metastasis is one of the major issues in diagnostic imaging of the liver.

The role of MRI with its high sensitivity and superb contrast resolution in the evaluation of metastases has been seen as pivotal in the development of abdominal MRI. Several controversial issues, such as better technique to evaluate metastases, varying results in diverse magnetic field strengths, role of MRI versus CT, and algorithm of imaging for staging patients with known malignancy, have been major issues since the early applications of MRI to the study of the abdomen. This section presents our approach to the use of MRI for evaluation of liver metastases.

DIAGNOSTIC CHALLENGES

Radiologists face several challenges in the evaluation of liver metastases (see accompanying box). The most common request to perform a liver MRI connected to metastatic disease is to stage oncologic patients that have known malignancy in the alimentary system or elsewhere, as the liver is one of the most common sites for visceral metastases in the body. Therefore, before surgery, chemotherapy, or radiation therapy and as a baseline pretreatment study, MRI of the liver may be used to establish the presence or absence of metastatic foci from a host of primary malignancies.

A second important challenge in metastatic disease is to establish resectability in patients that have solitary or few metastases, primarily from colonic cancer. Resectability should be established ideally by a noninvasive method such as MRI. Invasive diagnostic techniques, such as intraarterial CT and potentially hepatic artery perfusion scintigraphy, may be used as a second step to further assess resectability in these cases.[5]

A third important challenge for MRI is to characterize either single or multiple lesions detected by other imaging modalities. MRI may help characterize these lesions as nonhemangiomas and, therefore, particularly if multiple, suggest them as metastases requiring biopsy.

It is well recognized that the majority of metastases present as multiple gross foci.[2] However, 30% to 40% of metastases present grossly as single lesions; therefore, the diagnosis of metastases in the noncirrhotic liver should be considered for both multiple and single focal abnormalities.

Diagnostic challenges in liver metastases

1. Staging in patient with known malignancy
2. Noninvasive preoperative evaluation of resectability
3. Characterization of lesions detected by other imaging techniques
   a. Single
   b. Multiple

In short, the major diagnostic challenges for MRI of the liver are once again based on two major properties of MRI: (1) its superb sensitivity for lesions and (2) its potential for characterization of some benign focal liver lesions such as hemangioma and fatty change.

CLASSIFICATION

Grossly and microscopically the features of liver metastases vary, depending on the tumor of origin. Therefore, it is not possible to analyze the MRI findings of all metastatic lesions to the liver combined. Several gross and microscopic features may be used to classify liver metastases. Although the majority of metastases are hypovascular, some are hypervascular, such as hemorrhagic metastasis, choriocarcinoma, thyroid carcinoma, renal cell carcinoma, angiosarcoma, melanoma, and metastases from neuroendocrine tumors (carcinoid, islet cell tumor, etc.) (Fig. 10-31). Kaposi's sarcoma, although hypervascular, is not as hemorrhagic in the liver as the above-mentioned metastases (Table 10-3).

Fibrous reaction to the metastatic tumor is common for some metastases from breast and pancreatic carcinomas. "Fish flesh" texture is common for cellular and undifferen-

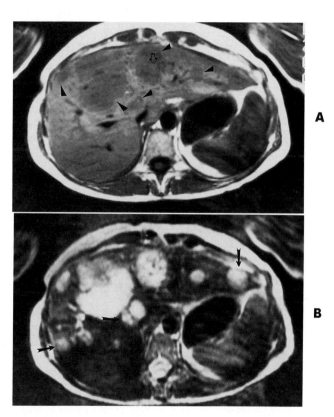

Fig. 10-31. Metastases from pancreatic insulinoma. **A,** T1WI using spin-echo technique demonstrates lesions throughout the liver. Some of the lesions have areas of decreased density *(arrowheads)* and other areas of increased density *(open arrow),* corresponding to areas of hemorrhage. **B,** T2-weighted spin-echo image demonstrates more lesions than in A *(arrows).*

Table 10-3. Morphologic patterns of hepatic metastases

Morphologic pattern	Primary tumor
1. Expansile	
• Massive (single large mass ± satellite nodules)	• Colon • Gallbladder • Testis
• Nodular (multiple nodules of similar size)	• Lung • Melanoma • Pancreas
2. Infiltrative	
• Massive	• Lung • Breast • Pancreas • Gallbladder • Melanoma
• Nodular	• Breast • Pancreas • Lung • Melanoma
• Diffuse	• Breast • Pancreas • Lymphoma • Colon
3. Subcapsular	• Colon • Ovary • Stomach (occasionally)
4. Miliary	• Prostate

Modified from Edmondson HA, Craig JR: Neoplasms of the liver. In Scniff L, Schiff ER, editors: Diseases of the liver, ed 6, New York, 1987, JB Lippincott.

tiated tumors such as small cell cancer and adenocarcinoma of the lung, non-Hodgkin lymphoma, some sarcomas, and melanoma. Except for hemorrhagic tumors, the overwhelming majority of metastases are hypovascular in relation to the normal liver parenchyma, particularly because they derive their blood supply from the hepatic artery, and they do not have vascular supply for the portal system.

Some morphologic patterns have been associated with the site of primary tumors such as expansile, infiltrative, surface spreading, and miliary. Within each of these categories, massive (large solitary mass with or without multiple satellites), nodular (multiple nodules of similar size), and diffuse have also been noted.

Table 10-3 summarizes the morphologic patterns of metastatic disease in liver tumors. It demonstrates significant overlap in the morphologic pattern of hepatic metastases, but still provides justification to few metastases, not as a single entity but as a conglomerate of focal lesions that vary in appearance both grossly and by MRI, depending on the site of origin.

TECHNICAL PRINCIPLES

The detection of liver cancer is based on differences in relaxation times between tumoral tissue and normal sur-

rounding liver. Therefore, the selection of a pulse sequence is critical for the detection of liver metastases, and several reports have been designed to identify the optimal technique to detect hepatic metastases.[19,25,27] A major problem with the initial reports on the appearance and sensitivity of MRI versus CT in the evaluation of hepatic metastases has been the magnetic field strength that seems to play a role for the detection of focal hepatic lesions. Although a study by Steinberg et al[29] demonstrated no significant difference in detection of hepatic metastases, when 0.5 versus 1.5 T units were compared, Reinig et al[20] in a prior study, demonstrated that inversion recovery technique was better in detecting hepatic lesions at 1.5 T in comparison with spin-echo sequences with a 0.5 T magnet.

A second crucial point for the evaluation of hepatic metastases is optimization of pulsing sequences, depending on magnetic field strength. This point has been controversial, as reflected in the recent literature, as the greatest SNR difference between normal liver and normal tissue is the paramount criterion for the selection of a particular technique.

The so-called "classic" sequences for liver MRI are T1WI (short TE), using spin-echo or gradient-echo with breath-holding, and T2-weighted spin-echo images. Both sequences have shown similar contrast discrimination for hepatic metastases.[24]

T2-weighted spin-echo images have been known to allow certain tissue specific characterization (i.e., hemangioma versus some metastases) from the initial applications of MRI to the liver.[28] This observation has been recently confirmed, indicating that heavily T2-weighted spin-echo images (TR 2350, TE 180) provide possible tissue characterization when both morphological and quantitative analyses are performed (Fig. 10-32).[3] Currently, the most universally accepted technique for detecting metastases is still based on T1- and T2-weighted spin-echo images.

Short time inversion recovery (STIR) also has been used for detection of liver metastases. With a STIR technique, respiratory artifacts from fat tissue are reduced, although artifacts from bowel and respiratory motion are increased. Imaging of the liver with a surface coil (i.e., Helmholtz coil) can also be used to increase contrast-to-noise ratio (CNR) between liver and metastases (Fig. 10-33). The application of other techniques for the detection of metastases, such as gradient-echo, has not been as fruitful as conventional spin-echo techniques. At this time, there is not enough experience with the use of fat suppression techniques for the evaluation of liver metastases (Fig. 10-34).

MRI APPEARANCE

Liver metastases are visible in MRI due to prolongation of the T1- and T2-relaxation times of the metastatic tissues. Therefore, in T1-weighted spin-echo images, the majority of metastases will appear as hypointense lesions.

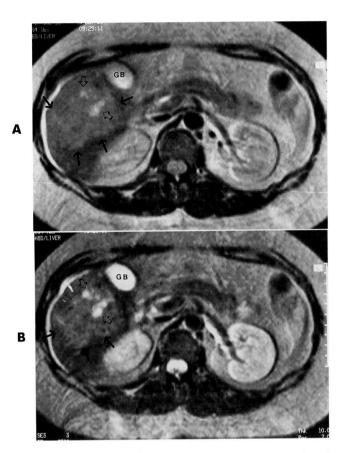

Fig. 10-32. Technique optimization, moderate versus heavily T2-weighted spin-echo images. **A,** T2-weighted spin-echo image (TR 2500 msec/TE 90 msec) demonstrates a subtle area of increased intensity in the right lobe of the liver *(arrows)* with areas of increased intensity *(open arrows)* within it. **B,** In the heavily weighted T2 image (TR 2500 msec/TE 120 msec) there is increased hyperintensity of the area of central necrosis *(open arrows),* similar to the increased intensity noticed in the gallbladder *(GB).* However, there is no significant difference in the appearance of the metastatic lesion itself *(arrows),* which maintains similar intensity in both images. This technique differentiates metastases from benign lesions in the liver, such as hemangioma or cyst, which would increase in intensity with prolonged TE.

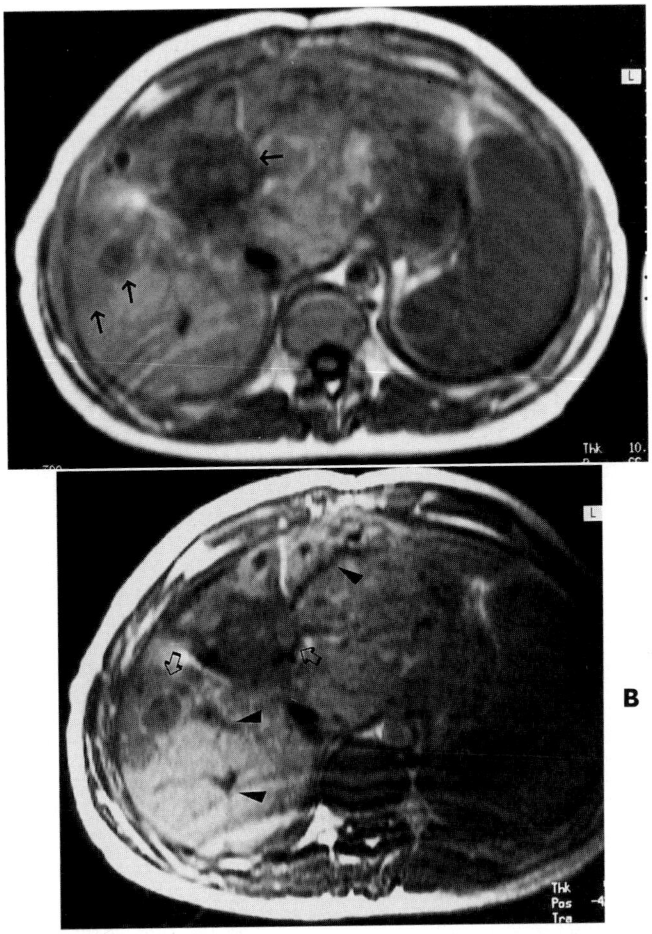

Fig. 10-33. Body coil versus Hemholtz coil for metastases. **A,** T1-weighted spin-echo image performed with a body coil demonstrates several liver metastases from colon cancer *(arrows).* **B,** Image performed with identical technique, but using a Hemholtz coil, demonstrates better delineation of the metastases, as well as a better relationship of the lesions to the hepatic vessels *(open arrows)* and better visualization of the portal and hepatic veins *(arrowheads).*

On STIR images, metastases appear hyperintense, even though the pulsing sequence is T1-weighted.[1]

T2-weighted spin-echo images demonstrate metastases as hyperintense areas compared to normal liver, but not as bright as the gallbladder, the spinal canal, or hemangiomas. T2-weighted spin-echo images are used to confirm suspicious lesions seen on T1-weighted spin-echo images. T2-weighted spin-echo images are able to confirm that these are lesions and not vessels. On T1-weighted spin-echo images, both small metastases and vessels appear hypointense, whereas on T2-weighted spin-echo images, vessels remain hypointense and metastases become hyperintense. Differentiation between vessels and small metastases can be performed reliably using gradient-echo techniques where vessels, but not metastases, have marked

hyperintensity (Fig. 10-35). With the use of flow compensation techniques in T2-weighted spin-echo images, vessels appear as bright as metastases. Therefore, differentiation between small metastases and vessels is based primarily on gradient-echo pulsing sequences, as well as on morphologic appearance.

As previously mentioned, although liver metastases are bright on T2-weighted spin-echo images, their intensity does not increase proportionately with T2 weighting. This criterion is important to differentiate between liver metastases and certain benign liver lesions, such as cysts or hemangiomas, which are not only markedly hyperintense, but increase in hyperintensity as TE is lengthened.

With the advent of gradient-echo images, it was initially thought that T2-weighted gradient-echo images would combine the sensitivity of SE T2-weighted images with the speed and, therefore, lack of motion artifact of gradient-echo. The disadvantage of T2-weighted gradient-echo images, despite reduced acquisition time, is poor SNR and CNR, resulting in poor depiction of small hepatic lesions (Fig. 10-36). Therefore, T2-weighted spin-echo images are still considered an important pulse technique in high field magnets to search for metastases.

It has been mentioned that metastases vary morphologically, depending on the primary tumor. MRI is capable of distinguishing some of the morphologic features that may help distinguish between benign and malignant liver lesions and potentially identify a metastatic lesion. Certain metastases that induce a fibrotic response, such as of breast or pancreatic origin, may be characterized due to hypointensity secondary to fibrosis within the mass in T2-weighted spin-echo images.

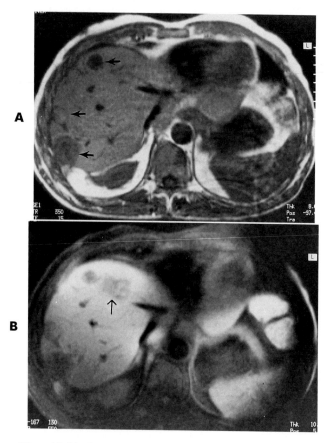

Fig. 10-34. Carcinoma metastases. **A,** Conventional T1-weighted spin-echo image (TR 350 msec/TE 15 msec) demonstrates multiple focal lesions with different patterns of intensity typical for colorectal carcinoma *(arrows)*. Note the inhomogeneous nature with central areas of further decreased intensity in the posterior segment of the liver. **B,** Fat suppression T1-weighted spin-echo image at the same level as **A** demonstates better demarcation of liver lesions. A lesion in the anterior segment of the liver *(arrow)* is identified, which can be seen only retrospectively on the T1-weighted spin-echo image.

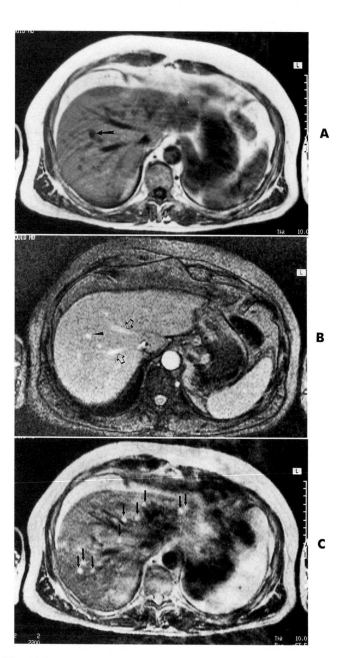

Fig. 10-35. Gradient-echo versus spin-echo to differentiate small vessels versus small metastases. **A,** T1-weighted spin-echo image demonstrates multiple hypointense lesions (throughout the liver). A round lesion between right and middle hepatic vein *(arrow)* is seen, perhaps larger than other surrounding vessels. **B,** T2-weighted gradient-echo image demonstrates that the lesion seen in **A** (as a potential area of metastases) corresponds to a vessel *(arrowhead)*. Other small vessels are seen (portal branches that have vertical orientation and are section transversally), as well as middle and right hepatic veins *(open arrows)*. **C,** T2-weighted spin-echo image confirms the presence of multiple metastatic foci *(arrows)* in this patient proven by biopsy to have adenocarcinoma metastases of unknown origin.

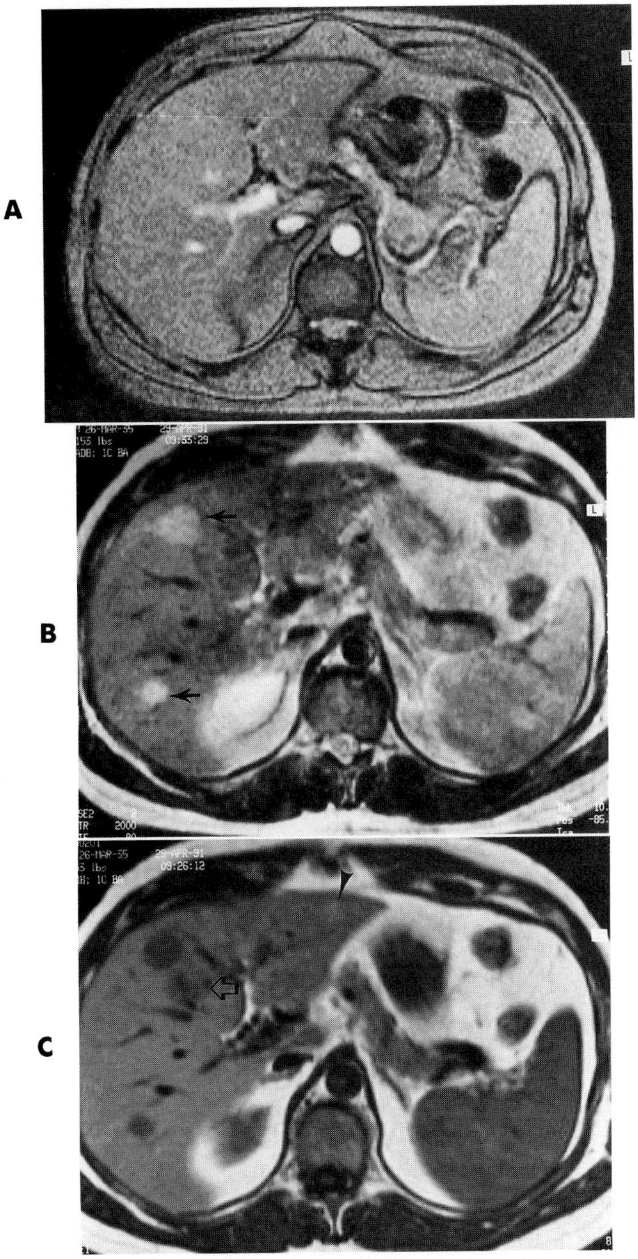

Fig. 10-36. Spin-echo versus gradient-echo in colon carcinoma metastases. **A,** T2-weighted gradient-echo image demonstrates no focal liver lesions but clearly depicts hepatic vessels. **B,** T2-weighted spin-echo image demonstrates at least two hyperintense areas *(arrows)* not seen in Fig. **A. C,** T1-weighted spin-echo image clearly demonstrates the two lesions seen in Fig. **B,** as well as a subtle third lesion *(open arrow)*. In the left lobe, a hyperintense area is seen, corresponding to an artifact from the aorta *(arrowhead)*.

Metastatic adenocarcinomas, particularly those of colonic origin, are recognized grossly by a large amount of mucin production. Mucin is demonstrated in MRI by hyperintensity in both T1-weighted and T2-weighted spin-echo images (Fig. 10-37).

Malignant melanoma, if rich in melanin, will be easily identified due to melanin content that was high intensity in T1-weighted spin-echo images. Melanoma metastasis may also have internal hemorrhage, as it is hypervascular.

DIFFERENTIAL DIAGNOSIS

A major point of controversy in the use of MRI to distinguish liver metastases is its differentiation from other, primarily nonsurgical, lesions. A major caveat in the diagnosis of metastases is the differentiation between hemorrhagic metastases and hemangioma of the liver. Because the diagnosis of hemangioma by MRI is based on the markedly hypervascular nature of this lesion (when gadolinium is not used and diagnosis is relied on nonenhanced images), it is easy to understand why hypervascular metastases may be difficult to distinguish from hemangioma. Even grossly, certain metastases may mimic hemangioma due to marked hypervascularity. Hypervascular/hemorrhagic metastases are listed in the box below.

In the differential diagnosis of metastases from other benign focal lesions such as hemangioma, it is important not only to use intensity criteria but also to observe morphologic features, such as margin sharpness, internal inhomogeneity, extension into the surface of the liver and/or beyond the liver into surrounding organs, characteristics of the liver surrounding the tumor, etc. (Fig. 10-38) (see discussion on hemangioma vs. metastasis in section two [p. 192]. In general, metastases would be inhomogeneous due to either central liquefactive necrosis (hyperintensity in T2-weighted spin-echo images), internal hemorrhage (hyper-intensity in T1-weighted spin-echo images), or fibrosis (hypointensity in T1- and T2-weighted spin-echo images). The margins of the metastases are irregular and ill-defined, as metastases have by definition no capsule and an infiltrative border. Typically, peritumoral edema surrounds metastases not seen in benign focal lesions of the

---

Hemorrhagic metastasis

- Melanoma
- Choriocarcinoma
- Thyroid carcinoma
- Renal cell carcinoma
- Angiosarcoma
- Neuroendocrine tumors
    Islet cell carcinoma
    Carcinoid
- Kaposi's sarcoma

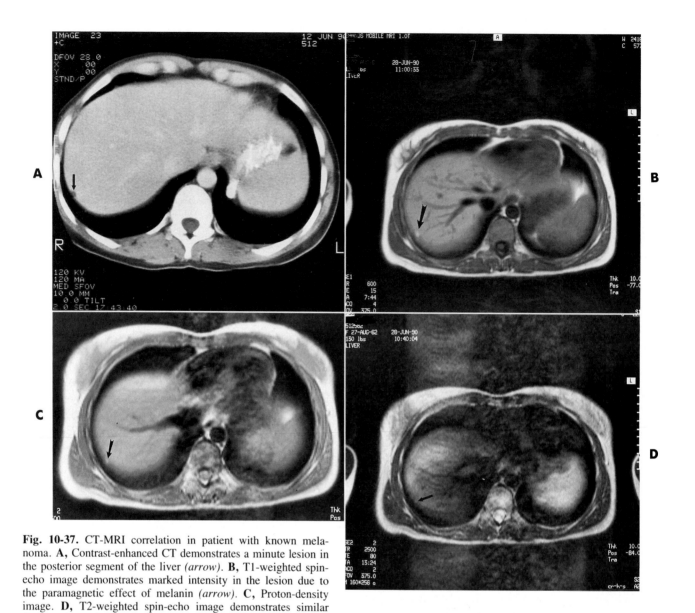

Fig. 10-37. CT-MRI correlation in patient with known melanoma. **A,** Contrast-enhanced CT demonstrates a minute lesion in the posterior segment of the liver *(arrow)*. **B,** T1-weighted spinecho image demonstrates marked intensity in the lesion due to the paramagnetic effect of melanin *(arrow)*. **C,** Proton-density image. **D,** T2-weighted spin-echo image demonstrates similar findings *(arrow)*.

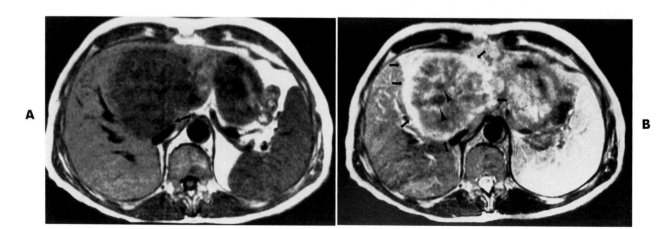

Fig. 10-38. Solitary metastases from adenocarcinoma of the colon. **A,** T1-weighted spin-echo image demonstrates a single lesion in this patient with a known colon cancer. The lesion appears inhomogeneous, with irregular margins, and extending into the inferior vena cava *(arrow)*. **B,** T2-weighted spin-echo image confirms that this lesion is not a hemangioma, and it is likely malignant. Criteria for malignancy include peritumoral edema *(arrows)* and marked inhomogeneity with hypointense areas, suggesting fibrosis *(arrowheads)*. Fibrosis is elicited in some metastases including adenocarcinoma of the colon.

mor metastases (Fig. 10-39). These morphologic features are best visualized on mild to moderate T2-weighted spin-echo images.[21]

Regarding the use of MRI versus CT in the diagnosis of hepatic metastases, a consensus opinion has not been found. In the early development of MRI, when CT was already a well-established technique, initial reports indicated that CT was the most useful examination for the evaluation of suspected hepatic metastases when compared with third-generation body MRI imagers.[6] Later, other investigators have demonstrated greater sensitivity of MRI for detecting individual metastatic foci, comparing unenhanced spin-echo MRI with contrast-enhanced CT.[10,26]

When MRI is compared with CT portography, the latter is more sensitive for lesions smaller than 1 cm in diameter.[13] However, intraarterial CT portography is an invasive technique that should be reserved for certain conditions (i.e., presurgical evaluation for resectability for metasta-

ses) and not used as a general screening method for metastatic disease, as discussed under Diagnostic Challenges in this section (p. 219).

CONTRAST AGENTS

The hepatic MR contrast agents can be divided into three major categories:

1. Contrast agents distributed in the interstitial-extracellular fluid compartment
2. Reticuloendothelial system-directed contrast agents
3. Hepatobiliary contrast agents.

Contrast agents can also be divided into two categories according to their susceptibility and interaction with the external magnetic field strength: (1) superparamagnetic agents, such as superparamagnetic iron oxide (i.e., SPIO or AMI-25 [Advanced Magnetics, Inc., Cambridge, Mass]), which decrease the intensity and thus "darken" the normal liver; and (2) paramagnetic contrast agents, such as gadopentate dimeglumine or manganese-DPDP, which increase the intensity of normal hepatocytes.

Extracellular enhancing agents, such as gadopentetate

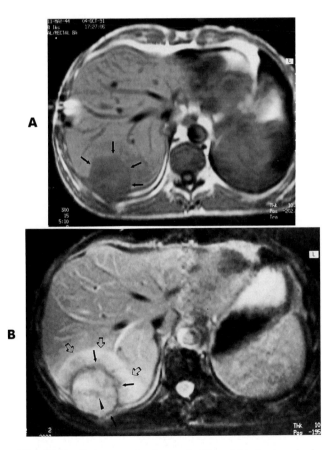

Fig. 10-39. Perimetastatic edema. **A,** T1-weighted spin-echo image in this patient with metastases from squamous cell carcinoma of the bladder demonstrates a lesion in the posterior segment *(arrows)*. **B,** T2-weighted spin-echo image demonstrates an area of hyperintensity surrounding the lesion (barely noticeable as a hypointense halo in **A**), corresponding to perimetastatic edema *(open arrows)*. Additional morphologic features noted are irregular margins *(arrows)* and lesion inhomogeneity *(arrowheads)*.

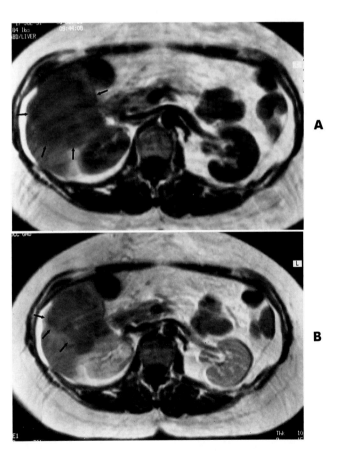

Fig. 10-40. Gadopentetate dimeglumine effect on metastases. **A,** Precontrast T1WI demonstrates a hypointense mass in the right lobe of the liver *(arrows)*. **B,** Post gadopentetate dimeglumine administration, there is improvement in the demarcation of the lesion when compared to **A** *(arrows)*.

dimeglumine or Gd-DOTA-meglumine, produce shortening of the T1-relaxation time of perfused tissue (Fig. 10-40). Because these contrast agents are distributed in the interstitial compartment of both metastases and normal liver, they cannot detect liver metastases. The imaging differences resulting after the injection of gadopenetate dimeglumine are based on the differences of blood flow between normal liver and metastatic disease. This difference is produced after the infusion of a bolus of contrast media followed by rapid dynamic imaging. This seems to have a limited value and little practical application for the study of metastatic disease.[18,22]

Conversely, reticuloendothelial agents, which are targeted to the Kupffer cells that line the hepatic sinusoids, appear to be effective for the evaluation of liver metastases. The best known of the reticuloendotheial agents is SPIO (ferrite or Feridex), which produces shortening of the T2-relaxation time of normal liver tissue. Because all metastases to the liver are by definition not hepatic tissue, all metastatic foci have no Kupffer cells and, therefore, are

incapable of sequestering particles of SPIO. After the intravenous administration of SPIO, the normal liver demonstrates a marked decrease in T2-relaxation time. However, there is no significant decrease in intensity in metastases, which appear bright and are consequently easy to identify qualitatively (Figs. 10-41 and 10-42).[8,9] Currently, the role of SPIO-enhanced liver MRI is being studied in clinical trials and compared with unenhanced MRI and CT. In the future, use of reticuloendothelial system contrast may be routine, particularly for the detection of hepatic metastases. Currently, efforts are being made to provide sequence optimization post-SPIO administration to allow even better metastases-liver contrast and higher sensitivity when compared with routine pulsing to detect small lesions sequences.[9]

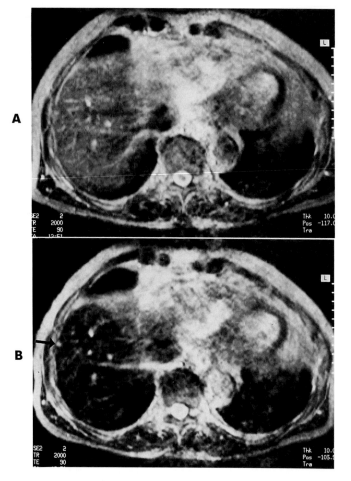

Fig. 10-41. SPIO enhancement. **A,** Pre-SPIO-enhanced T2WI demonstrates no definite focal lesions. **B,** Post-SPIO intravenous administration a peripheral lesion is clearly seen *(arrow)*.

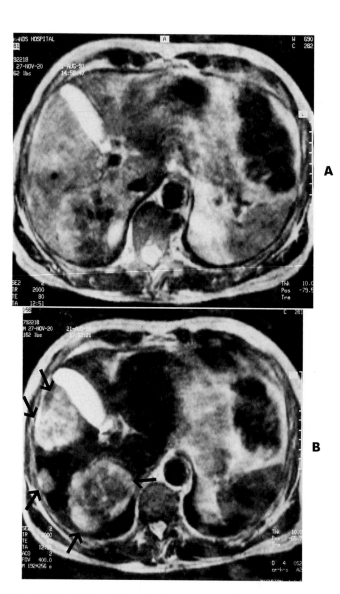

Fig. 10-42. SPIO enhancement. **A,** Pre-SPIO-enhanced T2WI demonstrates no obvious lesions. **B,** Multiple large metastases are identified post-SPIO intravenous administration *(arrows)*.

Hepatobiliary agents currently are paramagnetic contrast agents taken up primarily by hepatocytes and eliminated through the biliary system. They produce shortening of the T1 relaxation, and therefore, render "bright" the areas that they enhance. The first experimental studies were conducted with paramagnetic complexes, such as iron [Fe (III)] or gadolinium [Gd (III)]. More recently, complexes with relatively high hepatobiliary excretion (such as Gd-BOPTA and Gd-EOB-DTPA), have been evaluated in the United States and Europe in clinical trials as positive liver agents. Mn-DPDP, a chelate or pyridoxal-5'-phosphate and manganese is derived from vitamin B6 and is metabolized by hepatocytes. Therefore, it can be used as a biliary agent because it is excreted in the bile. Mn-DPDP is a positive contrast agent to evaluate hepatocyte activity, as well as biliary excretion.

In initial animal studies, a fivefold increase in tumor-to-liver CNR has been described after administration of manganese, or Mn-DPDP, versus unenhanced MRI.[4] Recent reports in the use of Mn-DPDP in humans demonstrate increase in the detection of liver lesions due to liver enhancement versus nonenhancement in metastases.[11,15] The use of these two groups of agents (reticuloendothelial system [SPIO] and biliary system [Mn-DPDP]) is similar to that of well-known nuclear medicine radionuclides, where both reticuloendothelial agents (sulfur colloid tagged with ^{99m}Tc) and hepatobiliary agents (aminodiacetic acid derivatives tagged with ^{99m}Tc) play a significant role in the evaluation of liver masses. The use of MRI contrast agents, as well as a multiplanar technique, will probably solve the well-known problem of differentiating small subcentimeter liver metastasis from small vessels.[22]

Additional information on hepatic contrasts can be found in Chapter 6.

SUMMARY

The use of MRI for the detection of liver metastases is one of the major indications for MRI of the liver and, in general, MRI of the abdomen. It appears that MRI is as sensitive, or perhaps even more sensitive, than contrast-enhanced CT, particularly with the use of reticuloendothelial contrast agents. This sensitivity, coupled with MRI's noninvasiveness, makes it the technique of choice for the noninvasive evaluation of the liver, particularly for staging of metastases.

MRI probably should be used as the first step to evaluate patients when resectability of hepatic metastases is considered. Resection of hepatic metastases is a well-established method to treat patients with a limited burden of metastatic disease to the liver in certain relatively slow progressing tumors, and typically adenocarcinoma of the colon. In these cases, MRI should be performed to assess resectability. If MRI demonstrates potential for resectability, it is not clear if an invasive technique, such as intraarterial CT portography with or without hepatic arterial perfusion scintigraphy, may be needed before surgery to assess the presence of small lesions.

Regarding characterization of single or multiple masses identified by other imaging modalities, recent evidence indicates that it is possible to differentiate hemangioma from metastases using qualitative and quantitative T2-relaxation times,[7,16] morphologic criteria, and behavior postcontrast administration.[12] Again, the major caveat—distinction between hemorrhagic hepatic metastases and hemangioma—may be less important than initially believed,[14] as the overwhelming majority of hemorrhagic metastases do not present as liver metastases, initially but later in the course of the disease when a patient is known to have a primary tumor.

Finally, with the advent of several contrast agents, the role of liver MRI will probably increase and become more complex. MRI will be able to select contrast agents to fit particular needs and, therefore, achieve a final diagnosis.

REFERENCES

1. Bydder GM, Steiner RE, Blumgart LH, et al: MR imaging of the liver using short T1 inversion recovery sequences, J Comput Assist Tomogr 9(6):1084-1089, 1985.
2. Craig JR, Peters RL, Edmondson HA: Tumors of the liver and intrahepatic bile ducts. In Craig, Peters, Edmonton, eds: Atlas of Tumor Pathology, Washington, DC, 1989, Armed Forces Institute of Pathology.
3. Egglin TK, Rummeny E, Stark DD, et al: Hepatic tumors: quantitative tissue characterization with MR imaging, Radiology 176:107-110, 1990.
4. Elizondo G, Fretz CJ, Stark DD, et al: Preclinical evaluation of Mn-DPDP: new paramagnetic hepatobiliary contrast agent for MR imaging, Radiology 178:73-78, 1991.
5. Fagien M, Drone W, Hawkins JF Jr, et al: Hepatic arterial perfusion scintigraphy for detection of hepatic metastases, Radiology 177(P):122, 1990.
6. Glazer GM, Aisen AM, Francis JR, et al: Evaluation of focal hepatic masses: a comparative study of MRI and CT, Gastrointest Radiol 11:263-268, 1986.
7. Goldberg MA, Saini S, Hahn PF, et al: Differentiation between hemangiomas and metastases of the liver and ultrafast MR imaging: preliminary results with T2 calculations, Am J Roentgenol 157:727-730, 1991.
8. Ferrucci JT, Stark DD: Iron oxide-enhanced MR imaging of the liver and spleen: review of the first 5 years, Am J Roentgenol 155:943-950, 1990.
9. Fretz CJ, Elizondo G, Weissleder, et al: Superparamagnetic iron oxide-enhanced MR imaging: pulse sequence optimization for detection of liver cancer, Radiology 172:393-397, 1989.
10. Fretz CJ, Stark DD, Metz GE, et al: Detection of hepatic metastases: comparison of contrast-enhanced CT, unenhanced MR imaging, and iron oxide-enhanced MR imaging, Am J Roentgenol 155:763-770, 1990.
11. Hamm B, Voge TJ, Branding G, et al: Focal liver lesions: MR imaging with Mn-DPDP—initial clinical results in 40 patients, Radiology 182:167-174, 1992.
12. Hamm B, Fischer E, Taupitz M: Differentiation of hepatic hemangiomas from metastases by dynamic contrast-enhanced MR imaging, J Comput Assist Tomogr 14(2):205-216, 1990.
13. Heiken JP, Weyman PJ, Lee JKT, et al: Detection of focal hepatic masses: prospective evaluation with CT, delayed CT, CT during arterial portography, and MR imaging, Radiology 171:47-51, 1989.

14. Li KC, Glazer GM, Quint LE, et al: Distinction of hepatic cavernous hemangioma from hepatic metastases with MR imaging, Radiology 169:409-415, 1988.

15. Lim KO, Stark DD, Leese PT, et al: Hepatobiliary MR imaging: first human experience with Mn-DPDP, Radiology 178:79-82, 1991.

16. Lombardo DM, Baker ME, Spritzer CE, et al: Hepatic hemangiomas vs metastases: MR differentiation at 1.5 T, Am J Roentgenol 155:55-59, 1990.

17. Melato M, Laurino L, Mucli E: Relationship between cirrhosis, liver cancer, and hepatic metastasis: an autopsy study, Cancer 64:455-459, 1989.

18. Mirowitz SA, Lee JKT, Gutierrez E, et al: Dynamic gadolinium-enhanced rapid acquisition spin-echo MR imaging of the liver, Radiology 179:371-376, 1991.

19. Paling MR, Abbitt PL, Mugler JP, et al: Liver metastases: Optimization of MR imaging pulse sequences at 1.0 T, Radiology 167:695-699, 1988.

20. Reinig JW, Dwyer AJ, Miller DL, et al: Liver metastases: detection with MR imaging at 0.5 and 1.5 T, Radiology 170:149-153, 1989.

21. Rummeny E, Saini J, Wittenberg J, et al: MR imaging of liver neoplasms, Am J Roentgenol 152:493-499, 1989.

22. Saini S: Contrast-enhanced MR imaging of the liver, Radiology 182:12-14, 1992.

23. Saini S, Stark DD, Brady TJ, et al: Dynamic spin-echo MRI of liver cancer using gadolinium-DTPA: animal investigation, Am J Roentgenol 147:357-362, 1986.

24. Saini S, Li W, Wallner B, et al: MR imaging of liver metastases at 1.5 T: similar contrast discrimination with T1- and T2-weighted pulse sequences, Radiology 181:449-453, 1991.

25. Stark DD, Wittenberg J, Edelman RR, et al: Detection of hepatic metastases: analysis of pulse sequence performance in MR imaging, Radiology 159:365-370, 1986.

26. Stark DD, Wittenberg J, Butch RJ, et al: Hepatic metastases: randomized, controlled comparison of detection with MR imaging and CT, Radiology 165:399-406, 1987.

27. Stark DD, Wittenberg J, Middleton MS, et al: Liver metastases: detection by phase-contrast MR imaging, Radiology 158:327-332, 1986.

28. Stark DD, Felder RC, Wittenberg J, et al: Magnetic resonance imaging of cavernous hemangioma of the liver: tissue-specific characterization, Am J Roentgenol 145:213-222, 1985.

29. Steinberg HV, Alarcon JJ, Bernardino ME: Focal hepatic lesions: comparative MR imaging at 0.5 and 1.5 T, Radiology 174:153-156, 1990.

Section six
Focal infectious processes

Deborah A. Allen

Pyogenic and fungal abscesses
Amebic abscess
Echinococcal cyst

PYOGENIC AND FUNGAL ABSCESSES

Abscesses of the liver may be caused by bacterial, amebic, or fungal infections, which result in a localized collection of inflammatory cells and destruction of surrounding parenchyma. Determining the etiology of a hepatic abscess is important, as the prognosis and treatment vary for different abscesses.

Pyogenic abscesses are usually caused by gram-negative bacteria from the GI tract. The bacteria reach the liver via the bile ducts, blood vessels, or lymphatics or by penetrating trauma or direct extension from perihepatic abscesses.

Fungi generally gain access into the liver or spleen via arterial circulation as the result of fungal septicemia. Multiple small abscesses (microabscesses) form in the parenchyma of the liver or spleen.

Clinical presentation of patients with a hepatic abscess includes fever, right upper quadrant abdominal pain, and hepatomegaly. The onset of symptoms may be acute (as in pyogenic abscess) or prolonged (as in amebic abscess). Hepatic abscesses may result in malnutrition, wasting, sepsis, shock, or rupture into nearby organs such as the lungs and heart.

Ultrasound and CT scan have been the primary imaging techniques in the evaluation of hepatic lesions such as abscesses. Ultrasound defines the internal composition of an abscess better than CT, but CT is able to delineate the anatomic relationship of an abscess with neighboring structures. Sonographically, abscesses have discrete borders and good through transmission; calcifications may also be detected. Fungal abscesses may have a target, or "wheel within wheel", appearance on ultrasonography.[1]

On CT scans, hepatic abscesses appear as hypodense lesions with an internal pattern of varying density compared with liver tissue. The "cluster sign" is suggestive of abscess and represents smaller lesions surrounding a larger abscess. Another CT sign, the "double target" is seen with early abscess and refers to a hypodense lesion surrounded by a hyperdense rim and outer low-density region.[1]

MRI has emerged as a valuable imaging modality in the evaluation of hepatic lesions. The advantage of MRI over other imaging techniques includes superior soft tissue contrast resolution and multiplanar imaging capabilities. The MR characteristics of pyogenic abscesses, hepatic and extrahepatic, have been described. An abscess appears as an

Fig. 10-43. **A,** Pyogenic abscess. Gradient-echo coronal MRI showing a hyperintense mass in the right lobe of the liver compressing the inferior vena cava. **B,** T-1 weighted gradient-echo MRI post-gadolinium injection. Note again the large hepatic mass now with peripheral enhancement after gadolinium *(arrows).* This area of enhancement corresponds to the capsule of the abscess.

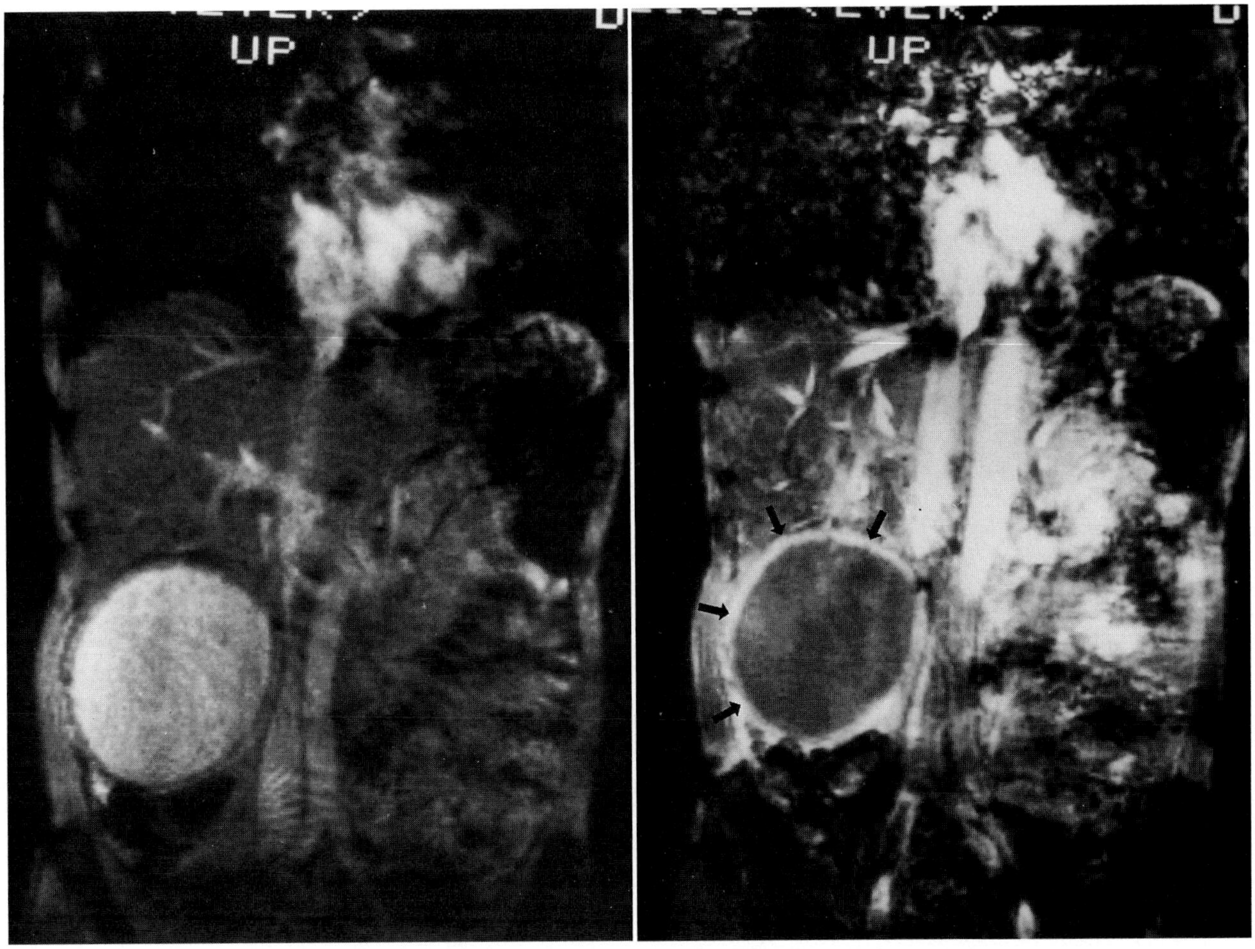

area of decreased signal intensity on T1WI and increased signal intensity on T2WI compared with surrounding tissue (Fig. 10-43, *A* and 10-43, *B*). The abscess cavity may be homogeneous or heterogeneous in signal intensity.[4,5] A low-intensity rim corresponding to the capsule is often seen. With use of gadopentetate dimeglumine (Gd-DTPA), the abscess wall will enhance rapidly, followed by a slower increase in signal intensity within the center of the abscess.[3,5]

A recent case report has described the MR findings of hepatosplenic candidiasis in patients with superimposed hemochromatosis secondary to repeated blood transfusions. The fungal microabscesses appear as diffuse small lesions of intermediate signal intensity on T1WI and increased signal intensity on T2WI compared with the hypointense parenchyma of the liver and spleen (Figs. 10-44 and 10-45). The decreased signal intensity of the liver and

spleen, due to hemochromatosis, improves contrast resolution of the microabscesses.[2]

No MR characteristics are specific to hepatic abscesses, and the patient's clinical history must be strongly considered when evaluating liver lesions. The differential diagnosis of a focal hepatic mass, which is hypointense on T1WI and hyperintense on T2WI, includes simple cysts and neoplasms of the liver.

AMEBIC ABSCESS

Amebiasis, caused by the parasite *Entamoeba histolytica,* is a disease endemic in tropical areas such as the southwestern United States, Mexico, Central and South America, Africa, and Asia. Amebic liver abscess is formed after infestation of colonic mucosa by the parasite, which lodges in the portal system. Necrosis of liver tissue then occurs with subsequent formation of an "anchovy

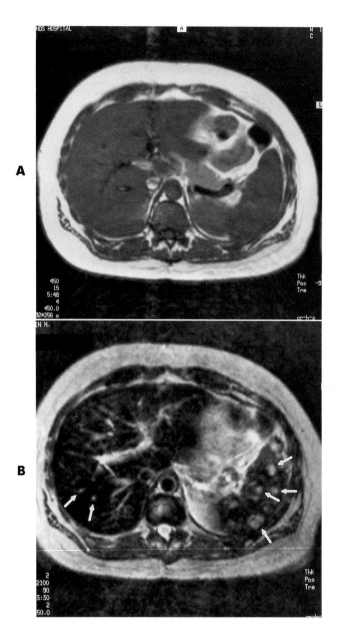

Fig. 10-44. Hepatosplenic candidiasis. **A,** Axial T-1 and **B,** T-2 weighted images showing numerous lesions in the liver and spleen *(arrows),* which appear isointense on T1WI and very hyperintense on T2WI.

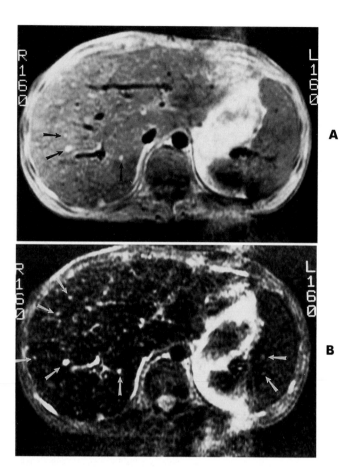

Fig. 10-45. Hepatosplenic candidiasis. **A,** Axial proton-density and **B,** T-2 weighted images showing multiple lesions in the liver and spleen *(arrows),* which again are better seen on T-2 images.

paste" abscess. The parasite may also gain access into the liver by direct extension from the hepatic flexure of the colon. Up to 25% of all carriers of amebiasis will develop hepatic abscess. Amebiasis may be detected by serologic examinations. Aspiration of an abscess is usually negative for the organism and is unnecessary, as the abscess is often responsive to amebicidal therapy.[6]

The detection of a liver abscess and the establishment of its etiology are important because therapy and prognosis vary among amebic, bacterial, and fungal abscesses. Untreated abscesses may cause severe malnutrition and wasting, sepsis, or infection of other organs. Moreover, the abscess can rupture or form fistulae into organs including the pericardium, pleura, GI tract, and peritoneum.[6]

Imaging studies such as nuclear medicine, ultrasound, and CT have been successful in distinguishing patients with amebic abscess from those with uncomplicated amebic infections of the intestine. MRI is a sensitive method for characterizing focal lesions of the liver, and findings in patients with known hepatic amebic abscess have been described.

On both T-1 and T-2 weighted MRI, amebic abscesses are well-defined structures with rimlike areas of varying signal intensity. Within the abscess cavity the signal intensity is decreased on T1WI compared with normal hepatic parenchyma (Fig. 10-46, *A*). On T2WI the lesion is hyperintense and often surrounded by an area of even higher signal intensity corresponding to edema within normal liver tissue.[1,8] There is no correlation between the signal intensity within the abscess on MRI and the density of the lesion on CT or the echogenicity on ultrasound.[8]

MR has been shown to be clinically useful in the evaluation of a patient's response to medical or surgical treat-

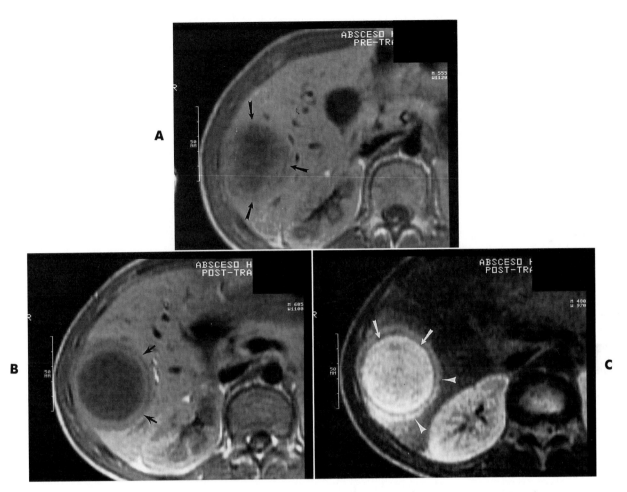

Fig. 10-46. Untreated amebic liver abscess. **A,** T1WI showing hypointense liver mass. Note the incomplete rim around the abscess cavity *(arrows)*. **B,** Same amebic abscess 10 days after initiation of medical treatment. T1WI shows that the signal intensity of the cavity has decreased and become more homogeneous. The cavity is now surrounded by a hyperintense ring and an outer hypointense rim *(arrows)*. **C,** On T-2 weighted image the cavity is hyperintense and surrounded by a hypointense ring *(arrows)* identical to that seen in the T1WI. An outer hyperintense zone surrounds the entire mass *(arrow heads)*. (From Elizondo G, Weissleder R, Stark DD, et al: Radiology 165:795, 1987.)

ment. Characteristic imaging findings have been described in amebic abscesses after successful therapy compared with pretreatment images.

With initiation of specific therapy (metronidazole), histologic changes representing healing of the amebic abscess can be detected with MRI. Liquefaction necrosis occurs in the center of the cavity as early as 4 days after treatment has begun. On T1WI this appears as a decrease in signal intensity within the abscess compared with pretreatment T1WI. Necrosis is followed by maturation of the abscess wall, which is seen as formation of concentric rings on MR. These rings correspond to discrete histologic zones that develop in response to antibiotic therapy. An inner layer of granulation tissue appears isointense to normal liver on T1WI. This inner margin is surrounded by collagen corresponding to a hypointense ring on both T1WI and

T2WI (Fig. 10-46, *B*). The outermost layer consists of inflammation and edema of hepatic parenchyma, which appears as the outer hyperintense ring on T2 (Fig. 10-46, *C*). As edema resolves with successful treatment, the hyperintense area seen around the cavity on T2WI before treatment becomes isointense to normal liver parenchyma.[7]

After surgical drainage of the abscess, the cavity collapses and the mass effect on surrounding normal liver resolves. The wall then matures and with concurrent antibiotic therapy, the rings will become distinct.[7]

MR has advantages over other imaging techniques in the evaluation of amebic liver abscess. With its multiplanar capabilities, MR is able to show the relationship of the abscess to vital structures and may detect occult lesions. MR is also helpful in following the response of an abscess to therapy and allowing a change in therapy if necessary.

ECHINOCOCCAL CYST

Though rare in the United States, hydatid disease, caused by the parasite *Echinococcus granulosus,* occurs frequently in Mediterranean countries.

Dogs are the normal host for the adult parasite, and hundreds of worms may exist in their intestinal tract. Sheep, cattle, other herbivores, and humans are intermediate hosts for the parasite after contact with dog feces. In heavily endemic areas, about 50% of dogs and up to 90% of sheep and cattle are infected with *E. granulosus.* Eggs are passed by the dogs and can be ingested by intermediate hosts.

Once inside the intermediate host, the parasitic eggs hatch, and embryos penetrate the intestinal mucosa to enter lymphatic and venous channels. Most of the embryos are filtered by the liver and lungs with the remaining parasites reaching other organs including the brain, spleen, kidneys, and musculoskeletal system. Viable embryos transform into cysts which grow 1 cm/year. The wall of the hydatid cyst is composed of two layers: the endocyst, a germinal layer, and the ectocyst, a proteinaceous membrane. A dense fibrous capsule containing collagen, the pericyst, is formed by the host (Fig. 10-47).

Echinococcal cysts usually develop in the liver (75% of cases) but may occur in any part of the body. The lesions are often asymptomatic for many years and are discovered incidentally by ultrasound or CT scans. Hydatidosis can also be detected by serologic tests. Classic symptoms of hepatic hydatid cyst include upper abdominal pain and hepatomegaly. Treatment consists of surgical removal of the cyst or antiparasitic drug therapy. If left untreated, a hepatic hydatid cyst may rupture into surrounding structures such as liver parenchyma, biliary system, peritoneum, GI tract, or pleura.

The appearance of hydatid cyst on CT and ultrasound have been described, and either imaging study can be used to establish the diagnosis of hydatidosis. Recently, several studies have characterized the MR findings in patients with known hepatic echinococcal cysts.

Hydatid cysts have decreased signal intensity on T1WI and increased signal intensity on T2 images compared with normal liver parenchyma (Fig. 10-48). A low-intensity rim around the cyst is present in most cases and is more conspicuous on T2WI than T1WI weighted sequences. This rim corresponds to the pericyst, which is rich in collagen and has a short T2-relaxation time. The rim is not merely caused by a chemical-shift artifact, as it completely surrounds the cyst and is not only present in the direction of the phase-encoding gradient.[9,11]

Some authors feel that the low-intensity rim around hepatic hydatid cyst is an inconsistent and nonspecific finding.[12,13] Similar walls can be seen on MRI of encapsulated liver masses such as hepatocellular carcinoma, Amebic abscess, hematoma, and hepatic adenoma; but differentiation from hydatid cyst is possible. Hydatid cysts are not surrounded by a hyperintense region of edema as are most malignant tumors of the liver. Moreover, hydatid cysts have a single hypointense rim, whereas treated amebic abscesses and resolving intraparenchymal hematoma have multiple rims of varying signal intensity. MR can distinguish between hydatid cyst and nonencapsulated masses of the liver including simple hepatic cysts, metastases, hemangiomas, and focal nodular hyperplasia, as these lesions do not have rims of MRI.[12]

MR demonstrates the internal structure and architecture of hepatic echinococcal cyst better than either ultrasound or CT.[5] Daughter cysts are isointense to hypointense on T1WI and isointense on T2WI compared with the hydatid fluid and internal debris (the "hydatid sand") of the mother cyst. Membranes within the hydatid cyst appear on MRI as

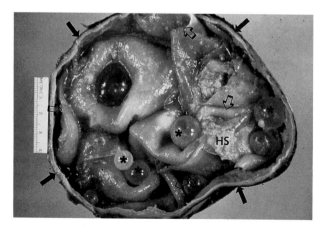

Fig. 10-47. Echinococcal cyst. Gross specimen. Cut section of echinococcal cyst demonstrates a thick pericyst *(arrows).* The germinal layer is peeled from the pericyst in some areas *(open arrows).* Multiple daughter cysts are present *(*).* Hydatid sand *(HS)* is seen between the daughter cysts and the crumpled germinal layer.

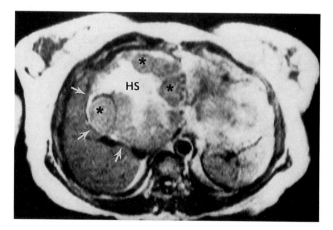

Fig. 10-48. Hepatic echinococcal cyst. Axial T2WI of hydatid cyst demonstrating hyperintense daughter cysts *(*)* in a well-defined mass. Note the hypointense pericyst *(arrows)* and very hyperintense hydatid sand *(HS).*

dark structures that float within the cavity when the cyst undergoes degeneration. Further destruction of the cyst results in intraparenchymal rupture of the wall, which appears as a defect in the low-intensity rim on MR images.[10,12] Rupture is followed by external rupture of the cyst and organ capsule, and MR is able to show the spillage of hydatid contents into the peritoneal cavity. Calcification within the cyst occurs as the final stage of degeneration. Though better seen on CT scan, calcifications may be seen on MRI as a signal void.[12]

It is possible to distinguish between a hepatic hydatid cyst and other well-circumscribed masses of the liver using the characteristic MR finding of a low-intensity rim. MR can also be used to monitor the response of a cyst to therapy, as it demonstrates the internal features of the cyst. Moreover, with its large field of view and multiplanar imaging capability, MR allows evaluation of the relationship proximity of hepatic and extrahepatic hydatid cysts with other organs and structures.

REFERENCES

1. Barreda R, Ros PR: Diagnostic imaging of liver abscess, Crit Rev Diagn Imaging 33:29-58, 1992.
2. Cho J, Kim EE, Varma DGK, Wallace S: MR imaging of hepatosplenic candidiasis superimposed on hemochromatosis, J Comput Assist Tomogr 14:774-776, 1990.
3. Schmiedl U, Paajanen H, Arakawa M, et al: MR imaging of liver abscesses; application of Gd-DTPA, Magn Reson Imaging 6:9-16, 1988.
4. Wall SD, Fisher MR, Amparo EG, et al: Magnetic resonance imaging in the evaluation of abscesses, Am J Roentgenol 144:1217-1221, 1985.
5. Weeissleder R, Saini S, Stark DD, et al: Pyogenic liver abscess: contrast-enhanced MR imaging in rats, Am J Roentgenol 150:115-120, 1988.
6. Barreda R, Ros P: Diagnostic imaging of liver abscess, Crit Rev Diagn Imaging 33:29-58, 1992.
7. Elizondo G, Weissleder R, Stark DD, et al: Amebic liver abscess: diagnosis and treatment evaluation with MR imaging, Radiology 165:795-800, 1987.
8. Ralls PW, Henley DS, Colletti PM, et al: Amebic liver abscess: MR imaging, Radiology 165:801-804, 1987.
9. Hoff FL, Aisen AM, Walden ME, Glazer GM: MR imaging in hydatid disease of the liver, Gastrointest Radiol 12:39-42, 1987.
10. Lupeti AR, Dash N: Intrahepatic rupture of hydatid cyst: MR findings, Am J Roentgenol 151:491-492, 1988.
11. Marani SAD, Canossi GC, Nicoli FA, et al: Hydatid disease: MR imaging study, Radiology 175:701-706, 1990.
12. von Sinner W, te Strake L, Clark D, Sharif H: MR imaging in hydatid disease. Am J Roentgenol 157:741-745, 1991.
13. Wojtasek DA, Teixidor HS: Echinococcal hepatic disease: magnetic resonance appearance, Gastrointest Radiol 14:158-160, 1989.

Section seven
Vascular diseases

Pablo R. Ros
Luis H. Ros Mendoza
Christophoros Stoupis

General principles and technique
Portal vein thrombosis
Portal hypertension
Budd-Chiari syndrome

Vascular diseases of the liver are in general, like all other vascular-related pathologies, an ideal area for MRI. The inherent MRI capabilities of multiplanar imaging, as well as visualization of vascular structures without contrast administration, are in themselves enough justification for the widespread use of MRI in vascular diseases of the liver. In addition, the recent capability of MRI to obtain not only anatomic information but also quantification of blood flow using bolus tracking technique may make MRI the imaging technique of choice to study vascular diseases of the liver (Fig. 10-49).[3,5,6]

GENERAL PRINCIPLES AND TECHNIQUE

Primary liver abnormalities (i.e., cirrhosis or hepatocellular carcinoma) can produce abnormalities in the portal vein and inferior vena cava. Conversely, primary abnormalities in these vessels (inferior vena cava [IVC] thrombosis, cavernomatous transformation of the porta) may result in liver abnormalities.

In general, all vascular structures in spin-echo imaging have lack of signal within its lumen due to the normal blood flow. However, due to artifacts (i.e., even-echo rephasing) or slow flow within intrahepatic vessels, particularly within the porta in cases of portal hypertension, there may be intraluminal signal.

In general, if a vessel has flow void (no signal), it is easy to confirm its patency. However, if there is intraluminal signal, a vessel may either be patent (signal due to artifact) or may have thrombus within it. To differentiate between artifact or slow flow and intraluminal thrombus within the IVC or portal vein, it is helpful to obtain images in two different planes (i.e., axial and coronal). True thrombi will be seen within a vessel in both planes; however, if there is signal due to slow flow, thrombi will only be present in one of the two planes because of the different factors that contribute to signal intensity of blood vary according to the orientation of the flow of blood and encoding gradient.[7,8]

MRI is becoming an alternative to hepatic angiography and dynamic CT to evaluate major hepatic vessels.[9] The major applications of MRI are to rule out intraluminal thrombus and to assess collateral circulation. Because both can be easily observed, MRI is preferable to angiography

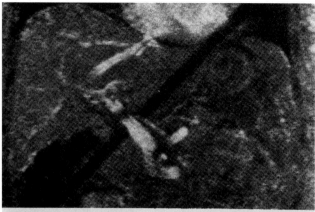

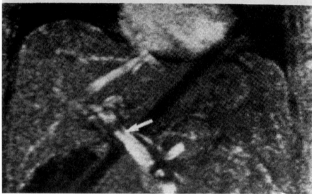

Fig. 10-49. Bolus tracking technique. Coronal MR angiogram (gradient-echo imaging) of the liver using bolus tracking technique, shows patent portal vein. With this technique, determination of the flow direction within the porta is also possible. Note the hepatopedal motion of the saturated *(tagged)* bolus within the portal vein *(arrow)*. (Reproduced with permission from Edelman RR, Zhao B, Liu CP, et al: Am J Roentgenol 153:755-760, 1989.)

because of its noninvasiveness and to dynamic CT, because it does not require contrast administration.

Recently, MR angiography (MRA) has become available for three-dimensional evaluation of the perihepatic vessels. (For additional information, see Chapter 7.) In addition, MRI can assess the direction and velocity of blood flow using the bolus tracking technique. This technique is a combination of gradient-echo cineangiography and flow presaturation. Initially, a bolus of blood is marked with a presaturation pulse that will be followed in time. The presaturated bolus, which is dark, is easily distinguished from the remaining blood, which is bright.[6] This technique allows direct demonstration of flowing blood, obviating potential errors due to phase changes unrelated to flow. In addition, it allows differentiation of thrombosis from slow flow.

Preliminary results in the portal vein with the bolus tracking technique indicate a tremendous potential in the study of portal thrombosis, portal hypertension, and patency of grafts.[5]

PORTAL VEIN THROMBOSIS

Portal vein thrombosis is usually due to one of the following:

1. Slow flow due to liver cirrhosis
2. Compression of the portal vein by porta hepatis lymphadenopathy
3. Direct invasion by neoplasm (HCC)
4. Portal vein thrombophlebitis due to inflammatory processes (pancreatitis or abdominal infection).

Conventional spin-echo technique allows the diagnosis of portal vein patency using the simple criterion of the presence or absence of signal within the portal vein (Fig. 10-50). When only spin-echo images are obtained in one plane, false-positive diagnosis of thrombosis is possible, as there is always some signal at the level of the spleno-portal confluence.[10]

Using morphologic criteria, it is not possible to differentiate between tumoral thrombus and regular blood clot. In the majority of reported cases, however, tumoral thrombi have similar signal characteristics as a main tumoral mass in the liver both in T1WI and T2WI. Additional criteria for identifying a tumoral thrombus within the portal vein are the following:

1. Nonvisualization of a portion of the wall of the porta
2. Vessel expansion due to tumor
3. Distortion of the normal circular morphology of the portal vein.

One of the most important signs of hepatocellular carcinoma is occlusion (invasion by tumor thrombus) of the intrahepatic portal vein. Occlusion is seen as a triangular shape within the liver, with its vertex located in a central position and its base adjacent to the hepatic periphery, having high signal intensity in T2WI that is likely due to edema or infarct of the liver.[12]

PORTAL HYPERTENSION

MRI is a useful method to evaluate portal dilation, as well as portal systemic collaterals in portal hypertension (Fig. 10-51). Dilated veins are seen as dilated tubular structures of low signal intensity in spin-echo images. Cavernous transformation of the portal vein due to chronic portal vein obstruction and the development of periportal collaterals is seen as a "bag of worms" (of low intensity) in the area of the porta.[1,2]

In patients with portosystemic shunts, either postsurgical or spontaneous, shunt patency is easily demonstrable with MRI as flow void in the anastomosed vessel. The presence of marked endoluminal signal intensity, indicating flow-related artifacts, also can be used to confirm permeability within a shunt. Areas of stenosis in the vessels that constitute the shunt, as well as persistence of collateral vessels, are, on the other hand, MRI signs that indicate an ineffective portal decompression.

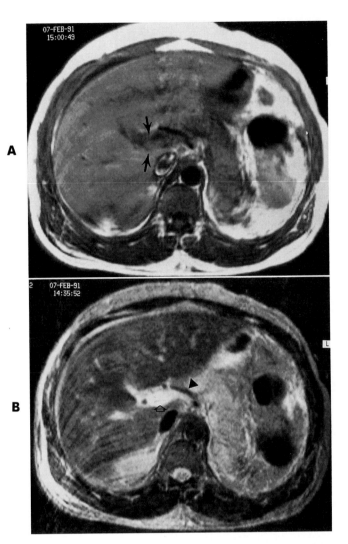

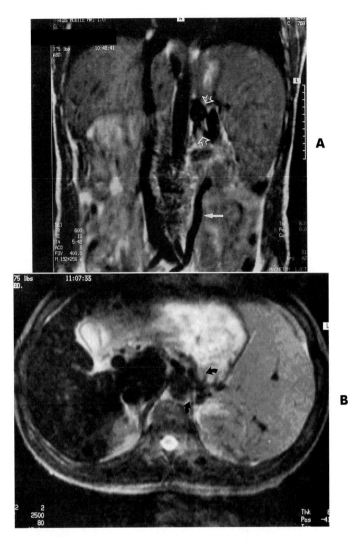

Fig. 10-50. Clot in the intrahepatic portion of the portal vein. **A,** Axial T1WI (TR 450 msec/TE 15 msec) shows the portal vein filled with material isointense to the liver *(arrows)*. **B,** Axial T2-weighted spin-echo image (TR 2200 msec/TE 90 msec) reveals hyperintense signal along the course of the main portal vein *(open arrow)*. Note the normal signal of the hepatic artery *(arrowhead)*.

Fig. 10-51. Portal hypertension. **A,** Coronal T1WI (TR 600 msec/TE 15 msec) demonstrates a markedly dilated left spermatic vein *(white arrow)* constituting one of the systemic sites of the portosystemic anastomoses. Splenomegaly and a network of collaterals at the spleen hilus *(open arrows)* are also noted. **B,** Same patient in axial plane T2-weighted spin-echo image (TE 2500 msec/TE 80 msec) reveals the collaterals at the spleen hilus *(curved arrows)*, splenomegaly, and cirrhotic liver with siderotic nodules.

The coronal plane is chosen to evaluate portocaval and splenorenal shunts. In addition, it is possible to determine the direction of flow in the portovenous system by observing the entry slice phenomenon and confirming whether it occurs in the cranial or caudal extreme of the scan volume.[11]

MRI can be used to evaluate the presence of ascites (low intensity in T1) and splenomegaly. In cases of splenomegaly, MRI is highly effective in detecting signal intensity changes within the enlarged splenic parenchyma, indicating areas of infarction due to venous congestion and slow flow.

In summary, MRI is becoming an alternative method to angiography in the presurgical evaluation for portocaval

shunt in patients with portal hypertension. An additional benefit of MRI as compared to angiography is its noninvasiveness, as coagulopathy frequently is present in patients with cirrhosis, making angiographic evaluation risky. MRI is also used to monitor the patency of portocaval shunts postsurgically.

With the advent of MRA with dynamic bolus tracking, MRI provides a new noninvasive option for the evaluation of anatomy, flow direction, and speed of blood in the portal system. Furthermore, MRA allows excellent demonstration of collateral circulation and status (patency) of portosystemic shunts.[5,6]

BUDD-CHIARI SYNDROME

Budd-Chiari syndrome is characterized clinically by the presence of portal hypertension, ascites, and progressive hepatic insufficiency.

Pathogenetically, Budd-Chiari syndrome is due to obstruction of venous flow at the hepatic sinusoid level and has multiple etiologies. Major etiologies of Budd-Chiari syndrome are the following:

1. Hepatic and/or renal neoplasms
2. Abnormal suprahepatic portion of the IVC (tumors, congenital membranes)
3. Right atrium anomalies with abnormal drainage of hepatic veins
4. Hypercoagulable states (e.g., polycythemia vera)

Severe hepatic cirrhosis can produce imaging abnormalities similar to those seen in Budd-Chiari syndrome due to the compression of hepatic veins by cirrhotic nodules and to the increase of the intracapsular pressure of the liver.

However, severe liver cirrhosis is not considered a cause of primary or secondary Budd-Chiari syndrome.

The major MRI signs in Budd-Chiari syndrome are as follows (Fig. 10-52):

1. Lack of visualization of hepatic veins confluence
2. Decrease in caliber of the major hepatic veins or lack of visualization of major hepatic vein branches
3. Decrease in the caliber of the intrahepatic IVC
4. Dilation of the azygous vein
5. Intrahepatic venous collaterals, which are transversely oriented and arch-shaped ("comma-shaped" intrahepatic varices) (Fig. 10-53). This finding is considered characteristic of this entity (see accompanying box).[11]

The caudate lobe, which has direct venous draining into the IVC, appears normal in size in acute cases of Budd-Chiari syndrome, but the rest of the liver enlarges due to vascular compression. The signal intensity in the enlarged

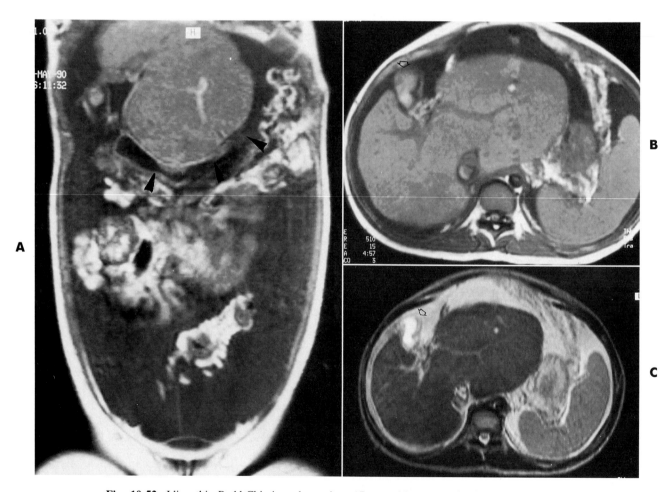

Fig. 10-52. Idiopathic Budd-Chiari syndrome in a 17-year-old woman. **A,** Coronal T1WI (TR 600 msec/TE 15 msec) reveals ascites and abnormal configuration of the liver. Note a markedly enlarged caudate lobe *(arrowheads).* **B,** Axial T1WI (TR 510 msec/TE 15 msec) demonstrates an enlarged caudate lobe. **C,** Axial T2WI (TR 2300 msec/TE 90 msec) reveals absent hepatic veins. A prominent draining vein is seen anterior to the liver *(open arrows).*

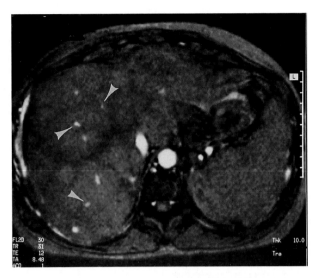

Fig. 10-53. Comma-shaped intrahepatic varices. Axial T2-weighted gradient-echo image (TR 31 msec/TE 12 msec/FLIP 30) reveals the intrahepatic venous, arch-shaped collaterals, in a patient with secondary Budd-Chiari syndrome *(arrowheads)*.

MRI signs in Budd-Chiari syndrome

- Nonvisualization of hepatic veins confluence
- Decrease in caliber of hepatic vein
- Nonvisualization of secondary hepatic veins
- Narrowing of intrahepatic IVC
- Azygous vein dilation
- Intrahepatic varices ("comma-shaped" collaterals)

---

liver is increased on T2WI due to increase in water content. In chronic Budd-Chiari syndrome, the liver becomes cirrhotic and hypointnese on T2WI, except in the caudate lobe, which appears markedly enlarged due to compensatory hypertrophy and with normal signal intensity. In many cases, MRI findings allow the establishment a specific diagnosis of Budd-Chiari syndrome. MRI is not only useful to establish the diagnosis of Budd-Chiari syndrome, but also to plan management.

REFERENCES

1. Bernardino ME, Steinberg HV, Pearson TC, et al: Shunts for portal hypertension: MR and angiography for determination of patency, Radiology 158:57-62, 1986.
2. Cohen JM, Weinreb JC, Redman HC: Postoperative assessment of splenorenal shunts with MRI: preliminary investigation, Am J Roentgenol 146:597, 1986.
3. Edelman RR, Zhao B, Liu CP, et al: MR angiography and dynamic flow evaluation of the portal venous system, Am J Roentgenol 153:755-760, 1989.
4. Edelman RR, Mattle HP, Kleefield J, et al: Quantification of blood flow with dynamic MR imaging and presaturation bolus tracking, Radiology 171:551-556, 1989.
5. Edman WA, Weinreb JC, Cohen JM, et al: Venous thrombosis: clinical and experimental MR imaging, Radiology 161:233-238, 1986.
6. Hricak H, Amparo E, Fisher MR, et al: Abdominal venous system: assessment using MR, Radiology 156:415-422, 1985.
7. Itai Y, Ontomo K, Kokubo T, et al: Segmental intensity differences in the liver on MR images: a sign of intrahepatic portal flow stoppage, Radiology 167:17-79, 1988.
8. Levy HM, Newhouse JH: MR imaging of portal vein thrombosis, Am J Roentgenol 151:283-286, 1988.
9. Moss AA, Goldberg HJ, Stark DD, et al: Hepatic tumors: magnetic resonance and CT appearance, Radiology 150:141-147, 1984.
10. Ros RR, Viamonte M Jr, Soila K, et al: Demonstration of cavernomatous transformation of the portal vein by magnetic resonance imaging, Gastrointest Radiol 11:90-92, 1986.
11. Stark DD, Hahn PF, Trey C, et al: MRI of the Budd-Chiari syndrome, Am J Roentgenol 146:1141-1148, 1986.
12. Williams DM, Cho KJ, Aiseu AM, et al: Portal hypertension evaluated by MR imaging, Radiology 157:703-706, 1985.

Section eight
Diffuse diseases

Pablo R. Ros
Luis H. Ros Mendoza
Christophoros Stoupis

Fatty liver
Hepatitis
Cirrhosis
Hemochromatosis—iron deposition liver disease
Copper deposition liver disease
Lymphoma
Summary

For the majority of diffuse diseases of the liver, MRI currently is no more effective than other imaging techniques, such as ultrasound, CT, or nuclear medicine. Although MRI provides important information to complement laboratory and biopsy findings for several diseases (fatty replacement, hepatitits, cirrhosis, copper deposition, and lymphoma), the major indication for MRI in diffuse liver diseases is iron deposition disease or hemochromatosis. MRI is also used when other imaging modalities cannot be performed due to special circumstances, or as a problem-solving modality when equivocal findings have been obtained by ultrasound or CT. This section covers the current applications of MRI to diffuse diseases of the liver and discusses its future potential.

FATTY LIVER

Fatty liver is defined as excessive accumulation of fat within the cytoplasm of hepatocytes. It is considered a nonspecific response of the liver to a variety of both metabolic injuries and liver toxins. The most common cause of fatty liver in the Western Hemisphere is alcoholism. Fatty liver is considered an intermediate stage between alcoholic hepatitis and alcoholic cirrhosis.[22]

Fatty liver can be either diffuse or focal. Focal fatty change produces a wide spectrum of findings both pathologically, and in imaging.[17] Focal fatty change has become one of the most frequent problems in the differential diagnosis of focal liver lesions in the daily practice of abdominal MRI, along with hemangioma and hepatic cyst.

Although focal fatty change itself is a common problem for the radiologist, the issue becomes more complex, as focal lesions (primary neoplasms, both benign and malig-

nant, as well as metastasis) may appear in a fatty liver. Furthermore, there may be areas of fatty change within primary neoplasms, such as adenoma and hepatocellular carcinoma.[11,14]

Conventional spin-echo pulse sequences are not very sensitive for diagnosing fatty change.[31] In animal models, extreme fatty change produced experimentally with high-lipid diets does not produce significant changes in either the T1- or T2-relaxation values of the hepatic parenchyma. There is only a minimal increment in liver intensity despite the dramatic shortening of T1 produced by fat. This minor increase in intensity in fatty liver occurs because most of the liver signal comes from water protons in the hepato-

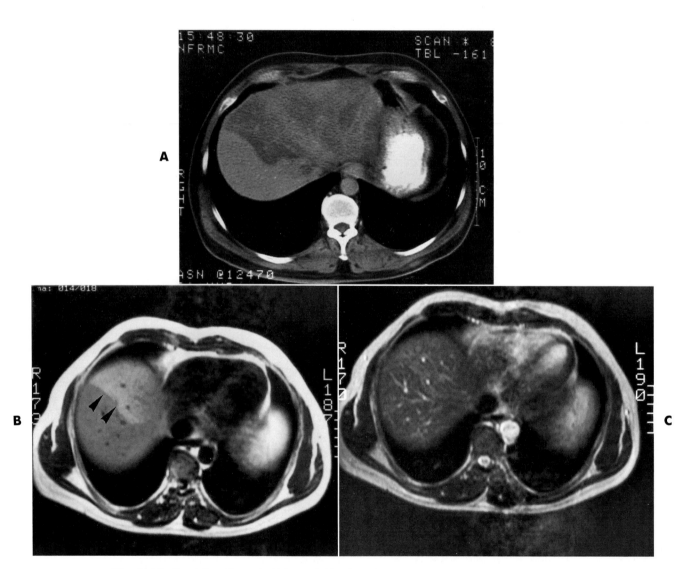

Fig. 10-54. Focal fatty liver. **A,** Enhanced CT of the liver confirmed a large, hypodense ill-defined lesion in this patient with prior colectomy for adenocarcinoma of the colon. **B,** Axial T1-weighted spin-echo image (TR 300/TE 40) reveals an area of increased intensity. Note the straight margin *(arrowheads)* and nondisplaced vessels. **C,** Axial T2-weighted spin-echo image (TR 2000/TE 80) reveals minimally brighter signal intensity and normal vessels without displacement or invasion.

Table 10-4. Fatty change versus neoplasm with fat (HCC and HCA): MRI appearance

	T1	T2	Vessels
Fatty change	Mild hyper-intensity	Isointense or slightly hyperintense to normal liver	Uninvolved
Neoplasm	Hyperintense	Hyperintense	Displaced

cytes, which are not altered by the presence of fat nearby.[4,27]

In some cases, when the degree of fatty change is high and heavily T1WI are used with a very short TR (less than 500 msec) and short TE, it is easy to identify an increase in signal because the relaxation time of fat is shorter than that of normal liver. In these cases, areas of fatty replacement have higher intensity than the spleen.[27] In many cases where fatty change is suspected by CT or ultrasound, despite the previously mentioned limitations, the spin-echo technique allows the diagnosis of fat as a hyperintense area crossed by nondisplaced vessels (Fig. 10-54).[11,31]

Fat suppression sequence is more sensitive than conventional spin-echo for the diagnosis of fatty change.[5,10,14] This technique has the potential to quantitate noninvasively the amount of fat in the liver.[16]

MRI is helpful to differentiate a space-occupying lesion (i.e., a neoplasm) from fatty change. In general, neoplastic processes are hypointense in T1WI, whereas fatty change produces an increase in signal intensity. On T2WI, neoplasms usually are hyperintense to normal liver, whereas fatty change is indistinguishable from normal tissue (Table 10-4).

There is recent evidence that patients who have fatty

liver may have some laboratory abnormalities, particularly an increase in the transaminase levels. In these cases, because the laboratory findings may mimic the presence of cirrhosis, it is important to differentiate between cirrhosis and fatty liver. Currently, the only method to distinguish between these two entities is liver biopsy. However, fat suppression MRI may prove to be helpful.

Fat can be seen in the liver in a number of circumstances (see box at bottom left). In addition, because fat is related to a host of products toxic to the liver such as alcohol or steroids, it is possible to find in the same liver areas of fat (either focal or diffuse) and neoplasms. This fact compounds the issue for the radiologist, and a clear understanding of the appearance of fat versus neoplasms is important. The box below summarizes the major causes of fatty liver. In the Western world, the three most common causes are alcoholism, obesity, and diabetes. Of particular mention are the rapid changes that occur in patients who receive portal hyperalimentation and those who have liver transplants. Livers that have been imaged before hyperalimentation or transplantation have become fatty and are replaced in a very short period of time, as little as a few days.

HEPATITIS

The usefulness of MRI in the evaluation of inflammatory processes of the liver is limited. In cases of acute hepatitis, there may be an increase in T1- and T2-relaxation times of the liver due to the marked increase in free water within the liver parenchyma. This phenomenon has been described only for focal changes of hepatitis, as normal liver surrounding the involved area remains as an internal control.[11] In general, MRI is not sensitive enough in cases of diffuse hepatitis due to the variability of signal in normal livers.

In chronic hepatitis, areas of increased signal have been noted in T2WI, corresponding to inflammatory changes. These areas most likely represent active hepatitis within chronic hepatitis and reflect the marked edema in these areas.[28]

The use of superparamagnetic iron oxide (SPIO) may

Fat in the liver

- Focal fatty change (mimics space-occupying lesion)
- Diffuse fatty change
- Diffuse fatty change with areas of normal liver (e.g., caudate lobe) (normal liver mimics a space-occupying lesion)
- Diffuse fatty change with synchronous neoplasm
- Focal fatty change with synchronous neoplasm
- Neoplasms rich in fat
  Hepatocellular carcinoma
  Hepatocellular adenoma
- Fatty neoplasms
  Lipoma
  Liposarcoma
  Angiomyolipoma
- Intrahepatic fat
  Periportal fat
  Pseudolipoma

Etiology of fatty liver

- Alcoholism
- Obesity
- Diabetes mellitus
- Hepatitis
- Drugs
  Steroids
  Chemotherapy
  Cholesterol-lowering agents
- Hyperalimentation
- Liver transplantation

be helpful to study patients with active hepatitis, as there is less uptake of SPIO particles by the inflamed tissue. This characteristic results in hyperintensity of the abnormal areas as compared with normal tissue.[6]

CIRRHOSIS

Because cirrhosis is defined as the substitution of the normal hepatic parenchyma by fibrosis, there was initial hope that MRI would play a significant role in its diagnosis and monitoring. Histologically, however, although there is increased fibrosis, there is no change in the volume of hepatic water within the cytoplasms of hepatocytes. Therefore, the signal intensity of the cirrhotic liver and even the relaxation times are indistinguishable from

the normal liver, particularly when there is no associated hepatitis.[26,27]

Therefore, the diagnosis of hepatic cirrhosis with MRI depends, as in CT and ultrasound, on the morphologic appearance of the liver and secondary findings of portal hypertension. The well-known findings of cirrhosis by other imaging techniques—such as increase in size of the left lobe and caudate, nodularity (hobnail appearance) of the surface of the liver, the relative decrease in size of the right lobe, splenomegaly, and portosplenic collateral circulation—are the major indicators for cirrhosis of the liver (Fig. 10-55).

Other signs, such as the distortion or compression of the intrahepatic vessels, indicative of regenerating nod-

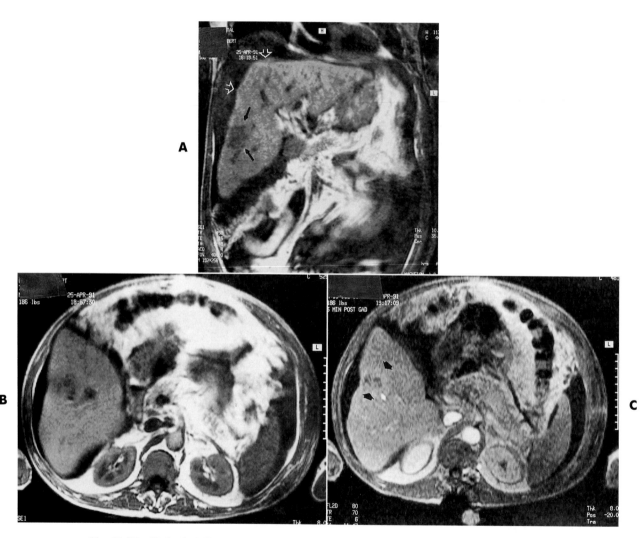

Fig. 10-55. Cirrhosis: MR appearance. **A,** Coronal T1-weighted spin-echo image (TR 450/TE 15) reveals an atrophic right lobe of one lung, nodular surface of the liver *(open arrows),* and ascites. Hypointensity in the inferoanterior segment of the right lobe with irregular margins, corresponding to hepatocellular carcinoma. **B,** Axial T1-weighted spin-echo image (TR 450/TE 15). **C,** Axial T1-weighted gradient-echo image after gadolinium (TR 70, TE 5, FLIP angle 80 degrees) demonstrates the irregular surface of the shrunken liver, ascites, and irregular enhancement of the hepatocellular carcinoma *(arrows).*

ules, can also be used to determine the presence of cirrhosis. Regenerating nodules in cirrhosis are generally of the same signal intensity as normal liver. However, they may appear hyperintense due to fatty change (Fig. 10-56).[8]

In cases of cirrhosis secondary to prior viral hepatitis, multiple small nodular areas with very low signal intensity in T2WI have been described, likely corresponding to regenerating nodules that contain either hemosiderin or are surrounded by fibrous walls.[12,21] These low intensity nodules are particularly well seen in gradient-echo images, due to susceptibility artifacts caused by the presence of iron and/or fibrous tissue within these nodules (Fig. 10-57).

In general, the cirrhosis findings due to portal hypertension, such as splenomegaly, increase in portal vein size, varices, ascites, etc., are very well studied with MRI.[20] In patients with chronic cirrhosis, one of the major uses of MRI is to determine the patency of the portal vein, the patency of portosystemic shunts, and the direction of the flow of blood in the portal vein.[1] (See Chapter 7 and the Vascular Disease section in this chapter.)

Regarding the use of some contrast agents in the study of cirrhosis, recent evidence indicates that intravenous SPIO may be helpful in the diagnosis of liver cirrhosis. In patients with cirrhosis, there is decrease in the uptake of SPIO particles by the cirrhotic liver, resulting in less hypointensity and more heterogeneity in the liver signal than is produced by SPIO in normal livers. Heterogenity is most likely due to the hepatic structural changes caused by cirrhosis. This pattern contrasts with the lack of uptake in patients with chronic hepatitis where there is also a decreased uptake, but the hepatic parenchyma appears homogeneous.[6]

HEMOCHROMATOSIS—IRON DEPOSITION LIVER DISEASE

Hemochromatosis is defined as an excessive deposit of iron in multiple tissues. A primary form (primary or "true"

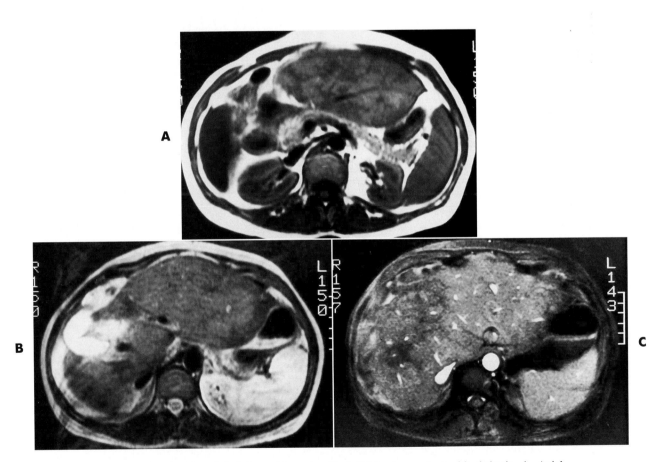

Fig. 10-56. Shrunken right lobe and hypertrophic left lobe in a patient with cirrhosis. **A,** Axial T1-weighted image (TR 500/TE 20) reveals multiple isointense to hyperintense nodules in the left lobe of the liver with distortion of the vessels. **B,** Axial T2-weighted spin-echo image (TR 2500/TE 80) with similar findings. **C,** Axial T2-weighted gradient-echo image (TR 22/TE 13/FLIP angle 30 degrees) with multiple comma-shaped intrahepatic varices mimicking Budd-Chiari syndrome. Due to compression of intrahepatic vessels by cirrhotic nuclei, a pattern identical to the one seen in Budd-Chiari syndrome can develop.

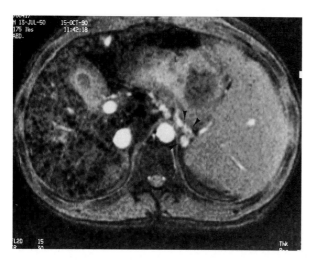

Fig. 10-57. Cirrhosis with siderotic regenerative nodules. Axial T2-weighted gradient-echo image (TR 30/TE 12/FLIP angle 15 degrees) shows multiple low-intensity nodules within this cirrhotic liver. Note susceptibility artifacts due to iron accumulation. Thickened gallbladder wall, splenomegaly, and splenic varices *(arrows)* can also be seen.

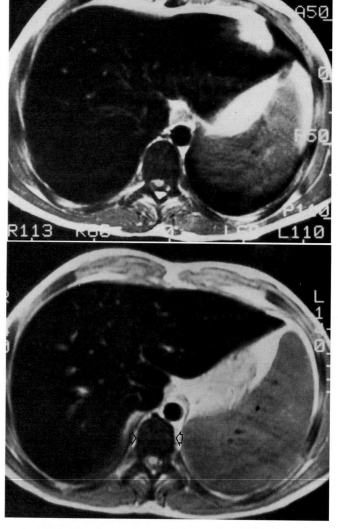

Fig. 10-58. Transfusional iron overload with liver involvement in this patient of Greek origin with thalassemia major. **A,** Axial T1WI (TR 789/TE 20) reveals marked decrease in hepatic signal, whereas the splenic signal remains normal. **B,** Axial proton-weighted image (TR 2308/TE 20) shows similar findings in the liver. No change in the intensity is noted. Note drop of signal in the bone marrow *(open arrows)*.

hemochromatosis) is due to the increased intestinal absorption of iron. A secondary form, resulting from multiple transfusions, is due to an increase in the turnover of red blood cells. In general, both primary and secondary forms of hemochromatosis are termed *iron deposition disease.*

Iron deposits are present in multiple organs, but primarily in the liver, pancreas, spleen, joints, heart, and skin. Deposition in the muscle fibers of the heart becomes critical. The cause of death of patients with hemochromatosis is usually myocardiopathy secondary to iron deposition.[7,9]

Iron deposition in the liver induces cirrhosis and eventually the appearance of hepatocellular carcinoma. Twenty percent of patients with hemochromatosis develop hepatocellular carcinoma. The normal levels of iron in the liver are less than 250 ng/g. In patients with chronic hemochromatosis, the levels of iron are higher than 2 mg/g. MRI is capable of detecting concentrations of iron in the liver by producing an abnormal low signal at 1.2 mg/g (Fig. 10-58).[27] Therefore, MRI is able to offer a specific diagnosis of iron deposition disease because iron deposited as ferritin, hemosiderin, or other molecular forms is paramagnetic, altering the relaxation times of tissue hydrogen. This alteration translates predominantly into shortening of the T2-relaxation time, reducing the signal intensity of the liver. This principle underlies the use of SPIO as a contrast agent in MRI.

Due to the susceptibility of hepatic iron deposits, T2WI are more sensitive than T1WI for hemochromatosis in the early stages of the disease. T1WI allows a gross estimation of the disease in the more advance stages when large amounts of iron are accumulated within the liver. Al-

though the pancreas and the spleen accumulate iron only in advanced stages of this disease, when they are involved, the findings are similar to those in the liver with decrease in the signal intensity, particularly in T2WI.

Because MRI can yield a specific diagnosis of iron deposition disease, it is no longer necessary to perform liver biopsies to diagnose hemochromatosis. In addition, MRI has been proposed as the ideal method to monitor the evolution and response to therapy in these patients.[2,3,15,18,27]

At this point, the quantification of tissue iron by MRI is a research area.[29] Preliminary results are limited, as conventional spin-echo techniques are not sufficiently sensitive to resolve significant differences when there is an iron level below 2 mg/g.

An added advantage of MRI for following patients with iron deposition disease is the ability to screen concurrently for hepatocellular carcinoma, a well-known complication of hemochromatosis. Because the malignant hepatocytes in hepatocellular carcinoma do not accumulate iron, hepatocellular carcinoma appears as a conspicuous area of very high intensity in T2WI against the very low signal background of liver hemochromatosis. MRI is the method of choice to evaluate hepatocellular carcinoma (and/or metastatic disease if a primary cancer is discovered elsewhere) in patients with primary or secondary hemochromatosis.

COPPER DEPOSITION LIVER DISEASE

The diseases characterized by copper deposition in the liver include Wilson's disease, chronic biliary obstruction, and primary biliary cirrhosis. In patients with Hodgkin's disease, there is also evidence of high concentrations of copper in the liver; therefore, hepatic involvement in

Hodgkin's disease may also be considered in the differential diagnosis of these processes.

The normal level of copper within the liver is 15-55 mg/g. In patients with Wilson's disease, the level of copper is higher than 250 mg/g.[24]

Copper deposited in the liver is superparamagnetic in its ionic form. Therefore, its effect on the MRI signal of liver should be similar to that of ferric iron deposited in patients with hemochromatosis. However, the MRI appearance of the liver in patients with Wilson's disease is unremarkable, with signal intensity on both T1WI and T2WI in the range of a normal liver (Fig. 10-59).

This lack of signal decrease in patients with copper deposition may be due to the proteinaceous conjugation of the copper ions within hepatocytes. One theory is that the mobile hydrogen ions are protected from the superparamagnetic effect of copper because the metal ions are buried deep within the structure of the copper-protein complexes. A second hypothesis postulates that the lack of decrease in signal is secondary to associated fatty change and/or underlying cirrhosis.[13]

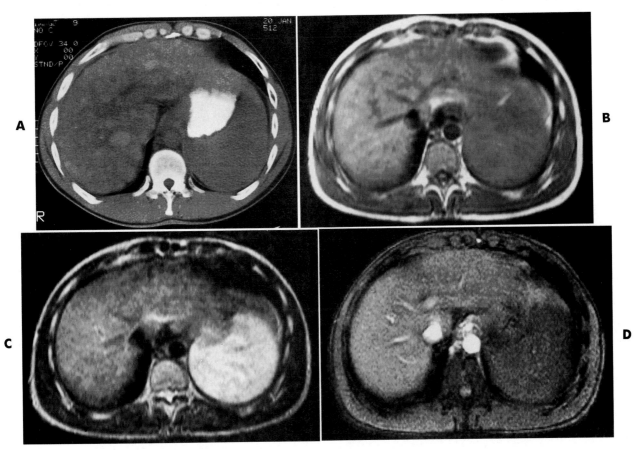

Fig. 10-59. Wilson's disease. **A,** Nonenhanced CT of the liver with obvious inhomogeneity of the liver due to multiple cirrhotic nodules caused by copper overload. **B,** T1WI (300/15). **C,** T2WI (2000/80). The nodular pattern seen in CT is obscured. **D,** Even a T1-weighted gradient-echo image (TR 31/TE 12/FLIP 80 degrees) is unable to show any hepatic tissue abnormalities or evidence of susceptibility artifacts due to copper deposition within the nodules.

LYMPHOMA

There are two types of lymphomatous involvement of the liver. The first, primary hepatic lymphoma, is rare. It usually presents as a solitary mass that corresponds histologically to large cell lymphoma.[30] The more common secondary involvement of the liver occurs with both Hodgkin's and non-Hodgkin's types, presenting in 23% and 16% of lymphoma cases, respectively.[23,34]

Overall, primary liver lymphoma is much less common than in other organs because the amount of lymphatic tissue in the liver is very small, present only in the periportal spaces. There are no lymphatics in the hepatocyte cords or in the centrolobular veins.

Morphologically, there are three patterns of hepatic involvement in lymphoma. The most common is the diffuse infiltrating form with microscopic invasion along the periportal tracks. The other two forms are a focal mass and a mixed form (combining a focal mass and infiltration).

Focal hepatic lymphoma is detected by MRI as a homogeneous mass characterized by prolonged T1- and T2-relaxation times when compared to a normal liver (Fig. 10-60). Therefore, the pattern is the usual one of focal neoplasms with hypointensity in T1WI and hyperintensity in T2WI, compared to normal parenchyma. Although lymphoma is readily distinguishable from normal liver, the difference in relaxation times from either metastases or hepatocellular carcinoma is not significant.

The diffuse form of lymphoma has not been detected by MRI. Neither morphologic nor quantitative criteria have been sensitive enough to detect diffuse lymphomatous infiltration. Changes in the T1- and T2-relaxation time of involved parenchyma are not sufficiently altered to detect infiltration by lymphomatous cells.[19,25,33] Experiments using SPIO intravenously as a contrast material also have not detected significant differences between normal liver and liver diffusely infiltrated with lymphoma.[32]

The mixed pattern, having focal lesions combined with diffuse infiltration, produces a mild decrease in signal in

T1WI and focal increase of signal in T2WI superimposed on a background of slight diffuse hyperintensity. In general, MRI may be slightly more sensitive than CT in the detection of hepatic lymphoma in its mixed form. MRI appears to have similar accuracy to contrast-enhanced CT to detect focal lymphoma.[25]

SUMMARY

The major current indication for the evaluation of diffuse diseases of the liver is the diagnosis of hemochromatosis. In this disease, MRI has obviated the use of a liver biopsy for its diagnosis. MRI is also useful for detecting the presence of secondary hepatocellular carcinoma in hemochromatosis and/or the occasional development of metastases in hemochromatic livers.

MRI is also helpful, particularly using fat suppression techniques, to detect fatty infiltration of the liver. In combination with other imaging modalities, MRI is helpful in the work-up not only of diffuse or focal fatty liver, but also in other fat-related situations where it may be important to distinguish fat from focal or diffuse space-occupying lesions in the liver.

MRI is of marginal help in the diagnosis and/or monitoring of other diffuse processes of the liver such as hepatitis, cirrhosis, copper deposition diseases, and lymphoma. The advent of tissue-specific contrast agents, such as SPIO and manganese-DPDP, may be of help to further evaluate these diseases. There is experimental evidence, and therefore hope, that MRI may be helpful to distinguish and/or quantify chronic active hepatitis from chronic cirrhosis based on the pattern and intensity of SPIO uptake (either diffuse or heterogeneous) by the liver.

Regarding the study of lymphoma of the liver, MRI is as useful as CT in the detection of focal lymphoma and may be slightly more useful than CT, particularly if combined with SPIO, in the detection of the mixed form of lymphoma. However, infiltrative lymphoma remains an elusive diagnosis for imaging in general and MRI in particular.

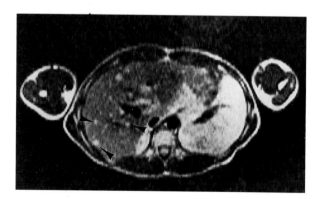

Fig. 10-60. One-year-old boy with Hodgkin's disease. T2-weighted spin-echo image (TR 2000/TE 80) shows multiple small focal areas of increased signal intensity in the liver (arrows). The spleen is moderately enlarged.

REFERENCES

1. Bernardino ME, Steinberg HV, Pearson TC, et al: Shunts for portal hypertension: MR and angiography for determination of patency, Radiology 158:57-61, 1986.
2. Brown DW, et al: Nuclear magnetic resonance study of iron overload in liver tissue, Magn Reson Imaging 3:275-282, 1985.
3. Brasch RC, Wesbey GE, Gooding CA, et al: Magnetic resonance imaging of transfusional hemosiderosis complicating thalassemia major, Radiology 150:767-771, 1984.
4. Buonocore E, et al: NMR imaging of the abdomen: technical considerations, Am J Roentgenol 141:1171-1178, 1983.
5. Dixon WT: Simple proton spectroscopic imaging, Radiology 153:189-194, 1984.
6. Elizondo G, Weissleder R, Stark DD, et al: Hepatic cirrhosis and hepatitis: MR imaging enhanced with superparamagnetic iron oxide, Radiology 174:797-801, 1990.

7. Finch SC, Finch CA: Idiopathic hemochromatosis, an iron storage disease, Medicine 34:381-430, 1955.

8. Goldberg HI, Moos AA, Stark DD, et al: Hepatic cirrhosis: magnetic resonance imaging, Radiology 153:737-739, 1984.

9. Grace ND, Powell LW: Iron storage disorders of the liver, Gastroenterology 67:1257-1283, 1974.

10. Heiken JP, Lee JRT, Dixon WT: Fatty infiltration of the liver: evaluation by proton spectroscopic imaging, Radiology 157:707-710, 1985.

11. Itai Y, Ohtomo K, Kokubo T, et al: CT and MR imaging of fatty tumors of the liver, J Comput Assist Tomogr 11(2):253-257, 1987.

12. Itai Y, Onishi S, Ohtomo K, et al: Regenerating nodules of liver cirrhosis: MR imaging, Radiology 165:419-423, 1987.

13. Lawler GA, Pennock JM, Steiner RE, et al: NMR imaging in Wilson disease, J Comput Assist Tomogr 7:1-8, 1983.

14. Lee JRT, Dixon WT, Ling D, et al: Fatty infiltration of the liver: demonstration by proton spectroscopic imaging: preliminary observations, Radiology 153:195-201, 1984.

15. Leung AW, Steiner RE, Young IR: NMR imaging of the liver in two cases of iron overload, J Comput Assist Tomogr 8:446-449, 1984.

16. Levenson H, Greensite F, Hoets J, et al: Fatty infiltration of the liver: quantification with phase-contrast MR imaging at 1.5T vs biopsy, Am J Roentgenol 156:307-312, 1991.

17. Lewis E, Bernadino ME, Barnes PA, et al: The fatty liver: pitfalls in the CT and angiographic evaluation of metastatic disease, J Comput Assist Tomogr 7:235-241, 1983.

18. Murphy FB, Bernardino ME: MR imaging of focal hemochromatosis, J Comput Assist Tomogr 10(6):1044-1046, 1986.

19. O'Neil J, Ros PR: Knowing hepatic pathology aids MRI of liver tumors, Diagn Imaging 58-65, 1989.

20. Ohtomo K, Itai Y, Makita K, et al: Portosystemic collaterals on MR imaging, J Comput Assist Tomogr 10:751-755, 1986.

21. Ohtomo K, Itai Y, Ohtomo Y, et al: Regenerating nodules of liver cirrhosis: MR imaging with pathologic correlation, Am J Roentgenol 154:505-507, 1990.

22. Pimstone NR, French SW: Alcoholic liver disease, Med Clin North Am 68:39-56, 1984.

23. Ros PR, Rasmussen JF, Li KCP: Radiology of malignant and benign liver tumors, Curr Prob Diagn Radiol 3:95-155, 1989.

24. Runge VM, et al: Nuclear magnetic resonance of iron and copper disease states, Am J Roentgenol 141:943-948, 1983.

25. Shirkhoda A, Ros PR, Farah J, et al: Lymphoma of solid abdominal viscera, Radiol Clin North Am 28(4):785-801, 1990.

26. Smith FW, Mallard JR: NMR imaging in liver disease, Br Med Bull 40:194-196, 1984.

27. Stark DD, Bass NM, Moss AA, et al: Nuclear magnetic resonance imaging of experimentally induced liver disease, Radiology 148:743-751, 1983.

28. Stark DD, Goldberg HJ, Moss AA, et al: Chronic liver disease: evaluation by magnetic resonance, Radiology 150:149-151, 1984.

29. Stark DD, Mosley ME, Bacon BR, et al: Magnetic resonance imaging and spectroscopy of hepatic iron overload, Radiology 154:137-142, 1985.

30. Weinreb JC, Brateman L, Muravilla RR: MRI of hepatic lymphoma, Am J Roentgenol 143:1211-1214, 1984.

31. Wenker JC, Baker MK, Ellis JH, et al: Focal fatty infiltration of the liver: demonstration by magnetic resonance imaging, Am J Roentgenol 143:573-574, 1984.

32. Weissleder R, Stark DD, Compton CC, et al: Ferrite enhanced MR imaging of hepatic lymphoma: an experimental study in rats, Am J Roentgenol 149:1161-1165, 1987.

33. Weissleder R, et al: MRI of hepatic lymphoma, Magn Reson Imaging 6:675-681, 1988.

34. Zornoza J, Ginaldi S: Computed tomography in hepatic lymphoma, Radiology 138:405-410, 1981.

Chapter 11

BILIARY

Stephen J. Kennedy

INDICATIONS

For most gallbladder and biliary tract disease, ultrasound and CT are superior to MRI, due mostly to low cost and ease of availability. MRI also produces motion artifact in the upper abdomen. Nevertheless, it is important to recognize biliary tract disease on MRI examinations obtained for other indications. In select circumstances of neoplastic disease, MRI is indicated for staging in cases where CT and ultrasound fail to delineate the extent of disease and spread to adjacent structures.

Common bile duct patency is best examined by a radionuclide study. However, MRI may be indicated for evaluating the concentrating ability of the gallbladder.

NORMAL ANATOMY

The normal gallbladder lies in the right upper quadrant of the abdomen in the gallbladder fossa, in the fissure between the right and left hepatic lobes. The gallbladder stores and concentrates bile and delivers it to the duodenum by contraction in response to appropriate chemical stimulation.

Concentrated gallbladder bile in fasting patients has high signal intensity in T1-weighted images (T1WI).[8] This high intensity is due to absorption of water during the bile concentration process in the normally functioning gallbladder, causing a shortening of the T1 relaxation time.[4] Normal hepatic bile is 3% solids; the rest is water.[14] The normal gallbladder selectively absorbs water, certain organic ions, and small amounts of bile salts.[14] The resultant volume is about five to ten times smaller than the original hepatic secretion.[14]

Sometimes, a layering effect can be seen in patients who have recently eaten, with low signal intensity hepatic bile layering above high intensity concentrated bile (Fig. 11-1).[8] In this respect, MRI gives us information about the physiology of the gallbladder.[11] Imaging a patient in the fasting and nonfasting state may give an indication of the concentrating ability of the gallbladder. Normal intrahepatic bile ducts are not seen on standard spin-echo MRI sequences, and extrahepatic bile ducts are seen only occasionally.[17]

CONGENITAL ANOMALIES
Choledochal cyst

There are three types of choledochal cysts: an aneurysmal dilation of the common bile duct (type I), diverticulum of the duct (type II), and a choledochocele (type III). As expected, the MR appearance of a choledochal cyst is low signal intensity on T1WI and high signal intensity on T2WI (Fig. 11-2).[1]

Other

The biliary tract can have a variety of anomalous connections and patterns. The most important anomaly is

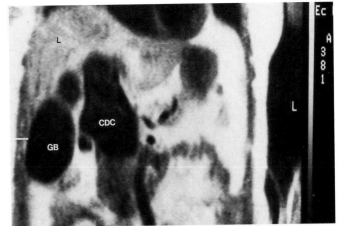

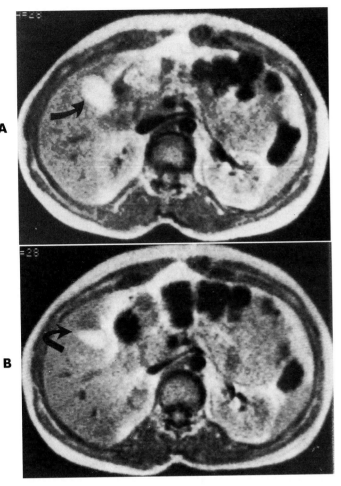

Fig. 11-1. A, T1WI of a fasting subject shows high signal concentrated gallbladder bile. **B,** T1WI in the same subject after gallbladder stimulation. Note the layering of dilute hepatic bile above the residual concentrated bile *(curved arrow)*. (From Hricak H, Filly RA, Margulis AR, et al: *Radiology* 147:481-484, 1983.)

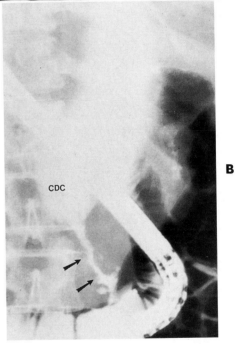

Fig. 11-2. A, Coronal T1WI of a choledochal cyst *(CDC)* showing low signal intensity fluid within the cyst. *(L* = liver, *GB* = gallbladder). **B,** ERCP from the same patient showing the choledochal cyst and the irregular mucosa of the common bile duct *(arrows)* in this patient with cholangiocarcinoma.

agenesis of all or any portion of the hepatic or common bile ducts, or duplication of these structures.[14] Variation of common bile duct or cystic duct anatomy important to the surgeon are not well depicted on MRI at present.

Dilation of biliary tree

Ultrasound, CT, and radionuclide scans are the modalities of choice for primary evaluation of the dilated biliary tract. However, it is important to recognize dilated biliary structures on MRI examinations performed for other indications. In general, dilated biliary ducts appear as low signal-intensity structures on T1WI and high signal-intensity structures on T2WI with respect to liver and pancreas.[5] Using both T1WI and T2WI together is important in the evaluation. T1WI gives superior anatomic detail. However, low signal biliary ducts tend to blend with the portal venous structures on T1WI.[17] T2WI offers the advantage

of high contrast of dilated biliary ducts with respect to liver and vascular structures, but gives poor spatial resolution.[17] Therefore, T2WI can detect the bright biliary structures, and T1WI can better show their relationship to the portal structures (Fig. 11-3).[17]

INFLAMMATORY DISEASE
Cholelithiasis

The vast majority of gallstones are composed mainly of cholesterol and bilirubin. Although cholesterol forms a large fraction of the total stone weight in many gallstones,

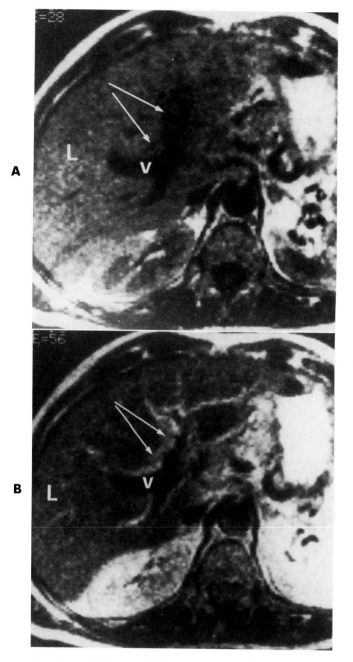

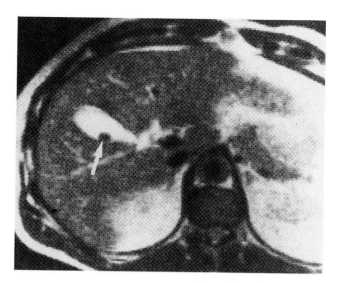

Fig. 11-4. T1WI of a subject with asymptomatic gallstones. High intensity bile outlines a low intensity stone *(arrow)*. (From McCarthy S, Hricak H, Cohen M, et al: *Radiology* 158:333-336, 1986.)

Fig. 11-3. T1WI and T2WI of dilated intrahepatic ducts *(arrows)*. **A,** With T1 weighting, the bile ducts are low signal intensity with respect to liver *(L)*, but blend with the venous structures *(v)*. **B,** The relative T2 weighting of shows the high signal intensity bile ducts distinguished from the portal venous structures. (From Dooms GC, Fischer MR, Higgins CB, et al: *Radiology* 158:337-341, 1986.)

it plays a relatively small role in determining its MR characteristics.[2] The behavior of water in the gallstone's crystalline matrix, not the chemical composition, determines its signal characteristics.[2]

Almost all gallstones produce little or no signal, despite having significant cholesterol and water content (Fig. 11-4).[12] Gallstones are brightest on T1WI and dark on T2WI.[2] A high intensity central signal sometimes is seen in the gallstone.[11] There is no correlation between MR signal intensity and solubility of stones in dissolution therapy.[3]

Cholecystitis

The normally functioning gallbladder will absorb fluids and electrolytes from the bile. However, an acutely inflamed gallbladder will not concentrate bile and may actually secrete fluid into its lumen.[12] Therefore, gallbladder bile in patients with acute cholecystitis will have low signal intensity on T1WI with respect to liver and fat.

Patients with chronic cholecystitis also have impairment of bile concentrating ability, which is not as severe as in patients with acute cholecystitis (Fig. 11-5).[9] Therefore, chronic cholecystitis patients will have more concentrated bile than patients with acute cholecystitis. Due to other factors, such as differences in protein content, however, there is no significant difference in T1 and T2 relaxation times of bile between acute and chronic cholecystitis. Therefore, MR signal characteristics cannot be used to differentiate acute from chronic cholecystitis reliably.

Cholangitis

Cholangitis refers to intraductal inflammation of the extrahepatic ducts, intrahepatic ducts, or both. Edema and inflammatory cell infiltration about the biliary ducts are the pathologic basis for intrahepatic periportal abnormal intensity (PAI) seen in patients with biliary disease including cholangitis and obstructive jaundice.[10] The finding generally is absent in patients without biliary disease. PAI is defined as abnormal intensity, seen as a periportal ring or tramline, surrounding the intrahepatic portal veins (Fig. 11-6). On T2WI, PAI appears as high signal intensity on both sides of intrahepatic portal vein branches. In normal patients, high signal intensity on T2WI is usually seen only on one side of the intrahepatic portal veins, in the region of the accompanying bile ducts.

NEOPLASMS
Biliary cystadenoma

Biliary cystadenoma is a rare tumor of biliary epithelial origin. It typically occurs in women over 30 years old. Most are intrahepatic.[7] On ultrasound, they appear to be cystic masses with irregular margins, septations, and papillary excrescences. CT shows a near-water-density mass with septations and occasional excrescences. MRI appearance is low signal intensity on T1WI and high signal inten-

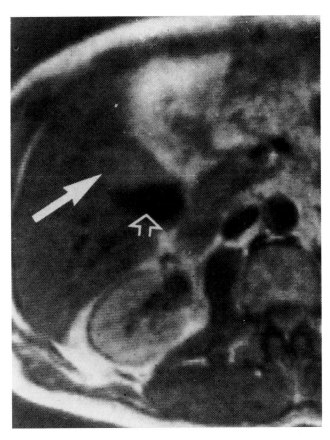

Fig. 11-5. This T2WI shows gallstones *(open arrow)* differentiated from gallbladder bile *(closed arrow)*. Note that the gallbladder bile is of lower signal intensity than would be expected in a normal fasting subject. This case demonstrates surgically proven chronic cholecystitis. (From McCarthy S, Hricak H, Cohen M, et al: *Radiology* 158:333-336, 1986.)

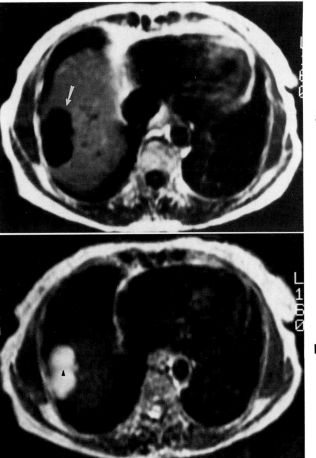

A

B

Fig. 11-7. A, Biliary cystadenoma. Note the low signal intensity mass on this T1WI. **B,** Biliary cystadenoma. The mass has a high signal intensity on T2WI with a lower signal intensity septation *(arrowhead)*.

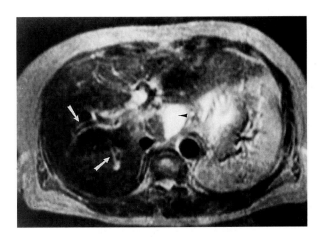

Fig. 11-6. Patient with clinically diagnosed cholangitis. Note the periportal ring *(lower arrow)* and the periportal tram line *(upper arrow)* on this T2WI. The patient has an abscess in the caudate lobe *(arrowhead)*. (From Matsui O, Kadoya M, Takashima T, et al: *Radiology* 171:335-338, 1989.)

sity on T2WI, except for the intervening low intensity septations (Fig. 11-7).[13] Different locules within the tumor may have variable signal intensity, according to the composition of the fluid within them (that is, hemorrhagic, thick proteinaceous, clear serous, etc). (See Chapter 10, section three, for more information about this tumor.)

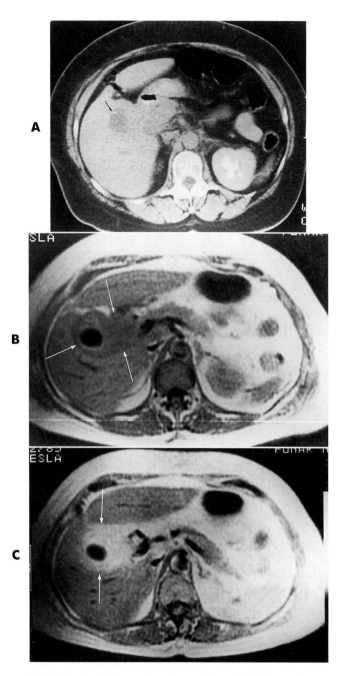

Fig. 11-8. A, CT scan of a patient with gallbladder carcinoma. Note the faintly calcified gallstone *(arrow)* surrounded by a small amount of fluid. **B,** T1WI (SE 500/28) shows the gallstone as a signal void, surrounded by high intensity bile and the low intensity mass *(arrows).* **C,** The mass increases in signal intensity with more relative T2 weighting (SE 2000/28). (From Rossman MD, Friedman AC, Radecki PD, et al: *Am J Roentgenol* 148:143-144, 1987.)

Gallbladder carcinoma

Gallbladder carcinoma appears as a low signal intensity vesicular mass on T1WI and high signal intensity on T2WI with respect to normal liver.[15] In very large tumors in which the organ of origin may be obscured, MRI can show gallstones trapped within the tumor, providing a clue to the diagnosis of gallbladder carcinoma (Fig. 11-8).[16] Direct liver invasion and distant liver metastasis can readily be seen on MRI, with MRI performing as well as CT in

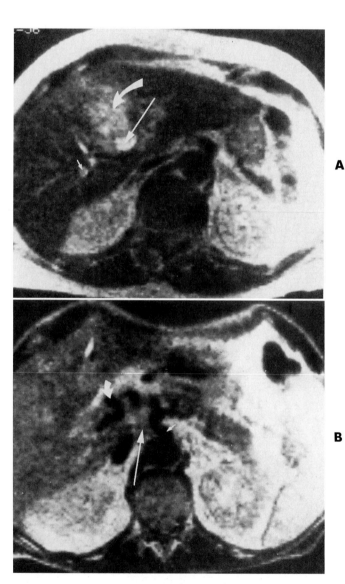

Fig. 11-9. A, T2WI of a cholangiocarcinoma at the level of the hepatic hilus. Note the high signal intensity mass *(long arrow)* with extension into the medial segment of the left lobe *(curved arrow)* and the dilated biliary ducts *(short arrow).* **B,** T2WI of cholangiocarcinoma at the level of the hepatic hilus. The soft tissue mass *(long arrow)* is seen to the right of the celiac trunk *(short arrow)* and extends to surround the hepatic artery *(curved arrow).* Note the intermediate signal intensity of this histologically confirmed scirrhous subtype of cholangiocarcinoma. (From Dooms GC, Kerlan RK, Hricak H, et al: *Radiology* 159:89-94, 1986.)

this respect. MRI has not been shown to accurately diagnose the presence or absence of duodenal involvement, probably due to motion artifacts, partial volume effects, and the lack of fat. MRI is effective in evaluating the spread of tumor to the hepatoduodenal ligament and paraaortic region because of high contrast between tumor and surrounding fat tissue. T2WI is helpful in differentiating nodal metastases from the caudate lobe of the liver.

Cholangiocarcinoma

The two major cell types of cholangiocarcinoma have different signal characteristics on MRI. The well-differentiated subtype shows high signal intensity on T2WI, which is typical for malignant masses.[6] The scirrhous subtype shows only slightly higher signal intensity than normal liver on T2WI because of its fibrous stroma.[6] Evidence shows that MRI is equal to CT in evaluating cholangiocarcinoma for feasibility of surgical resection. A major advantage of MRI is better detection of spread to adjacent organs (Fig. 11-9).[6] Although MRI does not detect biliary dilation as well as CT, most patients will have had an ultrasound, which will readily show biliary dilation. Correlation of ultrasound with MRI covers both duct patency and local extension of the neoplasm, without requiring an iodinated contrast injection.

SUMMARY

MRI is useful in the evaluation and staging of gallbladder carcinoma and cholangiocarcinoma. In some instances, it can be superior to CT and ultrasound. In the case of cholangiocarcinoma, the two major subtypes of can be differentiated based on their signal characteristics. Bile duct anomalies are better examined by ultrasound and CT. Common duct patency is best shown by a radionuclide scan.

In the future, MRI may be effective for evaluating gallbladder fuction. Low signal intensity gallbladder bile in fasting patients should indicate the possibility of acute or chronic cholecystitis. Periportal abnormal intensity (PAI) is generally seen in patients with inflammatory or obstructive biliary disease. Stones of varying signal intensity may be found incidentally on scans performed for other indications.

REFERENCES

1. Alexander MC, Hagga JR: MR imaging of a choledochal cyst, *J Comput Assist Tomogr* 9(2):357-359, 1985.
2. Baron RL, Schuman WP, Lee SP, et al: MR appearance of gallstones in vitro at 1.5T: correlation with chemical composition, *Am J Roentgenol* 153:497-502,1989.
3. Baron RL, Kuyper SJ, Lee SP, et al: In vitro dissolution of gallstones with MTBE: correlation with characteristics at CT and MR imaging, *Radiology* 173:117-121, 1989.
4. Demas BE, Hricak H, Moseley M, et al: Gallbladder bile: An experimental study in dogs using MR imaging and proton MR spectroscopy, *Radiology* 157:453-455, 1985.
5. Dooms GC, Fischer MR, Higgins CB, et al: MR imaging of the dilated biliary tract, *Radiology* 158:337-341, 1986.
6. Dooms GC, Kerlan RK, Hricak H, et al: Cholangiocarcinoma: Imaging by MR, *Radiology* 159:89-94, 1986.
7. Friedman AC, editor: *Radiology of the liver, biliary tract, pancreas and spleen,* Baltimore, 1987, Williams & Wilkins.
8. Hricak H, Filly RA, Margulis AR, et al: Work in progress: Nuclear magnetic resonance imaging of the gallbladder, *Radiology* 147:481-484, 1983.
9. Loflin TG, Simeone JF, Mueller PR, et al: Gallbladder bile in cholecystitis: In vitro MR evaluation, *Radiology* 157:457-459, 1985.
10. Matsui O, Kadoya M, Takashima T, et al: Intrahepatic periportal abnormal intensity on MR images: an indication of various hepatobiliary diseases, *Radiology* 171:335-338, 1989.
11. McCarthy S, Hricak H, Cohen M, et al: Cholecystitis: Detection with MR imaging, *Radiology* 158:333-336, 1986.
12. Moon KL, Hricak H, Margulis AR, et al: Nuclear magnetic resonance imaging characteristics of gallstones in vitro, *Radiology* 148:753-756, 1983.
13. Palacios E, Shannon M, Solomon C, et al: Biliary cystadenoma: ultrasound, CT, and MRI, *Gastrointest Radiol* 15:313-316, 1990.
14. Robbins SL, Cotran RS, Kumar V: *Pathologic basis of disease,* ed 2, Philadelphia, 1984, WB Saunders.
15. Rossman MD, Friedman AC, Radecki PD, et al: MR imaging of gallbladder carcinoma, *Am J Roentgenol* 148:143-144, 1987.
16. Sagoh T, Itoh K, Togashi K, et al: Gallbladder carcinoma: evaluation with MR imaging, *Radiology* 174:131-136, 1990.
17. Stark DD, Bradley WG: *Magnetic resonance imaging,* St Louis, 1988, Mosby–Year Book.

Chapter 12

PANCREAS

Sharon S. Burton

INDICATIONS

Imaging of the pancreas is usually performed for one of the following reasons: (1) to evaluate the severity of acute or chronic pancreatitis and detect complications from inflammatory disease, (2) to investigate the patient with jaundice, (3) to localize islet cell tumors in patients with endocrine symptoms, (4) to screen patients with abdominal pain and weight loss for suspected malignancy, and (5) to detect pancreatic injury after abdominal trauma.

Advances in radiologic and endoscopic techniques have produced numerous ways to diagnose pancreatic disease. The oldest and most nonspecific modalities are plain radiography and barium studies, which provide only indirect evidence of pancreatic disease. Cross-sectional techniques including ultrasound, computed tomography (CT), and magnetic resonance imaging (MRI) display much greater anatomic detail of both pancreas and peripancreatic organs. Of these three modalities, CT is generally recognized as the best initial test for evaluating the pancreas.[25,83] In an appropriate clinical setting, more invasive procedures such as endoscopic retrograde cholangiopancreatography (ERCP), endoscopic ultrasound, percutaneous aspiration and needle biopsy, angiography, and portal venous sampling procedures can be useful.[83]

The specific indications for MRI of the pancreas are still evolving. Most investigators suggest that MRI be used as a problem-solving modality when results of CT are equivocal, when surgical clips in the peripancreatic region obscure detail on CT scanning, or when patients cannot receive iodinated contrast for CT scanning because of severe contrast reaction or renal insufficiency.[66,69,80] The improvements being made in abdominal MRI using fat suppression, breath-hold imaging with intravenous contrast, and oral contrast agents for bowel opacification may allow MRI to play a greater role in pancreatic imaging in the future.

COMPARISON OF CT AND MRI

CT is currently the best single screening test for pancreatic disease.[25,50,83] Both inflammatory and neoplastic diseases of the pancreas are well demonstrated using CT scans performed with dynamic intravenous contrast enhancement and adequate oral contrast. Contrast-enhanced CT for detection of pancreatic necrosis has proved an important prognostic indicator in patients with severe acute pancreatitis.[3] Pancreatic calcifications and ductal dilation are well demonstrated in chronic pancreatitis.[7] The presence of peripancreatic invasion, adenopathy, vascular encasement, and metastatic disease are well evaluated in patients with pancreatic neoplasms.[26] Limitations of CT include indeterminate studies due to suboptimal bowel contrast opacification or lack of iodinated contrast, artifact from surgical clips in postoperative patients, and limited contrast resolution, making it difficult to detect small neoplasms that do not distort the pancreatic contour.[66]

Initial studies of pancreatic MRI using standard spin-echo pulse sequences concluded that MRI could demonstrate the normal pancreas and inflammatory and neoplastic lesions, but had no significant advantage over CT.[69,80] Major limitations of MRI were lack of a bowel contrast agent to aid differentiation of pancreas from adjacent bowel, respiratory and peristaltic motion artifacts, and inability to reliably detect calcifications.

More recently, however, the use of fat suppression, breath-hold FLASH imaging, and dynamic gadolinium enhancement has significantly improved the results of pancreatic MRI.[66] In a prospective study comparing CT, ERCP, and MRI at 1.5 T, MRI showed slightly greater accuracy than CT in detecting pancreatic neoplasm when the tumor did not distort the contour of the gland. More accurate diagnosis of chronic pancreatitis was also possible in contrast-enhanced MRI as compared with CT. Further investigations using these pulse sequence techniques, intravenous contrast, and oral contrast agents are needed to determine the true potential of MRI for pancreatic imaging.

TECHNIQUE
Oral contrast

Since the pancreas is bordered by stomach, duodenum and jejunum, a bowel contrast agent is essential for optimal pancreatic imaging. Collapsed loops of bowel show similar signal intensity to normal pancreas and can be confused with masses and adenopathy (Fig. 12-1, A).

Visualization of the pancreas has been improved using a wide variety of contrast agents. Superparamagnetic iron oxide (SPIO)[32] and high-density barium (Fig. 12-1, B)[14,51,62] are negative contrast agents that reduce the signal intensity of bowel contents. Carbon dioxide has been used in conjunction with glucagon.[87] Positive contrast agents that cause increased signal intensity in the lumen include gadopentetate dimeglumine mixed with mannitol,[43,46] ferric ammonium citrate,[87] and mixtures of corn oil emulsions.[1] Best results are obtained when an antiperistaltic agent such as glucagon (1 mg IV or IM) is administered with the oral contrast agent.[46,87]

Intravenous contrast

The primary intravenous contrast used for MRI of the pancreas is gadopentetate dimeglumine, a paramagnetic contrast agent with pharmacologic properties similar to iodinated contrast agents. When this agent is given as a rapid intravenous bolus in a dose of 0.1 mmol/kg, rapid scanning techniques such as FLASH imaging show maximum opacification of the pancreas within the first 2 minutes after bolus injection.[33] Enhancement of the normal pancreas is uniform and homogeneous. Pancreatic tumors

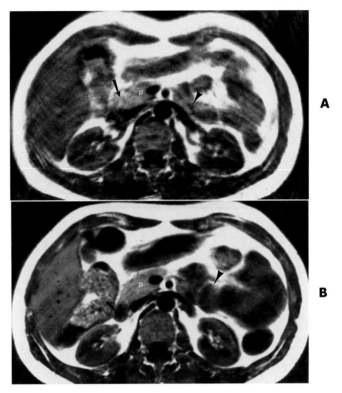

Fig. 12-1. Oral contrast for pancreatic imaging. **A,** Axial T1WI without contrast: The head of pancreas *(P)* has higher signal intensity than the adjacent collapsed duodenum *(arrow)* and has similar intensity as the posterior gastric wall. The structure with intermediate signal intensity anterior to the left renal vein could be pancreas or bowel *(arrowhead)*. **B,** Axial T1WI postbarium: The pancreatic head *(P)* is well delineated from the duodenum *(arrow)* and stomach, both of which are filled with contrast. Opacified loops of jejunum are seen anterior to the left renal vein *(arrowhead)*.

show decreased enhancement relative to normal parenchyma.[15,66]

Protocols

After a 4-hour fast, patients are given 400 to 600 ml of an oral contrast agent. Glucagon (1.0 mg IV or IM) may be given to patients without history of pheochromocytoma or suspected insulinoma. Standard spin-echo imaging is performed using a body coil with T1-weighted images (T1WI) and T2-weighted images (T2WI), 7 to 10 mm slice thickness and 1.5 mm gap. Improved contrast can be gained using shorter echo times (TE), reducing TE from 20 to 12 msec.[54] Fat suppression techniques provide good contrast between pancreas and surrounding tissues.[54,66] Breath-hold imaging using FLASH can be used dynamically in conjunction with intravenous contrast enhancement.[66] Surface coil imaging can improve depiction of the pancreas, with fewer motion artifacts but with a limited view of adjacent organs.[67]

ANATOMY

The pancreas is located in the retroperitoneum in the anterior pararenal space. Vascular landmarks that surround the pancreas include the splenic and portal veins, superior mesenteric artery and vein, aorta, and inferior vena cava. These structures are well demonstrated on MRI without an intravenous contrast agent.

The normal pancreas can be seen on T1WI as a medium signal intensity structure surrounded by higher intensity retroperitoneal fat (Fig. 12-2). The margins of pancreas may be smooth or lobulated. At low field strength (0.35 T), the signal intensity of normal pancreas is similar to that of liver.[69,80] On T1WI at high field strength (1.5 T), the signal intensity of the pancreas is slightly higher than liver in the majority of patients.[57] T2WI are best for demonstrating the common bile duct due to the high signal intensity within its lumen. With aging, the pancreas becomes more inhomogeneous due to parenchymal atrophy. The normal pancreatic duct is a low signal intensity structure on T1WI and measures < 2 mm.[85]

The efficacy of MRI in demonstrating the pancreas has improved over time. In an early study of pancreatic MRI at low field strength (0.35 T) using spin-echo and inversion recovery techniques, good delineation of the head, body, and tail of pancreas was achieved in 54%, 60%, and 64% of patients, respectively.[69] When retroperitoneal fat was sparse, there was difficulty differentiating bowel from pancreas. In a more recent study at high field strength (1.5 T), better visualization of the pancreas was obtained.[57] T1WI provided the greatest anatomic detail, showing the pancreas head, body, and tail in 81%, 100%, and 96% of cases, respectively. Blurring from motion artifact was present in 1% of T1WI and in 37% of T2WI. Delineation of the head, body, and tail of pancreas was 74%, 77%, and 54%, respectively, on T2WI.

Surface coil imaging improves anatomic definition of the pancreas. A study using a 0.6 T magnet, prone patient position, and a surface coil showed good visualization of the pancreas with improvement in signal-to-noise ratio (SNR) versus body coil images.[67] The normal pancreatic

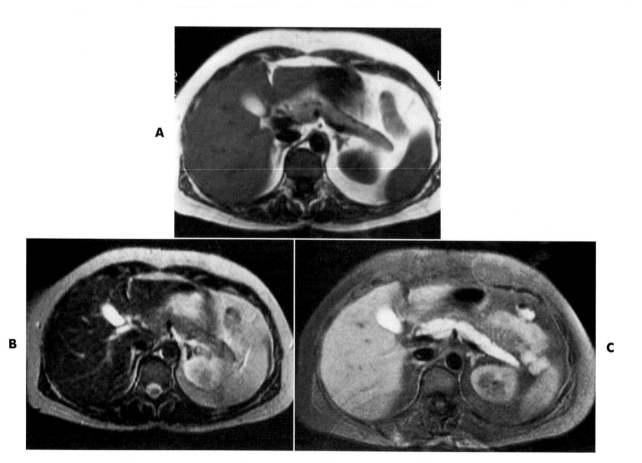

Fig. 12-2. Normal pancreas. **A,** Axial T1WI: Normal pancreas has intermediate signal intensity, higher than liver and spleen and less than adjacent retroperitoneal fat. **B,** Axial T2WI: Signal intensity of pancreas remains slightly higher than liver. There is high signal intensity from fluid in the stomach. **C,** Axial image with fat suppression: The normal pancreas has high signal intensity, and pancreatic margins are well defined. Bowel loops also contain high signal intensity.

duct was identified in five of eight normal volunteers and motion artifacts were significantly reduced. Possible disadvantages of surface coil imaging include limited field of view, inability to fully evaluate surrounding organs, and lack of widespread availability of appropriate surface coils.

Using fat suppression techniques, the normal pancreas shows homogeneous, high signal intensity that is greater than the signal intensity in any adjacent structure including bowel (Fig. 12-2, C).

CONGENITAL ANOMALIES
Pancreas divisum

Pancreas divisum is a developmental anomaly of the pancreas in which the dorsal and ventral pancreatic ducts fail to fuse. The dorsal duct drains via the accessory duct of Santorini into the minor duodenal papilla, and the ventral duct drains with the common bile duct into the papilla of Vater. This variant occurs in up to 11% of autopsy specimens[8,94] and is seen in up to 5.8% of patients undergoing ERCP.[53,94] Some reports indicate that pancreas divisum is associated with a higher incidence of pancreatitis.[18] Other studies have found no increased incidence of chronic pancreatitis in these patients.[21] Whether patients with pancreas divisum are predisposed to developing pancreatitis remains a controversial issue.

Using thin-section CT scanning with dynamic contrast enhancement, subtle changes can be seen in the pancreatic head in pancreas divisum.[94] Focal enlargement of the pancreatic head may occur, which can mimic tumor. The most reliable signs of pancreas divisum on CT scans are relatively uncommon: demonstration of a fat plane separating ventral and dorsal portions of the pancreas or demonstration of dorsal and ventral pancreatic ducts that fail to unite (Fig. 12-3). The lower spatial resolution of MRI may make diagnosis of these subtle findings in pancreas divisum more difficult. ERCP remains the most definitive test for this and other pancreatic ductal abnormalities.

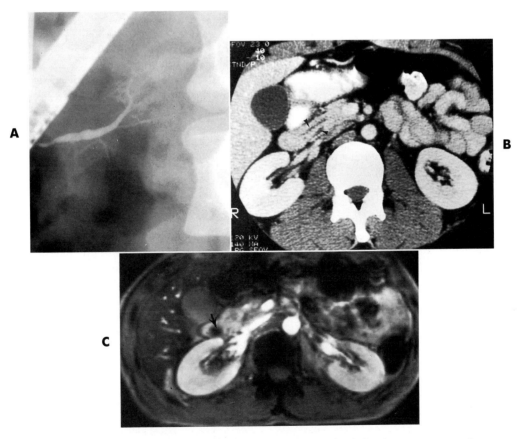

Fig. 12-3. Pancreas divisum. **A,** ERCP: Endoscopic retrograde cholangiopancreatogram shows filling of only the ventral pancreatic duct via the major papilla. **B,** CT scan: Axial scan through the level of the pancreatic head shows two distinct ducts *(arrowheads)* arranged in parallel fashion in the same patient with pancreas divisum. **C,** Axial proton density image after gadolinium enhancement: The duodenal lumen is defined by oral barium *(arrow),* and there is enhancement of the duodenal mucosa. The ducts in the head of pancreas are not as well defined compared with the CT scan.

Cystic fibrosis

Cystic fibrosis (CF) is an autosomal recessive disorder that has clinical manifestations in multiple organ systems, including lungs, gastrointestinal (GI) tract, reproductive system, and skeletal system.[34] The hallmark of the disease is the presence of abnormally thick secretions from exocrine or mucus glands. In the pancreas, viscous secretions precipitate in the ducts resulting in obstruction, atrophy, and fatty replacement of the parenchyma.[23] Pancreatic insufficiency develops in approximately 80% to 95% of patients,[55] being manifested by steatorrhea, azotorrhea (protein loss), malnutrition, and diabetes mellitus. Pancreatic enzyme replacement therapy is required.

The most common appearance of the pancreas in patients with CF is an enlarged, lobulated pancreas with complete fatty replacement.[78] Fatty replacement is seen as increased echogenicity of the pancreas on ultrasound,[24] septated fat density replacing pancreas on CT, and high signal intensity with lower intensity septations in the pancreas on T1WI. Other patterns of abnormality include pancreatic atrophy with partial replacement by fat tissue, diffuse atrophy of the pancreas without fatty replacement,[78] and formation of multiple pancreatic cysts.[35] MRI is slightly more sensitive than ultrasound[24] and is comparable to CT in detecting pancreatic disease in CF. The primary disadvantage of MRI in this setting is inability to define small pancreatic and renal calcifications that may be present in patients with CF.

PANCREATITIS

Acute pancreatitis

Acute pancreatitis is a common disease that results from a wide variety of causes including alcohol abuse, gallstones, hyperlipidemia, familial disorders, viral illness, drugs, blunt trauma, peptic ulcer disease and iatrogenic injury from ERCP, biopsy, or surgical procedures.[34] The initial diagnosis of acute pancreatitis is frequently based on clinical signs of nausea, vomiting, and elevated amylase and lipase without the aid of imaging studies.[83] Differentiation of the milder form of acute interstitial or edematous pancreatitis from the more severe necrotizing and hemorrhagic pancreatitis is often difficult based on clinical findings. Objective clinical criteria, the Ranson criteria, have been established to identify patients with severe pancreatitis who will be more likely to develop complications.[58,59]

Imaging studies have been extremely useful in assessing the extent of pancreatic injury and detecting complications of pancreatitis. The best imaging modality for evaluating acute pancreatitis to date is dynamic, contrast-enhanced CT. CT has been used to categorize pancreatic inflammatory disease into grades that correlate with prognosis of the patient.[4] In Grade A, the pancreas is normal in appearance. In Grade B, there is focal or diffuse pancreatic enlargement with contour irregularities, inhomogeneous attenuation patterns, or small fluid collections in the pancreas. Grade C includes haziness and inflammatory changes in the peripancreatic fat in addition to intrinsic abnormalities of the pancreas. Grade D indicates presence of a single ill-defined fluid collection or phlegmon, and Grade E includes presence of two or more poorly defined fluid collections or gas within or adjacent to pancreas.[4] In a series of 83 patients with acute pancreatitis, none with Grade A or B disease developed abscesses or died. Patients with phlegmons and peripancreatic fluid collections, Grade D or E, had a much higher incidence of superimposed bacterial infection or abscess, with resulting increased morbidity and mortality.

Perhaps the most important prognostic indicator in severe, acute pancreatitis is the presence of pancreatic necrosis.[3,4,10] Necrosis is currently best demonstrated with dynamic, intravenous contrast-enhanced CT.[10,42,44] The normal pancreas and inflamed pancreas without necrosis show homogeneous contrast enhancement during a rapid bolus injection of iodinated contrast. In pancreatic necrosis, the blood supply to involved portions of the pancreas is interrupted, and the necrotic regions appear as low-density regions within the remaining, normally enhancing pancreatic parenchyma.[10,42] Patients with large regions of necrosis of the pancreas in acute pancreatitis have the highest likelihood of development of pancreatic infection, abscess, with resulting morbidity and mortality.

MRI has been investigated as an imaging modality for acute pancreatitis[41,66,69,80] and shows morphologic changes similar to those demonstrated by CT. In early stages, the pancreas appears diffusely enlarged, with ill-defined margins on T1WI and T2WI. Inflammatory changes in peripancreatic fat are seen as low signal intensity strands and are best demonstrated on T1WI (Figs. 12-4 and 12-5)[67] or FLASH images.[66] Fat suppression reduces the contrast between inflammatory changes and fat, making these changes more difficult to detect.[66] Thickening of the renal fascia is seen as a low signal intensity linear structure on T1WI and medium to high signal intensity on T2WI.[80] Dynamic contrast enhancement using a rapid bolus of gadopentetate dimeglumine has been performed in patients with early stages of acute pancreatitis, showing homogeneous parenchymal enhancement. This technique has potential use in detecting pancreatic necrosis by MRI in the same way that iodinated contrast is used in dynamic enhanced CT.[66]

Chronic pancreatitis

In contrast to acute pancreatitis, which is a reversible condition, chronic pancreatitis results in permanent structural damage to the pancreas. Pathologically, fibrosis with periductal scarring and chronic inflammatory cell infiltration are demonstrated in chronic pancreatitis.[56] Based on clinical symptoms, patients are subdivided into those with chronic pancreatitis or relapsing chronic pancreatitis. Relapsing pancreatitis is characterized by recurring episodes

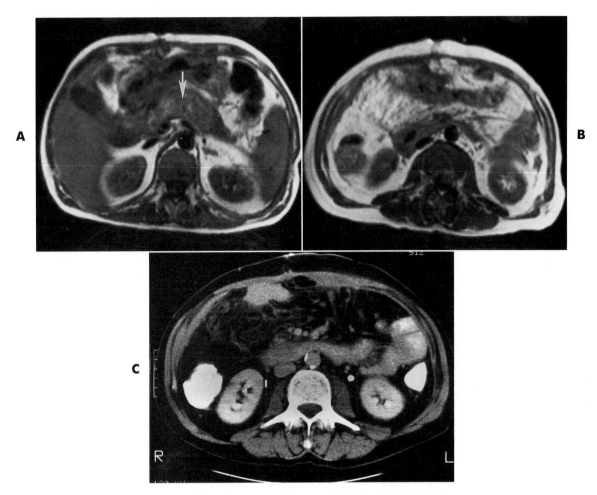

Fig. 12-4. Acute pancreatitis. **A,** Axial T1WI: The pancreas *(arrow)* is swollen and shows inhomogeneous signal intensity. There is poor delineation between the thickened gastric antral wall and pancreatic head and neck. **B,** Axial T1WI: Inflammatory changes in peripancreatic and mesenteric fat are seen as linear strands of low signal intensity within the high-intensity peripancreatic fat. **C,** CT scan: Linear strands of increased attenuation reflect edema and inflammatory changes in the peripancreatic and mesenteric fat.

of acute inflammation superimposed on chronic disease. The most common clinical symptom in chronic pancreatitis is abdominal pain. Exocrine pancreatic insufficiency develops if more than 90% of the exocrine function is destroyed[34]; these patients develop weight loss, abnormal stools, and other signs of malabsorption. Diabetes mellitus occurs less commonly. Predisposing conditions include alcohol abuse and familial pancreatitis.

Radiologic features of chronic pancreatitis include pancreatic ductal dilation, localized or diffuse intraductal calcifications, focal or diffuse pancreatic enlargement, pseudocyst, and atrophy.[37,48] The pancreas may also be normal in appearance by imaging studies. ERCP is the most accurate technique for demonstrating pancreatic duct pathology.[83] CT demonstrates abnormalities of the pancreatic duct with a high degree of accuracy, particularly when

5 mm contiguous sections and intravenous contrast are used.[7] CT also has a high accuracy for detection of pancreatic calcification, which is the most specific sign of chronic pancreatitis.

Early clinical evaluations of MRI in chronic pancreatitis have shown that most of the morphologic changes shown by CT can be demonstrated by MRI.[69,80] These changes include pancreatic enlargement, pseudocysts, and pancreatic ductal dilation (Fig. 12-6). A primary disadvantage of MRI compared with CT is in the detection of calcifications. Large calcifications greater than 1 cm can be seen as ill-defined, low-intensity regions on spin-echo sequences (Fig. 12-7),[69] but smaller calcifications are not apparent. These calcifications are particularly critical in differentiating focal pancreatitis from malignancy. The presence of diffusely scattered ductal calculi within a focal mass

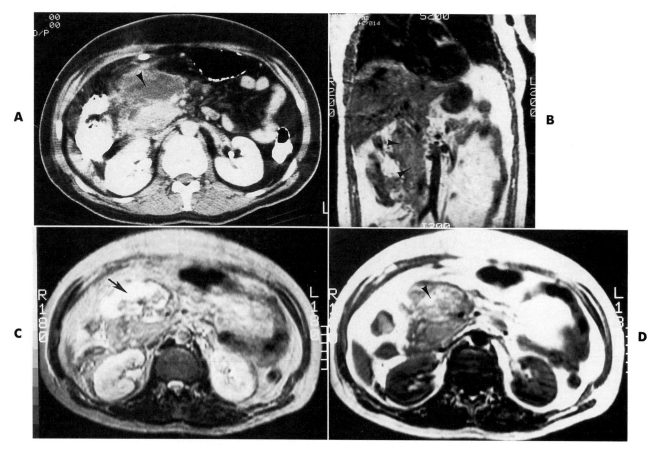

Fig. 12-5. Severe acute pancreatitis. **A,** CT scan: An ill-defined inflammatory mass with fluid collection *(arrowhead)* is seen in this patient with postcholecystectomy pancreatitis. **B,** Coronal T1WI: The inflammatory mass *(arrowheads)* extends from the head of pancreas inferiorly to just above the aortic bifurcation. **C,** Axial T1WI: Regions of high signal intensity *(arrowhead)* may represent hemorrhage, proteinaceous material, or residual fat. **D,** Axial T2WI: Very high signal intensity is seen within the fluid components of the inflammatory mass *(arrow).*

strongly favors focal inflammatory disease,[48] and inability to detect the calcifications with MRI is a distinct disadvantage.

Newer MRI techniques such as dynamic scanning with intravenous gadopentetate dimeglumine, fat suppression, and FLASH sequences have improved MRI diagnosis of chronic pancreatitis.[66] Features of chronic pancreatitis seen at 1.5 T using these techniques include pancreatic ductal dilation, low parenchymal signal intensity on nonenhanced images, and diminished contrast enhancement when compared with normal pancreatic parenchyma. In a small series of five patients with chronic pancreatitis, MRI accurately detected four of five cases and misclassified one patient with focal pancreatitis as having pancreatic cancer. These results were better than those obtained with CT: Two patients with chronic focal pancreatitis were misclassified as cancer and one case of surgically proven chronic pancreatitis was normal by CT. The decreased pancreatic enhancement in chronic pancreatitis is attributed to de-

creased vascularity related to fibrosis, which could prove to be a useful indicator of chronic pancreatitis.[66]

Complications of pancreatitis

Infection. Between 3% and 21% of patients with acute pancreatitis develop infected necrotic tissue or infected fluid collections in the pancreas or peripancreatic region.[5] Sepsis related to pancreatic infection is a major source of morbidity and mortality in pancreatitis with mortality rates up to 50%.[84] In a surgical study of 1090 patients operated for acute and chronic pancreatitis,[6] infection was found in 108 cases (9.9%), and the overall mortality rate was 15.7%. Patients with purulence mixed with necrotic tissue in a "spreading" pattern had a higher mortality rate, 23.6%, than patients with well-localized collections of pus contained within a wall, whose mortality rate was 7.5%. Multiple pus-containing collections were seen in 80% of cases.

The most specific criterion for diagnosis of infection

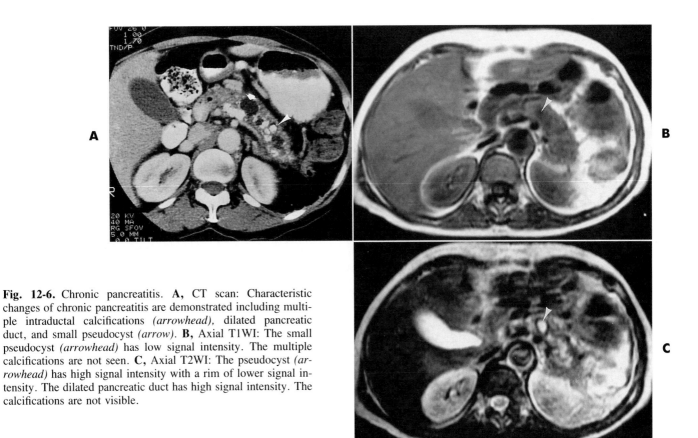

Fig. 12-6. Chronic pancreatitis. **A,** CT scan: Characteristic changes of chronic pancreatitis are demonstrated including multiple intraductal calcifications *(arrowhead)*, dilated pancreatic duct, and small pseudocyst *(arrow)*. **B,** Axial T1WI: The small pseudocyst *(arrowhead)* has low signal intensity. The multiple calcifications are not seen. **C,** Axial T2WI: The pseudocyst *(arrowhead)* has high signal intensity with a rim of lower signal intensity. The dilated pancreatic duct has high signal intensity. The calcifications are not visible.

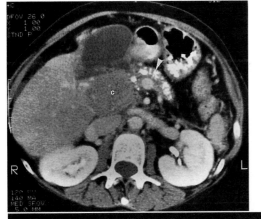

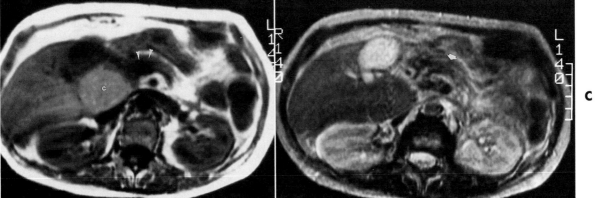

Fig. 12-7. Chronic pancreatitis. **A,** CT scan: The pancreas *(arrowhead)* is atrophic with numerous calcifications. There is low density in the caudate lobe of liver *(C)*. **B,** Axial T1WI: The pancreas has low signal intensity. The larger calcifications are faintly seen as regions of lower signal intensity *(arrowheads)*. The caudate lobe of the liver has higher signal intensity than adjacent liver, suggesting fatty change. **C,** Axial T2WI: The pancreas *(arrowheads)* shows low signal intensity and is more difficult to define compared with the T1WI.

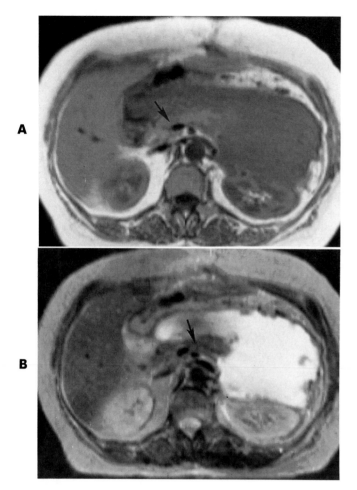

Fig. 12-8. Pancreatic abscess. **A,** Axial T1WI: A large, homogeneous fluid collection is present in the pancreatic region. Only a small segment of head and body of pancreas remains *(arrow)* and has increased signal intensity relative to adjacent fluid. **B,** Axial T2WI: The abscess has high signal intensity and irregular contours. The remaining pancreatic tissue *(arrow)* is easily identified in contrast with the high signal intensity fluid.

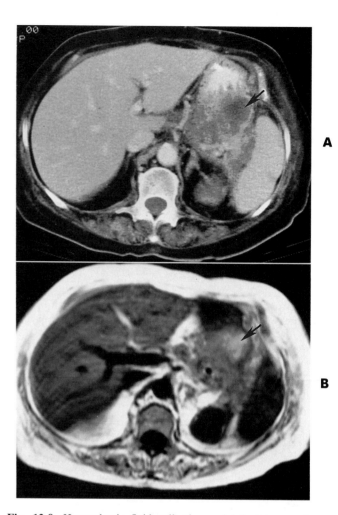

Fig. 12-9. Hemorrhagic fluid collection and infected necrosis. **A,** CT scan: Extensive inflammatory change is present in the tail of pancreas, splenic hilum, and lesser sac region. A low-density collection is seen posterior to the stomach *(arrow)*. **B,** Axial T1WI: This region has high signal intensity. Surgical exploration showed infected, hemorrhagic, and necrotic tissue.

within pancreatic necrosis, fluid collection, or pseudocyst is the presence of gas bubbles. The air bubbles are produced by gas-forming bacteria and have been seen by CT in up to 22% of abscesses.[3] The other potential source of gas in the retroperitoneum is an enteric fistula.[79] By MRI, pancreatic abscess typically shows characteristics of a fluid collection, with low signal intensity on T1WI and high signal intensity on T2WI (Fig. 12-8). Infected necrosis with hemorrhage may appear as a region of high signal intensity on T1WI (Fig. 12-9).

Hemorrhage and arterial complications of pancreatitis. Patients with acute or chronic pancreatitis may develop bleeding from a variety of causes. Nonpancreatic causes of bleeding in these patients include gastritis, stress ulcers, peptic ulcer disease, variceal bleeding, and Mallory-Weiss tears.[86]

Damage to arterial walls in pancreatitis results from autodigestion by proteolytic enzymes, particularly elastase.[31,47] Arterial complications include pseudoaneurysm formation and arterial rupture. Bleeding may result from oozing of small vessels in necrotic tissue or it may be massive, due to rupture of larger arteries or pseudoaneurysms in the peripancreatic region or within the walls of pseudocysts.

Acute, life-threatening hemorrhage can occur into the pancreatic bed, peritoneal cavity, GI tract, or into a pseudocyst cavity forming a large pseudoaneurysm. The splenic artery is most commonly involved, but gastroduodenal, pancreaticoduodenal,[68] left gastric, and colic arteries can also be affected.[73] Severe hemorrhage is seen in only 1.7% to 2.5% of patients with pancreatitis,[73] but carries a high mortality rate, ranging from 37%[68] to 53%.[73]

The highest survival rates are in patients with hemorrhage into pseudocysts. Patients with hemorrhage associated with necrotizing pancreatitis respond poorly to any medical or surgical management.[73]

The role of diagnostic imaging is to identify the hemorrhage, to localize the vessels involved, and, when possible, to palliate or stop bleeding by means of embolization procedures. Arteriography is useful both as a diagnostic and therapeutic tool for diagnosis and embolization of bleeding arteries or pseudoaneurysms. Arteriographic localization of the site of bleeding is recommended before operative intervention in stable patients with pancreatic hemorrhage.[68,86]

CT accurately demonstrates acute intraabdominal hemorrhage as regions of high density with attenuation values in the range of 60 to 80 Hounsfield units (HU).[74] The high density is due to the presence of hemoglobin in the retracted clot or sedimented blood.[92] A hematoma may contain localized or diffuse increased density or fluid-fluid levels. The density of blood decreases over time, becoming isodense with soft tissue as early as 1 week after acute hemorrhage,[38] and hypodense in the seroma stage. Thus, by CT, a subacute hemorrhage has a nonspecific appearance with differential diagnosis including hematoma, abscess, or evolving pseudocyst.

MRI has two advantages for investigation of vascular complications of pancreatitis. First, vessels are well demonstrated on gradient echo MRI with flow compensation. This sensitivity may allow noninvasive detection of large pseudoaneurysms. Second, hemorrhage is detectable, even in the subacute or chronic phase when CT is nonspecific. The predictable evolution of hemorrhage by MRI may improve accuracy of diagnosis of hemorrhage related to pancreatitis.

Acute hemorrhage has low signal intensity equal to or less than muscle on T1WI.[75] With time, breakdown of hemoglobin to methemoglobin results in shortening of T1 due to the paramagnetic effect of methemoglobin. After 4 days, most hematomas have high signal intensity within them on T1WI. This subacute phase of hemorrhage lasts from several days to several weeks (Fig. 12-10). Formation of a concentric ring appearance or halo sign within a subacute hematoma is characteristic.[75] Eventually, in the chronic phase of hemorrhage, hemosiderin deposition occurs, which causes decreased signal intensity on T2WI (Fig. 12-11).

Experiments using in vitro MR spectroscopy of fluids obtained from intraabdominal fluid collections showed that hematomas and abscesses have significantly shorter T1 values than those seen in pseudocysts, urinomas, bile, or other sources.[12] Hemorrhage had a mean T1 value of 859 ± 223 msec and abscesses had a mean value of 1222 ± 81 msec. The T1 values correlated with quantity of total protein present. Based on these in vitro data, the differential diagnosis of a region of high signal intensity on T1WI in-

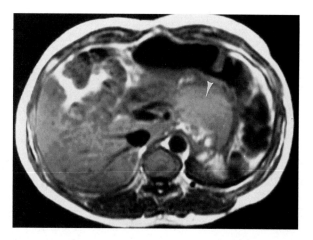

Fig. 12-10. Hemorrhagic pseudocyst. Axial T1WI: A well-defined fluid collection *(arrowhead)* in tail of pancreas is mildly hyperintense. Although this image could represent subacute hemorrhage or high protein content, surgical drainage yielded dark, thick fluid from old hemorrhage.

cludes hemorrhage or proteinaceous material including abscess.

Venous thrombosis. The primary venous complication of pancreatitis is thrombosis of peripancreatic veins, resulting in left-sided portal hypertension. Splenic vein thrombosis occurs in up to 45% of patients with pancreatitis.[86] The superior mesenteric vein and portal veins may also be effected. Splenic vein thrombosis results in the formation of gastric varices that direct flow from the spleen to the short gastric veins, right and left gastric veins, and into the portal vein. Other collateral pathways may lead to formation of colonic varices and retroperitoneal collaterals.[86]

Pseudocyst. Fluid collections in the peripancreatic regions are common in acute pancreatitis, and many resolve spontaneously. A pseudocyst is a persistent fluid collection, which is defined as "a fluid-filled cystic mass confined by a dense fibrous capsule."[5] The wall is composed of granulation tissue and fibrous tissue[84] without a true epithelial lining. Pseudocysts may occur in the pancreas, peripancreatic region, or in distant sites such as the mediastinum via proteolytic digestion of normal fascial planes.[90]

Complications resulting from pseudocysts include infection, hemorrhage, rupture, and obstruction of the biliary tract when the cyst is in the head of the pancreas.[61] Indications for treatment of pseudocysts include infection, persistence longer than 6 weeks, size greater than 4 or 5 cm, continued growth, or persistent clinical symptoms. Treatment of noninfected or infected pseudocysts can be initiated either by percutaneous catheter drainage[84] or internal or external surgical drainage.

Imaging of pseudocysts using ultrasound, CT, and MRI shows a mass containing fluid with variable wall thickness. The appearance of the internal structure of the

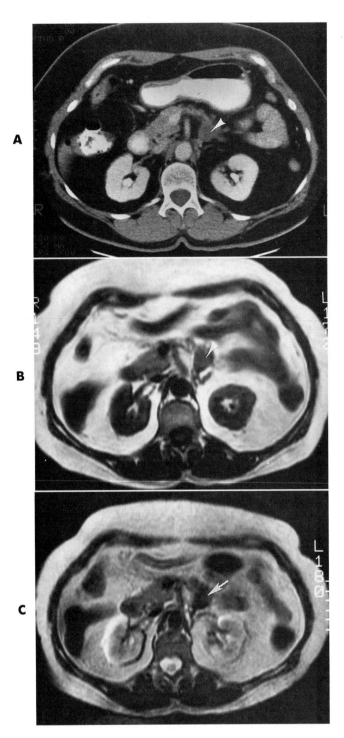

Fig. 12-11. Chronic abscess with hemosiderin deposition. **A,** CT scan: A small hypodense mass is present posterior to pancreatic tail *(arrowhead)*. **B,** Axial T1WI: The small mass *(arrowhead)* is well defined with low signal intensity relative to normal pancreas. The bowel is well opacified by oral contrast (superparamagnetic iron oxide). **C,** Axial T2WI: The mass *(arrowhead)* continues to have low signal intensity on T2WI. Surgical exploration revealed a chronic abscess with hemosiderin deposition.

pseudocyst depends on presence of fluid, debris, infection, or hemorrhage within the pseudocyst cavity.

Spin-echo MRI shows simple pseudocysts as having low signal intensity on T1WI (Fig. 12-11) and high signal intensity on T2WI. Pseudocysts containing proteinaceous fluid or hemorrhage show higher signal intensity on T1WI (Figs. 12-10 and 12-12). Using dynamic contrast enhancement, pseudocysts are seen as oval lesions of relative signal void compared with adjacent, enhancing pancreatic parenchyma.[66] The multiplanar capability of MRI is advantageous when imaging extensive pseudocysts in extrapancreatic locations.[90]

NEOPLASM
Ductal adenocarcinoma

Ductal adenocarcinoma is the most common pancreatic neoplasm and is the fourth leading cause of cancer death in

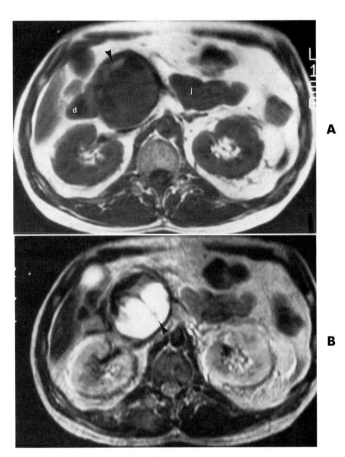

Fig. 12-12. Pseudocyst. **A,** Axial T1WI: A large cystic mass in the pancreatic head has a complex wall containing regions of higher signal intensity *(arrowhead)*. By CT, these regions were hyperdense, suggesting hemorrhage. The duodenum *(d)* and jejunum *(j)* are well opacified by oral contrast (superparamagnetic iron oxide). **B,** Axial T2WI: Fluid in the mass has high signal intensity and is subdivided by a septation *(arrowhead)*. The complex nature of the right anterolateral wall of the mass again is seen. Differential diagnosis includes cystic pancreatic neoplasm, but surgical exploration revealed only a pseudocyst.

the United States.[20] Approximately 60% to 70% of ductal adenocarcinomas occur in the pancreatic head. Obstruction of the common bile duct by tumor commonly results in painless jaundice, allowing diagnosis of pancreatic head tumors at a relatively early stage.[91] Carcinomas in the body and tail of pancreas are often clinically silent until more advanced local disease spread or metastatic disease develops. Pancreatic duct obstruction can lead to obstructive pancreatitis and cyst formation, which may be difficult to differentiate from benign pancreatitis.[39]

The most frequent radiographic appearance of ductal adenocarcinoma is that of a focal mass or localized pancreatic enlargement. Nonfocal enlargement of the pancreas due to tumor involving more than one region of pancreas is not uncommon.[91] Differentiation of focal pancreatitis from pancreatic neoplasm and diffuse pancreatitis from diffuse tumor is frequently difficult using clinical and imaging techniques. A comparative study using the serum marker CA 19-9, ultrasound, CT, and percutaneous needle biopsy found that biopsy was the most reliable diagnostic tool to differentiate benign from malignant disease.[22]

Staging of pancreatic cancer has been primarily based on CT or a combination of CT and angiography.[27] Based on CT criteria, a resectable tumor is less than 2 cm in diameter and is contained within the pancreatic parenchyma without evidence of local extension, vascular invasion, adenopathy, or liver metastases. In one series of 161 pancreatic tumors, only 13 tumors met these criteria.[26] Unresectable tumors are greater than 3 cm in diameter; extend to or beyond the surface of the pancreas; or show invasion of adjacent organs, vascular encasement, metastases, adenopathy, or ascites.[27] Signs of vascular involvement include venous or arterial occlusion or encasement. Although obliteration of the fat surrounding the celiac axis or superior mesenteric artery is relatively specific for adenocarcinoma, it has been seen in other tumors and rarely in pancreatitis.[2,49]

Pancreatic adenocarcinoma has been evaluated with multiple MRI techniques. Comparative studies have shown that most morphologic changes demonstrated by CT are also seen on MRI, ranging from focal mass with pancreatic ductal obstruction (Fig. 12-13) to diffuse pancreatic enlargement (Fig. 12-14). Reported advantages of MRI over CT in patients with neoplasms include good demonstration of vascular involvement, detection of liver metastases and liver invasion, and improved diagnosis in postoperative patients whose CT examinations are compromised by clip artifacts.[80]

The enhanced tissue contrast obtained with current MR techniques has improved detection of neoplasms. Early studies showed that T1 and T2 relaxation times are not useful to differentiate normal pancreas from pancreatitis or pancreatic neoplasm because of overlap between values.[41,80] The signal intensity of adenocarcinomas is variable depending on the techniques, ranging from isointense

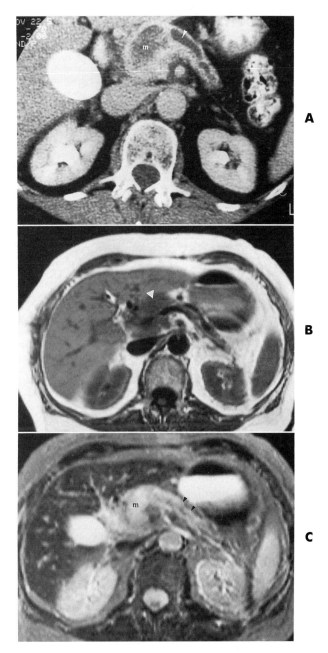

Fig. 12-13. Pancreatic ductal adenocarcinoma. **A,** CT scan: A hypodense mass *(m)* in the pancreatic head produces pancreatic ductal obstruction *(arrowhead)* and atrophy of the pancreatic tail. The right margin of the pancreatic head is indistinct. **B,** Axial T1WI: The pancreatic head mass *(arrowhead)* is hypointense. The dilated pancreatic duct is well seen as a low-intensity tubular structure in the atrophic pancreatic tail. **C,** Axial T2WI: The pancreatic head mass *(m)* is heterogeneous with predominantly high signal intensity. The dilated pancreatic duct *(arrowheads)* has high signal intensity.

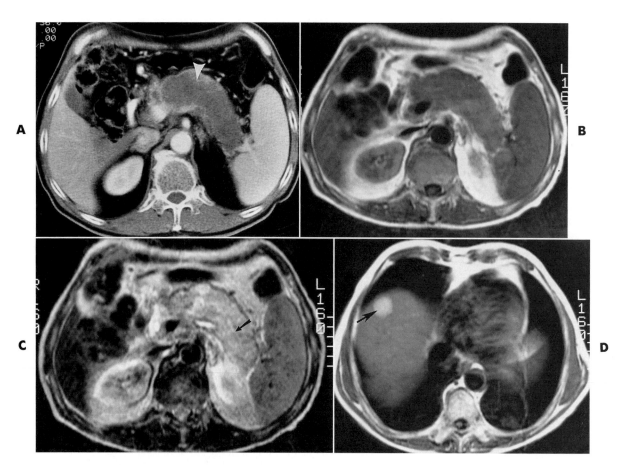

Fig. 12-14. Pancreatic adenocarcinoma, diffuse form. **A,** CT scan: The pancreas *(arrowhead)* is diffusely enlarged, showing low attenuation. Several round, hypodense lesions, representing cysts or solid masses, were shown within the liver on other scans. Differential diagnosis includes tumor, pancreatic necrosis, and fluid collection. **B,** Axial T1WI: The diffusely enlarged pancreas has intermediate signal intensity. **C,** Axial T2WI: The pancreatic mass has moderately high signal intensity consistent with a solid lesion. There are focal regions of higher signal intensity. The tubular, high intensity structure in the tail of pancreas *(arrow)* may represent the pancreatic duct. **D,** Axial T1WI: One of several hemorrhagic lesions in the liver *(arrow)* consistent with hemorrhagic metastases. Surgical exploration showed a "rock-hard" pancreatic adenocarcinoma with liver metastases.

to hyperintense with normal pancreas on T1WI at $0.35T^{80}$ to predominantly hypointense compared to normal pancreas on T1WI using high field strength (1.5 T)[85] or surface coil imaging.[67] Fat-suppression techniques provide a greater contrast difference between the low-intensity adenocarcinomas and the normal, high-intensity pancreatic parenchyma (Fig. 12-15).[54] Dynamic gadolinium enhancement also increases the contrast difference between normal, enhancing parenchyma and the hypovascular, poorly enhancing neoplasm.[15,66,85] The improvement in tissue contrast with MRI has made it possible to detect small, noncontour deforming neoplasms not visible with CT using both surface coil techniques[67] and fat-suppression techniques with dynamic enhancement.[66]

Islet cell tumors

The islets of Langerhans are responsible for the endocrine functions of the pancreas and contain four cell types. Beta cells produce insulin, alpha cells secrete glucagon, delta cells contain somatostatin and possibly gastrin, and PP cells produce pancreatic polypeptides.[60] Tumors in the islet cells can be functional or nonfunctional, benign or malignant. Although functional tumors may produce a variety of hormones, they are classified by the dominant endocrine effect. Islet cell tumors may occur sporadically or in association with multiple endocrine neoplasia or von Hippel-Lindau disease.[9]

The most common functional islet cell tumor is insulinoma. This benign neoplasm produces hyperinsulinism, a

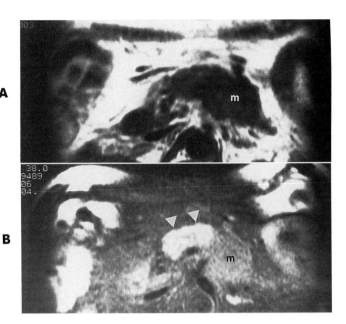

Fig. 12-15. Pancreatic adenocarcinoma: Use of fat-suppression. **A,** Axial T1WI: A mass *(m)* in the tail of the pancreas is hypointense on standard T1WI. **B,** Axial T1WI with fat suppression: The normal pancreas has high signal intensity *(arrowheads).* The mass *(m)* has intermediate signal intensity. Contrast difference between normal pancreas and tumor is enhanced using fat suppression. (From Mitchell DG, Vinitski S, Saponaro S, et al: *Radiology* 178:67-71, 1991.)

clinical syndrome consisting of recurrent attacks of hypoglycemia occurring in the morning or at night, unrelated to meals. Seizure disorder or psychiatric symptoms may also occur. Because patients are symptomatic, the tumors are often very small at the time of diagnosis. Surgical resection is curative in the majority of cases.[63]

The second most common functioning islet cell tumor, gastrinoma, produces the Zollinger-Ellison syndrome. Symptoms include recurrent ulcers due to persistent acid hypersecretion. Ulcers occur in the stomach and duodenum in 75% of cases and in the distal duodenum and jejunum in 25% of cases.[77] In contrast to insulinoma, 60% of gastrinomas are malignant and have metastasized to the liver, lymph nodes, or bones at the time of diagnosis. Localization of gastrinomas is more difficult because the tumors are frequently extrapancreatic, occurring in the duodenum, distal stomach, mesentery, splenic hilum, and elsewhere.[77]

Glucagonoma is a rare pancreatic tumor that can be diagnosed clinically by the presence of a skin rash (known as necrolytic migratory erythema), diabetes mellitus, weight loss, anemia, and thrombophlebitis.[11,63] These tumors tend to be fairly large at the time of diagnosis, with an average diameter of 4 cm in one series.[11] Tumoral calcifications are seen within malignant forms of islet cell tu-

mor,[70] including many glucagonomas. Like other islet cell tumors, glucagonomas are hypervascular and produce hypervascular metastases to the liver.

Vipomas arise from islet cells that produce vasoactive intestinal polypeptide (VIP). Excess VIP production results in a clinical syndrome of watery diarrhea, hypokalemia, and achlorhydria.[63,76] This condition is also referred to as the Verner-Morrison syndrome or WDHA syndrome.

Diagnosis of islet cell tumors depends on a combination of factors including clinical history, laboratory results including measurements of hormone levels in blood using radioimmunoassay techniques, and radiologic and surgical localization. Nonfunctional tumors are usually large and easily identified. Localization of functioning islet tumors is frequently difficult because many of the functional tumors are small (1 to 2 cm), frequently multiple, and located in extrapancreatic sites. Radiologic methods that have been used for localization of islet cell tumors include arteriography, portal venous sampling, ultrasound, intraoperative ultrasound, CT, and MRI.[63]

Studies on the efficacy of MRI in detecting islet cell tumors are limited, probably because the tumors are uncommon, making a large series of patients difficult to obtain. Several investigators have reported the MR appearance of islet cell tumors in few patients, stating that they characteristically have low signal intensity on T1WI and are very hyperintense to normal parenchyma on T2WI (Fig. 12-16).[69,70,77] In a retrospective study of patients with advanced Zollinger-Ellison syndrome, both CT and MRI identified one or more primary tumors in 8 of 13 (62%) patients. All seven patients with liver metastases were identified by MRI. The signal intensity of the primary tumors was variable on T1WI, but was always increased on T2WI except in the case of a calcified tumor. Lymph node and liver metastases had low signal intensity on T1WI and very high signal intensity on T2WI. The signal intensity of liver metastases on T2WI was similar to that seen in cavernous hemangiomas of the liver. Tissue contrast on T2WI was better with MRI than CT, which relied primarily on contour changes for tumor diagnosis (Fig. 12-17).

Less favorable results were obtained in a prospective study of 24 patients with gastrinomas.[30] Using spin-echo imaging at 0.26 T or 0.5 T, the sensitivity of MRI for detection of primary tumors was only 20%, and the sensitivity for detection of metastatic gastrinoma in the liver was only 43%. No tumors smaller than 1 cm were identified, no extrapancreatic tumors were seen, and only 50% of tumors equal to or greater than 3 cm were diagnosed. High signal intensity within small bowel on T2WI had potential for obscuring the hyperintense lesions. The optimal combination of tests for diagnosis of gastrinoma in this series was abdominal ultrasound, CT, and angiography, which detected 17 of 20 (85%) of gastrinomas without using MRI. Nevertheless, MRI is potentially useful for noninva-

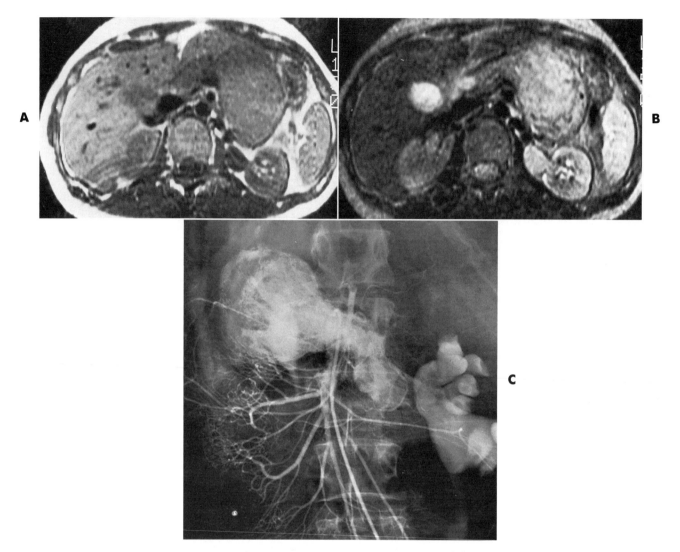

Fig. 12-16. Nonfunctioning islet cell tumor. **A,** Axial T1WI: A large, dumbbell-shaped mass is seen in the pancreatic tail with extension into the body. The signal intensity is similar to liver. **B,** Axial T2WI: The mass has predominantly high signal intensity, much less than liver. **C,** Arteriogram: The mass is hypervascular and has a dumbbell configuration.

sive follow-up in patients with inoperable lesions who undergo medical therapy.[30] Fat-suppression techniques may also permit diagnosis of smaller pancreatic neoplasms in the future.

Cystic neoplasms

Cystic tumors of the pancreas comprise between 5% and 15% of cystic lesions of the pancreas and less than 5% of pancreatic tumors.[19] The common cystic neoplasms discussed here include microcystic adenoma and mucinous cystic neoplasms. Other lesions included in the differential diagnosis of cystic masses of the pancreas are papillary cystic tumor, cystic islet cell tumor, mucinous ductal ectasia, pseudocyst, hemangioma, lymphangioma, and necrotic ductal cell tumors.[88]

Microcystic adenoma. Microcystic adenoma has also been called serous cystadenoma or glycogen-rich adenoma.[17] This benign neoplasm occurs in middle-aged or elderly women who are commonly asymptomatic but may present with abdominal pain or an abdominal mass. Pathologically, it is characterized by the presence of numerous tiny cysts separated by thin septa. The cysts contain thin, clear, fluid with glycogen and no mucin.[52] Hemorrhage may be present, as the lesions are often hypervascular.[29,17] Splenic vein occlusion and portal hypertension may occur.[13]

The classic radiologic appearance of a microcystic adenoma (Fig. 12-18) is a well-defined, lobulated mass with a honeycomb appearance[40] and frequently a central scar containing a sunburst calcification.[88] The tumor occurs in the

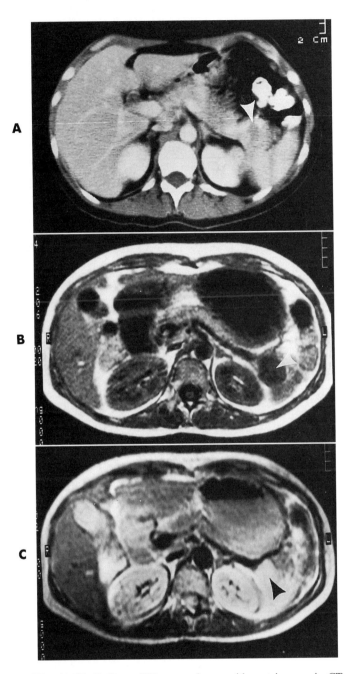

Fig. 12-17. Zollinger-Ellison syndrome with gastrinoma. **A,** CT scan: A focal mass is present in the pancreatic tail abutting the splenic hilum *(arrowhead).* There is little contrast difference between normal pancreas and mass. **B,** Axial T1WI: The tumor *(arrowhead)* is very well defined and shows much lower signal intensity than the normal pancreas. **C,** Axial T2WI: The tumor is very bright *(arrowhead)* and is closely related to the splenic vein. (From Tjon A, Tham RTO, Falke THM, et al: *J Comput Asst Tomogr* 13[5]:821-828, 1989.

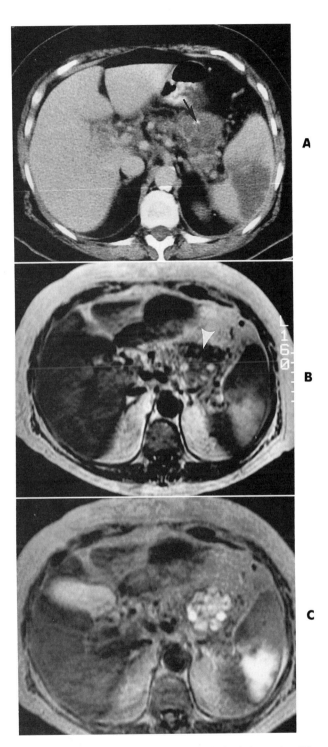

Fig. 12-18. Microcystic adenoma with splenic infarct. **A,** CT scan: A lobulated mass in the tail of pancreas has regions of low density as well as small calcifications *(arrow).* A wedge-shaped infarct in the spleen and collateral vessels around the pancreatic tail are secondary to splenic vein thrombosis. **B,** Axial proton density image: This shows a well-demarcated mass *(arrowhead),* which contains regions of high signal intensity, representing hemorrhagic cystic components found at surgery. The splenic infarct has high intensity as well. Collateral vessels are present in the splenic hilum. **C,** Axial T2WI: The mass is lobulated with septations and small heterogeneous cystic components. Pathology revealed a microcystic adenoma with hemorrhagic cysts, splenic vein thrombosis, and splenic infarct.

head, body, or tail of pancreas. In a study comparing MRI with CT for evaluation of cystic neoplasms,[52] MRI was equal to or superior to CT in demonstrating multilocularity and septations in cystic masses and was superior to CT in differentiating intensity differences between compartments in the masses. MRI did not demonstrate calcifications in masses as well as CT in four of five cases. The lobulated borders of microcystic adenomas are particularly well seen on T2WI, which shows very high signal intensity within the mass.[40,57] Although patients with a microcystic adenoma are predisposed to hemorrhage or hemoperitoneum[64] or mass effect on adjacent organs, the tumors are otherwise benign. In elderly or asymptomatic patients who have increased risk of surgical complications from resection, observation is warranted if the mass has the classic lobulated appearance with central calcification. Microcystic adenomas that lack these characteristic findings are difficult to differentiate from mucinous cystic neoplasms or other cystic masses and should be resected due to their malignant potential.[88]

Mucinous cystic neoplasms. Mucinous cystic neoplasms have also been termed macrocystic adenomas, mucinous cystadenomas, or mucinous cystadenocarcinomas. They occur in middle-aged women and predominantly involve the body and tail of the pancreas.[29] The tumor is composed of large, unilocular or multilocular cysts and may contain thickened septations and excrescences.

On MRI, mucinous cystic neoplasms[52] appear as rounded or oval masses with a mean diameter of 9 cm. They may contain septations with variable thickness including nodular excrescences. Multiple compartments are demonstrated within the tumors, and variations in signal intensity are seen between compartments. Pathologically proven hemorrhage within compartments appears as high-signal-intensity regions on T1WI and T2WI. Calcifications in walls and septa demonstrated by CT frequently are not visible by MRI but may be seen as regions of low signal intensity on T1WI and T2WI (Fig. 12-19).

Mucinous cystic neoplasms are potentially or frankly malignant at the time of diagnosis. In one series, 64% of mucinous tumors were malignant and 33% had metastases at the time of diagnosis.[88] Although previous reports indicated that these tumors have an improved prognosis over ductal adenocarcinoma of the pancreas, there may be two subcategories of mucinous neoplasms, with one group showing aggressive behavior with poor prognosis.[88] Surgical resection is warranted in masses suspected of being mucinous cystic neoplasms.

Other neoplasms

Pancreatoblastoma is a rare pancreatic tumor that occurs in children between 1 and 8 years of age. The tumor arises from pancreatic acinar cells and is usually large at the time of diagnosis, on the order of 7 to 12 cm in diameter. The differential diagnosis of pancreatoblastoma includes neuro-

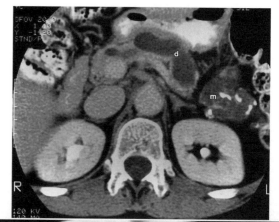

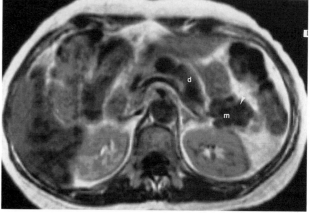

Fig. 12-19. Mucinous cystic neoplasm. **A,** CT scan: A low-density mass *(m)* with associated calcifications is present in the tail of pancreas. The pancreatic duct *(d)* is markedly dilated. This suggests the ductectatic form of mucinous cystic neoplasm. **B,** Axial T1WI: The mass *(m)* is hypointense. The dilated pancreatic duct *(d)* is easily seen. Coarse calcifications *(arrowhead)* are seen as lower signal intensity foci.

blastoma, hepatoblastoma, or lymphoma. On MRI, the primary tumor and metastatic liver lesions show low signal intensity on T1WI and bright, high signal intensity on T2WI.[72]

Pancreatic lymphangioma is a rare benign lesion that appears to arise from sequestration of lymphatic vessels. The abnormal lymphatics become fluid-filled, unilocular, or multilocular cystic masses, which can be located in the pancreas or elsewhere in the retroperitoneum. The mass may contain central calcification. In one case of pancreatic lymphangioma, MRI showed an inhomogeneous mass with low signal intensity on T1WI and predominantly high signal intensity within the venous lakes and cystic portions.[65]

Lymphoma commonly produces extensive abdominal lymphadenopathy, which can involve pancreas and peripancreatic regions. By MRI, lymphomatous masses are predominantly isointense with normal pancreatic parenchyma, making it difficult to define a discrete mass.[69] Only the presence of retroperitoneal adenopathy enables an accurate diagnosis of lymphoma.

PANCREATIC TRANSPLANTS

Pancreatic transplantation is performed in patients with diabetes mellitus in an attempt to restore normal glucose metabolism.[82] Methods for monitoring pancreatic graft function have included laboratory studies of urine chemistries and other parameters. The diagnosis of pancreatic rejection is difficult to make clinically, and percutaneous biopsy is not feasible because of the risk of subsequent pancreatitis. MRI has proved useful as a noninvasive means of assessing pancreatic grafts. Using coronal and axial T1WI and T2WI, the pancreatic graft is identified in the iliac fossa and can be compared with adjacent muscle, urinary bladder, and concomitant renal allograft, when present.

During acute rejection, regions of decreased signal intensity are seen within the pancreatic graft on T1WI, and T2WI show regions of increased signal intensity. The abnormalities may be diffuse or multifocal. The graft parenchyma shows decrease in signal intensity on T2WI after treatment for acute rejection. In chronic rejection, the pancreatic graft is reduced in size and shows low signal intensity on T1WI and T2WI. Measurements of T2 times of pancreatic transplants showed increased mean T2 times in patients with rejection compared with patients without rejection.[82] The improved tissue contrast of MRI compared with CT makes it a useful adjunct to other modes of clinical assessment in patients with pancreatic transplants.

REFERENCES

1. Ang PGP, Li KCP, Tart RP, et al: Geritol oil emulsion: ideal positive oral contrast agent for MR imaging, *Radiology* 173(P):522, 1989.
2. Baker ME, Cohan RH, Nadel SN, et al: Obliteration of the fat surrounding the celiac axis and superior mesenteric artery is not a specific CT finding of carcinoma of the pancreas, *Am J Roentgenol* 155:991-994, 1990.
3. Balthazar EJ, Ranson JHC, Naidich DP, et al: Acute pancreatitis: Prognostic value of CT, *Radiology* 156:767-772, 1985.
4. Balthazar EJ, Robinson DL, Megibow AJ, et al: Acute pancreatitis: Value of CT in establishing prognosis, *Radiology* 174:331-336, 1990.
5. Balthazar EJ: CT diagnosis and staging of acute pancreatitis, *Radiol Clin North Am* 27(1):19-37, 1989.
6. Bassi C, Vesentini S, Nifosi F, et al: Pancreatic abscess and other pus-harboring collections related to pancreatitis: a review of 108 cases, *World J Surg* 14:505-512, 1990.
7. Berland LL, Lawson TL, Foley WD, et al: Computed tomography of the normal and abnormal pancreatic duct: correlation with pancreatic ductography, *Radiology* 141:715-724, 1981.
8. Berman LG, Prior JT, Abramow SM, et al: A study of the pancreatic duct system in man by the use of vinyl acetate casts of postmortem preparations, *Surg Gynecol Obstet* 110:391-403, 1960.
9. Binkovitz LA, Johnson CD, Stephens DH: Islet cell tumors in von Hippel-Lindau disease: increased prevalence and relationship to the multiple endocrine neoplasias, *Am J Roentgenol* 155:501-505, 1990.
10. Bradley EL III, Murphy F, Ferguson C: Prediction of pancreatic necrosis by dynamic pancreatography, *Ann Surg* 210(4):495-504, 1989.
11. Breatnach ES, Han SY, Rahatzad MT, et al: CT evaluation of glucagonomas, *J Comput Asst Tomogr* 9(1):25-29, 1985.
12. Brown JJ, van Sonnenberg E, Gerber KH, et al: Magnetic resonance relaxation times of percutaneously obtained normal and abnormal body fluids, *Radiology* 154:727-731, 1985.
13. Buck JL, Hayes WS: Microcystic adenoma of the pancreas, *Radiographics* 10:313-322, 1990.
14. Burton SS, Ros PR, Otto PM, et al: Barium MR imaging of the pancreas: initial experience, *Radiology* 173(P):517, 1989.
15. Chezmar JL, Nelson RC, Small WC, et al: Magnetic resonance imaging of the pancreas with gadolinium-DTPA, *Gastrointest Radiol* 16:139-142, 1991.
16. Compagno J, Oertel JE: Microcystic adenomas of the pancreas (glycogen-rich cystadenomas): a clinicopathologic study of 34 cases, *Am J Clin Pathol* 69:289-298, 1978.
17. Compagno J, Oertel JE: Mucinous cystic neoplasms of the pancreas with overt and latent malignancy (cystadenocarcinoma and cystadenoma): a clinicopathologic study in 41 cases, *Am J Clin Pathol* 69:573-580, 1978.
18. Cotton PB: Congenital anomaly of pancreas divisum as cause of obstructive pain and pancreatitis, *Gut* 21:105-114. 1980.
19. Cubilla LA, Fitzgerald PJ: Classification of pancreatic cancer (nonendocrine), *Mayo Clin Proc* 54:449-458, 1979.
20. Cubilla AL, Fitzgerald PJ: Tumors of the exocrine pancreas. In *Atlas of Tumor Pathology,* Series 2, Fascicle 19, Washington, DC, 1983, Armed Forces Institute of Pathology.
21. Delhaye M, Engelholm L, Cremer M: Pancreas divisum: Congenital anatomic variant or anomaly? Contribution of endoscopic retrograde dorsal pancreatography, *Gastroenterology* 89:951-958, 1985.
22. DelMaschio A, Vanzulli A, Sironi S, et al: Pancreatic cancer versus chronic pancreatitis: diagnosis with CA 19-9 assessment, US, CT, and CT-guided fine-needle biopsy, *Radiology* 178:95-99, 1991.
23. Di Sant'Agnese PA, Davis PB: Research in cystic fibrosis, *N Engl J Med* 295:481, 1976.
24. Fiel SB, Friedman AC, Caroline DF, et al: Magnetic resonance imaging in young adults with cystic fibrosis, *Chest* 91(2):181-184.
25. Freeny PC, Marks WM, Ball TJ: Impact of high-resolution computed tomography of the pancreas on utilization of endoscopic retrograde cholangiopancreatography and angiography, *Radiology* 142:35-39, 1982.
26. Freeny PC, Marks WM, Ryan JA, et al: Pancreatic ductal adenocarcinoma: diagnosis and staging with dynamic CT, *Radiology* 166:125-133, 1988.
27. Freeny PC: Radiologic diagnosis and staging of pancreatic ductal adenocarcinoma, *Radiol Clin North Am* 27(1):121-128, 1989.
28. Freeny PC: Radiology of the pancreas, *Curr Opin Radiol* 1:81-93, 1989.
29. Friedman AC, Lichtenstein JE, Dachman AH: Cystic neoplasms of the pancreas: radiological-pathological correlation, *Radiology* 149:45-50, 1983.
30. Frucht H, Doppman JL, Norton JA, et al: Gastrinomas: comparison of MR imaging with CT, angiography, and US, *Radiology* 171:713-717, 1989.
31. Geokas MC: The role of elastase in acute pancreatitis, *Arch Pathol* 86:135-141, 1968.
32. Hahn PF, Stark DD, Lewis JM, et al: First clinical trial of a new superparamagnetic iron oxide for use as an oral gastrointestinal contrast agent in MR imaging, *Radiology* 175:695-700, 1990.
33. Hamed MM, Hamm B, Ibrahim ME, et al: Dynamic MR imaging of the abdomen with gadopentetate dimeglumine: normal enhancement patterns of the liver, spleen, stomach, and pancreas, *Am J Roentgenol* 158:303-307, 1992.
34. Isselbacher KJ, Adams RD, Braunwald E, et al: *Harrison's Principles of Internal Medicine,* ed 9, New York, 1980, McGraw-Hill.
35. Hernanz-Schulman M, et al: Pancreatic cystosis in cystic fibrosis, *Radiology* 148:629-631, 1986.

36. Housman JF, Chezmar JL, Nelson RC: Magnetic resonance imaging in hemochromatosis: extrahepatic iron deposition, *Gastrointest Radiol* 14:59-60, 1989.

37. Huntington DK, Hill MC, Steinberg W: Biliary tract dilatation in chronic pancreatitis: CT and sonographic findings, *Radiology* 172:47-50, 1989.

38. Isikoff MB, Hill MC, Silverstein W, et al: The clinical significance of acute pancreatic hemorrhage, *Am J Roentgenol* 136:679-684, 1981.

39. Itai Y, Moss AA, Goldberg HI: Pancreatic cysts caused by carcinoma of the pancreas: a pitfall in the diagnosis of pancreatic carcinoma, *J Comput Asst Tomogr* 6(4):772-776, 1982.

40. Itai U, Ohhashi K, Furui S, et al: Microcystic adenoma of the pancreas: spectrum of computed tomographic findings, *J Comput Asst Tomogr* 12(5):797-803, 1988.

41. Jenkins JPR, Braganza JM, Hickey DS, et al: Quantitative tissue characterization in pancreatic disease using magnetic resonance imaging, *Br J Radiol* 60:333-341, 1987.

42. Johnson CD, Stephens DH, Sarr MG: CT of acute pancreatitis: correlation between lack of contrast enhancement and pancreatic necrosis, *Am J Roentgenol* 156:93-95, 1991.

43. Kaminsky S, Laniado M, Gogoll M, et al: Gadopentetate dimeglumine as a bowel contrast agent: safety and efficacy, *Radiology* 178:503-508, 1991.

44. Kivisaari L, Somer K, Standertskjold-Nordenstam G-C, et al: A new method for the diagnosis of acute hemorrhagic-necrotizing pancreatitis using contrast-enhanced CT, *Gastointest Radiol* 9:27-30, 1984.

45. Kloppel G, Maillet B: Classification and staging of pancreatic nonendocrine tumors, *Radiol Clin North Am* 27(1):105-119, 1989.

46. Laniado M, Kornmesser W, Hamm B, et al: MR imaging of the gastrointestinal tract: value of Gd-DTPA, *Am J Roentgenol* 150:817-821, 1988.

47. Lee MJ, Saini S, Geller SC, et al: Pancreatitis with pseudoaneurysm formation: A pitfall for the interventional radiologist, *Am J Roentgenol* 156:97-98, 1991.

48. Leutmer PH, Stephens DH, Ward EM: Chronic pancreatitis reassessment with current CT, *Radiology* 171:353-357, 1989.

49. Leutmer H, Stephens DH, Fischer AP: Obliteration of periarterial retropancreatic fat on CT in pancreatitis: an exception to the rule, *Am J Roentgenol* 153:63-64, 1989.

50. Magnetic resonance imaging of the abdomen and pelvis: Council on Scientific Affairs, Report of the Panel on Magnetic Resonance Imaging, *JAMA* 261(3):420, 1989.

51. Marti-Bonmati L, Vilar J, Paniagua JC, et al: High density barium sulphate as an MRI oral contrast, *Magn Reson Imaging* 9:259-261, 1991.

52. Minami, Itai Y, Ohtomo K et al: Cystic neoplasms of the pancreas: comparison of MR imaging with CT, *Radiology* 171:53-56, 1989.

53. Mitchell CJ, Lintott DJ, Ruddell WST, et al: Clinical relevance of an unfused pancreatic duct system, *Gut* 20:1066-1071, 1979.

54. Mitchell DG, Vinitski S, Saponaro S, et al: Liver and pancreas: improved spin-echo T1 contrast by shorter echo time and fat suppression at 1.5 T, *Radiology* 178:67-71, 1991.

55. Murayama S, Robinson AE, Mulvihill DM, et al: MR imaging of pancreas in cystic fibrosis, *Pediatr Radiol* 20:536-539, 1990.

56. Neff CC, Simeone JF, Wittenberg J, et al: Inflammatory pancreatic masses: problems in differentiating focal pancreatitis from carcinoma, *Radiology* 150:35-38, 1984.

57. Piccirillo M, Bourque A, McCarthy S, et al: High field imaging of the normal pancreas, *Magn Reson Imaging* 7:457-461, 1989.

58. Ranson JHC, Pasternak BS: Statistical methods for qualifying the severity of clinical acute pancreatitis, *J Surg Res* 22:79-91, 1977.

59. Ranson JHC: Etiological and prognostic factors in human acute pancreatitis: a review, *Am J Gastroenterol* 9:633-638, 1982.

60. Robbins SL, Cotran RS: *Pathologic basis of disease,* Philadelphia, 1979, WB Saunders.

61. Rohrmann CA, Baron RL: Biliary complications of pancreatitis, *Radiol Clin North Am* 27(1):93-104, 1989.

62. Ros PR, Steinman RM, Torres GM, et al: The value of barium as a gastrointestinal contrast agent in MR imaging: a comparison study in normal volunteers, *Am J Roentgenol* 157:761-767, 1991.

63. Rossi P, Allison DJ, Bezzi M, et al: Endocrine tumors of the pancreas, *Radiol Clin North Am* 27(1):129-161, 1989.

64. Rubin GD, Jeffrey RB, Walter JF: Pancreatic microcystic adenoma presenting with acute hemoperitoneum: CT diagnosis, *Am J Roentgenol* 156:749-750, 1991.

65. Salimi Z, Fishbein M, Wolverson MK, et al: Pancreatic lymphangioma: CT, MRI, and angiographic features, *Gastrointest Radiol* 16:248-250, 1991.

66. Semelka RC, Kroeker MA, Shoenut JP, et al: Pancreatic disease: prospective comparison of CT, ERCP, and 1.5-T MR imaging with dynamic gadolinium enhancement and fat suppression, *Radiology* 181:785-791, 1991.

67. Simeone JF, Edelman RR, Stark DD, et al: Surface coil MR imaging of abdominal viscera, Part III. The pancreas, *Radiology* 157:437-441, 1985.

68. Stabile BE, Wilson SE, Debas HT: Reduced mortality from bleeding pseudocysts and pseudoaneurysms caused by pancreatitis, *Arch Surg* 118:45-51, 1983.

69. Stark DD, Moss AA, Goldberg HI, et al: Magnetic resonance and CT of the normal and diseased pancreas: a comparative study, Radiology 150:153-162, 1984.

70. Stark DD, Moss AA, Goldberg HI, et al: CT of pancreatic islet cell tumors, *Radiology* 150:491-494, 1984.

71. Steiner E, Stark DD, Hahn PF, et al: Imaging of pancreatic neoplasms: comparison of MR and CT, *Am J Roentgenol* 152:487-491, 1989.

72. Stephenson CA, Kletzel M, Seibert JJ, et al: Pancreatoblastoma: MR appearance, *J Comput Asst Tomogr* 14(3):492-494, 1990.

73. Stroud WH, Cullom JW, Anderson MC: Hemorrhagic complications of severe pancreatitis, *Surgery* 90(4):657-665, 1981.

74. Swensen SJ, Mcleod RA, Stephens DH: CT of extracranial hemorrhage and hematomas, *Am J Roentgenol* 143:907-912, 1984.

75. Swensen SJ, Keller PL, Berquist TH, et al: Magnetic resonance imaging of hemorrhage, *Am J Roentgenol* 145:921-927, 1985.

76. Tjon A, Tham RTO, Falke THM, et al: MR, CT, and ultrasound findings of metastatic Vipoma in pancreas, *J Comput Asst Tomogr* 13(1):142-144, 1989.

77. Tjon A, Tham RTO, Falke THM, et al: CT and MR imaging of advanced Zollinger-Ellison syndrome, *J Comput Asst Tomogr* 13(5):821-828, 1989.

78. Tjon A, Tham RTO, Heyerman HGM, et al: Cystic fibrosis: MR imaging of the pancreas, *Radiology* 179:183-186, 1991.

79. Torres WE, Clements JL Jr, Sones PJ Jr, et al: Gas in the pancreatic bed without abscess, *Am J Roentgenol* 137:1131-1133, 1981.

80. Tscholakoff D, Hricak H, Thoeni R, et al: MR imaging in the diagnosis of pancreatic disease, *Am J Roentgenol* 148:703-709, 1987.

81. Unger EC, Cohen MS, Gatenby RA, et al: Single breath-holding scans of the abdomen using FISP and FLASH at 1.5 T, *J Comput Tomogr* 12(4):575-583, 1988.

82. Vahey TN, Glazer GM, Francis IR, et al: MR diagnosis of pancreatic transplant rejection, *Am J Roentgenol* 150:557-560, 1988.

83. Van Dyke JA, Stanley RJ, Berland LL: Pancreatic imaging, *Ann Intern Med* 102:212-217, 1985.

84. van Sonnenberg E, Casola G, Varney RR, et al: Imaging and interventional radiology for pancreatitis and its complications, *Radiol Clin North Am* 27(1):65-72, 1989.

85. Vellet DA: Characterization of pancreatic adenocarcinoma by magnetic resonance imaging, *Can Assoc Radiol J* 42:180-184, 1991.

86. Vujic I: Vascular complications of pancreatitis, *Radiol Clin North Am* 27(1):81-91, 1989.

87. Wall SD, Brasch RC, Goldberg HI, et al: Improved imaging of the GI tract and pancreas, *MRI Decisions,* July/August:27-32, 1988.

88. Warshaw AL, Compton CC, Lewandrowski K, et al: Cystic tumors of the pancreas: new clinical, radiologic, and pathologic observations in 67 patients, *Ann Surg* 212(4):432-443, 1990.

89. Weinmann HJ, Brasch RC, Press W-R, et al: Characteristics of gadolinium-DTPA complex, a potential NMR contrast agent, *Am J Roentgenol* 142:619-624, 1984.

90. Winsett MZ, Amparo EG, Fagan CJ, et al: MR imaging of mediastinal pseudocyst, *J Comput Asst Tomogr* 12(2): 320-322, 1988.

91. Wittenberg J, Simeone JF, Ferrucci JT, et al: Non-focal enlargement in pancreatic carcinoma, *Radiology* 144:131-135, 1982.

92. Wolverson MK, Crepps LF, Sundaram M, et al: Hyperdensity of recent hemorrhage at body computed tomography: incidence and morphologic variation, *Radiology* 148:779-784, 1983.

93. Yuh WTC, Hunsicker LG, Nghiem DD, et al: Pancreatic transplants: evaluation with MR imaging, *Radiology* 170:171-177, 1989.

94. Zeman RK, McVay LV, Silverman PM, et al: Pancreas divisum: thin-section CT, *Radiology* 169:395-398, 1988.

Chapter 13

SPLEEN

Ali Shirkhoda

ANATOMIC CONSIDERATIONS

The spleen lies normally in the left upper quadrant almost entirely surrounded by peritoneum, which firmly adheres to its capsule. Twofolds of the peritoneum hold the spleen in position and come into contact between the stomach and the spleen, forming the gastrosplenic ligament, and between the left kidney and the spleen, forming the splenorenal ligament. Between the two ligaments are the splenic vessels. In addition the spleen is supported by the splenocolic ligament, on which its lower end rests. The spleen also has a bare area that is not covered by peritoneum.[62] This small, approximately 3 cm portion of the spleen is located between the anterior and posterior leaves of the splenorenal ligament. Recognition of this area helps in differentiating fluid in the peritoneal space from the pleural effusion.

The splenic artery is remarkable for its large size in proportion to the size of the organ and also for its tortuous course. Divided into six or more branches that enter the hilum of the spleen and ramify throughout the organ, the splenic artery carries approximately 150 ml of blood per minute (about 4% of the cardiac output). Abnormal and aged red and white blood cells, as well as platelets, are eliminated and sequestered from the circulation by the spleen. In addition, viruses, bacteria, nuclear remnants (Howell-Jolly bodies), and parasites are also removed by the spleen.

The size and weight of the spleen depend on the patient's age and in some individuals vary under certain circumstances. In the adult, the spleen weighs about 75 to 100 g and measures about 12 cm in length, 7 cm in diameter, and 4 cm in thickness.[29] Splenic dimensions are easily determined by using radiologic methods such as computed tomography (CT), ultrasound, and magnetic resonance imaging (MRI). The sum of the contiguous axial slices gives the length. The width is the longest anteroposterior diameter on any image, and the thickness is measured at the hilum. Because the position and configuration of the spleen vary significantly in humans, the splenic index has been used to determine splenomegaly. This index is the product of multiplying splenic thickness by width and length as seen on CT or MRI; its accuracy is said to be 90%.[60] The index should be 480 or less. A value of 500 or more is strong evidence of abnormality.

IMAGING TECHNIQUES

Evaluation of the spleen generally begins with palpation, which can often determine if a patient has splenomegaly. Also, in the case of trauma and infection, the spleen may be sensitive to motion. Numerous radiologic examinations can further determine the size and morphology of the spleen.

Plain film radiography

Plain radiographs are limited to demonstrating the size of the spleen in approximately 20% of cases.[35] However, because of variations in size and configurations, the spleen has to be large to be appreciated on plain film. The presence of splenic granulomas and other calcifications, such as those related to cysts and old hematoma, are also detectable on plain film. Occasionally, in cases of abscess, air is seen within the spleen on plain films.

Nuclear scintigraphy

Splenic scintigraphy is performed using technetium-99m sulfur colloid. Nearly 90% of this isotope goes to the liver, 5% to 10% to the spleen, and a smaller amount to the bone marrow. It is important to image approximately 20 to 30 minutes after intravenous injection of 5 mCi of isotope and obtain several views of the spleen, including anterior, posterior, lateral, and both obliques.[22] Although scintigraphy is a relatively sensitive technique, it remains nonspecific for pathologic conditions of the spleen. The sensitivity of this test has increased by using single photon emission computed tomography (SPECT). Its clinical indications are now limited to detecting congenital abnormalities, assessing the size and homogeneity of the spleen, and detecting an unknown mass such as a large accessory spleen or wandering spleen.[41]

Ultrasonography

Sonography is currently the most available and least expensive effective noninvasive modality for evaluating the spleen.[27] Gastric and colonic air and rib artifacts occasionally prohibit a thorough evaluation of the spleen by ultrasound because of the anatomic relationship of the colon, stomach, and spleen. However, by proper positioning of the patient (preferably left side up), intercostal scanning, and cephalic angulation of the transducer below the ribs, one can often achieve a good examination of the spleen. The spleen should be examined in coronal, sagittal, and axial planes. The best results are obtained during deep inspiration and occasionally after filling the stomach with water. The superior portion of the spleen is marked by the smoothly echogenic convex line representing the diaphragm. The medial and inferior portion is identified by the left kidney. Fine echogenicity of a normal spleen is similar to that of the liver. However, occasionally one may see bright echoes that represent blood vessels.

Computed tomography

Computed tomography of the abdomen identifies the spleen in virtually every patient who has one in the normal location. CT scanning demonstrates the size, configuration, location, and density of the spleen, as well as the presence of any focal or diffuse abnormalities.[29] On unenhanced CT, the spleen is homogeneous and slightly less dense than the normal liver. Slow intravenous injection of contrast agent usually results in a uniform increase in parenchymal density of a normal spleen.

Magnetic resonance imaging

Magnetic resonance imaging of the abdomen, like CT, consistently shows the normal spleen, regardless of the scanning parameters.[1] It has long T1 and T2 relaxation times. On T1-weighted spin echo images, the spleen is isointense with respect to liver; whereas on T2, it becomes hyperintense with respect to the liver. Splenic lesions have generally been evaluated by MRI without intravenous contrast agents.[1] However, the lesions and normal splenic parenchyma occasionally have similar T1 and T2 relaxation and proton density values. This may explain the insensitivity of conventional spin echo imaging in detecting focal splenic lesions, as reported by some who recommend gadolinium-enhanced studies in such patients.[39] Superparamagnetic iron oxide has been used by others to detect focal and diffuse splenic lesions.[66]

PITFALLS

Rapid delivery of intravenous contrast agent results in a heterogeneous pattern of splenic opacification during the

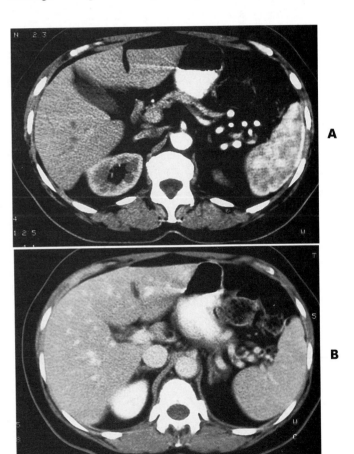

A

B

Fig. 13-1. CT pitfall. **A,** As the reuslt of rapid delivery of intravenous contrast, heterogeneous pattern of splenic enhancement appears in the early phase. **B,** In repeat scan at the same level, splenic enhancement is homogeneous and normal. MRI may be helpful in ruling out pathologic conditions if vascular phenomena are seen by CT, in cases such as this.

early phase of imaging (Fig. 13-1). This is a normal phenomenon and is related to variable rates of blood flow through the splenic red pulp.[18] This pattern is also seen in dynamic gadolinium-enhanced MRI of the spleen.[66] The temporary change in splenic density or intensity, lasting less than a minute, should not be mistaken for conditions such as tumor infiltration or infarct. Since splenic parenchyma achieves a uniform homogeneous appearance in less than 1 minute, a repeat scan is advised for those levels at which the spleen displays heterogeneity. MRI may also be used to rule out pathologic conditions in these cases. Other splenic pitfalls, as seen on CT, relate to its shape, position, and relationship with the left kidney.[52] On axial imaging, occasionally the medial aspect of the spleen is lobulated and extends to the region of the tail of the pancreas or into the left renal fossa. Following nephrectomy

on the left side, the spleen may rotate so that the lobulated surface faces anteriorly. All of these variations may be mistaken for tumors in the region of the pancreas, adrenal glands, or stomach. This is generally a less common pitfall for MRI because direct coronal images can be obtained. The CT pitfall generally can be avoided by coronal reformation of axial images or by additional thin slices.[51]

CONGENITAL ANOMALIES AND VARIATIONS

A splenic cleft is a congenital, normal variation usually seen in the anterior aspect of the midspleen and should not be mistaken for laceration in a traumatized patient. The term "wandering spleen" is generally used (Fig. 13-2) when the spleen is located in an abnormal position, such as the left lower quadrant or the upper pelvis. Aberrant position of the spleen probably relates to congenital abnormal fusion of the posterior mesogastrium, along with lack of fusion or maldevelopment of suspensory splenic ligaments.[21] It may also be an acquired condition; it has been seen commonly in multiparous women. Wandering spleen has higher incidence of torsion resulting in gastric varices or splenic infarction.[21,41]

Accessory spleens generally result from failure of embryologic splenic buds to unite within the dorsal mesogastrium. The incidence of accessory spleens in a large series of splenectomies in a pediatric population has been reported to be as high as 16%.[13] These small splenic tissue nodules are located usually in or near the hilum of the spleen but can be found in the abdomen or retroperitoneum, particularly near the pancreatic tail. Their blood supply and venous drainage are from and to the splenic artery and vein. They become hypertrophic following sple-

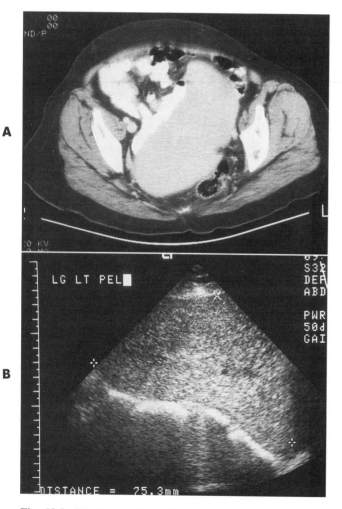

Fig. 13-2. Wandering spleen. **A,** Spleen was not seen in upper abdominal CT scan. Images in pelvis show spleen occupying most of the upper part of the left pelvis. **B,** Longitudinal sonogram shows bean-shape configuration of this pelvic spleen, which displays normal splenic echo pattern. (Courtesy Dr. Carol Bosanko, University of Michigan Hospital.)

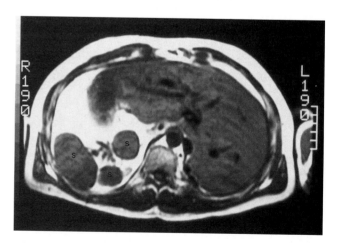

Fig. 13-3. Polysplenia. Patient with situs inversus has polysplenia, as seen on this upper abdominal T1-weighted (rate of repetition time to echo time is 500 to 25, indicated by TR/TE, 500/25) image. At least three spleens are seen in the right upper quadrant (*s*).

nectomy, can be a source of recurrent disease for conditions such as lymphoma or thrombocytopenic purpura.[2]

Other congenital abnormalities include asplenia and polysplenia, both of which are virtually always associated with a variety of congenital malformations. Intrathoracic and great vessel anomalies are most common with asplenia. Polysplenia is a multisystem congenital abnormality associated with multiple small spleens (Fig. 13-3), frequently having features of bilateral left-sidedness, often referred to as situs ambiguous with left isomerism.[48]

TRAUMA

Injury of the spleen is not uncommon and may result in rupture by blunt trauma, tear by a broken rib, or laceration by a gunshot wound or other penetrating injury. Between 50% to 80% of blunt splenic injuries are caused by car accidents, which may account for the high association between hepatic and splenic lacerations.[10] The great risk is hemorrhage, owing to the vascularity of the organ and the absence of a proper system of capillaries. Occasionally the splenic injury is spontaneous or iatrogenic, particularly when the organ is enlarged. Endoscopy, abdominal surgery, and inflammatory processes in the pancreas and other adjacent organs have also been reported to result in splenic injury.[32] As a result of splenic trauma, conditions such as subcapsular hematoma, intrasplenic hematoma, laceration, or combination of these may develop.

For many years splenic injury was an absolute indication for surgery because of the high degree of mortality without operative intervention.[10] However, it is now known that the contractile power of the splenic capsule can narrow the wound and prevent bleeding, reducing the risk of fatal bleeding. Vascularity of the spleen, which allows for extensive hemorrhage after injury, also provides a profound healing potential. Along with the high risk of postsplenectomy infection, these factors have prompted the use of conservative treatment approach in patients with splenic injury. CT has played an important role in the significant decrease of exploratory laparotomies and unnecessary splenectomies.[67] Therefore, a recent trend has developed toward clinical management of those patients who are hemodynamically stable to avoid and prevent the high incidence of future infection from splenectomy.[5] Whereas in some children, nonoperative treatment of splenic trauma is accepted,[11] such treatment in older patients is controversial.[36] This is primarily due to the high incidence of severe complications, including subphrenic abscess, pseudocyst formation, and delayed splenic rupture. For these reasons, sectional body imaging provides a reproducible technique for assessment of the result of conservative management (Fig. 13-4).[49]

CT is highly reliable in detecting splenic injury, providing proper protocol is used. It is important at the time of CT to move out of the scanning area electrocardiographic leads, tubes, and catheters that might be attached to the

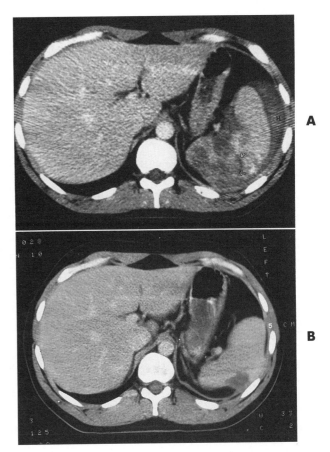

Fig. 13-4. Splenic laceration and subcapsular hematoma. **A,** Heterogeneous density in posterior aspect of the spleen is related to laceration *(arrows)* and intrasplenic hematoma. A large subcapsular hematoma *(H)* is visible in the lateral aspect of the spleen. **B,** After conservative management, a repeat CT scan at 2 months showed resolution of subcapsular hematoma, with a focal area of low density within the posterior aspect of the spleen, probably representing a small cyst, a sequela to hematoma.

left upper quadrant. It may be necessary to withdraw the nasogastric tube from the stomach and to recognize streak artifacts from air and fluid levels in the colon or stomach. If a study is done without using intravenous contrast agents, a subcapsular or perisplenic hematoma may be nearly isodense or hyperdense to the adjacent splenic parenchyma. In addition, without contrast media one may have difficulty identifying the normal part of the splenic parenchyma (Fig. 13-5). If the patient receives bolus contrast agent injection, then normal splenic parenchyma become significantly more dense than the adjacent blood.[1] Inadequate contrast or delayed scanning after intravenous contrast agent injection may result in obscuration of a hematoma since the splenic parenchyma may become enhanced to a density level equal to the adjacent blood. Splenic laceration or intrasplenic hematomas are seen as areas of inhomogeneous density within the splenic paren-

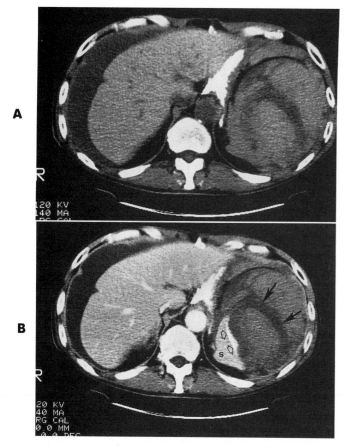

Fig. 13-5. Splenic laceration and intraperitoneal hemorrhage. **A,** On noncontrast CT study, a large globular mass in left upper quadrant contains bands of low density. Hematoma cannot be discriminated from normal splenic parenchyma. There is a large amount of intraperitoneal fluid. **B,** Repeat study with bolus intravenous contrast agent shows a small portion of splenic parenchyma *(s)* in the medial aspect. Contrast-enhanced blood is leaking from the spleen *(open arrows)* into the lacerated region. Bands of low density *(arrows),* as proven at surgery, represent lacerations.

chyma (see Fig. 13-4). A mottled, irregular pattern of contrast enhancement is characteristic of intraparenchymal hematoma.[14]

Splenic laceration is generally seen as linear areas of low density corresponding to fractures, along with splenic fragmentation (see Figs. 13-4 and 13-5). Resciniti and his colleagues[46] have developed a scoring system based on the CT findings of the severity of splenic parenchymal injury and the presence of free fluid. They have used this system to determine appropriate candidates for proper management.

Perisplenic hematoma or clot may be associated with peritoneal blood. The former is generally more dense than the latter.[14]

Occasionally, traumatized patients have normal findings on a CT scan obtained immediately after blunt abdominal trauma but develop a so-called delayed rupture of the spleen, manifested by left upper quadrant pain and a drop in hematocrit.[42] In such cases a repeat abdominal CT scan is always indicated.

MRI is not frequently used in splenic trauma, since patients are often studied on an emergency basis by CT. However, hematoma is easily detectable on MR images. The signal intensity depends on the age of the extravascular blood collection. Blood undergoes a complex transformation into deoxyhemoglobin and other paramagnetic products during the first 48 hours after extravasation. When deoxyhemoglobin is within intact red blood cells, a high field MR system is sensitive to its magnetic susceptibility effect and is able to identify a hematoma on T2-weighted images within a few hours after blood deoxygenation.[20] However, in subacute hematomas in which red cells undergo lysis, the paramagnetic effect is manifested as shortening of T1 and therefore as an area of bright signal on T1-weighted images (Fig. 13-6).

VASCULAR DISEASES

Changes of the spleen on CT, MRI, or ultrasound are seen secondary to obstruction of venous drainage or compromise of the arterial supply.

Splenic vein thrombosis is usually caused by pancreatic carcinoma, pancreatitis, trauma, polycythemia, or retroperitoneal fibrosis. The principle findings are splenomegaly and gastric varices.[40]

Blood supply to the spleen may be reduced almost completely by occlusion of the main splenic artery (Fig. 13-7). However, often one of its branches may become occluded, usually from thrombosis, leading to ischemia and infarction.[55] The parenchymal branches and end arteries within the spleen do not intercommunicate. Therefore, as a result of occlusion of one of the small branches, splenic infarct occurs. The most common cause is embolic disease, particularly in those patients with left side heart disease, sickle-cell disease, and myeloproliferative disorders. Other entities, such as arteriosclerosis, arteritis, splenic artery aneurysm, and (rarely) pancreatic diseases, may result in splenic infarct.[8] The spleen may be infarcted as a complication of hepatic embolization in the treatment of primary or metastatic liver disease.[61] Under these circumstances the particles delivered into the hepatic artery cause increased resistance to hepatic blood flow and may be refluxed into the celiac, gastroduodenal, right gastric, or pancreaticoduodenal arteries and thus eventually lodge in the spleen. In splenic infarct the patient's clinical history is that of a recent onset of left upper quadrant pain.

Different imaging methods may be used to assist diagnosis of splenic infarction. Scintigraphy has been advocated as an effective initial method; however, it is nonspecific. When there is total splenic artery occlusion, no radionuclide is carried to the spleen, which appears to be functionally absent. Otherwise, there may be focal decreased

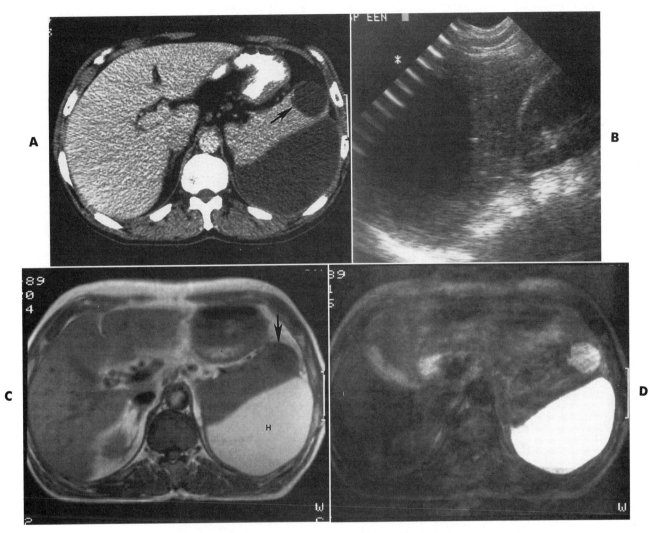

Fig. 13-6. Subcapsular hematoma and splenic cyst. **A,** CT scan in 55-year-old man demonstrates a large subcapsular hematoma, seen in superior and posterior aspects of the spleen. A well-defined area of low density *(arrow)* is visible in the anterior part of the spleen. **B,** Sagittal sonogram in left upper quadrant demonstrates the hematoma to be predominantly cystic and in the superior aspect of the spleen. **C,** T1-weighted axial MR image (TR/TE, 500/20) demonstrates subcapsular hematoma *(H)* as an area of bright signal intensity (extracellular methemoglobin) and fluid within the cyst *(arrow)* as an area of low signal intensity. **D,** Corresponding T2-weighted axial image (TR/TE, 2500/90) shows further enhancement of signal intensity of subacute bleeding. Fluid in the cyst is now an area of bright signal intensity.

uptake of techetium-99m sulfur colloid within the spleen, but no distinction is possible as to the solid or cystic nature of the lesion. Angiography may help to demonstrate the site of vascular occlusion.

Sonography adds specificity to the diagnosis[19]; the sonographic pattern generally depends on the time of the vascular insult. A fresh hemorrhagic infarct is more hypoechoic, whereas a headed infarct, because of development of fibrosis, is more echogenic. Old infarcts may become cystic; some splenic cysts are believed to be sequelae from infarction.

CT scanning with an intravenous contrast agent can be more specific. Usually one or several areas of decreased attenuation occur within the splenic parenchyma. Based on the size and number of arteries involved, the low attenuation area can be focal or diffuse (Figs. 13-7 and 13-8). Typically infarction is seen as a peripheral wedge-shaped defect; however, it often is seen as a round or irregular area of low attention (Fig. 13-9, *A*), occasionally occupying most of the splenic parenchyma.[3,55] The low attenuation is probably due to the presence of edema and sometimes results in cyst formation. According to Balcar, Selt-

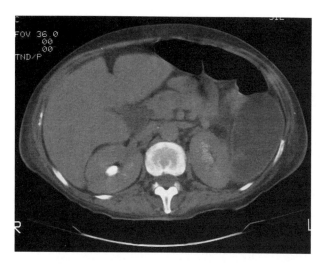

Fig. 13-7. Total splenic infarct. This axial contract-enhanced CT shows almost entire spleen as an area of low density. Complete occlusion of the splenic artery resulted in total splenic infarct.

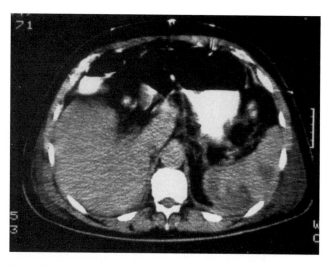

Fig. 13-8. Multiple infarcts in normal size spleen. Axial enhanced CT shows multiple peripheral wedge-shaped infarcts, some of which communicate in the posterior part of the spleen.

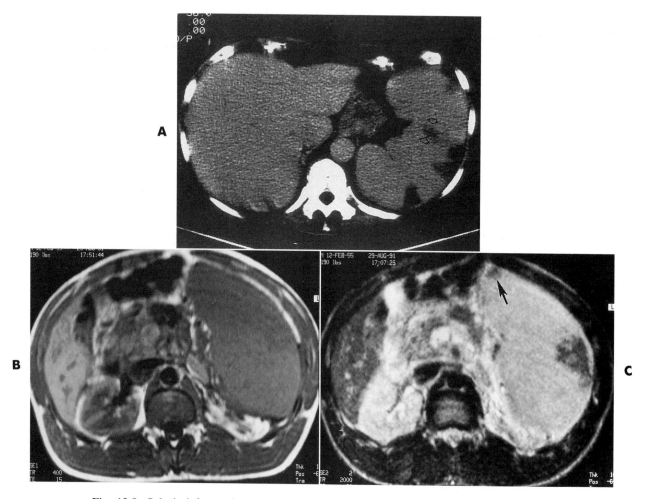

Fig. 13-9. Splenic infarcts. **A,** Multiple wedge-shaped infarcts are seen in the periphery of an enlarged spleen. Round infarcts *(open arrows)* are also seen within splenic parenchyma. **B** and **C,** Infarcts in 36-year-old man with thrombosis of the portal, superior mesenteric, and splenic veins. On T1-weighted image **(B),** the enlarged spleen has an area of intermediate signal intensity in its periphery. On T2-weighted image **(C),** the peripheral infarct is more conspicuous, and a second infarct *(arrow)* is found anteriorly. (**B** and **C** courtesy Dr. Pablo Ros, University of Florida, Gainesville, Fla.)

zer, Davis, and Geller,[3] CT appearance depends on the age of splenic infarct; however, if the lesions are followed, they decrease in size and may disappear.[61] In the acute and subacute phases of infarction, discrete focal low densities become progressively better demarcated and do not enhance. In the chronic phase the splenic density may return to normal with residual scarring or may remain as a wedge-shaped defect. Gas formation after transcatheter splenic infarction has been reported.[34]

On T1-weighted MR images the infarcted area may be seen as a wedge-shaped peripheral area displaying low or intermediate signal intensity (Fig. 13-9, *C*). On T2-weighted images the abnormality is usually more conspicuous because of the abnormal area displaying higher signal intensity (Fig. 13-9, *B*).

INFLAMMATORY DISEASES

Infectious processes such as histoplasmosis, tuberculosis, and brucellosis can cause changes in the spleen, result-

ing in multiple calcified granulomas. Most of these are incidentally found on plain abdominal radiographs or routine CT or ultrasound and have no clinical significance.

Splenic abscess is a rare condition with variable and often subtle clinical findings. The patient is often febrile, with left upper quadrant or left pleuritic chest pain. Radiographic findings may include elevation and fixation of the left hemidiaphragm, splenomegaly, and extraluminal gas in the left upper quadrant. Radionuclide studies, particularly those using gallium-67 citrate and indium-111, may provide specific diagnosis.[54] Without surgery the mortality of splenic abscess may reach 60%.[37] However, with early diagnosis and intervention the survival rate reverses to greater than 93%.[16]

Nowadays, earlier and more accurate detection is available using CT scanning, which can also be used for guided catheter drainage.[31] Therefore, MRI is usually not necessary, particularly since its application for interventional procedures is not well-established. When there is abscess,

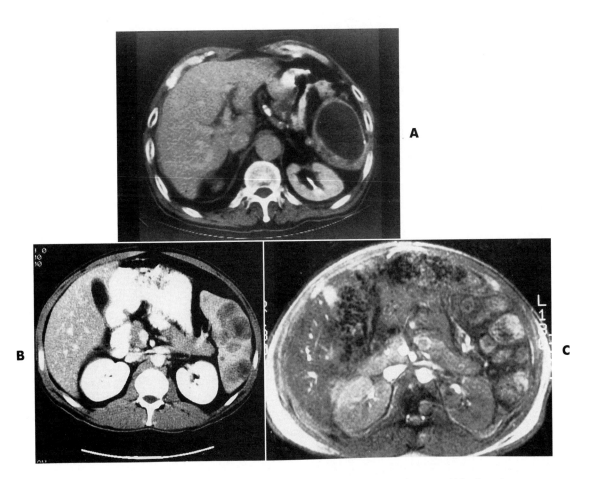

Fig. 13-10. Splenic abscess. **A,** A single well-defined low-density area is seen within the spleen. In this patient with fever and left pleural effusion, splenic abscess was suspected and drained. **B,** and **C,** CT scan of patient with AIDS shows multiple, well-defined, low-density lesions (**B**). Gradient echo T2-weighted MR image (**C**) shows lesions displaying high signal intensity but containing debris seen as areas of lower signal intensity at the center. Patient had splenic abscess from *Pneumocystis carini*. (**B** and **C** courtesy Dr. Kostaki Bis, William Beaumont Hospital.)

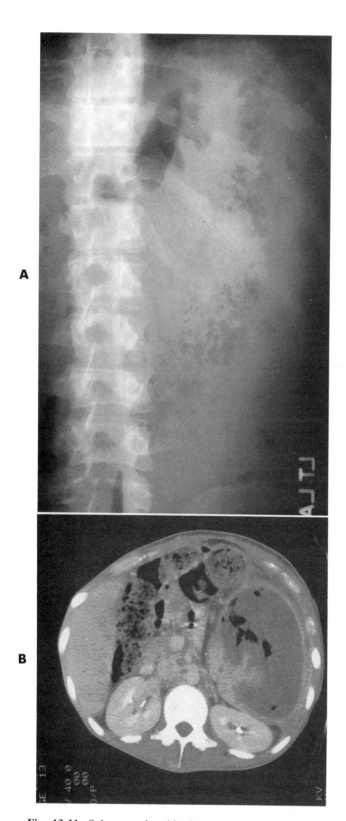

Fig. 13-11. Splenomegaly with abscess. **A,** Radiograph of 23-year-old man with melanoma shows large spleen extending to left upper pelvis. Numerous gas bubbles are seen within the spleen. **B,** CT scan shows diffuse area of low density in spleen, with multiple air bubbles proven to represent abscess.

typically CT shows a low density lesion (Fig. 13-10, *A,* and *B*) that is relatively well-defined and often displays some wall enhancement with intravenous contrast media. MRI reveals a low intensity on T1 that may have heterogeneous high signal intensity on T2 if the liquid abscess also contains fungus, calcium, or debris (Fig. 13-10, *C*). Occasionally an abscess may be multiloculated with septations and it may contain gas, as seen on a plain radiograph (Fig. 13-11). There may be layering of material of different densities within the cavity. In immune-compromised patients with lymphoma or other hematologic malignancies such as leukemia, numerous low density abscesses may be scattered throughout the spleen.[50] The size of these abscesses ranges between a few millimeters to more than 1 cm (Fig. 13-12). In most cases the infection is due to *Candida* organisms, although occasionally it is due to *Aspergillus* organisms.[50] Such patients are often treated with amphotericin, occasionally tagged with liposomes. The lesions in the liver and spleen may heal with residual calcification.[53] CT scanning is probably adequate for evaluation of such lesions. However, if MRI is done, one often sees microabscesses as areas of intermediate signal intensity in the liver and spleen. The conspicuity of detection may increase when the leukemic patient has underlying hemosiderosis from previous transfusions (Fig. 13-13).

Ultrasonography may demonstrate the splenic abscess as an area with mixed echo pattern, with septations mimicking a complicated cyst or even lymphoma or hematoma. Sonography can demonstrate disease processes extending from the splenic parenchyma to the adjacent left subphrenic and paranephric spaces.[44] In cases of candidiasis the lesion may have a bull's-eye or so-called wheel within wheel appearance (Fig. 13-14). This pattern is probably related to the presence of *Candida albicans* in the center of an abscess surrounded by inflammatory cells and fibrosis.[43] Ultrasound may also be used to guide for needle aspiration of the splenic lesion.

In sarcoidosis, about 25% of patients have hepatosplenomegaly. Splenic enlargement may be an isolated finding, without other lesions elsewhere. Occasionally, focal defects may be present (Fig. 13-15). These have been attributed to areas of sarcoid granulomas.[26] Other infectious causes of splenomegaly include malaria, infectious mononucleosis, schistosomiasis, tuberculosis, and histoplasmosis.

Hydatid disease represents 2% to 3% of inflammatory diseases of the spleen.[4] The typical picture of such disease on CT is a well-defined cystic mass in which occasionally one might see daughter cysts (Fig. 13-16). If a cyst ruptures in the gastrointestinal tract, such as in the colon, there may be gas extraluminally, within the splenic hydatid.

NEOPLASMS

Primary splenic neoplasms are rare and are usually benign conditions such as hemangioma, hamartoma, and

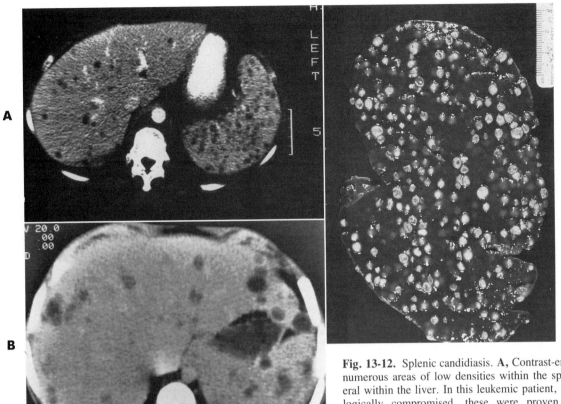

Fig. 13-12. Splenic candidiasis. **A,** Contrast-enhanced CT shows numerous areas of low densities within the spleen and also several within the liver. In this leukemic patient, who was immunologically compromised, these were proven to represent hepatosplenic abscesses from *Candida*. **B,** Another leukemic patient has larger abscesses within the liver and spleen. This patient also was immunologically compromised and had systemic candidiasis. **C,** Surgical specimen of patient with diffuse splenic candidiasis shows numerous candidal abscesses throughout the spleen.

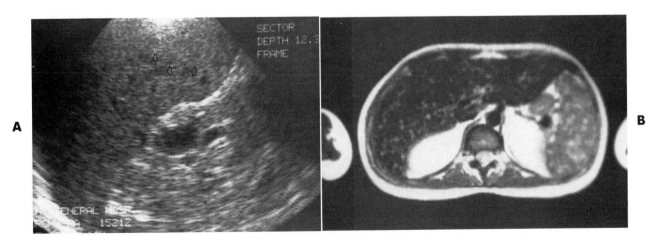

Fig. 13-13. Hepatosplenic aspergillosis. **A,** Ultrasound scan of 22-year old woman with Hodgkin's disease and on chemotherapy shows focal areas of low-intensity echoes *(open arrows)* within an enlarged spleen. **B,** On T2-weighted MR image (TR/TE, 2100/70) from a 0.5 Tesla magnet, several areas of bright signal intensity are seen in both the spleen and the liver. The diffuse low signal intensity of the liver, related to hemosiderosis, is a result of multiple transfusions.

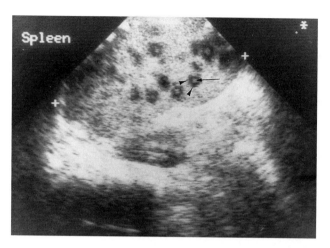

Fig. 13-14. Splenic candidiasis. Candidal abscesses in this patient's spleen are seen as "bull's eye," "target," or "wheels within wheels" lesions. The presence of *Candida albicans* in the central portions is seen as bright intensity echoes *(arrow)* surrounded by a halo of low-intensity echoes *(arrowheads)* probably caused by inflammatory cells and fibrosis.

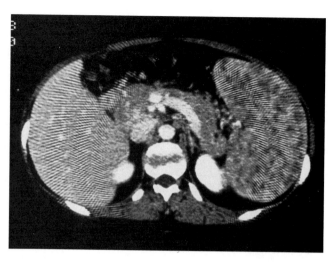

Fig. 13-15. Multiple defects are seen in this rather enlarged spleen. Patient was known to have sarcoidosis, and low-density areas seen in the spleen represent noncalcified sarcoid granulomas. Note computer artifacts in liver/spleen.

lymphangioma. Primary malignant tumors are even less common; they include angiosarcoma and lymphoma. In contrast, most common tumors of the spleen are secondary, with lymphoma being considered the most common malignant tumor of the spleen.[24]

Lymphoma. In the staging and treatment of Hodgkin's and non-Hodgkin's lymphoma, the diagnosis of splenic involvement is of considerable importance and is either microscopic or micronodular.[65] Splenic size may not change because of involvement by lymphoma. Both normal-sized and enlarged spleens can have a high rate of false-positive or false-negative diagnosis for lymphomatous infiltrate.[60] About 30% of enlarged spleens in patients with lymphoma are related to benign causes.[7] A large spleen on physical examination or on imaging study has a sensitivity of 36% and specificity of 61% in the diagnosis of splenic lymphoma.[17]

In addition to diffuse splenic infiltration, lymphoma can also involve the spleen as multiple nodules or as a single large lesion. These latter two forms of involvement are often detectable by imaging techniques.[54]

Technetium-99m sulfur colloid scintigraphy is often unreliable in evaluating the spleen, and it has an accuracy rate ranging from 54% to 64%,[56] often missing smaller lesions. Gallium-67 citrate is more specific in evaluating patients with lymphoma.[54]

Ultrasound can demonstrate splenomegaly and the presence of abnormalities within the splenic parenchyma as one or several focal areas of decreased echogenicity (Fig. 13-17). Rarely, lymphoma may be more echogenic than the surrounding normal spleen.[6] Sonography may not detect very small deposits, although in cases of splenomeg-

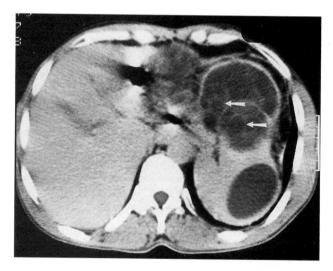

Fig. 13-16. Splenic hydatidosis. In 60-year-old man with splenomegaly, multiple hydatid cysts are seen within the spleen. In the largest, located in the anterior portion, one can see daughter cysts *(arrows)*. Another cyst is present within the left lobe of the liver. (Courtesy Dr Walter N Von Sinner, King Faisal Specialist Hospital and Research Center, Riyadh, Saudi Arabia.)

aly with marked lymphomatous involvement, the disease should be easily detectable.[27]

The size of most lymphomatous nodules in the spleen precludes detection by CT scanning. However, nodules in the proximity of 1 cm may be seen as areas of low density (Fig. 13-18, *A, B*).[12] CT studies should be done with intravenous contrast agents. The occasional pattern of early inhomogeneous splenic enhancement from bolus contrast media should be recognized and not mistaken for tumor in-

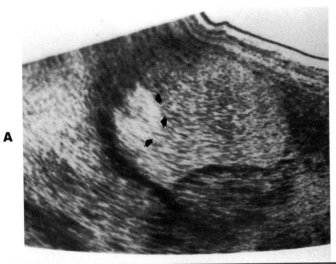

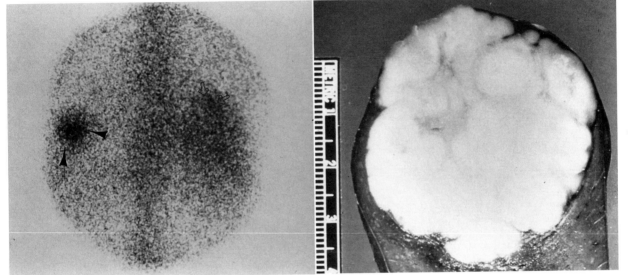

Fig. 13-17. Focal splenic lymphoma. **A,** Sagittal sonogram of spleen shows low echogenic mass in the superior aspect of the spleen *(arrows),* adjacent to the diaphragm. This 34-year-old man with right upper quadrant pain was searched and an identical lesion was seen in the upper portion of the liver. **B,** Posterior gallium-67 citrate image demonstrates two areas of increased uptake. One corresponds to the sonographic finding in **A** *(arrowheads);* the other is in the dome of the liver *(open arrows).* These were proven to represent hepatosplenic lymphoma. **C,** Surgical specimen of the spleen demonstrates the large lymphomatous deposit.

filtrate (see Fig. 13-1).[18,52] Numerous splenic lymphomatous nodules may be difficult to recognize on a T1-weighted MR image (Figs. 13-18, *C;* and 13-19, *B*). However, on T2-weighted images (Fig. 13-18, *D*), because of the short T2 relaxation time of normal spleen and long T2 relaxation time of focal lymphomatous areas, the nodules may be seen as focal high signal intensity regions (Fig. 13-19, *D*). When nodules are larger, they produce areas of low density on CT in a normal-sized or enlarged spleen (Fig. 13-19, *A*). With gadolinium enhancement (Fig. 13-19, *C*), the conspicuity of focal lesions may increase on T1-weighted images.

In Hodgkin's disease the spleen may be enlarged but not involved or may be normal sized yet infiltrated by tumor. The only way to be certain whether the spleen is involved by Hodgkin's disease is to remove it and examine it histologically, because the deposits of lymphoma may be tiny and diffuse. The presence of lymphoma in the liver almost always means that the spleen is involved as well. Therefore, a positive liver biopsy can be regarded as reflecting splenic involvement.[63]

Recent reports of the value of MRI for detection of diffuse splenic involvement by lymphoma suggest that

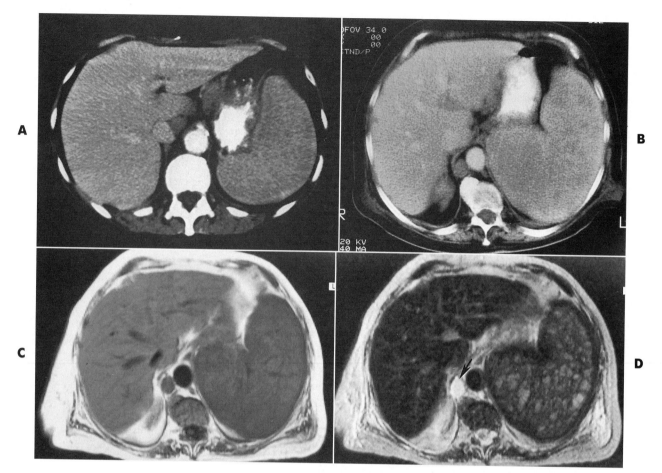

Fig. 13-18. Diffuse splenic lymphoma. **A,** On contrast-enhanced CT of patient with Hodgkin's disease and retroperitoneal adenopathy, spleen is large and contains punctate areas of low density throughout. This was proven to result from diffuse lymphomatous infiltrate. **B** to **D,** Contrast-enhanced CT scan (**B**) of 75-year-old woman with lymphoma shows inhomogeneous splenic enhancement with several areas of low density. On T1-weighted MR image (**C**), inhomogeneity of signal may be recognizable; however, no definite focal lesion is seen. On T2-weighted image (**D**), numerous focal areas of high signal intensity are present throughout the spleen. In addition to numerous focal lymphomatous infiltrates, patient also has splenomegaly, with an enlarged right retrocrural lymph node *(arrow)* displaying bright signal intensity on T2. (**B** to **D** courtesy Dr. Pablo Ros, University of Florida, Gainesville, Fla.)

MR imaging is not reliable, since both normal spleen and lymphomatous tissue may display similar signal intensities.[39,65] In cases of nodular involvement, conventional spin echo shows areas of low to intermediate signal intensity in short repetition and echo time (TR/TE) T1-weighted images. Because of prolongation of T2 relaxation, the signal intensity becomes bright on long TR/TE images (Fig. 13-19). Gadolinium may demonstrate minimal enhancement of such lesions. Super-paramagnetic iron oxide can significantly increase the rate of detectability of splenic involvement by lymphoma.[64] This contrast agent, which has a specific biodistribution to reticuloendothelial cells, does not concentrate in malignant tissues. Hence in cases of diffuse splenic involvement, no agent concentrates within the spleen. In cases of focal lesions, by concentrating in the normal parenchyma, ferrite (particulate iron oxide) effectively shortens the T2 of normal splenic tissue without altering the tissue characteristics of lymphomatous deposits or other focal splenic abnormalities.[64,66]

Hemangioma. Hemangioma is the most common primary neoplasm of the spleen.[47] It is usually a small tumor but sometimes attains a large size. Hemangiomas can be multiple (Fig. 13-20), so-called splenic hemangiomatosis, and occasionally are a part of generalized angiomatosis, with involvement of multiple organs by hemangiomas or lymphangiomas.[45]

Solitary splenic hemangioma is usually asymptomatic. Forty-five percent are associated with splenomegaly and 30% are found at autopsy. It has been reported that ap-

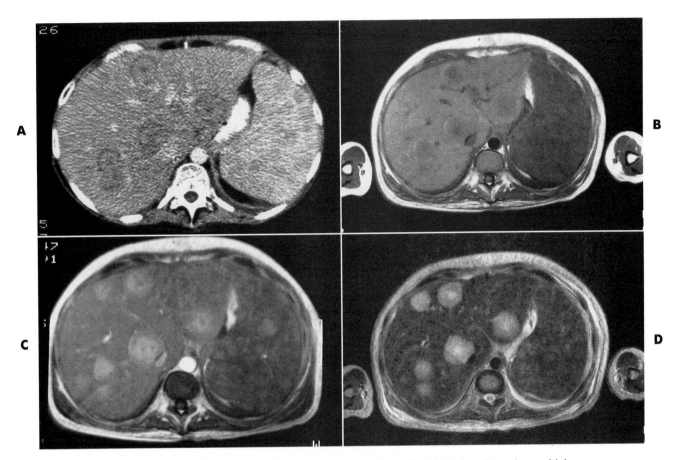

Fig. 13-19. Nodular splenic lymphoma. **A,** Patient with non-Hodgkin's lymphoma has multiple larger lymphomatous nodules in liver and spleen. Contrast-enhanced CT shows splenic lesions as areas of low density, whereas hepatic lesions are shown as target lesions. **B,** In a T1-weighted axial MR image (TR/TE, 650/25), splenic lesions are not well identified; however, inhomogeneity of signal within the splenic parenchyma is noticeable. Liver lesions are quite visible. **C,** Gadolinium-enhanced T1-weighted image (TR/TE, 650/25) increases conspicuity of lesion identified within the spleen and liver. Both organs display enhancement of the focal lesions, seen as areas of increased signal intensity. **D,** T2-weighted MR image (TR/TE, 2200/90) shows splenic lesions as numerous ill-defined bright signal-intensity areas.

proximately one-fourth of patients with splenic hemangiomas are brought to the emergency room because of rupture of the tumor.[25]

In sonographic studies the lesions are either echogenic (Fig. 13-20) or hypoechoic. CT features of splenic hemangioma may be similar to those seen in the liver. The lesion is hypodense or isodense to the normal spleen on noncontrast study and becomes either isodense or hyperdense (Fig. 13-20, *C*) following contrast agent injection (Fig. 13-21). The lesion may demonstrate a multicystic pattern, with areas of calcification and solid tissue. The solid portion enhances following contrast agent injection.[47]

MRI of splenic hemangioma often demonstrates features similar to hepatic hemangioma. The lesion is hypointense on T1-weighted and hyperintense on T2-weighted images (Fig. 13-20). This is due to the lack of solid tissue

architecture and the increased water content of these lesions, resulting in long T1 and T2 relaxation values.[33]

Hamartoma. These tumors, often incidentally found at autopsy, have been given different names, such as splenoma, fibrosplenoma, splenoadenoma, and nodular hyperplasia of the spleen. They are more common in women. Large hamartomas may cause vague left upper quadrant pain or may be found as palpable masses. They are usually solitary and may contain foci of hemosiderosis, calcification, and fibrosis.

A hamartoma is vascular as visualized in angiography and radionuclide studies.[58] CT scanning may show the lesion to be solid and isodense or hyperdense to the spleen (Fig. 13-22) or to have both cystic and solid components. It may be difficult to separate the tumor from the adjacent splenic parenchyma on conventional spin echo imaging.

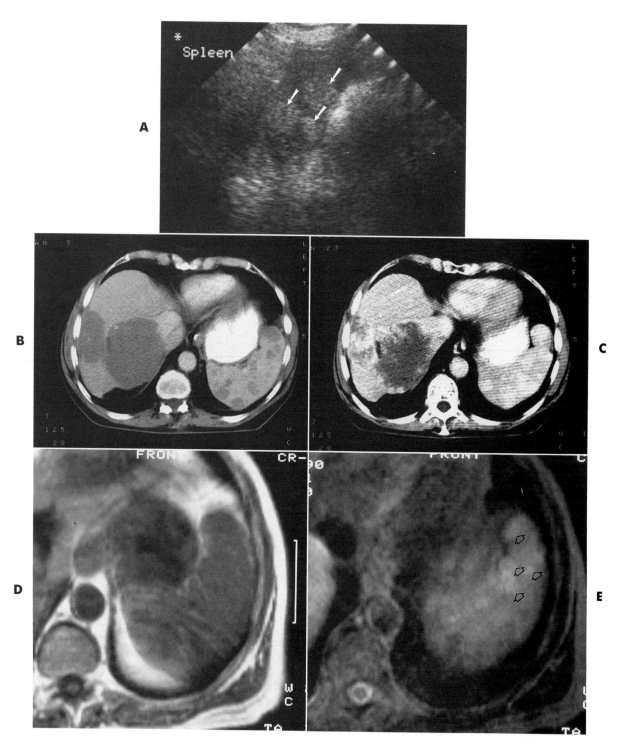

Fig. 13-20. Splenic hemangioma. This 78-year-old woman was examined because of the discovery of multiple splenic and hepatic lesions on routine abdominal sonogram. **A,** Ultrasound scan of the spleen shows multiple echogenic lesions; three of them are seen *(arrows)* on this longitudinal image. **B,** CT of the upper abdomen during early phase of contrast agent injection shows multiple splenic lesions and two large hepatic lesions. **C,** Repeat CT at the same level during late phase of contrast agent injection shows hepatic lesions partially filled in and splenic lesions completely filled in with contrast agent. **D,** On T1-weighted images (TR/TE, 600/25), splenic lesions are not conspicuous and appear to be isointense to adjacent normal parenchyma. **E,** On T2-weighted image (TR/TE, 2000/90), splenic lesions are seen as areas of increased signal intensity *(open arrows)*. A follow-up CT scan in 1 year showed no change, and these were presumed to represent multiple splenic and hepatic hemangiomas.

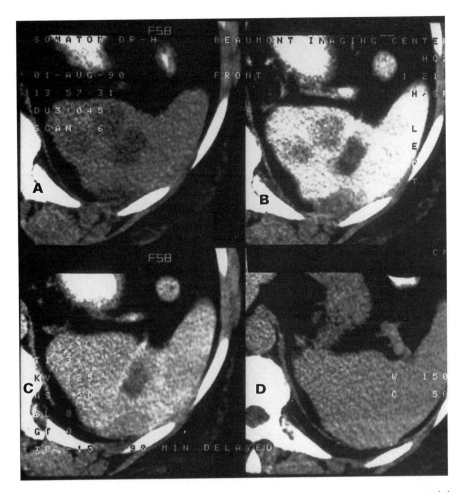

Fig. 13-21. Splenic hemangioma. Serial CT images during and after bolus contrast agent injection show at least four areas of low density in the spleen, best seen on the unenhanced image **(A)** and immediately during bolus injection **(B).** Ten minutes after contrast agent injection **(C),** most of these lesions were isodense to the spleen. Within 90 minutes **(D),** all lesions were isodense. This pattern, which also has been described in hepatic hemangiomas, is thought to be characteristic of multiple splenic hemangiomas.

However, when a hamartoma contains areas of calcification or hemosiderosis, it can be seen as a mass containing regions of low signal on MR images.

Metastasis. The spleen is not a common target for metastatic disease; however, carcinoma of the lung, breast, gastrointestinal tract, ovary, and prostate as well as melanoma may metastasize to the spleen.[15,28] Most metastases to the spleen are hematogenous: however, primary carcinoma of the pancreas, left kidney, splenic flexure of the colon, and stomach may directly extend into the splenic hilum.

Splenic metastasis is often evaluated by imaging modalities such as radionuclide study, sonography, CT, or MRI.[54,57] Filling defects in the spleen as shown in scintigraphy may appear as hypoechoic or echogenic lesions in ultrasound studies. CT scanning shows hypodense lesions

(Fig. 13-23) that may enhance following contrast injection. Contrast media are often necessary to illustrate the lesions, since the splenic metastasis may occasionally be isodense to the normal spleen on a nonenhanced CT study. CT scanning or sonography may also be used as a guide for biopsy of splenic metastasis. MRI usually shows the metastatic deposit as an area of low signal intensity on T1-weighted images, which becomes hyperintense on T2-weighted images. In cases of old hemorrhage within the metastatic deposit, the lesion displays low signal intensity on T2-weighted scans (Fig. 13-23, *C*). MRI with superparamagnetic iron oxide has proven to be superior to CT or conventional unenhanced spin echo imaging for determination of the size and number of splenic metastases (Fig. 13-24).[64]

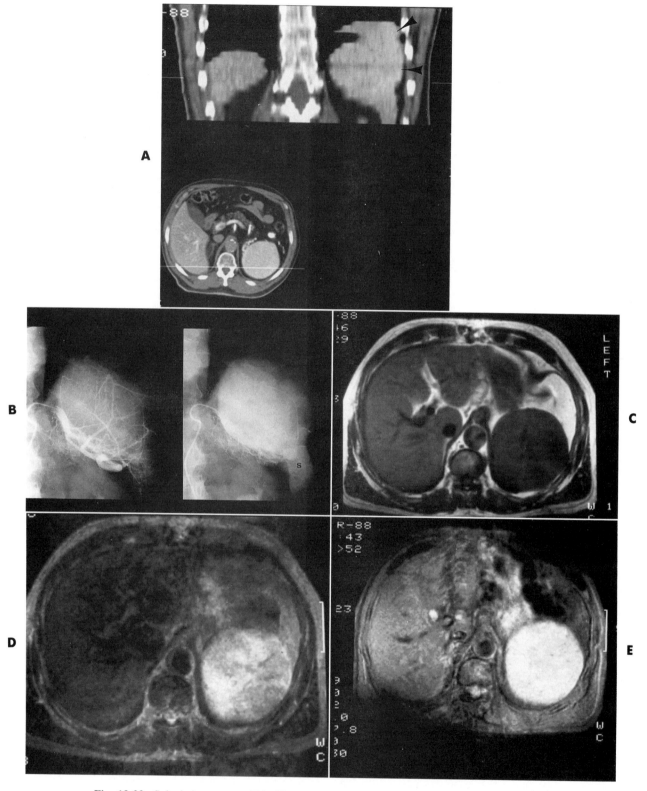

Fig. 13-22. Splenic hamartoma. This 68-year-old man was examined because of vague left upper quadrant pain. **A,** Intraarterial CT, with contrast injection in the celiac artery, demonstrates a globular appearance of the upper portion of the spleen. This is best seen on coronal reformation, in which a large bulge appears in the upper lateral portion of the spleen (*arrowheads*). Because of the suspected splenic mass, an angiogram was performed. **B,** Selective splenic arteriogram demonstrates that the vascular mass originates from the spleen. A normal portion of the spleen *(s)* is seen in the more caudal aspect. **C,** T1-weighted MR image (TR/TE, 550/22), shows round mass in left upper quadrant, with some vascular channels. **D,** On T2-weighted image (TR/TE, 2500/80), the mass displays some heterogeneous signal intensity, but overall its signal intensity increases in comparison to T1. **E,** On inversion recovery image (TR/TE, 500/22, TI, 99), signal intensity of this mass increases significantly. Surgery proved this to be a large splenic hamartoma.

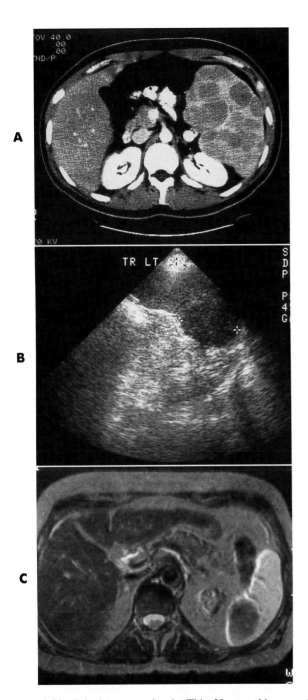

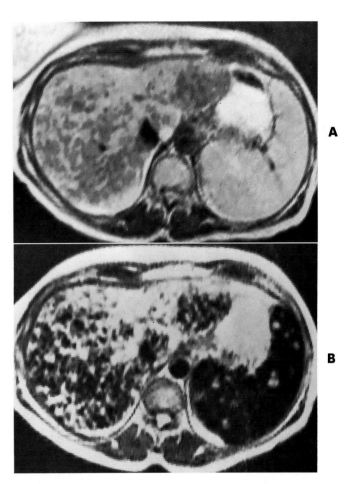

Fig. 13-24. Hepatosplenic metastasis. **A,** On T2-weighted MR image, multiple hepatic metastases are seen as areas of high signal intensity. However, spleen appears to be normal. **B,** Following intravenous administration of superparamagnetic iron oxide, because of T2 shortening induced in normal spleen by the contrast agent, splenic lesions are now identifiable and hepatic lesions better seen (From Hahn PF, Stark DD: MR imaging of the biliary system, spleen, and gastrointestinal tract. In Stark DD, Bradley WG, eds: *Magnetic resonance imaging,* ed 2, St Louis, 1991, Mosty–Year Book.)

Fig. 13-23. Splenic metastasis. **A,** This 23-year-old man with melanoma was found to have splenomegaly. Axial contrast-enhanced CT scan of the midabdomen shows multiple low-density lesions throughout the enlarged spleen. Patient received embolization of the spleen and later developed abscesses. **B,** Sonogram of 66-year-old woman who had been treated for cervical carcinoma and who had history of left upper quadrant pain shows a focal abnormal area of mixed echoes *(cursors)* in lower pole of spleen. **C,** On T2-weighted (TR/TE, 2200/90) image, lesion is of low signal intensity, probably because of old hemorrhage. Metastasis from carcinoma of cervix was proven by biopsy.

MISCELLANEOUS CONDITIONS

A splenic cyst is a benign condition, pathologically classified as a true cyst (epithelial) or pseudocyst. The former is usually congenital (Fig. 13-25), whereas the latter is secondary to trauma and is formed as a result of hemorrhage (see Fig 13-4, *B*). Splenic cysts may be single or multiple and often contain areas of calcification in their periphery (Fig. 13-26). On CT splenic cyst is seen as a well-defined low density mass, occasionally with septations (Fig. 13-25, *A*). MRI shows the simple cyst as a low signal mass on T1-weighted scans that has a bright signal on T2-weighted scans (Fig. 13-25, *B* to *D*).

The spleen may be involved in many other conditions, generally of systemic nature. Splenic enlargement has

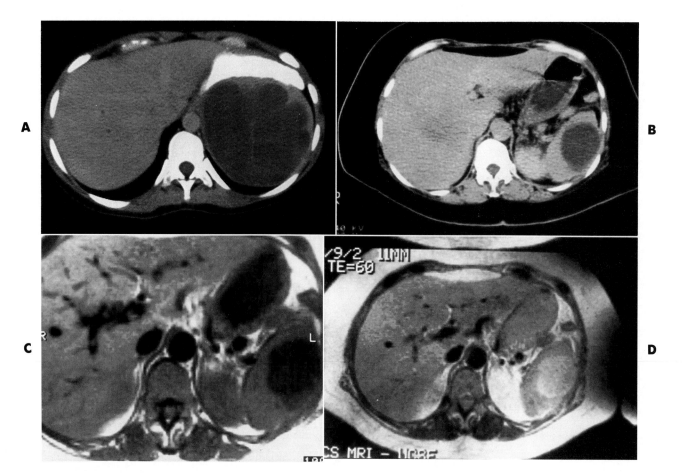

Fig. 13-25. Splenic cyst. **A,** CT scan of 43-year-old woman with left upper quadrant pain demonstrates a large low-density mass in left upper quadrant with lobulated anterior borders and internal septations. After diagnosis of splenic cyst, mass was percutaneously aspirated to decrease the patient's pain. However, shortly after aspiration, the size of cyst was the same on repeat CT scan. Eventually patient had splenectomy, and diagnosis of epithelial splenic cyst was confirmed. **B to D,** Enhanced CT scan shows a well-defined splenic cyst found incidentally in a woman. T1-weighted (TR/TE, 600/25) MR image (**C**) shows cyst as a well-defined low signal intensity lesion. **D,** On T2-weighted (TR/TE, 2000/60) image (**D**), cyst is of homogeneous high signal intensity. (**B to D** are courtesy of Dr. Kostaki Bis, William Beaumont Hospital.)

many underlying causes, including poor venous return (congestive splenomegaly), storage diseases, infectious causes, hemolytic anemias, collagen vascular diseases, extramedullary hematopoiesis, and neoplastic conditions. Leukemia (Fig. 13-27, *A*) and lymphoma are the leading causes of splenomegaly.[9] In most of these conditions, splenic enlargement is not associated with any focal lesion. However, as in lymphoma, leukemia may produce focal or diffuse areas of splenic infiltrate (Fig. 13-27, *B* to

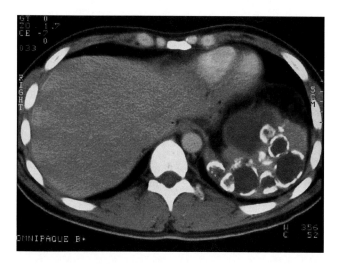

Fig. 13-26. Calcified splenic cysts. Multiple low-density lesions containing peripheral calcification are seen throughout the spleen. At splenectomy, multiple calcified splenic cysts were confirmed.

D). In congestive splenomegaly, such as with portal hypertension, MRI may show evidence of increased T1 and T2 relaxation times, probably as a result of increased blood content.[59] The presence of multiple low-intensity spots in the spleen in patients with portal hypertension is usually related to siderotic nodules (Gamna-Gandy nodules), which are best seen on examination with high field magnets.[38] The low intensity of these nodules is due to the paramagnetic effect of hemosiderin.

Amyloidosis is a rare condition characterized by deposition of extracellular fibrous protein in one or more sites. The liver is often involved, but splenic involvement is rare. If massive amyloid deposition occurs, the patient may experience spontaneous splenic rupture (Fig. 13-28).

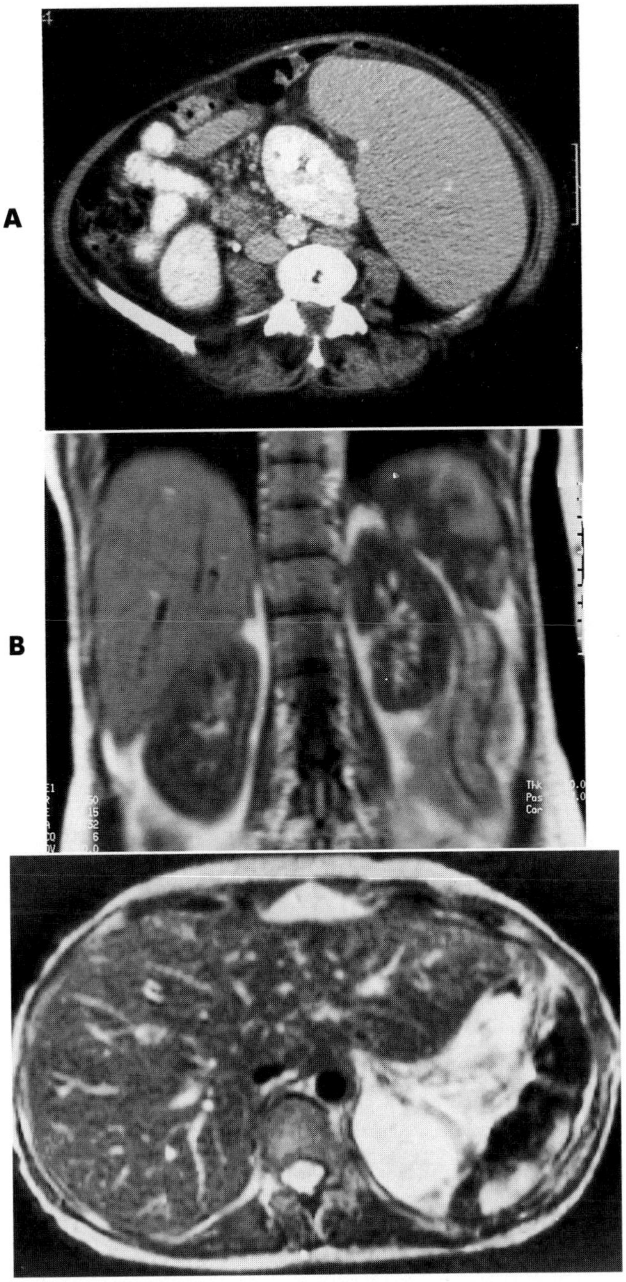

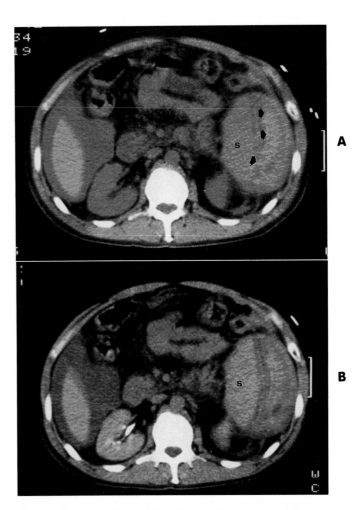

Fig. 13-27. Spleen and leukemia. **A,** This 64-year-old woman with fourth stage chronic lymphocytic leukemia and bone marrow involvement was treated for gastrointestinal bleeding, congestive heart failure, and splenomegaly. Abdominal CT shows enlarged spleen extended from left upper quadrant into the left iliac fossa, displacing the left kidney anteriorly. Splenic enlargement is homogeneous without any focal lesion. **B,** In a 41-year-old leukemic patient, spleen is not enlarged but displays a relatively well-defined area of intermediate signal intensity on T1-weighted image (TR/TE, 550/15). **C,** On axial T2-weighted image (TR/TE, 2000/90), the area with hemorrhagic leukemic infiltrate is in the periphery of the spleen of high signal intensity. (**B** and **C** courtesy of Dr. Pablo Ros, University of Florida, Gainesville, Fla.)

Fig. 13-28. Amyloidosis. This 49-year-old man with end-stage renal disease was treated for severe onset of left upper quadrant pain and a syncopal episode. **A,** On unenhanced CT, higher density subcapsular hematoma is seen lateral to the spleen *(s)*. There is a large amount of intraperitoneal fluid. **B,** On contrast-enhanced CT, normal splenic parenchyma *(s)* enhances slightly more than the adjacent bleeding. Patient had splenectomy, and diagnosis of amyloidosis with spontaneous splenic rupture was confirmed at surgery.

REFERENCES

1. Adler DD, Glazer GM, Aisen AM: MRI of the spleen: normal appearance and findings in sickle-cell anemia, *AJR* 147:843-845, 1986.

2. Ambriz P, Muñóz R, Quintanar E et al: Accessory spleen compromising response to splenectomy for idiopathic thrombocytopenic purpura, *Radiology* 155:793-796, 1985.

3. Balcar I, Seltzer SE, Davis S, Geller SC: CT patterns of splenic infarction: a clinical and experimental study, *Radiology* 151:723-729, 1984.

4. Bonakdarpour A: Echinococcus disease: report of 112 cases from Iran and a review of 611 cases from the United States. *AJR* 99:660-667, 1967.

5. Buntain WL, Gould HR, Maull KI: Predictability of splenic salvage by computed tomography, *J Trauma* 28:24-34, 1986.

6. Carroll BA, Ta HN: The ultrasonic appearance of extranodal abdominal lymphoma, *Radiology* 136:419-425, 1980.

7. Castellino RA: Imaging techniques for staging abdominal Hodgkin's disease, *Cancer Treat Rep* 66:697-700, 1982.

8. Cohen BA, Mitty HA, Mendelson DS: Computed tomography of splenic infarction, *J Comput Assist Tomogr* 8:167-168, 1984.

9. Crosby HW: Hypersplenism. In Williams WJ, Beutler E, Erslev AJ, Lictman MA, eds: *Hematology*, ed 3, New York, 1983, McGraw-Hill, pp 242, 660-666.

10. Delany HM, Jason RS: *Abdominal trauma: surgical and radiological diagnosis*, New York, 1981, Springer-Verlag.

11. Douglas GJ, Simpson S: The conservative management of splenic trauma, *J Pediatr Surg* 6:565-570, 1971.

12. Earl HM, Sutcliffe SBJ, Fry IK et al: Computerized tomographic (CT) abdominal scanning in Hodgkin's disease, *Clin Radiol* 31:149-153, 1980.

13. Eraklis AJ, Filler RM: Splenectomy in childhood: a review of 1413 cases, *J Pediatr Surg* 7:382-388, 1972.

14. Federle MP, Griffith B, Minagi H, Jeffrey RB Jr: Splenic trauma: evaluation with CT, *Radiology* 162:69-71, 1987.

15. Federle M, Moss AA: Computer tomography of the spleen, *CRC Crit Rev Diagn Imaging* 19:1-16, 1983.

16. Freund R, Pichl J, Heyder N et al: Splenic abscess—clinical symptoms and diagnostic possibilities, *Am J Gastroenterol* 77:35-38, 1982.

17. Glatstein E, Guernsey JM, Rosenberg SA et al: The value of laparotomy and splenectomy in the staging of Hodgkin disease, *Cancer* 24:709-718, 1969.

18. Glazer GM, Axel L, Goldberg HI, Moss AA: Dynamic CT of the normal spleen, *AJR* 116:651-656, 1981.

19. Goerg C, Schwerk WB: Splenic infarction: sonographic patterns, diagnosis, follow-up, and complications, *Radiology* 174:803-807, 1990.

20. Gomori JM, Grossman RI, Goldberg HI et al: Intracranial hematoma imaging by high field MR, *Radiology* 157:87-93, 1985.

21. Gordon DH, Burrell MI, Levin DC et al: Wandering spleen—the radiological and clinical spectrum, *Radiology* 125:39-46, 1977.

22. Gottschalk A, Potchen J: *Golden's diagnostic radiology section to diagnostic nuclear medicine*, Baltimore, 1976, Williams & Wilkins.

23. Hahn PF, Weissleder R, Stark DD, et al: MR imaging of focal splenic tumors, *AJR* 150:823-827, 1988.

24. Horm JW, Asire AJ, Young JL, Pollack ES: *Cancer incidence and mortality in the United States*, NIH Pub No 85-1837, Bethesda, Md, 1985, National Cancer Institute.

25. Hushi EA: The clinical course of splenic hemangioma, *Arch Surg* 83:681-685, 1961.

26. Iko BO, Chunwuba C, Anderson JE et al: Multifocal defects and splenomegaly in sarcoidosis: a new scintigraphic pattern, *J Natl Med Assoc* 74:739-741, 1982.

27. King DJ, Dawson AA, Bayliss AP: The value of ultrasonic scanning of the spleen in lymphoma, *Clin Radiol* 36:473-474, 1985.

28. Kissane JM, ed: *Anderson's Pathology*, ed 9, vol 2, St. Louis, 1990, Mosby–Year Book.

29. Koehler RE: Spleen. In Lee JKT, Sagel SS, Stanley RJ, eds: *Computed body tomography with MRI correlations*, New York, 1990, Raven Press, pp 521-538.

30. Lee VW, Caldarone AG, Falk RH et al: Amyloidosis of heart and liver: comparison of ^{99m}Tc-pyrophosphate and dyphosphonate for detection, *Radiology* 148:239-242, 1983.

31. Lerner RM, Spataro RF: Splenic abscess: percutaneous drainage, *Radiology* 153:643-645, 1984.

32. Levine E, Wetzel LH: Splenic trauma during colonoscopy: report of a case, *AJR* 149:939-940, 1987.

33. Levine E, Wetzel LH, Neff JR: MR imaging and CT of extrahepatic cavernous hemangiomas, *AJR* 147:1299-1304, 1986.

34. Levy JM, Wasserman PI, Weiland DE: Nonsuppurative gas formation in the spleen after transcatheter splenic infarction, *Radiology* 139:375-376, 1981.

35. MacPherson AIS, Richmond J, Stuart AE: *The spleen*, Springfield, Ill, 1973, Charles C Thomas.

36. Mahon PA, Sutton JE Jr: Nonoperative management of adult splenic injury due to blunt trauma: a warning, *Am J Surg* 149:716-721, 1985.

37. Miller FJ, Rothermel FJ, O'Neil MF, Shochat SJ: Clinical and roentgenographic findings in splenic abscess, *Arch Surg* 111:1156-1159, 1976.

38. Minami M, Itai Y, Ohtomo K et al: Siderotic nodulus in the spleen: MR imaging of portal hypertension, *Radiology* 172:681-684, 1989.

39. Mirowitz SA, Brown JJ, Lee JKT, Heiken JP: Dynamic gadolinium-enhanced MR imaging of the spleen: normal enhancement patterns and evaluation of splenic lesions, *Radiology* 179:681-686, 1991.

40. Muhletaler C, Gerlock AJ Jr, Goncharenko V et al: Gastric varices secondary to splenic vein occlusion: radiographic diagnosis and clinical significance, 132:593-598, 1979.

41. Nemcek AA Jr, Miller FH, Fitzgeral SW: Acute torsion of a wandering spleen: diagnosis by CT and duplex Doppler and color flow sonography, *AJR* 157:307-309, 1991.

42. Pappas D, Mirvis SE, Crepps JT: Splenic trauma: false-negative CT diagnosis in cases of delayed rupture, *AJR* 149:727-728, 1987.

43. Pastakia B, Shawker TH, Thaler M et al: Hepatosplenic candidiasis: wheels within wheels, *Radiology* 166:417-421, 1988.

44. Pawar S, Kay CJ, Gonzalez R et al: Sonography of splenic abscess, *AJR* 138:259-262, 1982.

45. Pinkhas J, Djaldetti M, deVries A et al: Diffuse angiomatosis with hypersplenism: splenectomy followed by polycythemia, *Am J Med* 45:795-801, 1968.

46. Resciniti A, Fink MP, Raptopoulos V et al: Nonoperative treatment of adult splenic trauma: development of a computed tomographic scoring system that detects appropriate candidates for expectant management, *J Trauma* 28:828-831, 1988.

47. Ros PR, Moser RP Jr, Dachman AH, et al: Hemangioma of the spleen: radiologic-pathologic correlation in ten cases, *Radiology* 162:73-77, 1987.

48. Rose V, Izukawa T, Moes CAF: Syndromes of asplenia and polysplenia: a review of cardiac and non-cardiac malformations in 60 cases with special reference to diagnosis and prognosis, *Br Heart J* 37:840-852, 1975.

49. Scatamacchia SA, Raptopoulos V, Fink MP, Silva WE: Splenic trauma in adults: impact of CT grading on management, *Radiology* 171:725-729, 1989.

50. Shirkhoda A: CT findings in hepatosplenic and renal candidiasis, *J Comput Assist Tomogr* 11:795-798, 1987.

51. Shirkhoda A: Pitfalls in abdominal and pelvic CT. In *Radiologic oncology of the abdomen and pelvis: an atlas and text*, Chicago, 1988, Year Book Medical Publishers, pp 1244-1252.

52. Shirkhoda A: Diagnostic pitfalls in abdominal CT, *Radiographics* 11:969-1002, 1991.

53. Shirkhoda A, Lopez-Berestein G, Holbert JM, Luna MA: Hepatosplenic fungal infection: CT and pathologic evaluation after

treatment with liposomal amphotericin B, *Radiology* 159:349-353, 1986.

54. Shirkhoda A, McCartney WH, Staab EV et al: Imaging of the spleen: a proposed algorithm, *AJR* 135:195-198, 1980.
55. Shirkhoda A, Wallace S, Sokhandan M: Computed tomography and ultrasonography in splenic infarction, *J Can Assoc Radiol* 36:29-33, 1985.
56. Silverman S, DeNardo GL, Glatstein E et al: Evaluation of the liver and spleen in Hodgkin's disease. II. The value of splenic scintigraphy, *Am J Med* 52:362-366, 1972.
57. Siniluoto T, Paivansalo M, Lahde S: Ultrasonography of splenic metastases, *Acta Radiol* 30(5):463-466, 1989.
58. Spalding RM, Jennings CV, Yam LT: Splenic hamartoma, *Br J Radiol* 53:1197-1200, 1980.
59. Stark DD, Goldberg, Moss AA, Bass NM: Chronic liver disease: evaluation by magnetic resonance, *Radiology* 150:149-151, 1984.
60. Strijk SP, Wagener DJT, Bogman MJJT et al: The spleen in Hodgkin disease: diagnostic value of CT, *Radiology* 154:753-757, 1985.
61. Takayasu K, Moriyama N, Muramatsu Y et al: Splenic infarction: a complication of transcatheter hepatic arterial embolization for liver malignancies, *Radiology* 151:371-375, 1984.
62. Vibhakar SD, Bellon EM: The bare area of the spleen: a constant CT feature of the ascitic abdomen, *AJR* 1412:953-955, 1984.
63. Warnke R, Dunnick NR et al: Clinical and surgical (laparotomy) evaluation of patients with non-Hodgkin's lymphomas, *Cancer Treat Rep* 61:1977, 1981.
64. Weissleder R, Elizondo G, Stark DD et al: The diagnosis of splenic lymphoma by MR imaging: value of superparamagnetic iron oxide, *AJR* 152:175-180, 1989.
65. Weissleder R, Hahn PF, Stark DD: MRI of the spleen. In Margulis AR, Burhenne JH, eds: *Alimentary tract radiology,* ed 4, St. Louis, 1988, CV Mosby, pp 1435-1448.
66. Weissleder R, Hahn PF, Stark DD et al: Superparamagnetic iron oxide: enhanced detection of focal splenic tumors with MR imaging, *Radiology* 169:399-403, 1988.
67. Wing VW, Federle MP, Morris JA Jr et al: The clinical impact of CT for blunt abdominal trauma, *AJR* 145:1191-1194, 1985.

Chapter 14

GASTROINTESTINAL TRACT: STOMACH, SMALL BOWEL, AND COLON

Sharon S. Burton

Radiologic evaluation of the gastrointestinal (GI) tract traditionally has been performed using barium as a contrast agent to opacify the bowel lumen. By this method, diagnoses are based on alterations in the mucosal lining, contour, and motility of the bowel. Clinical trials indicate that computed tomography (CT) of the GI tract is useful for detecting bowel wall thickening caused by inflammation or tumor, as well as for evaluating local disease extension and metastatic disease.[2,17] High resolution CT scanners with short scan times, combined with effective contrast agents for bowel opacification, provide optimal CT imaging of the GI tract. CT is now commonly used for diagnosis, staging, and therapeutic intervention in patients with GI disorders.

Magnetic resonance imaging (MRI) of the GI tract is still in the developmental stage. Although MRI has the potential advantages of multiplanar imaging and improved tissue contrast, technical problems with motion artifacts and adequate bowel opacification limit its usefulness for GI tract imaging. Applications of MRI in the GI tract include imaging of congenital anomalies such as esophageal duplications and malrotation, inflammatory bowel disease, and neoplasms. These topics are presented in this chapter. Chapter 18, on pediatric MRI, covers the use of MRI for evaluation of anorectal anomalies.

COMPARISON OF CT AND MRI

The primary advantages of MRI in the GI tract are multiplanar imaging including coronal and sagittal planes, lack of ionizing radiation or the need for iodinated contrast, and fewer artifacts from surgical clips. The primary limitations of MRI include motion artifacts related to respiratory and peristaltic motion and lack of an adequate, universally available bowel contrast agent.

Even if motion artifacts are eliminated on MRI scans by glucagon or rapid imaging, a primary advantage of CT over MRI is bowel opacification.[8] In a study comparing CT with MRI for detection of hepatic and extrahepatic lesions in patients with malignancy, CT alone detected 12 of 16 extrahepatic lesions. Failure of MRI scans to detect tumors was due to poor contrast between the extrahepatic tumor and adjacent bowel and stomach in five of seven cases. Although many oral contrast agents are under investigation for use in MRI to improve differentiation of normal and pathologic conditions in the bowel, no ideal contrast agent is available for universal use at this time.

Other advantages of CT for GI tract imaging include improved spatial resolution, generally shorter scan times, lower cost, and widespread availability. Considering all factors, CT is currently the preferred modality for cross-sectional imaging of the GI tract.

TECHNIQUE
Gastrointestinal contrast agents for MRI

A bowel contrast agent is needed to better delineate the normal bowel wall, distinguish bowel from other structures, and demonstrate pathologic lesions in the abdomen and pelvis. When the lumen is not distended, the bowel wall appears artificially thickened. Collapsed and unopacified loops of bowel have intermediate signal intensity that cannot be distinguished from the normal pancreas, lymph nodes, and many soft tissue masses in the abdomen (Fig. 14-1, *A*) or pelvis (Fig. 14-2, *A*). Gastric or enteric fluid produces high signal intensity on images weighted toward the spin-spin or transverse relaxation time (T2), which contributes to artifacts and reduces image quality (Fig.

14-3, *A* and *B*). High signal intensity in bowel loops may mimic or obscure pathologic processes in the abdomen or pelvis (Fig. 14-4, *A* and *B*). Although fecal material mixed with gas in the colon provides a fairly effective natural contrast agent for marking colonic loops, collapsed colon devoid of fecal content is not easily distinguishable from other normal structures or adjacent collapsed small bowel (Fig. 14-1, *A*).

One of the most active areas of research in abdominal MRI concerns GI contrast agents. Although many potential contrast agents have proved to be safe with adequate levels of patient acceptance and efficacy, no ideal GI contrast agent is commercially available at this time for use in MRI. Agents currently being investigated are classified

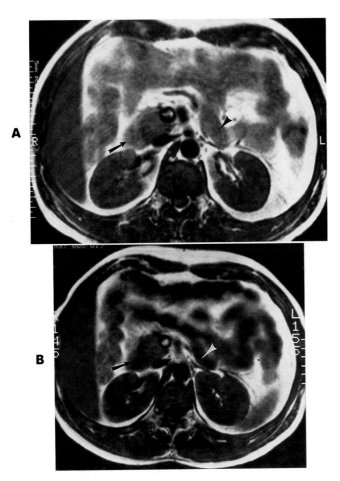

Fig. 14-1. Oral contrast agent (barium) in the upper abdomen. **A,** Axial T1-weighted image (T1WI) before contrast agent ingestion. Duodenum *(arrow)* and jejunum are collapsed, show intermediate signal intensity, and are poorly delineated from collapsed ascending and transverse colon. Adenopathy or masses may have similar signal characteristics. Structure anterior to the left kidney *(arrowhead)* could be the pancreas or bowel. **B,** Axial T1WI after barium administration. Excellent delineation of duodenum *(arrow);* jejunum and colon are seen with low signal intensity in bowel lumen. There is clearly no mass or adenopathy, and the structure anterior to the left kidney is a loop of opacified jejunum *(arrowhead).*

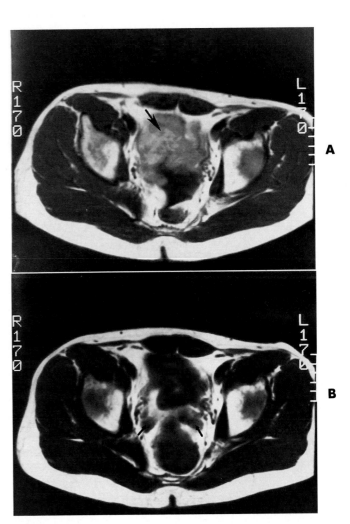

Fig. 14-2. Barium administered orally and rectally for pelvic imaging. **A,** Axial T1WI before contrast agent ingestion. Small bowel loops *(arrow)* are collapsed in the pelvis, show intermediate signal intensity, and are poorly delineated from adjacent, posterior structures. **B,** Axial T1WI after barium administration. Scan at same level after contrast agent administration shows low signal intensity in small bowel lumen, clearly defining margins of bowel. Rectal contrast agent produces rectal distension, making normal seminal vesicles visible *(arrows).*

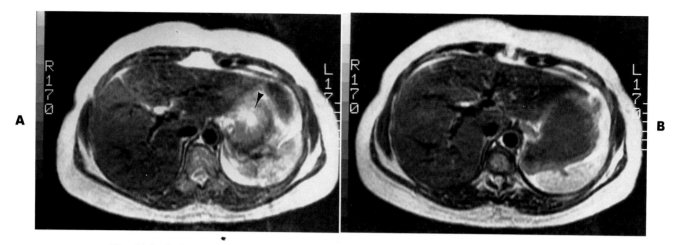

Fig. 14-3. Oral contrast agent (barium) used for gastric delineation. **A,** Axial T2-weighted image (T2WI) before barium is given. Stomach *(arrowhead)* is collapsed, making walls appear thickened. Gastric fluid has high signal intensity, which can contribute to artifacts. Margins of the spleen are not well defined. **B,** Axial T2WI after barium is given. Stomach is distended, and intraluminal contrast has low signal intensity. Splenic margins are better defined.

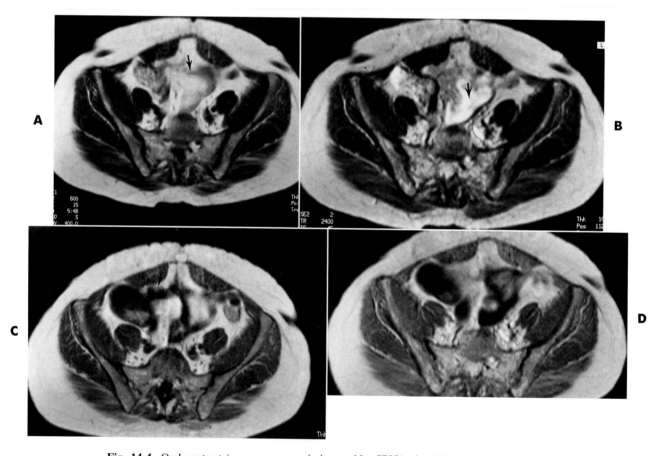

Fig. 14-4. Oral contrast (superparamagnetic iron oxide, SPIO). **A,** Axial T1WI before ingestion of SPIO. Small bowel is not distended and is ill defined *(arrow)*. **B,** Axial T2WI before ingestion of SPIO. Fluid in small bowel lumen *(arrow)* has high signal intensity, which can mimic or obscure a mass or abnormal fluid collection. **C,** Axial T1WI after SPIO ingestion. Small bowel is moderately distended with low intraluminal signal intensity. Terminal ileum *(arrow)* is well defined. **D,** Axial T2WI after ingestion of SPIO. Intra-luminal contrast agent maintains low signal intensity with good definition of bowel loops. There is no mass or pelvic fluid collection.

into four groups based on their effect on intraluminal contrast and degree of mixing with bowel contents: miscible and immiscible agents with a positive contrast effect, and miscible and immiscible agents with a negative contrast effect.[53] These are reviewed briefly here; Chapter 6, on contrast agents, contains a more complete discussion.

Miscible agents with positive contrast effects. Gadopentetate dimeglumine[26,32] and ferric ammonium citrate[64] are water soluble and mix with bowel contents to produce increased intraluminal signal intensity because of T1 (spin-lattice or longitudinal relaxation time) shortening. Gadopentetate dimeglumine has been used in combination with mannitol,[32] and in one clinical series[26] it produced uniform hyperintense bowel marking in 81% of the patients. Compared with scans made before contrast agent administration, lesion delineation was improved in 62% of the patients (Fig. 14-5, *A* and *B*). A potential disadvantage of positive contrast agents is the increase in noise or "ghosting" in the upper abdomen caused by movement of opacified bowel from respiratory motion or peristalsis. Use of intravenous scopolamine or glucagon significantly reduces artifacts from ghosting.[26]

Immiscible agents with positive contrast effects. Fats and oils do not mix with bowel contents, and because they must be given in sufficient quantity to replace intraluminal contents, there is potential for inhomogeneous bowel opacification. Combinations of agents such as corn oil emulsion mixed with Geritol have been useful in both gradient echo and spin echo imaging.[1]

Miscible agents with negative contrast effects. Superparamagnetic iron oxides, barium sulfate, oral magnetic particles,[50] and clays such as kaolin or Kaopectate[53] mix with bowel contents and produce decreased signal intensity in the bowel lumen. Superparamagnetic iron oxide (SPIO) particles have been investigated in vitro[20] and in clinical trials,[21,36] and have consistently produced a noticeable decrease in signal intensity in the bowel lumen (Fig. 14-4, *C* and *D*). Magnetic susceptibility artifacts limit the use of SPIO particles for gradient echo imaging.[34] Bowel opacification using SPIO has improved delineation of normal anatomic structures[21] and aided evaluation of pancreatic and retroperitoneal diseases.[62] Commercial availability of SPIO is contingent on completion of clinical trials.

Barium sulfate has been commercially available as a GI contrast agent for many years. In vitro and in vivo data have shown that barium sulfate provides a moderate negative contrast effect in MRI when used in concentrations of 60% to 70% weight per volume (w/v).[34,35,56] Bowel marking and delineation of normal anatomic structures in the abdomen (Figs. 14-1, *B,* and 14-3, *B*) and pelvis (Fig. 14-2, *B*) improved significantly using oral barium sulfate (60% w/v) and rectal administration of 400 ml of barium enema (Fig. 14-2, *B*).[51] High density barium (220% w/v) further reduces signal intensity and in clinical use has proved useful in delineation of the stomach and

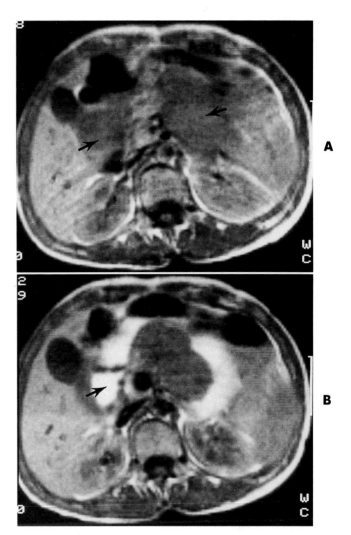

Fig. 14-5. Oral contrast (gadopentetate dimeglumine). **A,** Axial T1WI. Image of 39-year-old woman with islet cell tumor of the pancreas before contrast agent administration. Two areas of low signal intensity *(arrows)* are located medial to right lobe of the liver and ventral to the kidneys, which could represent bowel or mass lesions. **B,** Axial T1WI. With intraluminal gadopentetate dimeglumine, one "lesion" *(arrow)* is identified as the duodenum. Contrast agent in the jejunum surrounds a large mass in the pancreas. Presence of intraluminal contrast agent improved lesion delineation. (From Kaminsky S et al: *Radiology* 178:503-508, 1991.)

duodenum.[38] Other preliminary clinical studies indicate that barium is beneficial for MRI of the pancreas[4] and pelvis.[46]

Immiscible agents with negative contrast effects. Carbon dioxide gas and perfluoro-carbons do not mix with bowel contents. Carbon dioxide[64] given in the form of oral effervescent granules has no mobile protons and therefore has no signal on MRI. Its effectiveness as a contrast agent is somewhat limited because the distribution of gas in the bowel cannot be controlled. Perfluorocarbons[39,52] are tasteless, odorless liquids that decrease signal intensity by replacing bowel contents. When used in conjunction with an antiperistaltic agent, they improve delineation of the bowel and aid in detection of bowel wall abnormalities.

Glucagon

Because of the relatively long scanning times for spin echo imaging, peristalsis of bowel loops can contribute significantly to motion artifacts in the abdomen, making the margins of the bowel ill-defined and blurred.[65] Antiperistaltic agents such as scopolamine[26] or glucagon are used to decrease bowel motility.

Glucagon is a polypeptide produced by alpha cells of the islets of Langerhans in the pancreas.[63] When given intravenously (IV) or intramuscularly (IM) in doses ranging from 0.1 to 2.0 mg, glucagon induces transient atonicity or hypotonicity of the GI tract. The duodenum is most sensitive, followed by the proximal and distal jejunum, stomach, and colon.[42,43] The duration of hypotonicity varies with the dose, mode of injection, and portion of the GI tract examined, but it ranges from 18 to 26 minutes.

Since the 1970s glucagon has been used in low doses (0.1 to 0.2 mg IV) for barium studies of the upper GI tract and in moderate doses (0.5 to 1.0 mg IV) for barium enemas. Recently, glucagon has been administered (1 to 2 mg IV or IM) to improve MRI of the abdomen, usually in combination with an oral contrast agent or with effervescent granules that produce carbon dioxide.[64,65] The hypotonic effect of glucagon has improved delineation of the bowel from adjacent structures and has reduced artifacts from ghosting from positive oral contrast agents such as gadolinium and ferric ammonium citrate. Glucagon administration is contraindicated in patients with pheochromocytoma,[40] in whom it can induce life-threatening reactions, and in patients with an insulinoma.[41] Because the most common side effects of rapid IV injection of glucagon are nausea and vomiting, the dose should be given slowly over 1 minute for IV injection and over 15 seconds for IM injection.[6] Delayed adverse reactions to glucagon have occurred in patients receiving glucagon IM for abdominal MR (magnetic resonance) scanning. These reactions, which developed 1.5 to 2 hours after the IM dose, included symptoms of weakness, nausea, dizziness, and vomiting. The symptoms may be due to hypoglycemia resulting from glucagon administration.[6,7] Such reactions can be prevented by giving patients juice mixed with sugar at the completion of the MRI study.[6]

Protocol

The protocol chosen for MRI of the abdomen depends on the area of interest, reason for the study, and type of scanner and coils available. Esophageal imaging is typically performed with cardiac gating using axial T1- and T2-weighted imaging. Evaluation of the stomach, duodenum, and small bowel optimally follows a 4- to 6-hour fast using 400 to 600 cc of an oral contrast agent with an anti-

peristaltic agent such as glucagon (1 mg IV or IM).

Colorectal imaging has been performed with body or surface coils using axial, sagittal, and coronal imaging. The coronal plane is essential in patients with perirectal and perineal inflammatory disease for determining involvement of the levator ani. Patients being evaluated for primary colo-rectal cancer optimally undergo cleansing of the colon to improve detection of rectal lesions. Intraluminal contrast media (air, barium, other negative or positive contrast agent, or rectal balloon) improve detection of intraluminal lesions and delineation of adjacent structures in the pelvis and pelvic sidewalls. Oral contrast agents are also helpful in pelvic imaging since unopacified pelvic small bowel loops can mimic or obscure pathologic processes in the pelvis and pelvic sidewalls.

Dynamic studies of the GI tract are performed using an ultrafast technique called MBEST, or modulus blipped echo planar single pulse technique.[55] Images obtained have inherent T2-weighting with bright intraluminal fluid. Sequential, rapid images demonstrate peristalsis in the antrum and duodenum. Such techniques are used to obtain quantitative measurements of GI tract motion.

ANATOMY

Evaluation of the normal esophagus by MRI has been reported using a 0.35 T magnet.[48] The upper and distal esophagus were visible in all 20 patients evaluated, but the midesophagus was compressed by the left atrium and difficult to see in 6 of 20 cases. Single wall thickness averaged 3 mm and could only be evaluated in 3 of 20 patients who had air in the esophagus. The signal intensity of the esophageal wall was similar to skeletal muscle. No fat plane was found between the esophagus and trachea in 19 of 20 patients. Only two patients had a complete fat plane between the esophagus and aorta. The remaining patients had 10 to 80 degrees of effacement of the fat plane.

Imaging characteristics of the normal rectum[58] and anatomy of the normal anorectum as visualized with dynamic imaging[31] have been reported. However, standards for normal bowel wall thickness throughout the remainder of the GI tract have not been established for MRI. Based on experience with CT,[2] the normal thickness of the bowel wall varies with the degree of distension. The wall thickness is 1 to 2 mm in a well-distended loop of bowel and 2 to 3 mm in a partially distended loop of bowel. The stomach has the widest range of normal thickness, from 1 to 2 mm when distended to up to 2 cm when collapsed. The ability to assess bowel wall thickness on MRI is frequently limited by inadequate bowel distension. Care must be taken to avoid overdiagnosing bowel wall lesions in the absence of adequate distension.

CONGENITAL ABNORMALITIES

Esophageal duplication cysts are included in the spectrum of bronchopulmonary foregut malformations[22] and develop in the embryo when the solid esophagus fails to vacuolate completely. The duplication cyst thus formed can be lined with either respiratory or enteric epithelium.[23] The clinical manifestation occurs in childhood in 75% of patients; only 25% to 30% are diagnosed in adulthood.[67] Symptoms in adults may include dysphagia, nausea, weight loss, and anorexia. A more acute manifestation may occur when a cyst is complicated by hemorrhage or infection.[37]

In a case report describing a duplication cyst occurring in a 61-year-old woman,[37] T1-weighted imaging showed homogeneous high signal intensity within the central portion of the cyst and low signal intensity in the cyst wall. The fluid obtained from the cyst at surgery was viscous

and contained debris from hemorrhage and inflammation. In another case a large esophageal duplication cyst had predominantly low signal intensity because of the absence of hemorrhagic or fat content (Fig. 14-6).

Malrotation of the bowel is the second congenital anomaly that has been studied with MRI.[54] In normal fetal development, the bowel rotates in a counterclockwise direction along the long axis of the superior mesenteric artery. When normal rotation is completed, the superior mesenteric vein (SMV) resides to the right of the superior mesenteric artery (SMA), as demonstrated on axial CT or MRI. In midgut malrotation, the SMV lies to the left of the SMA on cross-sectional images. This has been referred

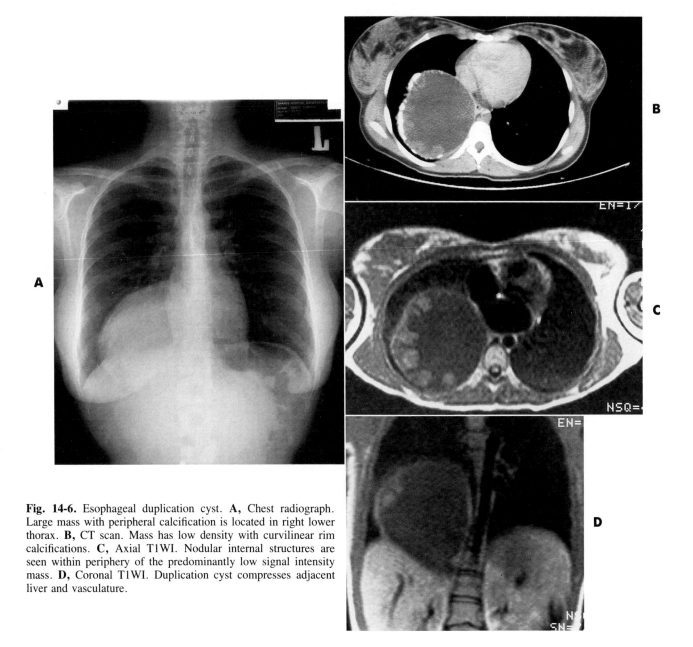

Fig. 14-6. Esophageal duplication cyst. **A,** Chest radiograph. Large mass with peripheral calcification is located in right lower thorax. **B,** CT scan. Mass has low density with curvilinear rim calcifications. **C,** Axial T1WI. Nodular internal structures are seen within periphery of the predominantly low signal intensity mass. **D,** Coronal T1WI. Duplication cyst compresses adjacent liver and vasculature.

to as the SMV rotation sign.[44] Although malrotation is frequently an incidental finding, it may be associated with other complications of midgut malrotation such as volvulus, obstruction, and ischemia.[14,44] MRI performed in the axial or coronal plane provides excellent demonstration of

vascular anatomy, including the SMV rotation sign (Fig. 14-7, A-C), and is a diagnostic aid for malrotation. A mass displacing the head of the pancreas or complete situs inversus produces a pseudopositive SMV sign in the absence of malrotation.[54]

INFLAMMATORY DISEASE

The primary application of MRI in inflammatory disease of the GI tract has been in the study of Crohn disease. Thickening of involved segments of bowel wall can be shown, particularly with the aid of an intraluminal contrast agent (Fig. 14-8, A).[26] Fistulae and sinus tracts in the abdomen and pelvis in patients with Crohn disease are well demonstrated.[29] On coronal and axial images, sinus tracts appear as linear or tubular structures with low signal intensity on T1-weighted images (T1WI) and relatively high signal intensity on T2-weighted images (T2WI) (Fig. 14-9, A to C). In 13 of 17 patients studied in one series, MRI showed the orifice of the fistula or sinus tract in the bowel wall, as well as connections to adjacent bowel, muscle, or skin.[29]

MRI is also useful in patients with perirectal or perianal abscesses because of excellent visualization of perirectal fat and the levator ani muscles in the coronal imaging plane (Fig. 14-10).[15,29]

NEOPLASMS
Esophagus

Benign esophageal tumors are rare, and reports of the MRI characteristics of these lesions are few. One benign neoplasm that has been studied with MRI is a giant fibrovascular polyp of the esophagus. This tumor arises from the wall in the upper one-third of the esophagus and is

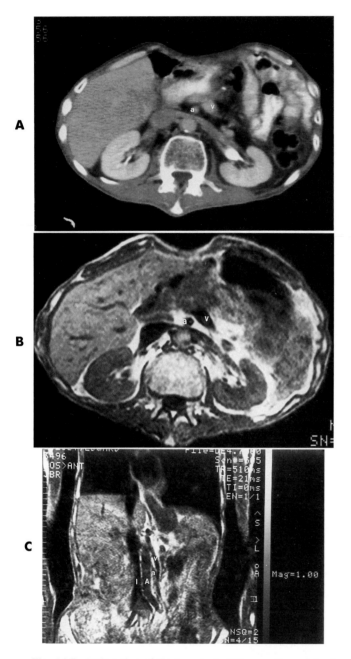

Fig. 14-7. Malrotation of the bowel. **A,** CT scan. Scan at level of left renal vein shows larger superior mesenteric vein (v) to the left of superior mesenteric artery (SMA, a). **B,** Axial T1WI. Malrotation of vessels is confirmed. **C,** Coronal T1WI. SMV (v) is to the left of SMA (a). Vascular anatomy is well-defined without the need for contrast media (inferior vena cava, I, and aorta, A). (From Schatzkes D et al: *J Comput Assist Tomogr* 14[1]:93-95, 1990.)

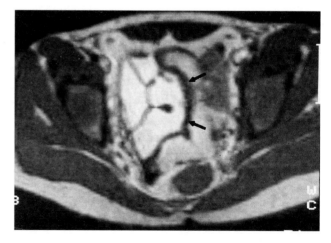

Fig. 14-8. Bowel wall thickening in Crohn's disease. Axial T1WI in 20-year-old patient with Crohn's disease shows asymmetric wall thickening in distal small bowel *(arrows)*. Bowel lumen is well-opacified by gadopentetate dimeglumine, permitting diagnosis of wall thickening. (From Kaminsky S et al: *Radiology* 178:503-508, 1991.)

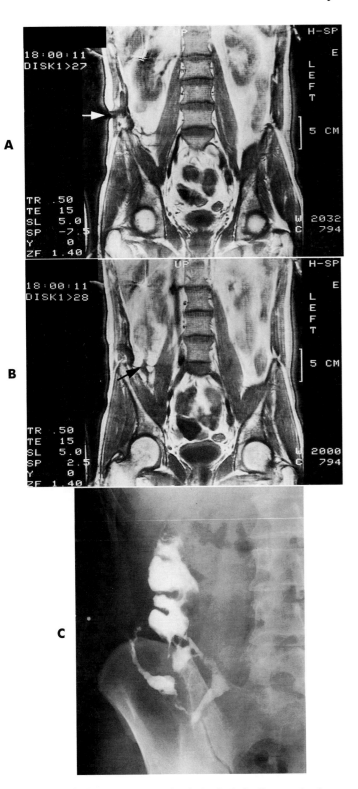

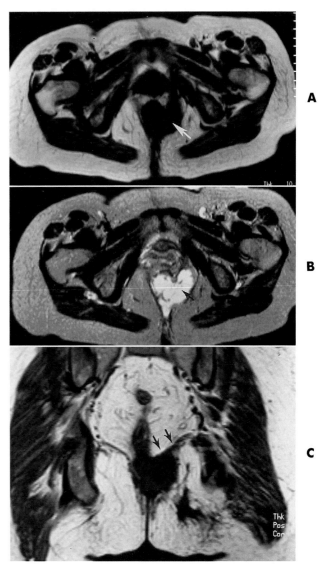

most commonly a pedunculated mass that occurs in adult men.[47] Surgical removal of larger lesions is performed since asphyxiation may occur from regurgitation of large, pedunculated tumors.[68] In a case report of CT and MRI of a giant fibrovascular polyp, on T1WI the polyp had a high signal intensity, which correlated with lipid attenuation on a CT scan. A histologic examination showed that the polyp contained myxomatous fibroadipose tissue.[68]

Imaging of esophageal cancer is performed to assess whether the tumor is resectable. Two studies have com-

Fig. 14-9. Enterocutaneous fistula in Crohn's disease. **A,** Coronal T1WI. Patient with recurrent Crohn's disease involving ileocolic anastamosis. Note cutaneous opening of the fistula in right lateral flank *(arrow)*. **B,** Coronal T1WI. Fistula terminates in region of anastamosis between new distal ileum and ascending colon *(arrow)*. **C,** Sinogram. Enterocutaneous fistula *(arrow)* communicates with distal ileum and ascending colon. Cutaneous opening of the fistula is marked with a lead marker. (From Koelbel G et al: *AJR* 152:999-1003, 1989.)

Fig. 14-10. Perirectal abscess in Crohn's disease. **A,** Axial T1WI. Low signal intensity mass represents an abscess in perirectal fat on the left *(arrow)*. **B,** Axial T2WI. Fluid within perirectal abscess *(arrow)* produces very high signal intensity on T2WI and improves differentiation of abscess from remaining perirectal fat. **C,** Coronal T1WI. Perirectal abscess extends up to level of the levator sling *(arrows)*. Note the fistula extending into adjacent fat of the buttocks.

pared CT and MRI in patients with esophageal cancer. In 13 patients with esophageal carcinoma,[48] the primary tumor was seen in 10 of 13 patients using a 0.35 T magnet, T1-weighted imaging, and cardiac gating. Staging was accurate in only 4 of 10 patients using MRI and 7 of 10 patients using CT. On MRI studies, one patient was overstaged and five were understaged because of inaccurate assessment of tumor invasion into periesophageal fat. Celiac adenopathy demonstrated by CT was missed or not clearly visible on MRI examinations. Based on the low staging accuracy of MRI at 0.35 T, the authors did not recommend MRI for routine preoperative evaluation of esophageal carcinoma.

A second study using a 1.5 T magnet showed more favorable results comparing MRI with CT in 35 patients with esophageal carcinoma.[59] Two criteria were used to assess tumor resectability: (1) the presence of tracheobronchial invasion, seen as a tumor extending into the lumen of the airway and (2) the presence of aortic invasion in which the triangular fat space between the esophagus, aorta, and spine adjacent to the aorta was obliterated. In the 35 patients studied, two MRI examinations were not adequate because of motion artifacts. Six unresectable tumors were correctly diagnosed by both MRI and CT based on aortic invasion in three cases and tracheobronchial invasion in three cases. The diagnosis of aortic invasion was indeterminate by MRI in three patients and by CT in four patients because of lack of a normal fat plane. In this series of patients, MRI was equivalent to CT in preoperative staging of esophageal carcinoma.

Stomach

Gastric neoplasms have not been extensively studied with MRI. Gastric wall thickening can be demonstrated by MRI but is a nonspecific finding that may be due to inflammatory, infiltrative, or neoplastic processes. Gastric adenocarcinoma (Fig. 14-11, *A* and *B*) can appear as a localized mass or wall thickening with low signal intensity on T1WI and high signal intensity on T2WI. In a case report of a patient with diffusely infiltrating gastric adenocarcinoma, MRI showed concentric thickening of the stomach wall, with low signal intensity in the thickened wall on both T1-weighted and T2-weighted images. These signal characteristics suggest the presence of fibrous tissue. Histologic findings showed that the submucosa was thickened and replaced by fibrous tissue because of the desmoplastic nature of the gastric adenocarcinoma.[69]

Small bowel

The differential diagnosis of a mass in the duodenum or small bowel includes benign and malignant neoplasms, congenital abnormalites, inflammatory lesions, and hematoma (see the following section, "Duodenal hematoma"). Imaging of small bowel masses usually includes barium studies, endoscopy, or CT scanning. Evaluation of small

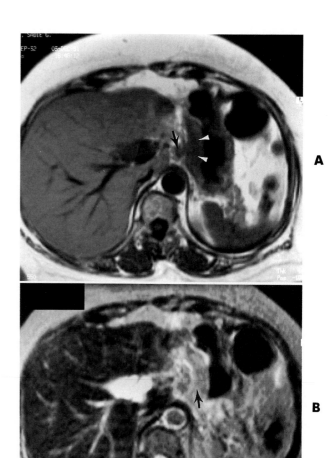

Fig. 14-11. Gastric adenocarcinoma. **A,** Axial T1WI. Wall thickening *(arrowheads)* is localized along lesser curvature of the stomach. Enlarged node is present in gastrohepatic ligament *(arrow)*. **B,** Axial T2WI. Tumor *(arrow)* has relatively high signal intensity on T2WI.

bowel neoplasms by MRI is still in the investigational stage. However, with adequate bowel contrast, intraluminal and mural lesions of the small bowel can be detected and characterized with MRI.

Lipomas of the small bowel (Fig. 14-12, *A* and *B*) have MRI characteristics similar to the more common colonic lipoma.[60,70] These benign tumors have a density similar to fat on CT and high signal intensity similar to subcutaneous or retroperitoneal fat on T1WI. They may be found incidentally or may produce pain, diarrhea, intussusception, or acute hemorrhage.[13]

Adenocarcinoma of the duodenum is in the differential diagnosis of masses involving the pancreatic head region. The improved tissue contrast of MRI aids differentiation of pancreatic head mass from duodenal mass when there is adequate duodenal contrast opacification (Fig. 14-13, *A*

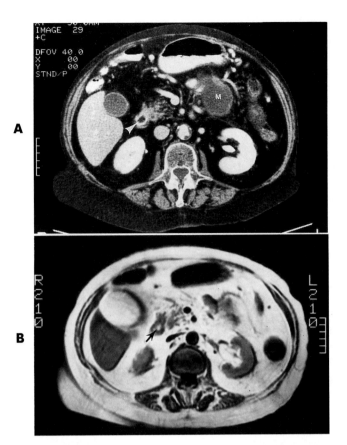

Fig. 14-12. Duodenal lipoma. **A,** Axial CT. Mass with the density of fat *(arrowhead)* is seen within lumen of the descending duodenum, adjacent to uncinate process of pancreas. Cystic mass *(m)* in tail of the pancreas is a mucinous cystic neoplasm. **B,** Axial T1WI. High signal intensity is seen within lumen of the duodenum, representing the small lipoma.

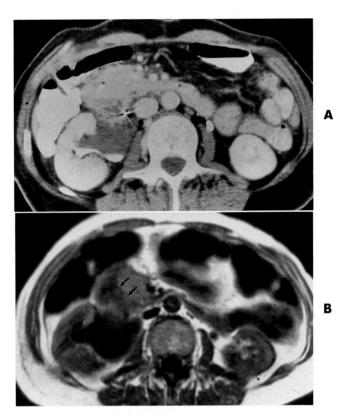

Fig. 14-13. Duodenal adenocarcinoma. **A,** CT scan. An ill-defined mass is in the region of pancreatic head. Duodenum is poorly opacified. Right hydronephrosis is present and the soft tissue mass abuts the renal pelvis. **B,** Axial T1WI after contrast (oral SPIO) administration. Margins of pancreatic head *(arrows)* are well-defined without evidence of a pancreatic mass. With contrast in the duodenal lumen, thickening of duodenal wall and tumor extension into periduodenal tissues are evident. Pathologic examination showed duodenal adenocarcinoma extending to, but not invading, the renal pelvis.

and *B*). Reported data offer no specific MRI features that would differentiate small bowel adenocarcinoma from lymphoma, metastatic disease, or localized inflammatory bowel disease.

Colon and rectum

The most common indication for MRI of GI tract neoplasms is the evaluation of colorectal cancer. The feasability of MRI for colonic neoplasms was investigated in vitro[24] using 1.5 T and 1.9 T systems to examine 15 resected colonic specimens containing elevated lesions. As with endoscopic ultrasound, normal layers of the bowel wall were identified on the in vitro specimens. Intramural tumor invasion limited to the bowel wall was best visualized with T2WI, and invasion of pericolonic fat tissues was best visualized with T1WI.

Preoperative staging of colorectal cancer. The key prognostic factors in colorectal cancer are the presence or absence of lymph node metastasis and the fixation of the tumor by direct invasion of adjacent tissues.[61] Two primary limitations of CT for preoperative staging of colorectal cancer are (1) the high prevalence of metastatic disease in normal-sized lymph nodes and (2) difficulty detecting minimal perirectal or pericolonic tumor infiltration. The staging accuracy of CT for colorectal cancer has been estimated to range from 17% for Dukes B lesions to 8% for Dukes D lesions.[3] Preoperative imaging is not routinely recommended in all cases but is used to identify patients with more advanced lesions who may benefit from preoperative or postoperative radiation therapy.

As a preoperative staging method, MRI has limitations similar to those of CT. One of the larger studies correlating histopathology with MR staging[10] in 29 patients with rectal cancer showed low accuracy in nodal assessment. Only four of seven cases of metastatic node involvement were detected, and two patients with enlarged inflammatory nodes were overstaged. Assessment of the local extent of the tumor was accurate in patients without a history of prior surgery or radiation therapy, and the T1WI was best for demonstrating local extension. Using the modified Astler-Coller staging classification, a correct staging diagnosis was made in 9 of 12 patients with Stage A (tumor limited to mucosa; no nodal involvement) and Stage B_1 (tumor in deeper layers but limited to bowel wall; no nodal involvement) tumors (Fig. 14-14, *A* and *B*). Three patients with Stage A or B_1 tumors who had prior radiation therapy or surgery were overstaged by MRI because of changes in the perirectal fat. Eleven patients with Stage B_2 (tumor infiltrating into perirectal fat; no nodal involvement) (Fig. 14-15) and six patients with Stage B_3 tumors (tumor invading adjacent organs or muscles; no nodal involvement) were correctly staged (Fig. 14-16, *A* and *B*). Therefore, MRI allowed differentiation of tumors limited to the rectal wall from those invading perirectal fat, except in patients with prior radiation therapy or surgery.

Additional studies have shown two advantages of MRI over CT in preoperative imaging. First, MRI provides better visualization of the extension of the tumor into bone or adjacent muscle because of improved tissue contrast.[5,18] Second, coronal imaging with gadolinium enhancement is useful for detecting tumor involvement of the levator ani, which changes the surgical approach from a low anterior resection to an abdominoperineal resection.[61]

Imaging of recurrent colorectal cancer. Following surgery for rectosigmoid cancer, local recurrence of tumors in the pelvis occurs in 30%-50% of patients.[45,66] The likelihood of recurrence varies with the site of the primary tumor, stage, and histologic type.[61] Patients are monitored

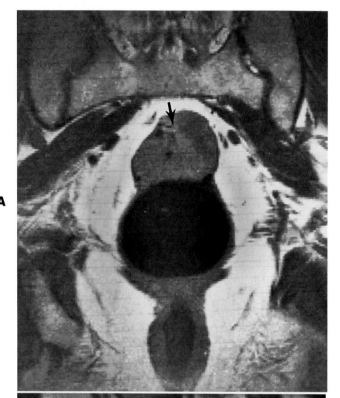

A

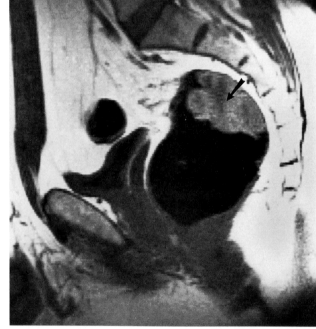

B

Fig. 14-14. Villous adenoma with stage B_1 carcinoma. **A** and **B,** Coronal and sagittal T1WI. Tumor *(arrow)* on posterior wall of the rectum is limited to bowel wall. Note sharp margins between the mass and perirectal fat. (From de Lange E et al: *Radiology* 176:623-628, 1990.)

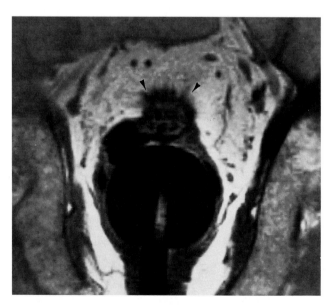

Fig. 14-15. Stage B_2 rectal carcinoma. Coronal T1WI. Small tumor on posterior wall of the rectum has ill-defined margins. Streaking of perirectal fat *(arrowhead)* adjacent to lesion indicates tumor invasion. Histologic examination confirmed strands of adenocarcinoma invading the perirectal fat. (From de Lange E et al: *Radiology* 176:623-628, 1990.)

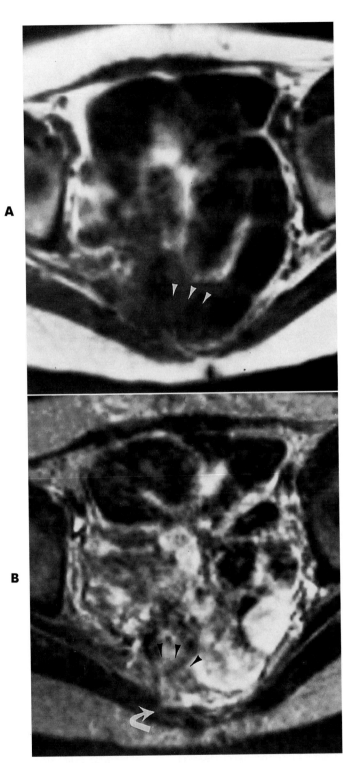

Fig. 14-16. Stage B$_3$ rectal carcinoma. **A,** Axial T1WI. Large tumor is on posterior rectal wall *(arrowheads)*. Fat plane between the lesion and right gluteus muscle is partially obliterated. **B,** Axial T2WI. Focal areas of higher signal intensity are in the gluteus muscle, indicating tumor invasion *(arrow)*. Tumor *(arrowheads)* displays inhomogeneous signal intensity. (From de Lange E et al: *Radiology* 176:623-628, 1990.)

with cross-sectional imaging studies to detect recurrent disease before the onset of clinical symptoms. However, a presacral mass is commonly seen after an abdominoperineal resection has been performed. The differential diagnosis of a presacral soft tissue mass includes postoperative fibrosis, unopacified small bowel, normal but displaced structures such as seminal vesicles or uterus,[33] or recurrent tumors. Benign masses from postoperative fibrosis become better defined and often decrease in size over time but may persist up to 2 years after surgery.[28] Signs suggesting recurrent tumor include growth of the mass; development of indistinct, ill-defined, or nodular margins; lymphadenopathy; or invasion of adjacent organs. A postoperative imaging study obtained 2 months after surgery can serve as a good baseline with which to compare subsequent examinations.

Early studies comparing MRI with CT for evaluating recurrent colorectal cancer proposed that MRI could provide a more specific diagnosis of tumor versus fibrosis based on signal intensity characteristics.[16,25,30,49] Theoretically, fibrosis has low signal intensity on both the T1WI and T2WI and can be differentiated from tumors, which generally show high signal intensity on the T2WI. This postulate has been helpful in differentiating tumors from fibrosis in other primary tumors.[58] However, signal intensity on the T2WI cannot be used to distinguish benign from malignant disease in rectosigmoid cancer.[9] The desmoplastic reaction associated with adenocarcinomas of the GI tract leads to formation of reactive fibrous tissue. Regions of low signal intensity on the T1WI and T2WI can therefore represent either benign fibrosis or fibrosis mixed with tumor and desmoplastic reaction. (Fig. 14-17) Likewise, regions of high signal intensity on T2WI can indicate tumor recurrence but may also represent edema, necrosis, inflammatory tissue, early phases of radiation fibrosis, or rarely a spermatic granuloma.[11]

In summary, MRI is useful as a sensitive test for demonstrating the location and extent of postoperative masses but cannot be used to make a histologic diagnosis in recurrent colorectal cancer. Another imaging study that may be useful in the future is positron emission tomography (PET) using fluorine-18-deoxyglucose, which has shown good results in differentiating tumors from fibrosis in lesions larger than 1.5 cm in diameter.[57] Percutaneous biopsy is ultimately required in many cases to make a definitive diagnosis of recurrent disease.

MISCELLANEOUS LESIONS
Small bowel ischemia

Experimental data in rabbits have shown that MRI is sensitive for detection of changes in the small bowel mucosal pattern in mesenteric ischemia.[27] After ligation of the arterial supply to the small bowel, the bowel wall thickens and signal intensity increases on the T2WI, reflecting the presence of edema. Application of MRI to in

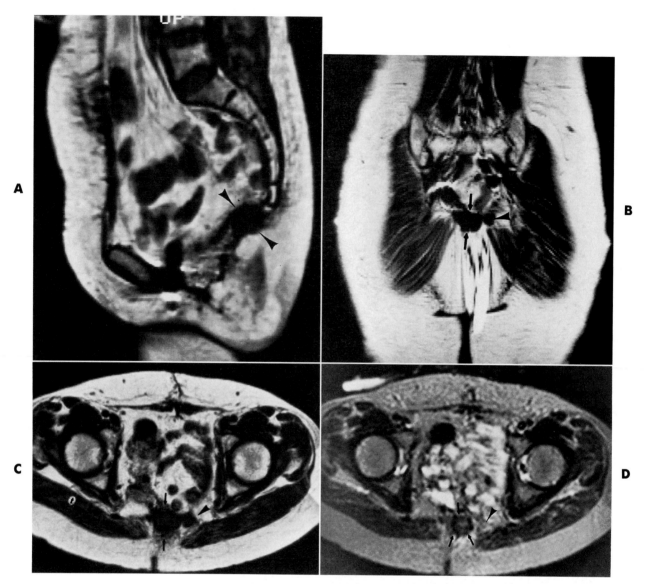

Fig. 14-17. Recurrent rectosigmoid carcinoma. **A,** Sagittal T1WI. Presacral mass *(arrowheads)* has low signal intensity. **B,** Coronal T1WI. Bilobed, presacral mass consists of large nodular mass *(arrows)* on the right and smaller nodule *(arrowhead)* on the left. **C,** Axial T1WI. Low signal intensity is seen within larger mass *(arrows)* on the right and smaller nodule *(arrowhead)* on the left. **D,** Axial T2WI. Most of the mass on the right shows signal intensity similar to that of muscle, with areas of low signal intensity seen in and around the lesion. Histologic findings show that this mass contained desmoplastic tissue with moderate amounts of tumor. Mass on the left *(arrowhead)* had high signal intensity and contained a necrotic tumor without desmoplastic tissue. Note high signal intensity within small bowel loops in the pelvis. (From de Lange E, Fechner RE, Wanebo HJ: *Radiology* 170:323-328, 1989.)

vivo imaging for ischemic bowel disease would likely have limited clinical value because of the non-specificity of mucosal edema.

Duodenal hematoma

MR findings are highly specific for the diagnosis of a duodenal hematoma.[19] Duodenal hematomas are most often caused by trauma but can arise spontaneously in pa-

tients on anticoagulant therapy. Barium studies may show a duodenal mass with crowding of the circular folds or a "picket fence sign" with perpendicular spiculated folds[12] or may be nonspecific. CT shows a hyperdense mass acutely, but in later stages the mass becomes lower density, with ring enhancement that may mimic abscess, a necrotic tumor, or pseudocyst. Using MRI, typical signal characteristics of hemorrhage with a ring sign are seen

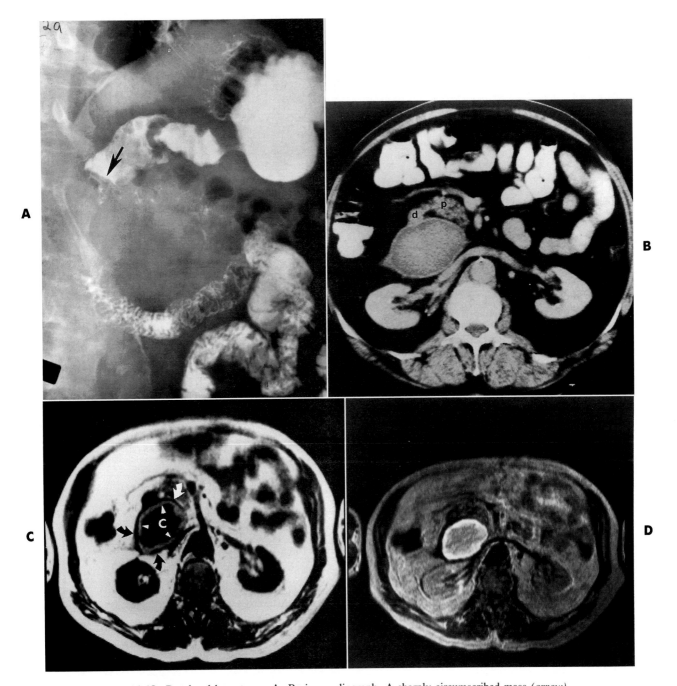

Fig. 14-18. Duodenal hematoma. **A,** Barium radiograph. A sharply circumscribed mass *(arrow)* partially obstructs descending duodenum. **B,** CT scan. A 10 cm mass compresses the duodenum *(d)* and displaces and elevates the pancreatic head *(p)*. A thin, soft tissue rim surrounds a region of lower density. **C,** Axial T1WI. Concentric ring appearance *(arrowheads)* is demonstrated. The middle, high intensity ring is thin and sharply demarcated from the core *(c)*. Large arrows show a low intensity peripheral rim. **D,** Axial T2WI. Middle ring is coarser and not as sharply differentiated from the core. (From Hahn PF et al: *Radiology* 159:379-382, 1986.)

within a subacute hematoma, allowing differentiation from other pathologic conditions of the small bowel. Since duodenal hematomas are usually managed conservatively, an accurate, noninvasive diagnosis with MRI can make further intervention unnecessary (Fig. 14-18).

REFERENCES

1. Ang PGP, Li KCP, Tart RP, et al: Geritol oil emulsion: ideal positive oral contrast agent for MR imaging, *Radiology* 173(P):522, 1989.
2. Balthazar EJ: CT of the gastrointestinal tract: principles and interpretation, *AJR* 156:23-32, 1991.
3. Balthazar EJ, Megibow AJ, Hulnick, et al: Carcinoma of the colon: detection and preoperative staging by CT, *AJR* 150:301-306, 1988.
4. Burton SS, Ros PR, Otto PM, et al: Barium MR imaging of the pancreas: initial experience, *Radiology* 173(P):517, 1989.
5. Butch RJ, Stark DD, Wittenberg J, et al: Staging rectal cancer by MR and CT, *AJR* 146:1155-1160, 1986.
6. Chernish SM, Maglinte DDT: Glucagon: common untoward reactions—review and recommendations, *Radiology* 177:145-146, 1990.
7. Chernish SM, Maglinte DDT, Brunelle RL: The laboratory response to glucagon dosages used in gastrointestinal examinations, *Invest Radiol* 23:847-852, 1988.
8. Chezmar JL, Rumancik WM, Megibow AJ, et al: Liver and abdominal screening in patients with cancer: CT versus MR imaging, *Radiology* 168:43-47, 1988.
9. de Lange EE, Fechner RE, Wanebo HJ: Suspected recurrent rectosigmoid carcinoma after abdominoperineal resection: MR imaging and histopathologic findings, *Radiology* 170:323-328, 1989.
10. de Lange EE, Fechner RE, Edge SB, et al: Preoperative staging of rectal carcinoma with MR imaging: surgical and histopathologic correlation, *Radiology* 176:623-628, 1990.
11. Feaster SH, Kinard RE, Yancey JM, et al: Spermatic granuloma complicating abdominoperineal resection of the rectum: diagnosis by CT, MR imaging and percutaneous biopsy, *AJR* 149:529-530, 1987.
12. Felson B, Levin EJ: Intramural hematoma of the duodenum: a diagnostic roentgen sign, *Radiology* 68:823-831, 1954.
13. Fernandez MJ, Davis RP, Nora PF: Gastrointestinal lipomas, *Arch Surg* 118:1081-1083, 1983.
14. Fisher JK: Computed tomographic diagnosis of volvulus in intestinal malrotation, *Radiology* 140:145-146, 1981.
15. Fishman-Javitt MC, Lovecchio JL, Javors B, et al: The value of MRI in evaluating perirectal and pelvic disease, *Magn Reson Imaging* 5:371-380, 1987.
16. Gomberg JS, Friedman AC, Radecki PD, et al: MRI differentiation of recurrent colorectal carcinoma from postoperative fibrosis, *Gastrointest Radiol* 11:361-363, 1986.
17. Gore RM, guest ed: CT of the gastrointestinal tract, *Radiol Clin North Am* 27(4), xi, 717-729, 1989.
18. Guinet C, Buy JN, Ghossain MA, et al: Comparison of magnetic resonance imaging and computed tomography in the preoperative staging of rectal cancer, *Arch Surg* 125:385-388, 1990.
19. Hahn PF, Stark DD, Vie L-G, et al: Duodenal hematoma: the ring sign in MR imaging, *Radiology* 159:379-382, 1986.
20. Hahn PF, Stark DD, Saini S, et al: Ferrite particles for bowel contrast in MR imaging: design issues and feasibility studies, *Radiology* 164:37-41, 1987.
21. Hahn PF, Stark DD, Lewis JM, et al: First clinical trial of a new superparamagnetic iron oxide for use as an oral gastrointestinal contrast agent in MR imaging, *Radiology* 175:695-700, 1990.
22. Heithoff KB, Shashikant MS, Williams HJ, et al: Bronchopulmonary foregut malformations—a unifying etiological concept, *AJR* 126:46-55, 1976.
23. Hocking M, Young DC: Duplications of the alimentary tract, *Br J Surg* 68:92-96, 1981.
24. Imai Y, Kressel HY, Saul SH, et al: Colorectal tumors: an in vitro study of high-resolution MR imaging, *Radiology* 177:695-701, 1990.
25. Johnson RJ, Jenkins JPR, Isherwood I, et al: Quantitative magnetic resonance imaging in rectal carcinoma, *Br J Radiol* 60:761-764, 1987.
26. Kaminsky S, Laniado M, Gogoll M, et al: Gadopentetate dimeglumine as a bowel contrast agent: safety and efficacy, *Radiology* 178:503-508, 1991.
27. Kaufman AJ, Tarr RW, Holburn GE, et al: Magnetic resonance imaging of ischemic bowel in rabbit model, *Invest Radiol* 23:93-97, 1988.
28. Kelvin FM, Korobkin M, Heaston DK, et al: The pelvis after surgery for rectal carcinoma: serial CT observations with emphasis on non-neoplastic features, *AJR* 141:959-964, 1983.
29. Koelbel G, Schmiedl U, Majer MC, et al: Diagnosis of fistulae and sinus tracts in patients with Crohn disease: value of MR imaging, *AJR* 152:999-1003, 1989.
30. Krestin GP, Steinbrich W, Friedmann G: Recurrent rectal cancer: diagnosis with MR imaging versus CT, *Radiology* 168:307-311, 1988.
31. Kruyt RH, Delemarre JBVM, Doornbos J, et al: Normal anorectum: dynamic MR imaging anatomy, *Radiology* 179:159-163, 1991.
32. Laniado M, Kornmesser W, Hamm B, et al: MR imaging of the gastrointestinal tract: value of Gd-DTPA, *AJR* 150:817-821, 1988.
33. Lee JKT, Stanley RJ, Sagel SS, et al: CT appearance of the pelvis after abdominoperineal resection for rectal carcinoma, *Radiology* 141:737-741, 1981.
34. Li KCP, Ho-Tai PCK: The search for the ideal enteric MR contrast agent, *Diagn Imaging* pp 110-114, March 1990.
35. Li KCP, Tart RP, Fitzsimmons JR, et al: Barium sulfate suspension as a negative oral contrast agent for MR imaging: in vitro and human optimization studies, *Radiology* 173(P):160, 1989.
36. Lonnemark M, Hemmingsson A, Bach-Gansmo T, et al: Effect of superparamagnetic particles as oral contrast medium at magnetic resonance imaging, *Acta Radiol* 30:193-196, 1989.
37. Lupetin AR, Dash N: MRI appearance of esophageal duplication cyst, *Gastrointest Radiol* 12:7-9, 1987.
38. Marti-Bonmati L, Vilar J, Paniagna JC, et al: High density barium sulphate as an MRI oral contrast, *Magn Reson Imaging* 9:259-261, 1991.
39. Mattrey RF, Hajek PC, Gylys-Morin VM, et al: Perfluorochemicals as gastrointestinal contrast agents for MR imaging: preliminary studies in rats and humans, *AJR* 148:1259-1263, 1987.
40. McLaughlin MJ, Langer B, Wilson DR: Life-threatening reaction to glucagon in a patient with pheochromocytoma, *Radiology* 140:841, 1982.
41. Miller RE, Chernish SM, Brunelle RL: Gastrointestinal radiology with glucagon, *Gastrointest Radiol* 4:1-10, 1979.
42. Miller RE, Chernish SM, Brunelle RL, et al: Dose response to intramuscular glucagon during hypotonic radiography, *Radiology* 127:49-53, 1978.
43. Miller RE, Chernish SM, Brunelle RL, et al: Double-blind study of dose response to intravenous glucagon for hypotonic duodenography, *Radiology* 127:55-59, 1978.
44. Nichols DM, Li DK: Superior mesenteric vein rotation: a CT sign of midgut malrotation, *AJR* 141:707-708, 1983.
45. Olson RM, Perencevich P, Malcom AW, et al: Patterns of recurrence following curative resection of adenocarcinoma of the colon and rectum, *Cancer* 45:2969-2974, 1980.
46. Panaccione, Ros PR, Torres GM, et al: Rectal barium in pelvic MR imaging: initial results, *JMRI* 1:605-607, 1991.
47. Patel J, Kieffer RW, Martin M, et al: Giant fibrovascular polyp of the esophagus, *Gastroenterology* 87:953-956, 1984.
48. Quint LE, Glazer GM, Orringer MB: Esophageal imaging by MR and CT: study of normal anatomy and neoplasms, *Radiology* 156:727-731, 1985.

49. Rafto SE, Amendola MA, Gefter WB: MR imaging of recurrent colorectal carcinoma versus fibrosis, *J Comput Assist Tomogr* 12(3):521-523, 1988.

50. Rinck PA, Smevik O, Nilsen G, et al: Oral magnetic particles in MR imaging of the abdomen and pelvis, *Radiology* 178:775-779, 1991.

51. Ros PR, Steinman RM, Torres G-M, et al: The value of barium as a gastrointestinal contrast agent in MR imaging: a comparison study in normal volunteers, *AJR* 157:761-767, 1991.

52. Rubin DL, Mueller HH, Nino-Murcia M, et al: Intraluminal contrast enhancement and MR visualization of the bowel wall: efficacy of PFOB, *JMRI* 1:371-380, 1991.

53. Saini S, Modic MT, Hamm B, et al: Advances in contrast-enhanced MR imaging, *AJR* 156:235-254, 1991.

54. Schatzkes D, Gordon DH, Haller JO, et al: Malrotation of the bowel: malalignment of the superior mesenteric artery-vein complex shown by CT and MR, *J Comput Assist Tomogr* 14(1):93-95, 1990.

55. Stehling MK, Evans DF, Lamont G, et al: Gastrointestinal tract: dynamic MR studies with echo-planar imaging, *Radiology* 171:41-46, 1989.

56. Storm BL, Li KCP, Tart RP, et al: Barium sulfate suspension as an oral contrast agent in MR imaging: initial clinical results, *Radiology* 173(P):522, 1989.

57. Strauss LG, Clorius JH, Schlag P, et al: Recurrence of colorectal tumors: PET evaluation, *Radiology* 170:329-332, 1989.

58. Sugimura K, Carrington BM, Quivey JM, et al: Postirradiation changes in the pelvis: assessment with MR imaging, *Radiology* 175:805-813, 1990.

59. Takashima S, Takeuchi N, Shiozaki H, et al: Carcinoma of the esophagus: CT vs MR imaging in determining resectability, *AJR* 156:297-302, 1991.

60. Taylor AJ, Steward ET, Dodds WJ: Gastrointestinal lipomas: a radiologic and pathologic review, *AJR* 155:1205-1210, 1990.

61. Thoeni RF: Colorectal cancer: cross-sectional imaging for staging of primary tumor and detection of local recurrence, *AJR* 156:909-915, 1991.

62. Torres, Erquiaga E, Ros PR, et al: Preliminary results of MR imaging with superparamagnetic iron oxide in pancreatic and retroperitoneal disorders, *Radiographics* 11:785, 1991.

63. Trenkner SW, Maglinte DDT, Lehman GH, et al: Esophageal food impaction: treatment with glucagon, *Radiology* 149:401-403, 1983.

64. Wall SD, Brasch RC, Goldberg HI, et al: Improved imaging of the GI tract and pancreas, *MRI Decisions,* pp 27-32, July/August 1988.

65. Weinreb JC, Maravilla KR, Redman HC, et al: Improved MR imaging of the upper abdomen with glucagon and gas, *J Comput Assist Tomogr* 8:835-838, 1984.

66. Welch JP, Donaldson GA: Detection and treatment of recurrent cancer of the colon and rectum, *Am J Surg* 135:505-511, 1978.

67. Whitaker JA, Deffenbaugh LD, Cooke AR: Esophageal duplication cyst, *Am J Gastroenterol* 73:329-332, 1980.

68. Whitman GJ, Borkowski GP: Giant fibrovascular polyp of the esophagus: CT and MR findings, *AJR* 152:518-520, 1989.

69. Winkler ML, Hricak H, Higgins CB: MR imaging of diffusely infiltrating gastric carcinoma, *J Comput Assist Tomogr* 11(2):337-339, 1987.

70. Younathan CM, Ros PR, Burton SS: MR imaging of colonic lipoma, *J Comput Assist Tomogr* 15(3):492-494, 1991.

Chapter 15

RETROPERITONEUM AND MESENTERY

W. Dean Bidgood, Jr.
Mark L. Schiebler

The retroperitoneum and mesentery have always posed difficult challenges in clinical evaluation and radiologic diagnosis. Pathologic lesions in both areas fortunately are infrequent. Since the regions are contiguous anatomically and their pathophysiology is strongly interrelated, they are combined for study here.

The five categories of retroperitoneal abnormality most likely to be encountered are vascular, inflammatory, traumatic, congenital, and neoplastic.[63,79,85,105] Mesenteric abnormalities most commonly are inflammatory, neoplastic, or congenital. Symptoms and signs may be obscure, delayed, nonspecific, or misleading.[79] Even neoplastic diseases of these tissues manifest with deceptive fever, leukocytosis, and neutrophilia.[34] For a retroperitoneal mass, plain films of the chest may show an elevated hemidiaphragm, atelectasis, ipsilateral pneumonia, or pleural effusion (Fig. 15-1, *A*).[105] Abnormalities are seen on intravenous pyelography in about 69% of cases of retroperitoneal abscess, but the false positive rate is approximately 30%.[32] Diagnosis and clinical management have been improved by CT,[32,63,79,105] and MRI is frequently useful as a secondary imaging modality.*

COMPARISON OF MRI AND CT

In the retroperitoneum, multiplanar imaging is a significant advantage of MRI over CT for a variety of lesions (Fig. 15-1, *B* and *C*).† The soft tissue contrast resolution of MRI is helpful.[9,34,50,67,94] Blood vessel recognition,[27] evaluation of blood flow,[31] and detection of thrombosis[1] are often improved by MRI,[18,49] even without intravenous

---

*References 29, 46, 47, 49, 63, 92.
†References 10, 23, 35, 44, 53, 59, 67, 94.

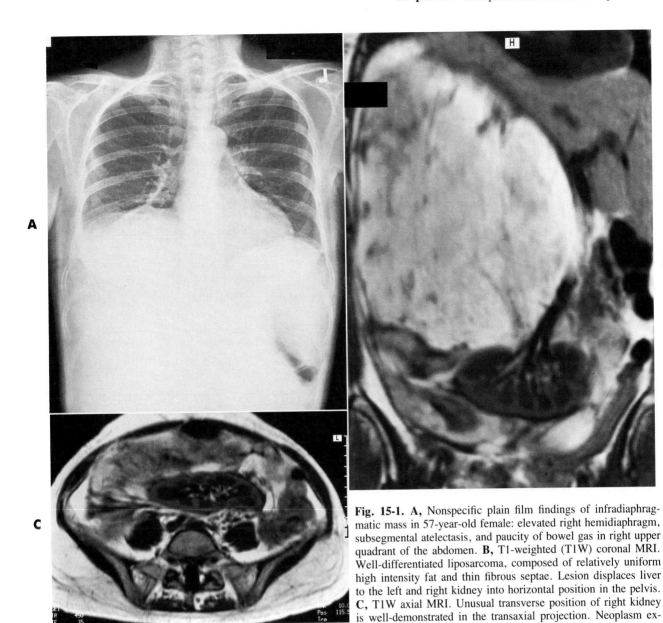

Fig. 15-1. A, Nonspecific plain film findings of infradiaphragmatic mass in 57-year-old female: elevated right hemidiaphragm, subsegmental atelectasis, and paucity of bowel gas in right upper quadrant of the abdomen. **B,** T1-weighted (T1W) coronal MRI. Well-differentiated liposarcoma, composed of relatively uniform high intensity fat and thin fibrous septae. Lesion displaces liver to the left and right kidney into horizontal position in the pelvis. **C,** T1W axial MRI. Unusual transverse position of right kidney is well-demonstrated in the transaxial projection. Neoplasm extends to ventral abdominal wall.

iodine contrast agents (Fig. 15-2, *B*).[23,53,67] Avoiding ionizing radiation is particularly advantageous for pediatric and obstetric examinations.[10,23,102] CT had superior spatial resolution in the early years of MRI,[25,33,44] but multicoil MRI now has better resolution than CT in some patients. Calcifications and abnormal gas collections are reliably detected by CT,[17,43,48,75] whereas they are frequently difficult or impossible to distinguish on MRI (Fig. 15-2, *A*).[56,63,102] For many lesions, CT and MRI offer comparable accuracy. Overall, CT still is preferred for acute trauma and for inflammatory lesions,[63] but MRI increasingly is chosen for congenital, vascular, and neoplastic lesions.*

*References 6, 37, 40, 46, 52, 56, 70.

ANATOMY

The system of compartmental organization popularized by Meyers[79] and further refined by others[61,77,84] has been useful in the differential diagnosis of retroperitoneal lesions by CT. In spite of its widespread recognition in the CT literature, compartmental analysis of the retroperitoneum has not been emphasized in standard MRI textbooks[29,47,92] or in major review articles.[32,46,52,62,65]

Retroperitoneum

Hartman[46] describes the retroperitoneum as "the space between the parietal peritoneum anteriorly and the transversalis fascia posteriorly." Within the retroperitoneum, Meyers[79] defines three compartments (Fig. 15-3, *A* and *B*). The anterior pararenal space (APRS) contains the ex-

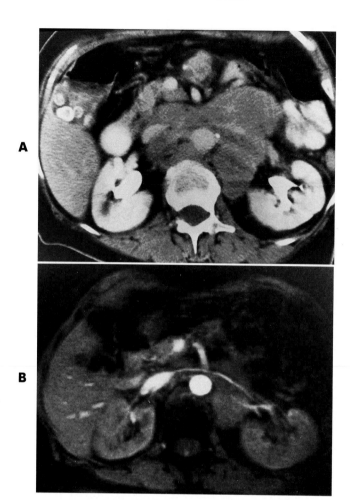

Fig. 15-2. Axial CT and MRI of lymphoma. **A,** Conglomerate mass of nodes envelopes aorta and inferior vena cava *(IVC)*. Incidental gallstones are clearly delineated in right upper quadrant. Bowel contrast and intravenous (IV) contrast agents have been given. **B,** Single breath-hold, fat-suppressed gradient echo sequence. Vessels encased by lymphadenopathy are demonstrated better than on CT. However, low intensity signal of gallstones is indistinguishable from that of bowel gas and suppressed fat.

traperitoneal portions of the ascending and descending colon and the duodenum. The right and left perirenal spaces (PRS) contain the kidneys, blood vessels, lymph nodes, and adrenal glands. The posterior pararenal space (PPRS) contains fat and vessels, but no solid organs. Lee and Glazer[64] describe the vectors of lesions involving the psoas muscles (and the lymph nodes interposed between them and the spine) according to the pattern of displacement of the muscular investing fascia.

The aorta, inferior vena cava, paraaortic lymph nodes, lymphatic vessels, and autonomic nerves are loosely bounded by fascia at the root of the mesentery.[79] For the purpose of this chapter, the loosely defined perivascular compartment is called the aorticocaval space (ACS) (Fig. 15-3, *A*). The psoas (and quadratus lumborum) compartments together are called the muscular space (MS).

The APRS is bounded anteriorly by the posterior parietal peritoneum and posteriorly by the anterior renal fascia.[79] The APRS is bounded laterally by the lateroconal fascia and cranially by the fused anterior and posterior renal fasciae. Toward the caudal region, the APRS, PRS, and PPRS have the potential for communication (Figs. 15-3, *B*, and 15-30).[77,79] The APRS is continuous across the midline; however, Meyers has observed that collections of fluid tend to remain ipsilateral to the side of origin (Fig. 15-3, *A* and *C*).[79]

Each PRS is bounded by anterior and posterior renal fascias (which as a unit are commonly called Gerota's fascia).[77] The multilaminar posterior renal fascia splits lateral to each PRS to form the anterior renal fascia and the lateroconal fascia.[84] The potential space between the layers of the posterior renal fascia can serve as a pathway for APRS effusions to migrate laterally and posteriorly to the kidney without actually entering the PPRS.[84] Bridging septa traversing the right and left PRS divide them into multiple subcompartments and connect each renal capsule to the ipsilateral renal fascia (see Fig. 15-31, *B*).[61] Each PRS is bounded medially by the fascias of the MS and ACS. No communication occurs across the midline between the right and left PRS.[79,84]

The PPRS is bounded anteriorly by the posterior renal fascia (Zuckerkandl's layer) and the lateroconal fascia.[77,84] The PPRS is bounded posteriorly by the fascias of the MS and transversalis fascia. The PPRS is in continuity with the properitoneal compartment.[79,84]

Determination of the compartmental center of a retroperitoneal mass is an aid to differential diagnosis in MRI just as it is in CT. Thickening of bridging septa and fascias is demonstrable by CT.[43,61] Similar pathologic conditions are likewise demonstrable by MRI (Figs. 15-4 and 15-5).[61]

Mesentery

The small bowel mesentery is a translucent suspensory ligament about 12 to 25 cm in length that attaches the jejunum and ileum to the dorsal wall of the abdomen (Fig. 15-6). Meyers[79] states that the mesentery "is composed of fatty *extraperitoneal* connective tissue, blood vessels, nerves, lymphatics, and an investment of peritoneum that reflects from the posterior parietal peritoneum." Its attachment (the root of the mesentery) extends from the ligament of Treitz to the cecum (Fig. 15-7). This course places the root of the small bowel mesentery into contiguity with the left side of the APRS, the ACS, right side of the PPRS, right side of the MS, and right side of the properitoneal fat compartment.

The mesentery is folded into soft pleats so that all six meters of small intestine attach to a 15 to 17 cm root (Figs. 15-6, and 15-8). The transverse colon is suspended from the dorsal wall of the abdomen by the transverse mesocolon (Fig. 15-8). Similar peritoneal reflections also suspend portions of the ascending and descending colon

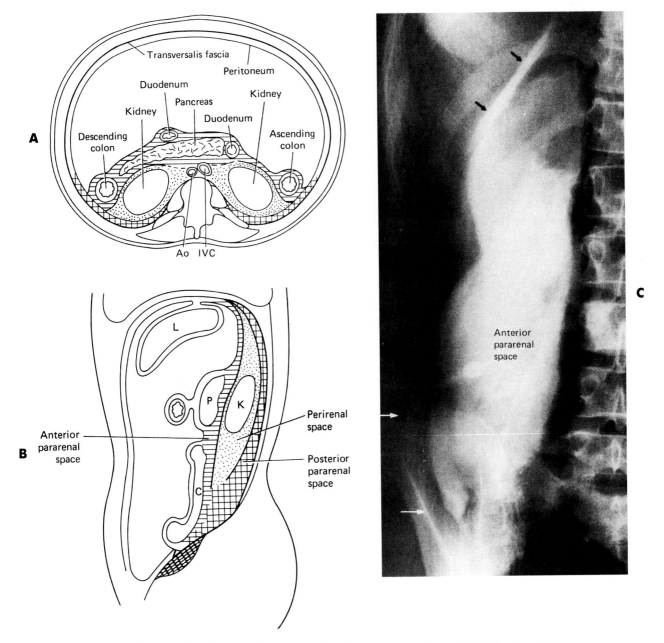

Fig. 15-3. A, Axial diagram of the retroperitoneal compartments shows APRS *(horizontal line shading),* PRS *(stippled shading),* and PPRS *(square cross hatch shading).* **B,** Sagittal diagram of retroperitoneal compartments shows liver *(L),* pancreas *(P),* kidney *(K),* descending colon *(C).* Shading of APRS, PRS, and PPRS is same as in **A.** Note confluence of all three major compartments caudally and potential communication of APRS with bare area of the liver. **C,** Postmortem contrast injection into right side of APRS. Contrast agent is distributed ipsilaterally, although potential left-right communication exists in APRS. Note extension of contrast agent into coronary ligament *(black arrows).* The properitoneal fat stripe is preserved *(white arrows).* (APRS, anterior pararenal space; PRS, perirenal space; PPRS, posterior pararenal space.) (**A,** from Meyers MA: *Dynamic radiology of the abdomen,* New York, 1976, Springer Verlag.)

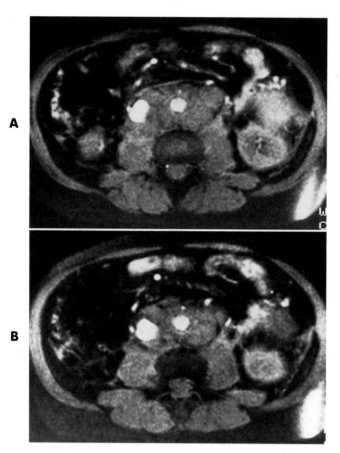

Fig. 15-4. Carcinoma of the left kidney; exophytic mass and retroperitoneal adenopathy. **A,** Axial single breath-hold, fat-suppressed gradient echo MRI. Neoplasm extends into PRS, anterior to left kidney. Posterior left renal fascia is thickened irregularly by tumor infiltration. **B,** Axial MRI using same technique as **A** and caudal to **A.** Thickening of bridging septae in left PRS and neoplastic extension to the lateroconal fascia and posterior renal fascia are well-demonstrated. Note anterior displacement of the aorta and IVC by infiltrated retrovascular nodes.

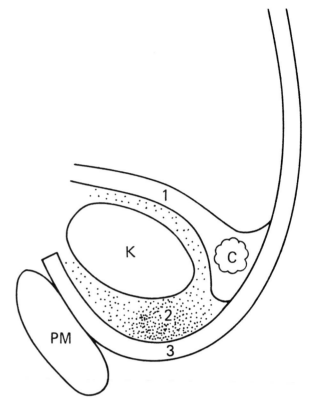

Fig. 15-5. Drawing of left renal fasciae and retroperitoneal compartments shows APRS *(1)*, PRS *(2)*, PPRS *(3)*, descending colon *(C)*, left kidney *(K)*, and psoas muscle *(PM)*. Posterior renal fascia (between *2* and *3*) divides to form anterior renal fascia and lateroconal fascia. Effusions in APRS can dissect layers of the posterior renal fascia to migrate posterior to the left kidney without entering PPRS. (From Meyers MA: *Dynamic radiology of the abdomen,* New York, 1976, Springer Verlag.)

(Figs. 15-7 and 15-10). Mesenteric attachments restrict the avenues of fluid flow along the dorsal wall of the peritoneal cavity (Fig. 15-7). The folded shape and large surface area of the small bowel mesentery tend to trap peritoneal effusions, making it vulnerable to drop metastasis from intraperitoneal malignancy (Fig. 15-9).[79] The relatively high arterial inflow and the rich lymphatic drainage of the mesentery are additional pathways for the deposition and dissemination of neoplasms (Fig. 15-10).

The mesentery is vulnerable to any permeative pathologic process involving the tissue to which it is attached. Effusions from pancreatitis or direct extension of pancreatic or renal carcinoma can invade the mesentery through its root . The converse is also true. Granulomatous enteritis, lymphoma, and carcinoma of the colon or stomach can invade the retroperitoneum by way of the mesentery (Figs. 15-10 to 15-12).[79]

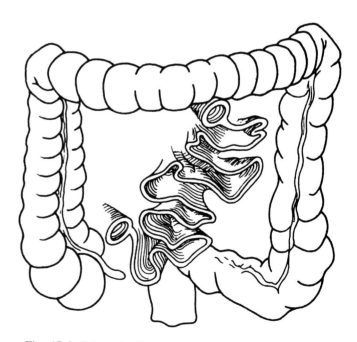

Fig. 15-6. Schematic diagram of the root of the mesentery. (From Meyers MA: *Dynamic radiology of the abdomen,* New York, 1976, Springer Verlag.)

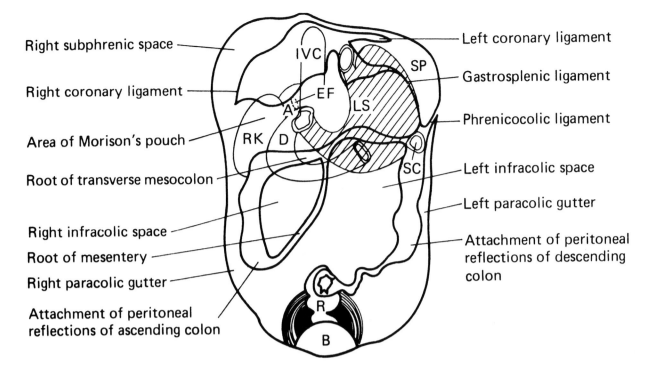

Right subphrenic space

Right coronary ligament

Area of Morison's pouch

Root of transverse mesocolon

Right infracolic space

Root of mesentery

Right paracolic gutter

Attachment of peritoneal
reflections of ascending colon

Left coronary ligament

Gastrosplenic ligament

Phrenicocolic ligament

Left infracolic space

Left paracolic gutter

Attachment of peritoneal
reflections of descending
colon

Fig. 15-7. Diagram of attachments of small bowel mesentery and colon demonstrates relationships to major organs; adrenal gland *(A)*, duodenum *(D)*, epiploic foramen *(EF)*, inferior vena cava *(IVC)*, lesser sac *(LS)*, right kidney *(RK)*, splenic flexure of the colon *(SC)*, and spleen *(SP)*. Mesenteric and colonic attachments divide intraperitoneal space into functional compartments and determine distribution and pattern of flow of intraperitoneal fluid. (From Meyers MA: *Dynamic radiology of the abdomen*, New York, 1976, Springer Verlag.)

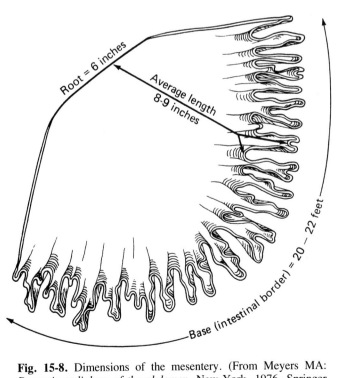

Root = 6 inches

Average length 8-9 inches

Base (intestinal border) = 20 – 22 feet

Fig. 15-8. Dimensions of the mesentery. (From Meyers MA: *Dynamic radiology of the abdomen*, New York, 1976, Springer Verlag.)

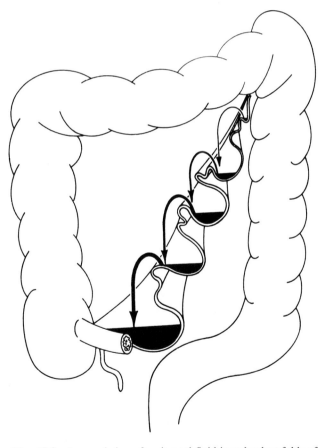

Fig. 15-9. Accumulation of peritoneal fluid in redundant folds of mesentery. Risk of focal neoplastic invasion or abscess formation is increased by relatively prolonged tissue contact afforded by these small locations. (From Meyers MA: *Dynamic radiology of the abdomen*, New York, 1976, Springer Verlag.)

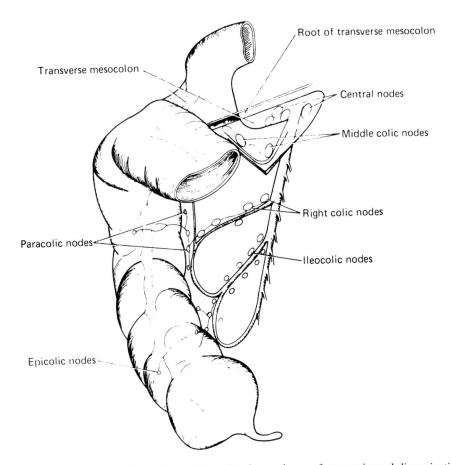

Fig. 15-10. Lymphatic drainage of ascending colon is a pathway of retroperitoneal dissemination of colon carcinoma and other diseases. (From Meyers MA: *Dynamic radiology of the abdomen,* New York, 1976, Springer Verlag.)

TECHNIQUES

Because of the rapid advances in MRI equipment and software, details of pulse sequence parameters are quickly supplanted by improved technology. Although they are destined soon to be replaced by faster sequences, the techniques used at the time of this writing have proven to be highly effective clinically. Therefore, specific parameters are presented as a reference guide. As improvements become available, they should be substituted for appropriate elements of the sample protocol.

The examination protocol for retroperitoneal MRI is highly dependent on the condition of the patient, specific region of interest, provisional diagnosis, and available scan techniques. A typical survey of the retroperitoneum begins with a coronal sequence weighted to the spin-lattice or longitudinal relaxation time (T1W) (TR 450 msec, TE 15 msec, FOV 50 cm, ST 8 mm, matrix 128 × 256, 6 NEX, 5:48 TA), with TR being the repetition time; TE, echo time; FOV, field of view; ST, slice thickness; Matrix, the resolution of the image; NEX, the number of signals averaged; and TA, total acquisition time of the sequence). An axial T1W sequence (TR 450 msec, TE 15 msec, FOV 40 cm, ST 8 mm, Matrix 192 × 256, 4 NEX,

5:48 TA) and an axial sequence weighted to the spin-spin or transverse relaxation time (T2W) (TR 2500 msec, TE 80 msec, FOV 40 cm, ST 10 mm, Matrix 128 × 256, 2 NEX, 10:44 TA) follows. If necessary for demonstration of vasculature or improvement of tissue contrast, a fat-suppressed, single breath-hold coronal or axial FLASH CHESS sequence (TR 60 msec, TE 12 msec, FA 30 degrees, ST 10 mm, Matrix 192 × 256, 1 NEX, with GMR, 0:12 TA), with FA being flip angle and GMR being gradient moment reduction—flow compensation) completes the examination.[73,74] Newer, fast techniques relying on partial echoes are also used in survey exams.

Respiratory motion suppression is recommended,[7,30,69,106] and fat suppression further reduces motion artifacts and improves the effective dynamic range of soft tissue intensity.[73,74,80,88,89] Combined gadolinium-enhanced and fat suppression imaging improves the demonstration of renal masses.[89] Oral contrast agents (barium sulfate or superparamagnetic iron oxide particulate suspension) improve the depiction of the pancreas and other retroperitoneal tissues.[15,45,97] In the future, an intravenous ultrasmall superparamagnetic iron oxide (USPIO) contrast

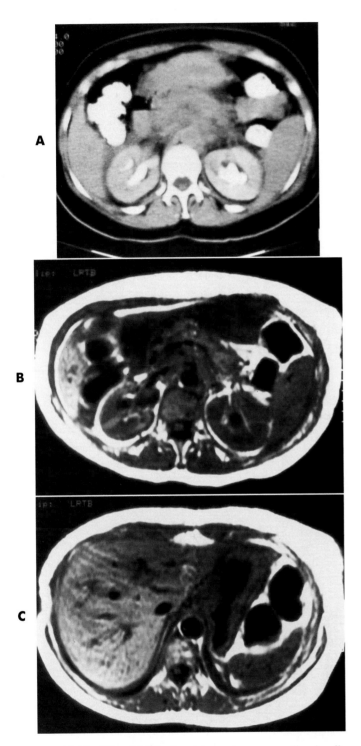

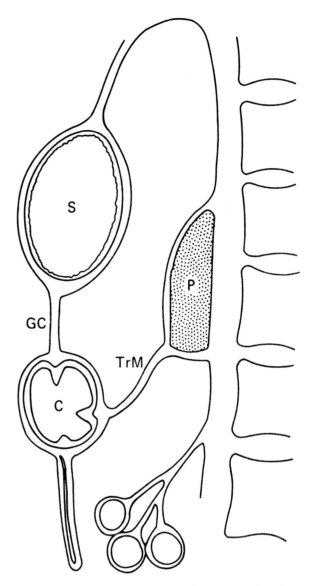

Fig. 15-12. Pathway of spread of gastric carcinoma into the retroperitoneum. Figure shows stomach *(S)*, gastrocolic ligament *(GC)*, transverse mesocolon *(TrM)*, and pancreas *(P)*. (From Meyers MA: *Dynamic radiology of the abdomen*, New York, 1976, Springer Verlag.)

Fig. 15-11. CT and MRI of gastric carcinoma spreading locally to the retroperitoneum. **A,** Axial CT at level of the superior mesenteric artery (SMA) using IV and oral contrast agents demonstrates widespread retroperitoneal lymphadenopathy. **B,** Axial T1W MRI at same level as **A.** Normal fat plane surrounding the SMA is obliterated by conglomerate mass of infiltrated lymph nodes. Splenic vein is displaced anteriorly. Low intensity fluid is present in the stomach and duodenum. **C,** Axial MRI at level of the splenic flexure. Wall of the stomach is thickened by carcinoma.

agent may be available for human use. Intravenous USPIO decreases the signal intensity of normal lymph nodes in rats, but does not decrease the signal intensity of tumor-infiltrated nodes.[103] MRI lymphangiography using USPIO may be doubly useful since conventional oil-based lymphangiographic contrast agents increase the signal intensity of lymph nodes, making them invisible against the background of retroperitoneal fat.[14]

PITFALLS FROM NORMAL VARIANTS
Diaphragmatic crura

The ligamentous crura form the diaphragmatic hiatus and blend with the anterior longitudinal ligament to attach

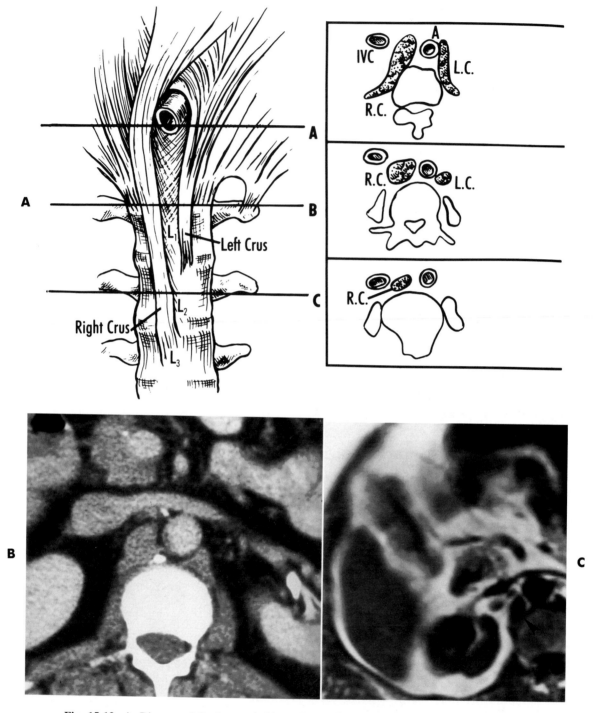

Fig. 15-13. A, Diagram of diaphragmatic hiatus. Insets depict transaxial projections of the crura at levels *A, B,* and *C.* **B,** CT with IV contrast agent with level similar to *B* of **A.** Crura are hypodense to the iodine-enhanced blood vessels. **C,** T1W MRI. Prominent right crus of the diaphragm *(black arrowhead)* has lower signal intensity than two nearby small retrocaval lymph nodes. In this patient with metastatic melanoma, it is impossible to determine from this section whether these 7 to 12 mm nodes are infiltrated by neoplasm. Image also shows mesenteric vessels leading to ascending colon.

the diaphragm to the spine.[90] The right crus extends farther caudally than the left crus.[15] Progressing caudally, the crura in cross section have an increasingly nodular appearance (Fig. 15-13, *A*). In transaxial sections on CT and MRI, the crura can mimic adenopathy (Figs. 15-13, *B* and *C*, and 15-33). This pitfall is avoided by review of serial transverse sections or by correlation with coronal sections. The lower signal intensity of the crus versus lymphadenopathy on T2W images is another helpful sign in MRI (Fig. 15-13, *C*).

Psoas minor

The psoas minor muscles arise at the level of the twelfth thoracic or first lumbar vertebra (Fig. 15-14, *A*).[90] Normal variation in thickness produces right-left asymmetry that can be a diagnostic pitfall in CT (Fig. 15-14, *B*) and MRI (Fig. 15-19, *A*). Slight hyperintensity of the psoas minor on MRI (Fig. 15-19, *A*) contributes to the

misdiagnosis of adenopathy. This appearance may be due to volume averaging with adjacent fat.

CONGENITAL ANOMALIES
Inferior vena cava and renal vein

Four of the most common venous anomalies are persistent left inferior vena cava (IVC), duplication of the IVC, circumaortic left renal vein, and retroaortic left renal vein (Figs. 15-15 to 15-17).[19,90] A circumaortic venous ring (a category that includes some cases of retroaortic left renal vein) occurs in 8.7% of the general population.[19] An isolated retroaortic left renal vein occurs in 1.8% to 2.4% of the population (Fig. 15-17).[21] Persistent left IVC occurs in 0.2% to 0.5% (Fig. 15-16) and duplication of the IVC occurs in 1% to 3% of the population.[19] These four, usually insignificant developmental anomalies most often are discovered incidentally.[37]

A more significant finding is interruption of the IVC

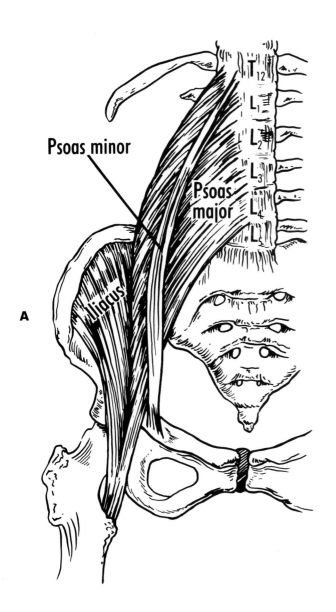

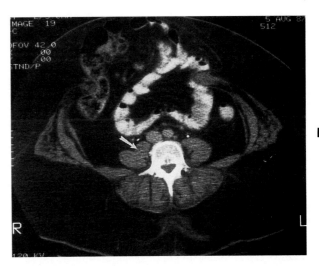

Fig. 15-14. A, Diagram of relationship of the psoas minor muscle to psoas major and iliacus muscles. **B,** Transaxial CT scan showing psoas minor, which could be mistaken for enlarged lymph node. Compare with the T1W transverse MRI of Fig. 15-19, *A*. Left psoas minor muscle in that section *(small white arrow)* has slightly higher signal intensity than the psoas major. (From Shirkhoda A: *Radiographics* 11:969-1002, 1991.)

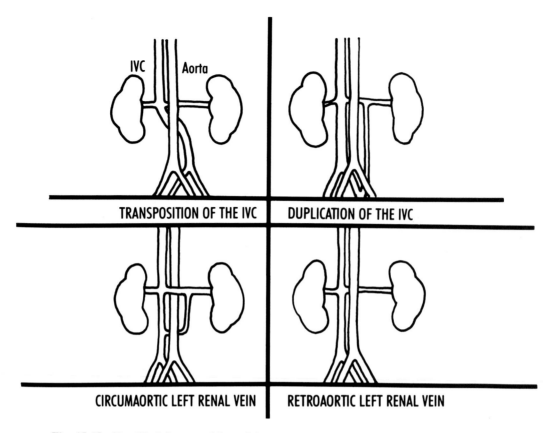

IVC Aorta

TRANSPOSITION OF THE IVC   **DUPLICATION OF THE IVC**

CIRCUMAORTIC LEFT RENAL VEIN   **RETROAORTIC LEFT RENAL VEIN**

Fig. 15-15. Simplified diagram of four of the most common retroperitoneal venous anomalies. (From Shirkhoda A: *Radiographics* 11:969-1002, 1991.)

with azygous continuation of the vein into the liver (Fig. 15-18).[19,87] This anomaly, resulting from failure of development of the hepatic segment of the IVC, is associated with congenital heart disease, asplenia, polysplenia, and situs anomalies.[87] The incidence in the general population is approximately 0.6%.[19]

CT provides a less invasive diagnostic alternative to angiography, athough an iodinated contrast agent is required for vascular examination.[21] Several authors have reported that spin echo MRI (with low intensity flowing blood) is as good as or better than CT for evaluation of abdominal vascular anomalies.[21,87,37] Single-breath gradient echo images with flow compensation often render flowing blood more clearly with high signal intensity (see Fig. 15-2, *B*). Breath-hold two-dimensional time-of-flight techniques also work well in the evaluation of abdominal venous disease.

Other anomalies

Renal anomalies such as horseshoe kidney (Fig. 15-19) and crossed-fused ectopia simulate pathologic masses in the retroperitoneum. Genitourinary tract anomalies as a group are relatively frequent. Other anomalies are relatively rare (with the possible exception of vascular malformations—see the following discussion). A recently pub-

lished example is the case of an accessory spleen occurring in the retroperitoneum. Vassilopoulos et al.[99] reported concerning a patient who had low back pain radiating to the left testicle and a mass deviating the left ureter laterally. At surgery a retroperitoneal accessory spleen was found in addition to the normal intraperitoneal spleen. Neurenteric cysts, lateral meningoceles, and duplication cysts of extraperitoneal portions of the alimentary tract are some other examples of uncommon congenital lesions that may occur as retroperitoneal masses.

BENIGN NEOPLASMS
Hemangiomatosis

According to Cohen, Weinreb, and Redman,[20] vascular malformations of the extremities fall into three classes: arteriovenous malformations, venous malformations, and hemangiomas. Enzinger and Weiss[34] state that "hemangiomas are benign neoplasms that closely resemble normal vessels . . . but could just as appropriately be considered malformations." Considered by many to be congenital malformations, the soft tissue hemangioma is a common lesion, occurring in all parts of the body.[20,34,57,67] Enzinger and Weiss[34] write about two types of hemangiomas: localized lesions (hemangiomatosis) and diffuse angioma-

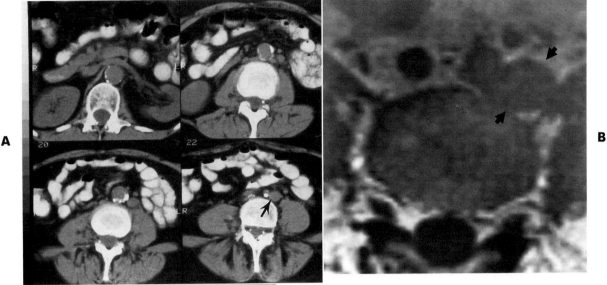

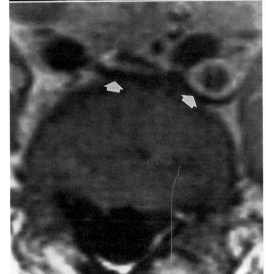

Fig. 15-16. Transposition of the inferior vena cava. **A,** CT with no IV contrast agent. Black arrows indicate anomalous IVC on the left side. **B,** Axial T1W noncontrast MRI of different patient. Slice location is similar to **A.** Black arrows denote IVC. **C,** T1W MRI in more caudal location in same patient as **B.** Note entry-slice flow-related enhancement *(white arrows)* of transposed common iliac veins. (**A** From Shirkhoda A: *Radiographics* 11:969-1002, 1991.)

tosis involving large regions of the body (Fig. 15-20).[34] Although these are indolent lesions, they may have devastating effects.

MRI and CT are useful for determining the extent of abnormality of soft tissue hemangiomas.[67] Levine, Wetzel, and Neff[67] report that MRI is more accurate than CT because of greater contrast between lesions and surrounding soft tissues. Kaplan and Williams state that CT underestimated the margins of 2 of 11 of their cases and showed the boundary of the lesions less distinctly than MRI. Hemangiomas are slightly hyperintense to muscle on T1W spin echo pulse sequences and sharply hyperintense on T2W spin echo sequences. Small lesions are typically homogeneous, with smooth contours.[67] Larger lesions have an inhomogeneous signal distribution (particularly on T2W images) and more irregular contour.[57,67] Serpiginous low

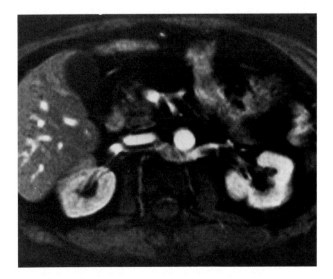

Fig. 15-17. Retroaortic left renal vein. Transaxial gradient echo, single breath-hold, fat-suppressed MRI with flow compensation. Anomalous vessel dorsal to the aorta is depicted with high contrast against suppressed signal of retroperitoneal fat.

intensity vascular channels may be seen, and phleboliths are plainly evident on CT and plain radiographs but may be confused with cross sections of vessels on MRI.[57]

Arteriovenous malformations (AVMs) have serpiginous vascular channels, T2W hyperintensity, and an inhomogenous signal pattern. They may enlarge spontaneously because of arterovenous fistulas, thrombosis, vascular ectasia, and pregnancy.[20] Hemangioendotheliomas (vascular tumors of intermediate malignancy) and malignant vascular tumors (angiosarcoma and Kaposi's sarcoma) are readily distinguished histologically from benign hemangiomas and other AVMs.[34]

Lymphangioma

Lymphangiomas are benign lymphatic vascular neoplasms that most often are seen in children. Seventy-five percent of lymphangiomas occur in the neck, 20% occur in

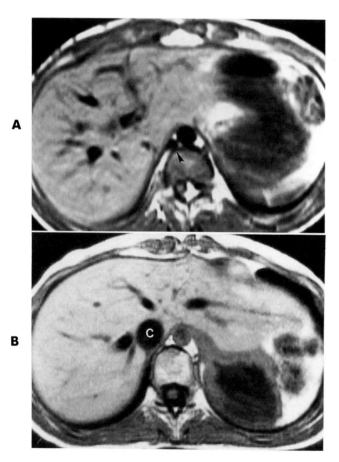

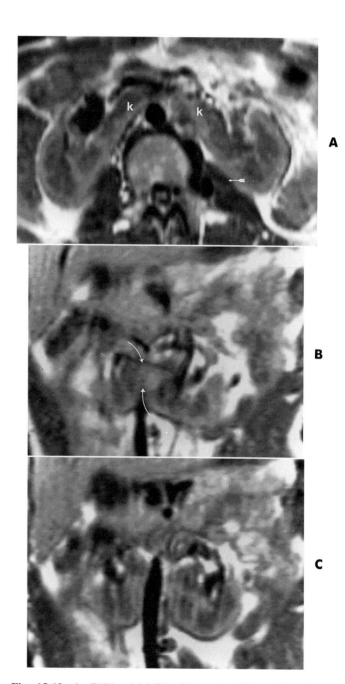

Fig. 15-18. Interruption of IVC with azygous continuation. **A,** T1W MRI reveals absence of hepatic segment of the IVC. Prominent azygous vein *(black arrowhead)* is remnant of cranial portion of embryonic supracardinal vein. This persisted as a dominant vessel because the prerenal (craniad) segment of the subcardinal vein did not anastomose with hepatic veins to produce the hepato-subcardinal channel, precursor of the hepatic segment of the IVC. **B,** T1W MRI of normal IVC *(white C)* for comparison. Note flow-related enhancement of the aorta.

Fig. 15-19. **A,** T1W axial MRI of horseshoe kidney. Note incomplete medial rotation of kidneys and fusion of renal tissue *(white k's)* across the midline. This tissue could be mistaken for a conglomerate nodal mass. Psoas minor muscle asymmetry *(white arrow)* on left is an incidental normal variant (see Fig. 15-14). **B,** Coronal T1W MRI. White curved arrows indicate small zone of cortical fusion. **C,** T1W MRI section of same patient, posterior to that of **B,** for comparison. Note abnormal renal axis, confirmed in the coronal plane.

the axilla, and the remaining 5% are found in many locations, including the retroperitoneum and mesentery (Fig. 15-21).[50] Hovanessian et al.[50] state that "they are classified histologically into simple, cavernous, and cystic" tumors. CT may reveal the low attenuation value of chyle. Signal intensity less than or moderately greater than surrounding muscle on T1W images becomes intense on T2W. Low intensity septations are visible within the high intensity fluid on T2W images (Fig. 15-21, *A* and *B*).

Other benign neoplasms

Leiomyomas occur occasionally in the gastrointestinal and genitourinary tracts but are rare in the retroperitoneum. Rhabdomyomas are extremely rare in adults; in all they constitute 2% or less of all neoplasms of striated muscle.[34] Benign lipomas typically have homogeneous high signal intensity similar to subcutaneous fat.[27] The soft tissue myolipoma is a mixed lesion of benign smooth muscle and mature fat. These tumors can be confused with more common liposarcomas of the retroperitoneum but are distinguishable by their distinctive histologic pattern.[78] Benign fibroblastic proliferations of idiopathic, reactive, or reparative etiologies are mimicked by some malignant tumors that produce collagen. Fibrous histiocytoma, fibrous mesothelioma, and neurofibroma (the most frequent of this group of lesions) can be mistaken for benign fibrous tumors.[34] Mature teratomas commonly remain following chemotherapy of primary or secondary malignant nonseminomatous germ cell tumors of the retroperitoneum (Fig. 15-22).[96] Although these are indolent lesions, they require regular follow-up examinations by MRI or CT throughout one's life. Primary benign cystic teratomas of the retroperitoneum are rare tumors thought to arise from vestigial embryonic totipotent cells.[9] They contain elements derived from any or all of the three primordial tissues: mesoderm, ectoderm, or endoderm. Several reports of their MRI appearance agree that CT and MRI are valuable for diagnosis of these lesions.[9,18,94] Advantages of MRI include sensitive demonstration of lipoid bone marrow elements and multiplanar imaging.[9,94] In the reported cases, MRI demonstrates the lack of invasion of adjacent organs and the relationship to major vessels.[9,18] The primary disadvantage of MRI is its lower sensitivity for calcifications, which frequently are present in these lesions.[9]

ACQUIRED VASCULAR LESIONS
Arterial lesions

MRI serves an increasingly important role in the evaluation of aortic dissection (Fig. 15-23, *D* and *E*).[3,24,107] MRI also is useful for diagnosis of complications of aortic surgery. The utility of CT and MRI following vascular surgery has been reviewed by several authors.[6,40,48,56,75] MR angiography is covered in detail in Chapter 7.

Bowel ischemia from arterial obstruction or insufficiency produces mucosal edema that is indistinguishable

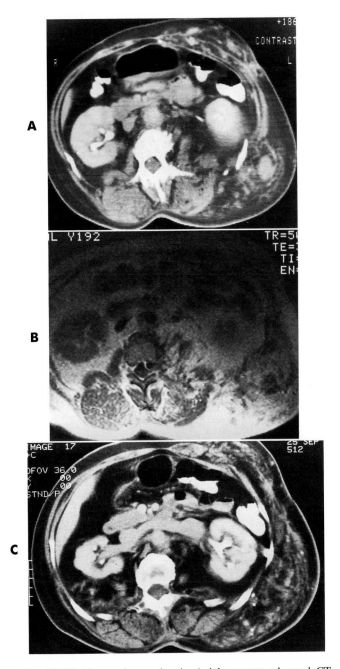

Fig. 15-20. Hemangiomatosis. **A,** Axial contrast-enhanced CT of 38-year-old patient demonstrates serpiginous and globular vascular structures (isodense to muscle) in right and left PPRS, left MS, left PRS, and abdominal wall. **B,** Axial 0.15 T MRI with elliptical surface coil. Findings on same patient, now 43, are similar to CT. Little change in 5 years. **C,** Follow-up CT on same patient, now 47, using iodine contrast agent. Image is located a few centimeters more craniad than **A** and **B**. Extensive multicompartmental deformity indicates slow progression over 9 years of follow-up. Note phleboliths in left flank soft tissues.

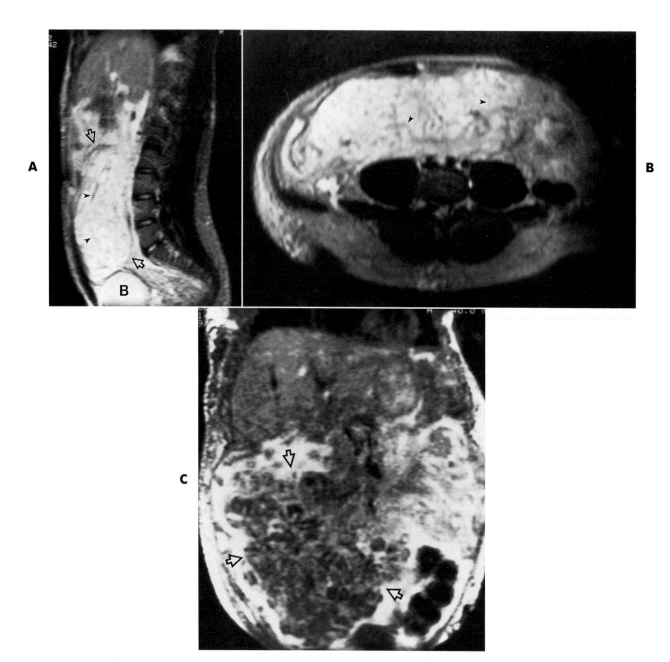

Fig. 15-21. Lymphangioma of the mesentery. **A,** Sagittal T2W (TR 2500/TE 80) MRI of abdominal mass immediately superior to the bladder *(B)*. Open arrows denote approximate margins of the mass. Low intensity septations *(arrowheads)* are present within the mass. **B,** Axial T2W MRI of same patient. Extensive high signal intensity mass merges imperceptibly with small bowel in lower abdomen. Septations *(arrowheads)* again are visible. **C,** Coronal T1W MRI. Multiple loops of small bowel are clumped in right lower quadrant among low intensity cystic masses of mesenteric lymphangioma *(arrows)*. Patient had a history of chronic lymphangitis involving the torso and lower extremities.

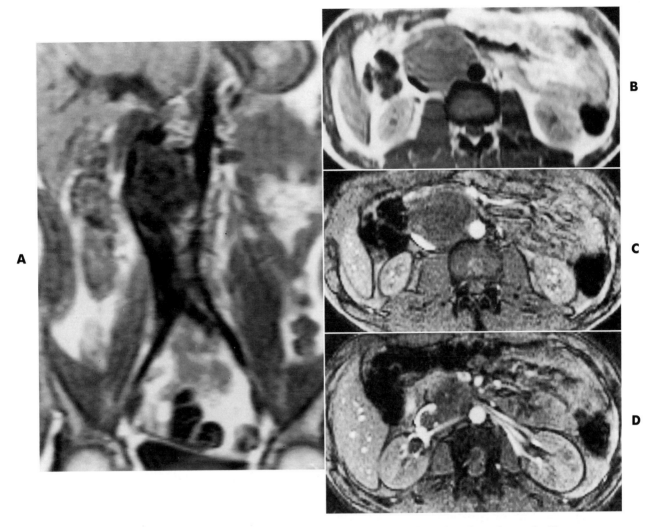

Fig. 15-22. Mature teratoma residual of mixed germ cell tumor following chemotherapy in 18-year-old male. Following right orchiectomy for a small mixed germ cell tumor, highly elevated tumor markers returned to normal. Bulky retroperitoneal mass did not decrease in size after chemotherapy. Surgery revealed only benign tissue. No change in 15 months of postoperative follow-up. **A,** Coronal T1W MRI. Heterogenous mass (slightly hypointense to muscle) displaces the IVC laterally. **B,** Axial TR 2200/TE 22 MRI. Signal of mass is intermediate to muscle and fat. **C,** FLASH TR 30/TE 12 with flow compensation. Note high intensity of flowing blood in the IVC and aorta. **D,** Same technique, slightly cephalad to **C.** Focal invasion of IVC. Histologic examination revealed no malignant tissue elements.

from mucosal injury of other etiologies.[58] However, MRI can be valuable in cases of intestinal angina (see Fig. 15-45). (For further discussion of ischemic bowel disease, also see Chapter 14.)

The incidence of abdominal aortic aneurysm (AAA) is approximately 2% in elderly individuals and is more common in males than in females.[39] Sonography is the most often used screening procedure for AAAs. Flak et al.[39] report that both MRI and ultrasound measurements of AAAs provide accurate dimensions. However, they report that MRI is more sensitive for evaluation of renal and iliac ar-

tery involvement, since intestinal gas does not obscure the vessels. CT provides accurate measurements of vessel cross sections, but requires iodinated contrast agents to confirm the absence of fresh intraluminal thrombi (Fig. 15-23). In their discussion, Flak et al. also state that on CT, perivascular lymphadenopathy may not be distinguishable from extravasated blood.[39] MRI clearly is superior to CT for characterization of extraperitoneal fluid collections and soft tissues (see Fig. 15-24, *E* to *G*).[26]

Spontaneous arteriovenous (A-V) fistulization complicates the rupture of an AAA. The incidence of A-V fistula

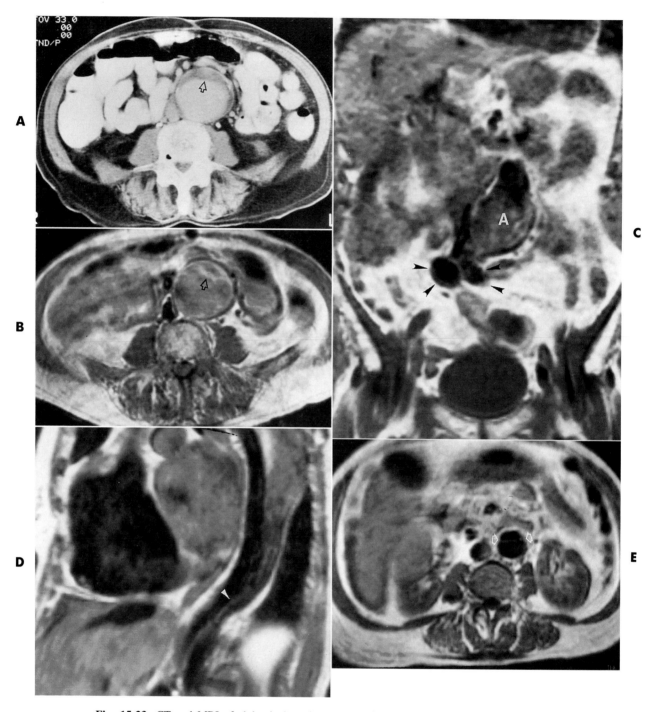

Fig. 15-23. CT and MRI of abdominal aortic aneurysm in a 77-year-old male. Compare with MRI of aortic dissection (**D** and **E**). **A,** CT with iodinated contrast agent demonstrates 6 cm AAA. Mural plaque and thrombus are visible *(open arrow)*. **B,** Proton density axial MRI reveals high intensity margin of mural thrombus *(open arrow)* without contrast agent. **C,** Coronal T1W MRI documents absence of renal artery involvement and distal extension of the aneurysm *(A)* into the common iliac arteries *(arrowheads)*. **D,** Sagittal T1W MRI demonstrates intimal flap of aortic wall dissection spiraling down the abdominal aorta from the thoracic aorta *(white arrow)*. **E,** Axial T1W MRI with signal void in both false and true lumens. Intimal flap *(open arrows)* is slightly hyperintense to flowing blood. (**D** and **E** courtesy of DC Rappaport, MD, Toronto, Ontario.)

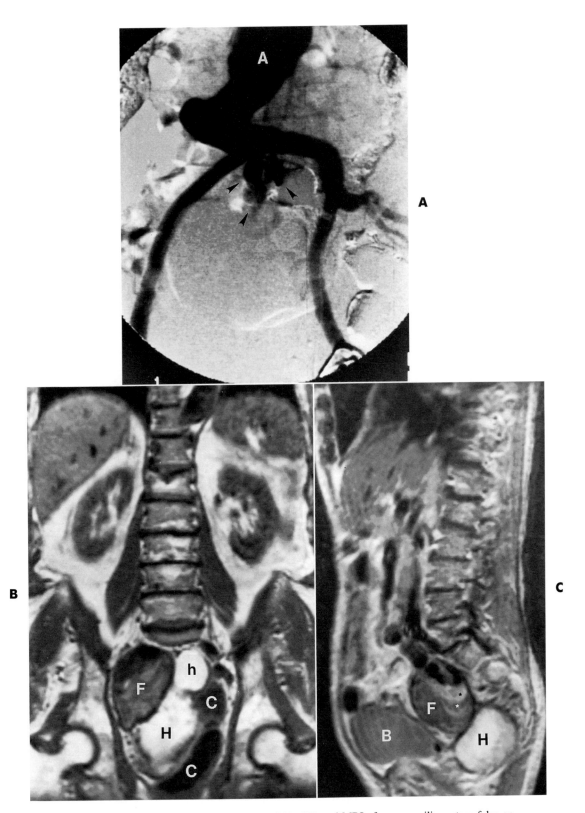

Fig. 15-24. Digital subtraction angiogram (DSA), CT, and MRI of common iliac artery false aneurysm and retroperitoneal hematoma. Same case as Fig. 15-23. **A,** DSA reveals "jet" of contrast agent into proximal portion of the false aneurysm *(arrowheads)*. Note fusiform aortic aneurysm *(white A)*. **B,** Coronal T1W MRI. False aneurysm *(F)*; a small, homogeneous retroperitoneal hematoma *(h)*; a large, inhomogeneous retroperitoneal hematoma *(H)*; and barium contrast-enhanced rectosigmoid colon *(C)* are depicted. **C,** Sagittal T1W MRI. Lamellated hemorrhage of varying age and intensity *(*)* is directly visible within false aneurysm *(F)*. Large hematoma *(H)* again is visible, as is the bladder *(B)*.

Continued.

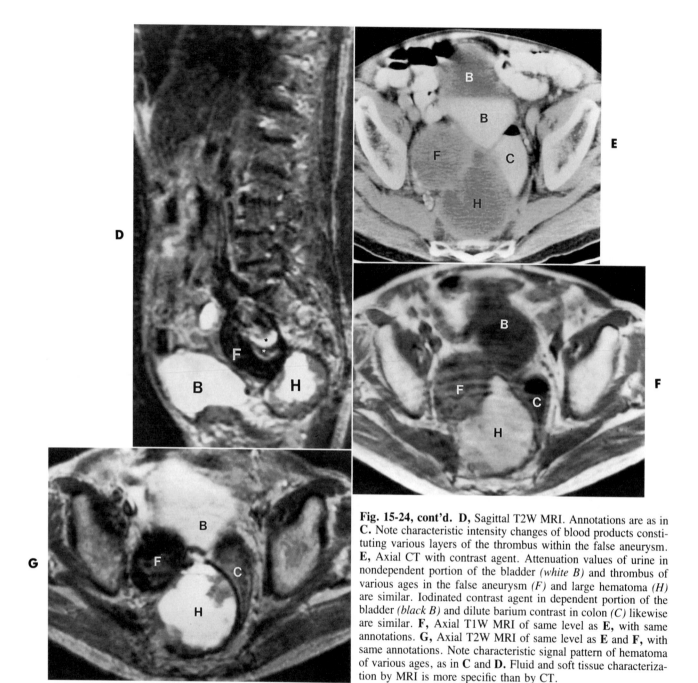

Fig. 15-24, cont'd. **D,** Sagittal T2W MRI. Annotations are as in **C.** Note characteristic intensity changes of blood products constituting various layers of the thrombus within the false aneurysm. **E,** Axial CT with contrast agent. Attenuation values of urine in nondependent portion of the bladder *(white B)* and thrombus of various ages in the false aneurysm *(F)* and large hematoma *(H)* are similar. Iodinated contrast agent in dependent portion of the bladder *(black B)* and dilute barium contrast in colon *(C)* likewise are similar. **F,** Axial T1W MRI of same level as **E,** with same annotations. **G,** Axial T2W MRI of same level as **E** and **F,** with same annotations. Note characteristic signal pattern of hematoma of various ages, as in **C** and **D.** Fluid and soft tissue characterization by MRI is more specific than by CT.

formation is increased by the presence of a retroaortic left renal vein. Renal and iliac veins are also potential fistula sites. The finding of an anomalous left renal vein on a preoperative scan or the absence of a normally situated left renal vein at surgery alerts the surgeon to the possibility of an A-V fistula.[16]

False aneurysms of major abdominal vessels are readily detectible by MRI. Lamellar distribution of signal intensities is sometimes seen. When present, this sign is evidence of incremental enlargement by recurrent bleeding (Fig. 15-24, *C* and *D*). Although angiography with iodinated con-

trast agents demonstrates extravasation from the arterial lumen, MRI better depicts the extent of false aneurysms and associated retroperitoneal hematomas (Fig. 15-24, *A* and *B*). For another example of specific characterization of retroperitoneal hematomas by MRI, see the discussion of traumatic duodenal hematomas in Chapter 14.

Venous lesions

Venous thrombosis is recognizable on CT by identification of a dilated vessel containing a filling defect with a low attenuation value. MRI has the advantage of sensitivity to at least two complementary physical properties associated with vascular thrombosis. First, the high signal intensity of a subacute intravascular thrombus on T1W images (or the low intensity of hemosiderin) often is detectable with good contrast against the background tissue. (However, the signal intensity of a thrombus in the IVC is highly variable.) Second, distortion of the normal signal pattern of flowing blood (loss of respiratory variation and of phase encoding ghosts) is a diagnostic sign even in the absence of characteristic signal intensity abnormalities (Fig. 15-25).[31,35,53]

The most common etiologies of renal vein thrombosis are dehydration, extension of the thrombus from the IVC, obstruction or invasion by a renal or extrarenal tumor, and idiopathic causes.[85] Transaxial and sagittal MRI readily demonstrates the involvement of the IVC by extrarenal neoplasms.[52] Fein[35] could not confirm that tumor thrombus (intravascular extension of renal carcinoma) could be

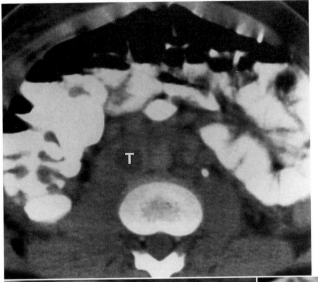

Fig. 15-25. Posttraumatic thrombosis of the IVC in 21-year-old female shown on CT and MRI examinations. **A,** CT with iodinated contrast agent demonstrates thrombus *(T)* in dilated IVC. **B,** On T1W coronal MRI, thrombus *(T)* has plainly visible high intensity in distal IVC. Aorta, superior mesenteric vein, and portal vein have typical low intensity from the flow void effect of the spin echo technique. **C,** On this gradient echo scan with flow compensation, flowing blood has high signal intensity. Note absence of intense signal in expected course of the IVC *(white arrows 1-3).*

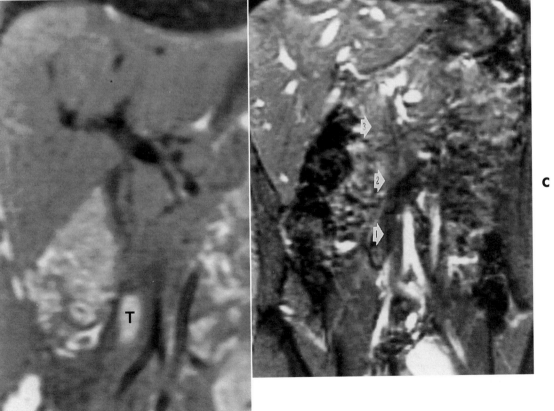

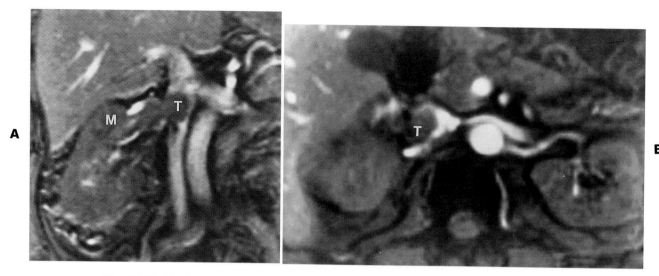

Fig. 15-26. Single breath-hold, fat-suppressed gradient echo MRI of renal cell carcinoma with intravascular extension to the IVC. **A,** Coronal section. CHESS fat suppression with an optimized presaturation pulse. Note contrast between low intensity of the tumor thrombus *(T)* and high intensity of the flowing blood in the IVC and left renal vein. Primary mass *(M)* in upper pole of the right kidney is not well-delineated by this pulse technique. **B,** Axial section with same technique. Tumor thrombus partially occludes dilated right renal vein and IVC. Abnormality of the right renal vein is striking in comparison to normal diameter and signal intensity of left renal vessels.

distinguished reliably from bland thrombus in his series of patients. Although its signal pattern may not be a reliable discriminator from bland thrombus, tumor thrombus is detectable by MRI with high sensitivity and specificity (Fig. 15-26).[52] Detection is possible without iodinated contrast agents, even in the presence of renal insufficiency.

Puerperal ovarian vein thrombosis (POVT) is encountered approximately once in every 600 to 2000 deliveries.[86] POVT is associated with postpartum endometritis, cesarean section, gynecologic surgery, and pelvic inflammatory disease. Fever, abdominal pain, distention, and nonspecific systemic signs occur 2 to 4 days postpartum or postoperatively. Eighty to ninety percent of cases are unilateral right-sided; 14% are bilateral.[76,86] CT signs of POVT are low attenuation filling defects in the ovarian vein (ultimately also in the IVC) and a permeative inflammatory mass in the aorticocaval space and the anterior pararenal space. The lesions are detectible by ultrasound, if bowel distention permits an acoustic window to the ACS and APRS.[76] MRI has confirmed the diagnosis of POVT in at least one patient for whom CT findings were nonspecific.[86] Coronal sections depict the tubular, distended thrombosed veins so that the diagnosis is readily perceived.[76,86] The characteristic intensity pattern of blood products is a confirmatory sign, as it is in the assessment of other thrombotic lesions by MRI.

Duplex Doppler ultrasonography, because of its convenience and relatively low cost, is the preferred initial imaging modality for evaluation of the portal vein thrombo-

sis.[1,31] However, ultrasound evaluation of the mesenteric and splenic veins frequently is limited by bowel gas artifacts. In these seriously ill patients, the risk of arteriography is avoided whenever possible. Even the risk of an iodinated contrast agent is unacceptably high in a significant number, precluding the use of CT. Thrombosis of the superior mesenteric, splenic, and portal veins is demonstrated noninvasively by MRI (Fig. 15-27). With the addition of magnetic resonance angiography (MRA), blood flow direction also is determinable.[31] MRA or a gradient echo, single breath-hold technique provides better resolution of small collateral veins than conventional spin echo imaging. Appropriately located varices are occasionally essential indirect evidence of abnormality in the major vessels (Fig. 15-28).

INFLAMMATORY DISEASES
Pancreatitis

In pancreatitis, exudate from an inflamed pancreas permeates the APRS and can separate the leaves of the posterior renal fascia to approach the PPRS.[84] Exudate crosses the midline within the APRS (Figs. 15-28; and 15-3, *A*) and extends craniad to the bare area of the liver (Figs. 15-3, *C*, and 15-30).[79] At its caudal margin the APRS freely communicates with the PPRS and PRS (Fig. 15-3, *B*).[77,79] APRS effusions, limited laterally by the lateroconal fascia, dissect into the left pericolic fat and simulate primary colonic inflammatory or neoplastic disease (Fig. 15-29). Infiltration of the fat surrounding the celiac axis

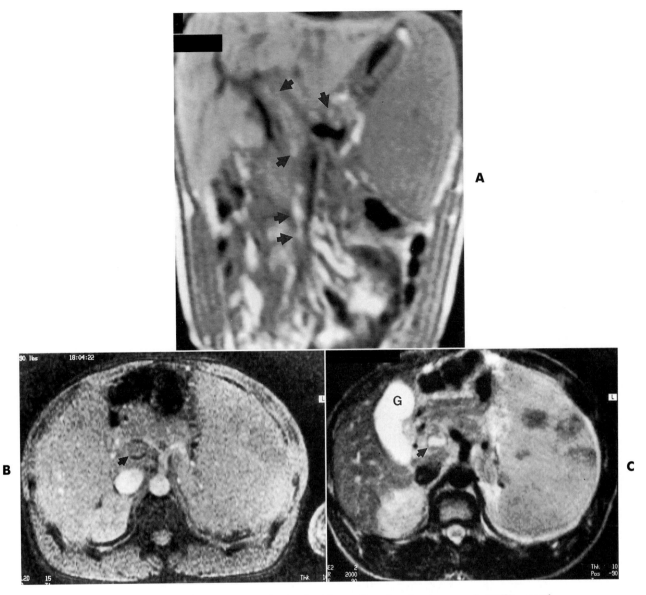

Fig. 15-27. MRI of 36-year-old professional athlete with polycythemia vera. **A,** T1W coronal section demonstrates abnormal high intensity in superior mesenteric, portal, and splenic veins *(arrows)*. Note marked enlargement of the spleen. **B,** On this transaxial gradient echo MRI, thrombosed portal vein *(arrow)* is isointense with liver parenchyma. High intensity signal of flowing blood is visible in the celiac axis and IVC. **C,** T2W scan at same level reveals high intensity of extracellular methemoglobin in lumen of the portal vein *(arrow)*. Thrombosed vein is isointense with gallbladder *(G)*. Low intensity (flow void) is observed in the normal vessels.

and the superior mesenteric artery is not a specific sign of pancreatic carcinoma (see Fig. 15-11, *A* and *B*).[8] This focal involvement of the APRS and mesenteric fat also is present in some cases of chonic pancreatitis. (See Chapter 12 for further discussion of pancreatitis.)

Abscess

Among the many etiologies of prolonged febrile illness (infections, neoplasms, connective tissue diseases, granu-lomatous diseases, metabolic diseases, thermoregulatory disorders, and others), infection is by far the most common. The physical and laboratory findings of retroperito-neal abscess are relatively nonspecific. Only 55% with perirenal abscess are febrile on first examination.[32] An abdominal mass or tenderness is present in 62%; leukocyto-sis (greater than 12,000/mm[3]) is present only in 57%; and pyuria is found in 74% of patients with perirenal abscess.[32] Failure to diagnose a retroperitoneal abscess can

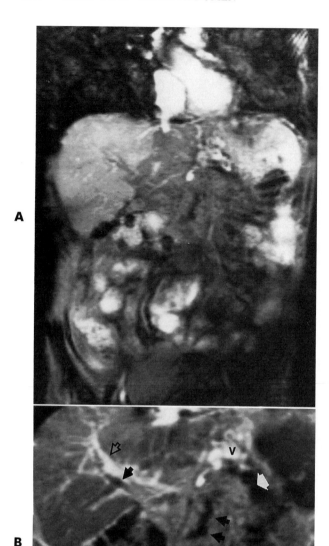

Fig. 15-28. MRI of pancreatitis. **A,** Coronal GRE breath-hold, fat-suppressed MRI with no contrast agent. Ill-defined mass of intermediate intensity (hypointense to liver) extends from diaphragm to subcostal region and from porta hepatis to hilum of the spleen. Short gastric varices are present. **B,** Coronal GRE breath-hold, fat-suppressed MRI with intravenous gadolinium-DTPA contrast agent and oral barium suspension. Right portal vein signal is intense *(open arrow)*. With gadolinium enhancement, inflamed pancreas is hyperintense to the liver. Its margins are sharply delineated by bowel containing low intensity barium contrast agent *(closed white arrows)*. Dilated low intensity biliary and pancreatic ducts *(single and double closed black arrows)* are best seen on this contrast-enhanced sequence. Splenic and proximal portal veins are visible on none of the coronal or axial sections (axials not shown here). Collateral vessels *(v)* confirm diagnosis of splenic and portal vein thrombosis.

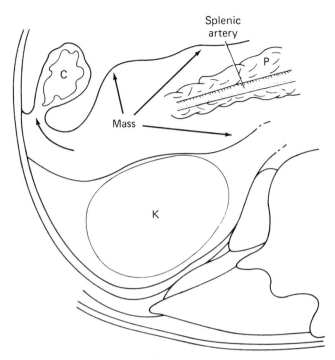

Fig. 15-29. Pathway of pericolonic fat infiltration by pancreatic exudate via APRS. Figure shows descending colon *(C)*, left kidney *(K)*, and pancreas *(P)*. Left side of drawing represents left side of the abdomen (mirror-image reversal of conventional orientation). Diffuse inflammation (similar to Fig. 15-28), neoplasm, pseudocyst, pancreatic abscess, or hematoma of the tail of the pancreas could similarly affect the descending colon. Epicenter of abnormality is readily identified as the pancreas by knowledge of compartmental anatomy. (From Meyers MA: *Dynamic radiology of the abdomen*, New York, 1976, Springer Verlag.)

result in a fatal or permanently disabling outcome.[105] Therefore, ultrasonography, CT, and MRI play major roles in the diagnostic evaluation of deep soft tissue infections.

Detection of abnormal intraperitoneal and soft tissue gas collections is one of the major indications for conventional radiography and CT examinations.[17,68,108] MRI is relatively unsuited for this application.[63] For detection and localization of soft tissue inflammatory masses and abscesses, however, MRI is a powerful tool.[59,63,105] Using compartmental anatomy as a guide, the source of retroperitoneal abscesses frequently can be determined.[79]

Rupture of retrocecal appendix. Finer and Merritt[36] state that acute appendicitis occurs in about 7% to 12% of the population in the western hemisphere and is the most common indication for emergency laparotomy. When used by experienced examiners, graded compression ultrasonography has sensitivity and specificity of about 90% for appendicitis.[12,36,98] In contrast, plain films reveal a radiopaque appendicolith in only 7% to 15% of cases.[36] Diagnosis of appendiceal perforation by ultrasound is more difficult. A sensitivity of 86% and specificity of only 60%

Fig. 15-30. Sagittal drawing of retroperitoneal relationships of the right colon and appendix shows APRS *(horizontal crosshatching)*, PRS *(stippled shading)*, and PPRS *(grid pattern)*. Inflammatory exudate from appendicitis (or bowel contents after appendiceal rupture) enter the peritoneum or APRS. Other retroperitoneal spaces are vulnerable to direct extension of the inflammatory process. (From Meyers MA: *Dynamic radiology of the abdomen,* New York, 1976, Springer Verlag.)

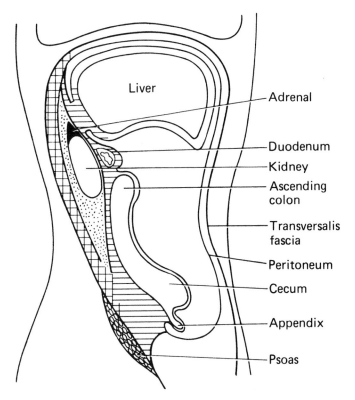

Fig. 15-31. MRI of appendiceal abscess. **A,** T1W coronal scan demonstrates fluid collection *(fl)* at caudal margin of the liver. Gerota's fascia appears thickened. Streaks of low intensity edema are visible in the retroperitoneal fat. **B,** T1W axial scan demonstrates fluid dividing layers of the posterior renal fascia *(open arrow)*. Fluid is present in region of the lateroconal fascia *(fl)*. Thickened, bridging septum *(arrowhead)* extends from posterior renal fascia to lower pole of the right kidney *(K)*. Fat is infiltrated posterior to the cecum *(C)*. **C,** T2W axial scan confirms pericolic edema and retroperitoneal abscess. Fluid *(fl and f)* has breached properitoneal fat compartment and has dissected into intermuscular fat planes of the abdominal wall. Figure shows kidney *(K)* and cecum *(C)*.

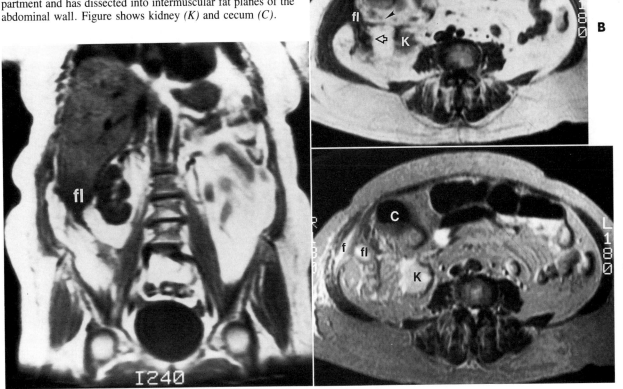

are reported by Borushok et al.[12] CT reliably demonstrates pericecal fat infiltration and fluid collections.[12,98] MRI also demonstrates edema of the APRS fat, dissection of fluid between the layers of the posterior renal fascia, and extension of an appendiceal abscess into the properitoneal fat compartment and abdominal wall (Figs. 15-30 and 15-31).

Enteric fistulization. Transmural inflammation produces internal fistulas in 16% of patients with Crohn's disease. Fistulization leads to the formation of intraperitoneal, mesenteric, and retroperitoneal abscesses. MRI shows fistulas and extramucosal inflammatory abnormalities in 14 of 17 cases reviewed by Koelbel et al.[59] Both MRI and CT are useful in the evaluation of mesenteric abscess caused by Crohn's disease (Fig. 15-32).

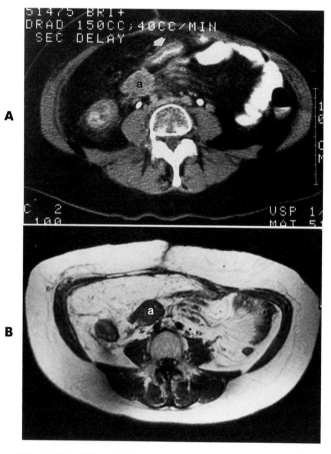

Fig. 15-32. CT and MRI of mesenteric abscess from Crohn's disease. **A,** Transaxial CT with intravenous and oral contrast agents. Mesenteric mass *(a)* is present in right lower quadrant anterior to the iliac vessels. Thickening of the bowel wall *(white arrow)* is evident. Note stranding edema in the mesenteric fat. **B,** Transaxial T1W MRI (same level as **A**) demonstrates low intensity fluid within mesenteric abscess *(a).* T2W scan (not shown) reveals abscess fluid to be hyperintense to fat. Note proximity of the mesenteric abscess to ACS and APRS. Infection could extend into the retroperitoneum by direct contiguity or by transmesenteric infiltration.

AIDS-related infections

Unusual pathogens such as *Mycobacterium tuberculosis* (MTB), *Mycobacterium avium-intracellulare* (MAI), and *Pneumocystis carinii* are most commonly encountered in patients with immune deficiency, especially in patients with AIDS acquired immunodeficiency syndrome.[71,83,95,105] These infections provoke retroperitoneal adenopathy, in addition to producing lesions in mesenteric lymph nodes, intraperitoneal solid organs, and the peritoneum. Necrotic nodes are observed in 93% of patients with abdominal involvement by MTB. MAI produces necrotic nodes in only 14% of cases. Lubat et al.[71] found calcification of abdominal lymph nodes (including retroperitoneal nodes) involved by *Pneumocystis carinii* in two of three AIDS patients on CT follow-up. Calcification developed also on the surface of the parietal peritoneum and in mesenteric lymph nodes in these patients.

Sarcoidosis. A retrospective study of biopsy-proven abdominal sarcoid lesions conducted by Britt et al.[13] reveals that 73% of the selected patients have retroperitoneal adenopathy and 55% have mesenteric adenopathy. Other nodal sites involved in more than 50% of the patients are the celiac artery axis, the porta hepatis, and the gastrohepatic ligament. The lymph nodes typically are discrete rather than conglomerate masses. Their size ranges from 1.1 to 7.5 cm, with a mean of 2.6 cm.[13]

Amyloidosis. Sueoka et al.[93] have reported one case of perirenal amyloidosis in a 76-year-old male with multiple myeloma. The amyloid infiltrate enhances with iodinated contrast agent on CT examination, and is hypointense to the renal cortex on a T1W MRI sequence. Gadolinium contrast produces only slight enhancement. On a T2W sequence the abnormal tissue is slightly less intense than the renal cortex.

Angioimmunoblastic lymphadenopathy. An unusual cause of lymph node hyperplasia, angioimmunoblastic lymphadenopathy (AIBL) can be confused with lymphoma. Armstrong, Wilson, and Dee[4] report that paratracheal, anterior mediastinal, and hilar adenopathy are commonly seen in AIBL. Retroperitoneal adenopathy also occurs (see Fig. 15-34). Other signs of AIBL are fever, rash, organomegaly, and immunologic abnormalities. Approximately one third of cases eventually develop a hematologic malignancy.

Retroperitoneal fibrosis (RPF). This is an uncommon fibroproliferative lesion that often causes ureteral or vascular obstruction.[5] About two thirds of RPF cases are idiopathic. Twelve percent of reported cases are caused by chronic use of methysergide; 8% to 10% of cases have a desmoplastic reaction to malignancy (malignant RPF); and other cases follow infection and hemorrhage. MRI of a typical benign case reveals a relatively well-marginated, homogeneous midline mass encasing the aorta and extending no farther than approximately 1 cm lateral to the ureters. In rare cases, fibrosis obstructs the common bile duct, portal vein, or bowel.[2] Structures engulfed by RPF are encased smoothly. MRI demonstrates RPF vascular compression without contrast agents.[51] The MRI signal intensity of mature benign RPF typically is low on T1W and T2W sequences.[2,5,51] High intensity on T2W scans is seen in a few benign cases (typically in the immature, formative stage and restricted to the paraaortic region).[2] As in the scenario of radiation-induced versus malignant fibrosis, T2W hyperintensity in RPF is not specific for malignancy.[2,41] Heterogeneity on T2W sequences is suggestive of malignant RPF[5]; however, definitive diagnosis is obtainable only by tissue biopsy.

Sclerosing mesenteritis. This benign lesion involves varying degrees of fatty degeneration, inflammation, and fibrosis. Bowel wall edema, retraction, and mesenteric thickening are observed. The principal differential diagnoses are carcinoid, secondary neoplasm, and mesenteric desmoid. Kronthal et al.[60] report a case having a well-demarcated mesenteric mass of intermediate intensity on T1W and low intensity on T2W imaging.

LYMPHADENOPATHY
Size

Adenopathy is roughly categorized by size as benign versus malignant, following guidelines based on experience with CT. Lymph nodes less than 10 mm are considered benign. An unknown percentage of these small nodes contain malignancy that is below the threshold of detectability. According to Hartman,[46] nodes in the 10 to 15 mm range are suspicious; cross-sectional diameters greater than 15 mm are abnormal. Three general patterns of adenopathy have been observed. First, the simplest pattern is enlargement of one or more discrete nodes (Fig. 15-33). Second, fusion of several abnormal nodes produces a focal mass (Fig. 15-34). Third, the most complex, and most likely malignant, configuration is the bulky, permeative conglomerate mass (Fig. 15-35).[62]

Signal intensity

The best contrast between lymph nodes and fat is usually achieved on T1W sequences (Fig. 15-34, *A*). Between lymph nodes and muscle, the best contrast is achieved on T2W sequences (Fig. 15-34, *B*).[25,66] Weiner et al.[101] state that nodes infiltrated with carcinoma often are hyperintense to fat on T2W; their T2 relaxation time is "longer than that of any other type of lymph node." Dooms et al.[26] report that acute inflammatory nodes have higher intensity on T2W images than nodes infiltrated with neoplasm or chronic granulomatous disease. They further report, as do others, that the signal patterns of various malignancies are similar on MRI (Figs. 15-34, 15-35).[26,62,63] Hyperintensity of lymphadenopathy on T2W images is not specific evidence of malignancy in general, nor is it evidence of a particular type of neoplasm. The spin density image (long TR, short TE) should not be used to evaluate for lymphadenopathy, since fat and lymph nodes may have the same signal intensity.

MRI vs CT detection

MRI compares favorably with CT regarding detection of adenopathy.[25,26,62,66] MRI is more specific than CT in the distinction of adenopathy from blood vessels, lymphoceles (Fig. 15-36, *C, D,* and *F*), retroperitoneal fibrosis, and retroperitoneal hematoma.[25,66] Although Lee et al.[65] suggested in 1981 that CT could discriminate recurrent rectal carcinoma from postoperative fibrosis, subsequent study has shown otherwise.[22] MRI is no better than CT at discriminating between benign fibrosis and recurrent carcinoma (note that some authors disagree about this); however, MRI demonstrates the extent of recurrent tumor and points out areas of desmoplastic reaction within masses.[22]

MALIGNANT PRIMARY NEOPLASMS

Primary retroperitoneal neoplasms are those that arise from the mesenchyme, neurogenic tissue, or embryonic rests of the retroperitoneum.[34,46] Neoplasms arising from the organs of the retroperitoneum (lymph nodes, kidneys, ureters, adrenal glands, vessels, duodenum, pancreas, and ascending and descending colon) are not included among the primary retroperitoneal lesions.[46] In this system of classification, lymphoma is considered a secondary neoplasm of the retroperitoneum.

The most common causes of kidney displacement by abnormal masses are abdominal aortic aneurysm, intracapsular extrarenal mass, intrarenal neoplasm, lymphoma, metastatic lymphadenopathy, other lymph node diseases, retroperitoneal neoplasm, and adrenal masses.[85] When evaluating an unknown retroperitoneal mass, one should

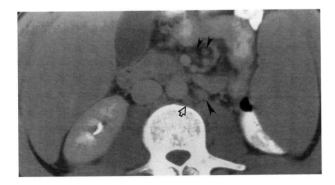

Fig. 15-33. CT of angioimmunoblastic lymphadenopathy shows retroperitoneal and mesenteric lymph node involvement. A 15 mm left paraaortic node *(large arrowhead)* and multiple small mesenteric nodes *(small arrowheads)* are present. This young man had signs of inflammatory illness, adenopathy, splenomegaly, and diffuse reticular pulmonary infiltrate. Pulmonary infiltrate cleared and all of his inflammatory symptoms resolved completely after a brief course of steroids. Note nodular-appearing left crus of the diaphragm *(open arrow),* which could be mistaken for a lymph node.

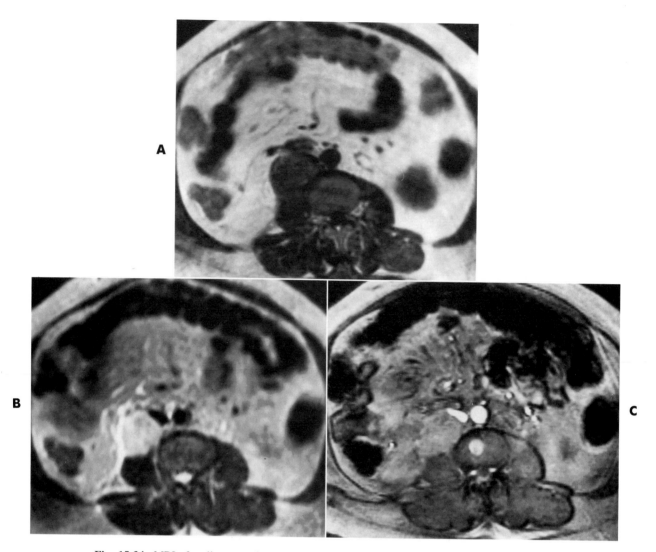

Fig. 15-34. MRI of malignant melanoma showing focal lymph node mass. **A,** Axial T1W. Adenopathy is slightly hyperintense to muscle. Node-fat contrast is good, but node-muscle and node-vessel contrast is poor. **B,** Axial T2W (same level as **A**). Adenopathy is slightly hyperintense to fat. Node-fat contrast is poor and node-muscle contrast is good. Node-vessel contrast is good, but vessel margins are indistinct. **C,** Axial gradient echo (same level as **A** and **B**). Adenopathy is nearly isointense with fat. Node-fat contrast is poor; node-muscle contrast is moderate; and node-vessel contrast is good, with well-defined vessel margins.

first consider benign treatable lesions, metastatic neoplasm, and lymphoma. It is reasonable to consider primary extraperitoneal malignancies only after the common lesions have been excluded.[46]

Malignant fibrous histiocytoma

Malignant fibrous histiocytoma (MFH) is the most common soft tissue sarcoma in patients over 50 years old.[34] The retroperitoneum (site of approximately 16% of cases) is the third most common location of MFH, after the lower and upper extremities (Figs. 15-36 and 15-37).[34,55] On MRI examination, MFH typically exhibits a heterogeneous signal pattern with low intensity on T1W and higher intensity on T2W sequences (Figs. 15-36, *A* and *B*, and 15-37, *B* and *C*).

Enzinger and Weiss[34] divide MFH into five subtypes: storiform-pleomorphic (more than 50%), myxoid (25%), giant cell, inflammatory (most of these are the retroperitoneum), and angiomatoid (seen in children and young adults). The inflammatory subtype is manifested by fever and leukocytosis.[34] The site of origin of a large mass may be obscure, since MFH can arise in retroperitoneal organs and the soft tissues.[55,82] The primary mass almost always is discovered before distant metastasis occurs.[55] The neoplasm typically has a well-circumscribed appearance (Fig. 15-37, *A* and *C*) but spreads insidiously along fascial

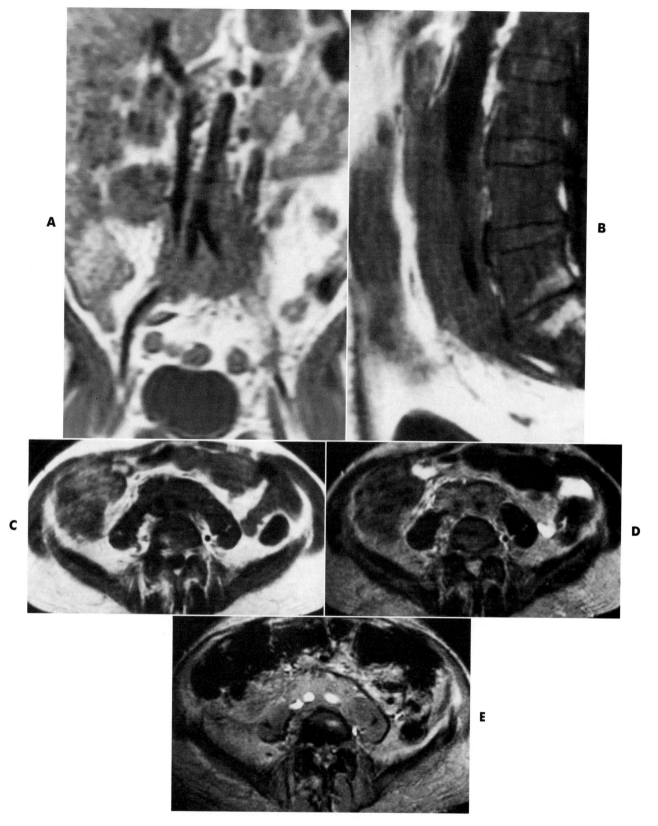

Fig. 15-35. MRI of lymphoma shows bulky conglomerate mass. **A,** Coronal T1W. Aorta and IVC have been engulfed by adenopathy. **B,** Sagittal T1W. Aorta is encased by confluent adenopathy. Note displacement of aorta from the spine by interposed nodes. This is usually evidence of malignancy, although occasionally displacement occurs in benign retroperitoneal fibrosis.[2] **C,** Axial T1W. Compare with Fig. 15-34, *A*. Contrast is poor between mass and muscle. **D,** Axial T2W. Compare with Fig. 15-34, *B*. Contrast is good between mass and muscle. Vessels are indistinct. **E,** Axial gradient echo. Compare with Fig. 15-34, *C*. Contrast is fair between mass and muscle. Vessels are well-demonstrated.

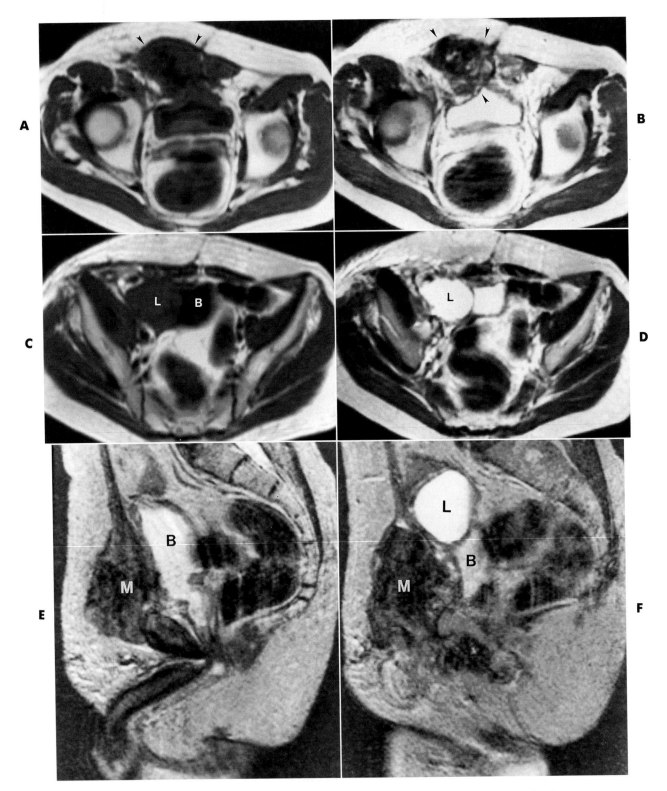

Fig. 15-36. MRI of malignant fibrous histiocytoma of rectus muscle sheath. Postoperative lymphocele was incidental finding. **A,** Axial T1W section through the neoplasm *(arrowheads)* demonstrates its inhomogeneous composition. Its signal is isointense with muscle. **B,** Axial T2W at same level as **A.** Mixed intensity lesion *(arrowheads)* displaces and invades anterior bladder wall. **C,** T1W axial section craniad to **A** and **B.** Low intensity mass *(L)* adjacent to MFH at dome of the bladder *(B)* mimics primary neoplasm or adenopathy. **D,** T2W axial section at same level as **C** reveals homogeneous hyperintense signal. Lymphocele *(L)* was surgically proven. See Fig. 15-43. **E,** Sagittal T2W midline section. Center of MFH *(M)* and its relationship to bladder *(B)* are demonstrated better than in the axial projection. **F,** Sagittal T2W right paramedian section shows mass *(M)* and lymphocele *(L)*. Signal intensity of lymphocele is greater than that of bladder *(B)*.

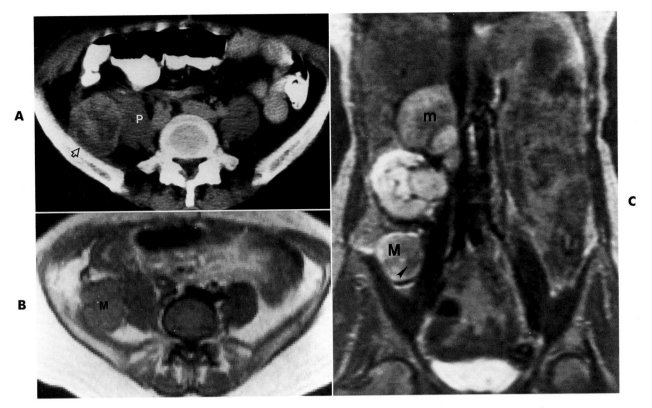

Fig. 15-37. CT and MRI of malignant fibrous histiocytoma. **A,** Transaxial CT with contrast demonstrates heterogeneous soft tissue mass *(open arrow)* in PPRS, abutting right psoas muscle *(P).* **B,** Axial T1W MRI at same level as **A.** Mass *(m)* is slightly hyperintense to muscle. **C,** Coronal T1W MRI. Note persistent low intensity *(arrowhead)* in dense fibrous region of the caudal portion of the mass *(M).* Mass *(m)* has extended toward the head within the PRS, greatly rotating kidney in the sagittal plane.

planes and among muscle fibers (Figs. 15-36, *E,* and 15-37, *C*). A few tumors bleed and appear as cystic hematomas. Hodgkin's disease and pleomorphic liposarcoma may have histologic patterns similar to MFH.[34] Meticulous histopathologic analysis is required to distinguish MFH from diverse other sarcomas occurring in the retroperitoneum, such as malignant mesenchymoma and dedifferentiated chondrosarcoma, which may have sharply different prognoses.[81]

Liposarcoma

Liposarcoma is the most common of the primary retroperitoneal malignancies and ranges from highly aggressive (Fig. 15-40) pleomorphic, dedifferentiated, and unclassified types to the more indolent, well-differentiated (atypical lipomatous tumors) (Fig. 15-38) and myxoid tumors (Fig. 15-39).[70] The overall 5-year survival in one series was 39%.[34] London et al.[70] report that the well-differentiated lesions have irregular nodular configuration on T1W sections. Their signal intensity is similar to subcutaneous fat and high intensity septa are present. On T2W images the septa become low intensity and the nodular tissue becomes hyperintense.[70] The extent of low intensity on T1W images is roughly proportional to the degree of cellularity of the neoplasm (Fig. 15-38). Multiplanar MRI demonstrates the extent of the neoplasm better than CT.[27,70] Vascular involvement is readily determined by MRI (Fig. 15-40). More recent reviews reaffirm the superiority of MRI over CT for characterization of soft tissue masses, including liposarcomas.[34,70]

Unusual cystic neoplasms

Malignant hemangiopericytoma is a rare malignancy in the retroperitoneum. Ultrasonography, CT, and MRI show it as a multiloculated cystic mass with areas of solid tissue.[54] This morphology, combined with ascites, can mislead the examiner to a presumptive diagnosis of ovarian malignancy and intraperitoneal seeding[42,100] (as in a recent case report of a malignant hemangiopericytoma of the omentum).[54]

Multilocular cysts and cystic neoplasms of the prostate are also rare lesions that present potentially confusing cys-

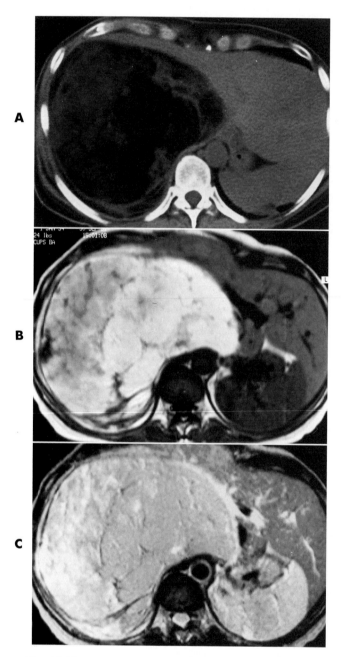

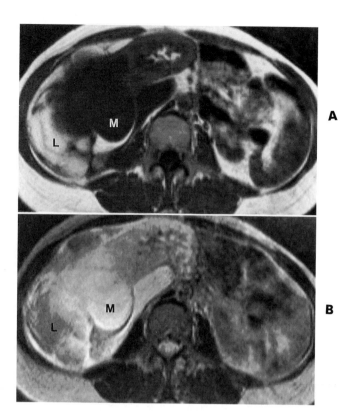

Fig. 15-39. Myxoid type of liposarcoma. **A,** Axial T1W MRI. High intensity, well-differentiated lobules of lipoid tissue *(L)* are demarcated by thin septations. Myxoid regions *(M)* have homogeneous low intensity typical of their high fluid content. Kidney is displaced anteromedially by the mass. **B,** Axial T2W MRI. Relative intensities of lipoid *(L)* and myxoid *(M)* components of the neoplasm are reversed on the TE 90 msec echo scan.

Fig. 15-38. Retroperitoneal liposarcoma. Contrasting regions of well-differentiated and less well-differentiated neoplasm. **A,** Axial CT. Better differentiated regions of neoplasm contain low density typical of fat. Areas of more aggressive tumor infiltration contain a greater proportion of tissue the density of water. **B,** Axial T1W MRI. Same slice location as **A.** High intensity lobules of well-differentiated fat tissue are present in well-differentiated region. Lower intensity is observed in more cellular region of the tumor. **C,** Axial T2W MRI at same location as **A** and **B.** Intense signal in lateral aspect of the mass is due to high water content of less well-differentiated region of the tumor.

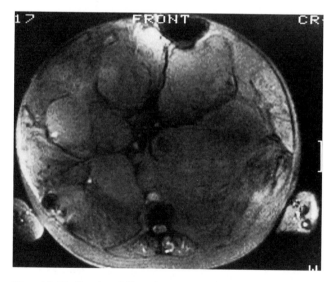

Fig. 15-40. Poorly differentiated (anaplastic) liposarcoma as shown on transaxial gradient echo MRI. This patient entered hospital emergency room with massive distention of the abdomen. MRI revealed infiltrative neoplasm throughout the retroperitoneum and peritoneal cavity. At autopsy the tumor weighed 35 kg.

tic morphology. Their appearance can be misleading on MRI, since macrocystic prostatic neoplasia are so uncommonly encountered. They should be considered in the extended differential diagnosis of retroperitoneal cystic and cyst-like lesions in men.[72] All of the previously mentioned cystic neoplasms must be differentiated from common benign lymphoceles, which either regress spontaneously or are treatable by percutaneous drainage (Figs. 15-36 and 15-43).[104]

METASTATIC NEOPLASMS
Lymphoma

Regarding detection of lymphoma, using a 0.15 T magnet, Skillings et al.[91] found that MRI and CT results were in agreement in 21 of 32 patients. In their experience, MRI had a lower false-negative rate than CT for identification of sites of disease. Adenopathy from lymphoma is detected at least as well by MRI as by CT. Lymph node necrosis, present in 26% of 125 patients with abdominal lymphoma, does not predict a poor clinical response or a decreased survival rate.[38] No consistent difference in the signal pattern of adenopathy is present between lymphoma

and metastatic carcinoma (Figs. 15-41 and 15-44).[26,62,63]

Lymphoma presents only rarely as a solitary mesenteric mass. The morphology of mesenteric lymphoma ranges from well-circumscribed masses to permeative infiltration and stellate lesions with desmoplastic distortion of contiguous tissues. Mesenteric lymphoma usually is encountered in immunocompromised hosts or late in the course of disseminated disease.[38]

Testicular malignancies

Testicular neoplasms are the most common malignancy in males from ages 15 to 34. Most of them are either nonseminomatous germ cell (NSGC) tumors, seminomas, or a combination of multiple cell types. Seminomas occur in an older age group than the NSGC tumors. Since seminomas typically respond to chemotherapy, they do not require the formal surgical staging that is customary for NSGC neoplasms.[33] The morphology of metastatic testicular neoplasms is similar to that of the primary NSGC tumors that occasionally occur in the retroperitoneum (Fig. 15-42).[11,33,96]

MRI and CT accurately predict the presence or absence

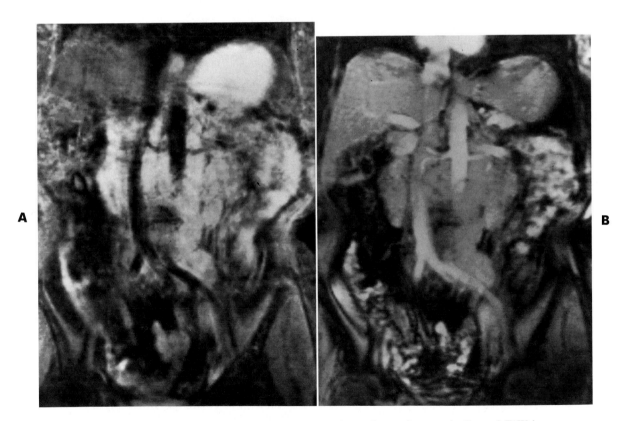

Fig. 15-41. Lymphoma as conglomerate nodal mass in aorticocaval space. **A,** Coronal T1W inversion recovery MRI. This sequence achieves good contrast among perivascular lymphadenopathy, liver, and vessels, but poor contrast between adenopathy and bowel. Anatomic margins are blurred by respiratory motion. **B,** Coronal gradient echo breath-hold, fat-suppressed MRI. Good contrast is achieved among perivascular nodal mass, bowel, and vessels. Anatomic margins are distinct. Adenopathy encircles aorta, extends bilaterally to renal hila, and follows iliac vessels distally.

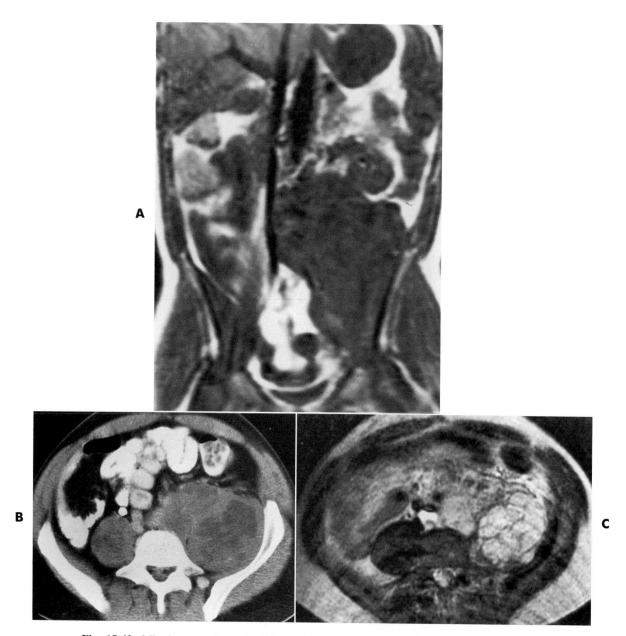

Fig. 15-42. Mixed germ cell tumor of testis. **A,** Coronal T1W MRI. Conglomerate nodal mass extends from the left iliac fossa to IVC. **B,** Axial CT with contrast agent. Left muscular space *(MS)* and posterior pararenal space *(PPRS)* are occupied by neoplasm that has infiltrated the psoas and posterior pararenal nodes. Areas of the mass are nearly isodense to normal right psoas muscle. **C,** Axial T2W MRI at same location as **B.** Heterogeneous, lobulated high intensity of the mass contrasts sharply with low intensity of the normal right psoas muscle.

of adenopathy from NSGC testicular neoplasms in 80% to 88% of cases.[33] Therefore, patients are divided into two groups preoperatively by CT or MRI. Those without bulky metastatic disease undergo a staging laparatomy for radical lymph node dissection. Those with bulky retroperitoneal metastases and those with evidence of distant metastasis undergo chemotherapy and subsequent CT or MRI reevaluation (Fig. 15-42). Only CT or MRI follow-up is required for patients who have a complete initial response to chemotherapy.[33,96] Anything less than a complete response is indication for staging laparotomy (Fig. 15-43). Some tumors regress to indolent mature teratomas following chemotherapy (see Fig. 15-22).[96]

Other metastatic neoplasia

Tumors from distant sites, such as melanoma, frequently metastasize to retroperitoneal lymph nodes (Fig. 15-13, *C*). Massive retroperitoneal adenopathy also can be observed with renal cell carcinoma and rectal, cervical, prostatic, and bladder carcinoma (Fig. 15-44).

Lymphatic metastasis from prostatic carcinoma typically occurs first in the pelvic region, with downstream extension to the retroperitoneum later in the course of the disease; however, mesenteric nodal metastases may rarely be seen, even in the absence of pelvic adenopathy. An unexpected location can obscure the diagnosis of an otherwise obvious disease (Fig. 15-45).

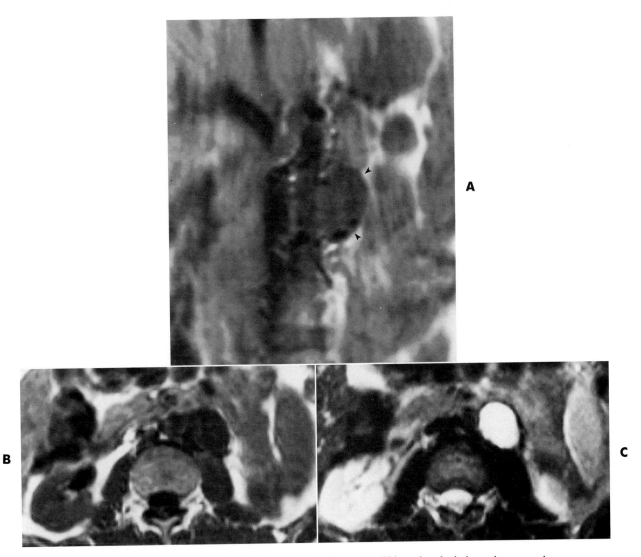

Fig. 15-43. Iatrogenous lymphocele. **A,** Coronal T1W MRI. This patient had chemotherapy and radical retroperitoneal lymph node dissection for metastatic nonseminomatous germ cell tumor of the testis. Left paraaortic mass mimics recurrent adenopathy. **B,** Axial T1W MRI. Mass is nearly isointense to muscle and aorta. **C,** Axial T2W MRI. Mass has homogeneous high intensity. Differential diagnosis is lymphocele, mature teratoma, and necrotic adenopathy. Postoperative diagnosis was lymphocele.

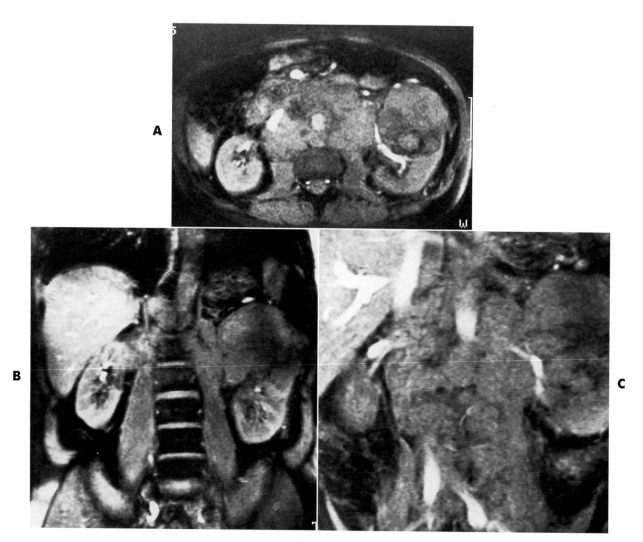

Fig. 15-44. Renal cell carcinoma with massive retroperitoneal adenopathy. **A,** Fat-suppressed, single breath-hold gradient echo MRI. APRS and ACS are filled with coalescent adenopathy. Aorta is engulfed and IVC is displaced. Upper pole left renal mass is visible, although the contrast with normal parenchyma is limited. **B,** Coronal MRI. Left renal carcinoma is demonstrated better than in the axial projection. No hyperintense metastasis is present in lumbar vertebrae. **C,** Anterior to **B.** Massive conglomerate nodal mass. Compare with Fig. 15-41.

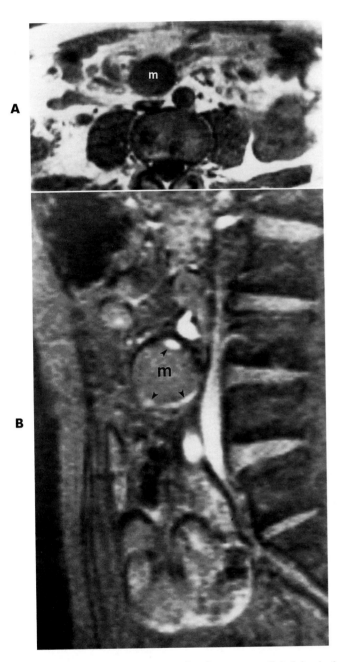

Fig. 15-45. Mesenteric mass. Patient has postprandial abdominal pain. **A,** Axial T1W MRI. Nonspecific, round, low intensity mass is present in the mesentery. **B,** Sagittal gradient echo MRI. Displacement of mesenteric vessels is evident on this flow-compensated, single breath-hold scan. Preoperative diagnosis was lymphoma. In spite of absence of typical regional adenopathy, this mass proved to be metastatic carcinoma of the prostate.

ACKNOWLEDGMENTS

MRI technologists: Bill Bell, Mary Ellen Bentham, David Damm, Larry Hoyle, and Michelle Werner. Research and manuscript preparation: Michael Cushman. Photographs: The University of Florida College of Medicine Learning Resources Center.

REFERENCES

1. Al Karawi MA, Quaiz M, Clark D, et al: Mesenteric vein thrombosis, non-invasive diagnosis and follow-up (US + MRI), and non-invasive therapy by streptokinase and anticoagulants, *Hepatogastroenterology* 37:507-509, 1990.
2. Amis ES: Retroperitoneal fibrosis, *AJR* 157:321-329, 1991.
3. Amparo EG, Higgins CB, Hricak H, et al: Aortic dissection: magnetic resonance imaging, *Radiology* 155:399-406, 1985.
4. Armstong P, Wilson AG, Dee P: *Imaging of diseases of the chest*, Chicago, 1990, Year Book Medical.
5. Arrive L, Hricak H, Tavares NJ, et al: Malignant versus nonmalignant retroperitoneal fibrosis: differentiation with MR imaging, *Radiology* 172:139-143, 1989.
6. Aufferman W, Olofsson P, Stoney R, et al: MR imaging of complications of aortic surgery, *J Comput Assist Tomogr* 11(6):982-989, 1987.
7. Bailes DR, Gilderdale DJ, Bydder GM, et al: Respiratory ordered phase encoding (ROPE): a method for reducing respiratory motion artifacts in MR imaging, *J Comput Assist Tomogr* 9:835-838, 1985.
8. Baker ME, Cohan RH, Nadel SN, et al: Obliteration of the fat surrounding the celiac axis and superior mesenteric artery is not a specific CT finding of carcinoma of the pancreas, *AJR* 155:991-994, 1990.
9. Bellin MF, Duron JJ, Curet PH, et al: Primary retroperitoneal teratoma in the adult: correlation of MRI features with CT and pathology, *Magn Reson Imaging,* 9:263-266, 1991.
10. Belt TG, Cohan MD, Smith JA, et al: MRI of Wilms tumor: promise as the primary imaging method, *AJR* 146:955-961, 1986.
11. Blomlie V, Lien HH, Fossa SD, et al: CT in primary malignant germ cell tumors of the retroperitoneum, *Acta Radiol* 32:155-158, 1991.
12. Borushok KF, Jeffrey RB Jr, Laing FC, et al: Sonographic diagnosis of perforation in patients with acute appendicitis, *AJR* 154:275-278, 1990.
13. Britt AR, Francis IR, Glazer GM, et al: Sarcoidosis: abdominal manifestations at CT, *Radiology* 178:91-94, 1991.
14. Buckwalter KA, Ellis JH, Baker DE, et al: Pitfall in MR imaging of lymphadenopathy after lymphangiography, *Radiology* 161:831-832, 1986.
15. Burton SS, Ros PR, Otto PM, et al: Barium MR imaging of the pancreas: initial experience, *Radiology* 173(P): 517, 1989.
16. Calligaro KD, Savarese RP, DeLaurentis DA, et al: Unusual aspects of aortovenous fistulas associated with ruptured abdominal aortic aneurysms, *J Vasc Surg* 12(5):586-590, 1990.
17. Cho KC, Baker SR: Air in the fissure for the ligamentum teres: new sign of intraperitoneal air on plain radiographs, *Radiology* 178:489-492, 1991.
18. Choi BI, Chi JG, Kim SH, et al: MR imaging of retroperitoneal teratoma: correlation with CT and pathology, *J Comput Assist Tomogr* 13(6):1083-1086, 1989.
19. Chuang VP, Mena CE, Hoskins PA: Congenital anomalies of the inferior vena cava: review of embryogenesis and presentation of a simplified classification, *Br J Radiol* 47:206-213, 1974.
20. Cohen JM, Weinreb JC, Redman HC: Arteriovenous malformations of the extremities: MR imaging, *Radiology* 158:475-479, 1986.
21. Cory DA, Ellis JH, Bies JR, et al: Retroaortic left renal vein demonstrated by nuclear magnetic resonance imaging, *J Comput Assist Tomogr* 8(2):339-340, 1984.
22. de Lange I, Fechner RE, Wanebo HJ: Suspected recurrent rectosigmoid carcinoma after abdominoperineal resection: MR imaging and histopathologic findings, *Radiology* 170:323-328, 1989.
23. Dietrich RB, Kangarloo H: Diagnostic oncology case study. Retroperitoneal mass with intradural extension: value of magnetic resonance imaging in neuroblastoma, *AJR* 146:251-254, 1986.
24. Dinsmore RE, Wedeen VJ, Miller SW, et al: MRI of dissection of

the aorta: recognition of the intimal tear and differential flow velocities, *AJR* 146:1286-1288, 1986.

25. Dooms GC, Hricak H, Crooks LE, et al: Magnetic resonance imaging of the lymph nodes: comparison with CT, *Radiology* 153: 719-728, 1984.

26. Dooms GC, Hricak H, Boseley ME, et al: Characterization of lymphadenopathy of magnetic resonance relaxation times: preliminary results, *Radiology* 155:691-697, 1985.

27. Dooms GC, Hricak H, Sollitto RA, et al: Lipomatous tumors and tumors with fatty component: MR imaging potential and comparison of MR and CT results, *Radiology* 157:479-483, 1985.

28. Dooms GC, Fisher MR, Hricak H, et al: MR imaging of intramuscular hemorrhage, *J Comput Assist Tomogr* 9(5):908-913, 1985.

29. Edelman RR, Hesselink JR: *Clinical magnetic resonance imaging,* Philadelphia, 1990, WB Saunders.

30. Edelman RR, Hahn PF, Buxton R, et al: Rapid MR imaging with suspended respiration: clinical application in the liver, *Radiology* 161:125-132, 1986.

31. Edelman RR, Zhao B, Liu CP, et al: MR angiography and dynamic flow evaluation of the portal venous system, *AJR* 153:755-760, 1989.

32. Edelstein H, McCabe RE: Perinephric abscess: modern diagnosis and treatment in 47 cases, *Medicine* 67:118, 1987.

33. Ellis JH, Bies JR, Kopecky KK, et al: Comparison of NMR and CT imaging in the evaluation of metastatic retroperitoneal lymphadenopathy from testicular carcinoma, *J Comput Assist Tomogr* 8(4):709-719, 1984.

34. Enzinger FM, Weiss SW: Soft tissue tumors, ed 2, St. Louis, 1988, Mosby–Year Book.

35. Fein AB: Diagnosis and staging of renal cell carcinoma: a comparison of MR imaging and CT, *AJR* 148:749-753, 1987.

36. Finer RM, Merritt CRB: Ultrasonography of the appendix, *Appl Radiol* pp 29-32, Aug 1991.

37. Fisher MR, Hricak H, Higgins CB: Magnetic resonance imaging of developmental venous anomalies, *AJR* 145: 705-709, 1985.

38. Fishman EK, Kuhlman JE, Jones RJ: CT of lymphoma: spectrum of disease, *Radiographics* 11(4):647-669, 1991.

39. Flak B, Li DKB, Ho BYB, et al: Magnetic resonance imaging of aneurysms of the abdominal aorta, *AJR* 144:991-996, 1985.

40. Geisinger MA, Risius B, O'Donnell JA, et al: Thoracic aortic dissections: magnetic resonance imaging, *Radiology* 155: 407-412, 1985.

41. Glazer HS, Lee JKT, Levitt RG, et al: Radiation fibrosis: differentiation from recurrent tumor by MR imaging, *Radiology* 156:721-726, 1985.

42. Goerg C, Schwerk WB: Peritoneal carcinomatosis with ascites, *AJR* 156:1185-1187, 1991.

43. Goodman P, Raval B: CT of the abdominal wall, *AJR* 154:1207-1211, 1990.

44. Guz BV, Wood DP, Montie JE, et al: Retroperitoneal neural sheath tumors: Cleveland clinic experience, *J Urol* 142: 1434-1437, 1989.

45. Hahn PF, Stark DD, Lewis JM, et al: First clinical trial of a new superparamagnetic iron oxide for use as an oral gastrointestinal contrast agent in MR imaging, *Radiology* 175:695-700, 1990.

46. Hartman DS: Retroperitoneal tumors and lymphadenopathy, *Urol Radiol* 12:132-134, 1990.

47. Higgins CB, Hricak H: *Magnetic resonance imaging of the body,* New York, 1987, Raven Press.

48. Hilton S, Megibow AJ, Naidich DP, et al : Computed tomography of the postoperative abdominal aorta, *Radiology* 145: 403-407, 1982.

49. Hohenfellner M, Steinbach F, Schultz-Lampel D, et al: The nutcracker syndrome: new aspects of pathophysiology, diagnosis and treatment, *J Urol* 146:685-688, 1991.

50. Hovanessian LJ, Larsen DW, Raval JK, et al: Retroperitoneal cystic lymphangioma: MR findings, *Magn Reson Imaging* 8:91-93, 1990.

51. Hricak H, Higgins CB, Williams RD: Nuclear magnetic resonance imaging in retroperitoneal fibrosis, *AJR* 141:35-38, 1983.

52. Hricak H, Amparo E, Fisher MR, et al: Abdominal venous system: assessment using MR, *Radiology* 156:415-422, 1985.

53. Hricak H, Demas BE, Williams RD, et al: Magnetic resonance imaging in the diagnosis and staging of renal and perirenal neoplasms, *Radiology* 154:709-715, 1985.

54. Imachi M, Tsukamoto N, Tsukimori K, et al: Malignant hemangiopericytoma of the omentum presenting as an ovarian tumor, *Gynecol Oncol* 39:208-213, 1990.

55. Joseph TJ, Becker DI, Turton AF: Renal malignant fibrous histiocytoma, *Urology* 37(5):483-489, 1991.

56. Justich E: Infected aortoiliofemoral grafts: magnetic resonance imaging, *Radiology* 154:133-136, 1985.

57. Kaplan PA, Williams SM: Mucocutaneous and peripheral soft-tissue hemangiomas: MR imaging, *Radiology* 163:163-166, 1987.

58. Kaufman AJ, Tarr RW, Holburn GE, et al : Magnetic resonance imaging of ischemic bowel in rabbit model, *Invest Radiol* 23:93-97, 1988.

59. Koelbel G, Schmiedel U Majer MC, et al: Diagnosis of fistulae and sinus tracts in patients with Crohn's disease: value of MR imaging, *AJR* 152:999-1003, 1989.

60. Kronthal AJ, Kang YS, Fishmann EK, et al: MR imaging in sclerosing mesenteritis, *AJR* 156:517-519, 1991.

61. Kunin M: Bridging septa of the paranephric space: anatomic, pathologic, and diagnostic considerations, *Radiology* 158:361-365, 1986.

62. Lawson TL, Foley WD, Thorsen MK, et al: Magnetic resonance imaging of discrete and conglomerate retroperitoneal lymph node masses, *Radiographics* 5(6):971-984, 1985.

63. Lee JKT: Magnetic resonance imaging of the retroperitoneum, *Urol Radiol* 10:48-51, 1988.

64. Lee JKT, Glazer HS: Psoas muscle disorders: MR imaging, *Radiology* 160:683-687, 1986.

65. Lee JKT, Stanley RJ, Sagel SS, et al: CT appearance of the pelvis after abdominoperineal resection for rectal carcinoma, *Radiology* 141:737-741, 1981.

66. Lee JKT, Heinken JP, Ling D, et al: Magnetic resonance imaging of abdominal and pelvic lymphadenopathy, *Radiology* 153:181-188, 1984.

67. Levine E, Wetzel LH, Neff JR: MR imaging and CT of extrahepatic cavernous hemangiomas, *AJR* 147:1299-1304, 1986.

68. Levine MS, Scheiner JD, Rubesin SE, et al: Diagnosis of pneumoperitoneum on supine abdominal radiographs, *AJR* 156:731-735, 1991.

69. Li KCP, Ho-Tai P: MR imaging of the liver: technique considerations, *Appl Radiol* 19(12):10-15, 1990.

70. London J, Kim EE, Wallace S, et al: MR imaging of liposarcomas: correlation of MR features and histology, *J Comput Assist Tomogr* 13(5):832-835, 1989.

71. Lubat E, Megibow AJ, Balthazar EJ, et al: Extrapulmonary *Pneumocystis carinii* infection in AIDS: CT findings, *Radiology* 174:157-160, 1990.

72. Maluf HM, DeLuca FR, Talerman A: Giant multilocular prostatic cystadenoma: a distinctive lesion of the retroperitoneum in men—a report of two cases, *Am J Surg Pathol* 15(2):131-135, 1991.

73. Mao J, Bidgood WD Jr, Ang GP et al: A clinically viable technique of fat suppression for abdomen and pelvis, *Magn Reson Med* 21:320-326, 1991.

74. Mao J, Yan H, Bidgood WD Jr: Fat suppression with an improved selective presaturation pulse, *Magn Reson Imaging* 10:49-53, 1992.

75. Mark A, Moss AA, Lusby R, et al: CT evaluation of complications of abdominal aortic surgery, *Radiology* 145:409-414, 1982.

76. Martin B, Mulopulos GP, Bryan PJ: MRI of puerperal ovarian-vein thrombosis (case report), *AJR* 147:291-292, 1986.

77. Marx WJ, Patel SK: Renal fascia: its radiographic importance, *Urology* 13:1-7, 1979.

78. Meis JM, Enzinger FM: Myolipoma of soft tissue, *Am J Surg Pathol* 15(2):121-125, 1991.

79. Meyers MA: *Dynamic radiology of the abdomen,* New York, 1976, Springer Verlag.

80. Mitchell DG, Vinitski S, Rifkin MD, et al: Liver and pancreas: improved spin-echo T1 contrast by shorter echo time and fat suppression at 1.5 T, *Radiology* 178:67-71, 1991.

81. Newman PL, Fletcher CDM: Malignant mesenchymoma, *Am J Surg Pathol* 15(7):607-614, 1991.

82. Oesterling JE, Epstein JI, Brendler CB: Myxoid malignant fibrous histiocytoma of the bladder, *Cancer* 66(8):1836-1842, 1990.

83. Radin DR: Intraabdominal mycobacterium tuberculosis vs *Mycobacterium avium-intracellulare* infections in patients with AIDS: distinction based on CT findings, *AJR* 156:487-491, 1991.

84. Raptopoulos V, Kleinmann PK, Marks S Jr, et al: Renal fascial pathways: posterior extension of pancreatic effusions within the pararenal space, *Radiology* 158:367-374, 1986.

85. Reeder MM, Felson B: *Gamuts in radiology,* ed 1, Cincinnati, 1975, Audiovisual Radiology of Cincinnati.

86. Savader SJ, Otero RR, Savader BL: Puerperal ovarian vein thrombosis: evaluation with CT, US, and MR imaging, *Radiology* 167:637-639, 1988.

87. Schultz CL, Morrison S, Bryan PJ: Azygos continuation of the inferior vena cava: demonstration by NMR imaging, *J Comput Assist Tomogr* 8(4):774-776, 1984.

88. Semelka RC, Chew W, Hricak H, et al: Fat-saturation MR imaging of the upper abdomen, *AJR* 155:1111-1116, 1990.

89. Semelka RC, Hricak H, Stevens SK, et al: Combined gadolinium-enhanced and fat-saturation MR imaging of renal masses, *Radiology* 178:803-809, 1991.

90. Shirkhoda A: Diagnostic pitfalls in abdominal CT, *Radiographics* 11:969-1002, 1991.

91. Skillings JR, Bramwell V, Nicholson RL, et al: A prospective study of magnetic resonance imaging in lymphoma staging, *Cancer* 67:1838-1843, 1991.

92. Stark DD, Bradley WG: *Magnetic resonance imaging,* ed 2, St. Louis, 1992, Mosby–Year Book.

93. Sueoka BL, Kasales CJ, Harris RD, et al: MR and CT imaging of perirenal amyloidosis, *Urol Radiology* 11:97-99, 1989.

94. Terada Y, Kato A, Kishi H, et al: Nuclear magnetic resonance imaging of a benign cystic teratoma in the retroperitoneum, *J Urol* 137:106-108, 1987.

95. Timins ME, Nemcek AA JR: Extrapulmonary *Pneumocystis carinii* infection: another cause of splenic "bull's-eye" lesions, *Radiology* 178(2):584, 1991.

96. Toner GC, Geller NL, Lin SY, et al: Extragonadal and poor risk nonseminomatous germ cell tumors, *Cancer* 67(8):2049-2057, 1991.

97. Torres GM, Erquiaga E, Ros PR, et al: Preliminary results of MR imaging with superparamagnetic iron oxide in pancreatic and retroperitoneal disorders, *Radiographics* 11(5):785-791, 1991.

98. Townsend RR, Jeffrey RB, Laing FC: Cecal diverticulitis differentiated from appendicitis using graded-compression sonography, *AJR* 152:1229-1230, 1989.

99. Vassilopoulos PP, Apostolikas NG, Papajoglu I, et al: Ectopic spleen in the retroperitoneum, *Acta Chir Scand* 156:655-658, 1990.

100. Wahl RL, Gyves J, Gross BH, et al: SPECT of the peritoneal cavity: method for delineating intraperitoneal fluid distribution, *AJR* 152:1205-1210, 1989.

101. Wiener JI, Chako AC, Merten CW, et al: Breast and axillary tissue MR imaging: correlation of signal intensities and relaxation times with pathologic findings, *Radiology* 160:299-305, 1986.

102. Weinreb JC, Cohen JM, Maravilla KR: Iliopsoas muscles: MR study of normal anatomy and disease, *Radiology* 156:435-440, 1985.

103. Weissleder R, Elizondo G, Wittenberg J, et al: Ultrasmall superparamagnetic iron oxide: an intravenous contrast agent for assessing lymph nodes with MR imaging, *Radiology* 175:494-498, 1990.

104. White M, Mueller PR, Ferrucci JT Jr, et al: Percutaneous drainage of postoperative abdominal and pelvic lymphoceles, *AJR* 145:1065-1069, 1985.

105. Wilson JD, Braunwald E, Isselbacher KJ, et al: *Harrison's principles of internal medicine,* ed 12, New York, 1991, McGraw-Hill.

106. Winkler ML, Thoeni RF, Luh N, et al: Hepatic neoplasia: breath-hold MR imaging, *Radiology* 170:801-806, 1989.

107. Yamada T, Tada S, Harada J: Aortic dissection without intimal rupture: diagnosis with MR imaging and CT, *Radiology* 168:347-352, 1988.

108. Zweig GJ, Li YP, Srinantaswamy S, et al: Gas-forming infections of the abdomen: plain film findings, *Appl Radiol* 2:37-42, 1990.

Chapter 16

ADRENAL

Sharon S. Burton

Three primary reasons for imaging the adrenal glands are (1) to detect metastatic disease in patients with a known malignancy, (2) to evaluate patients with clinical evidence of adrenal hormone excess or insufficiency, and (3) to follow up or characterize adrenal masses discovered incidentally in patients being evaluated for unrelated symptoms.

COMPARISON OF CT AND MRI

Computed tomography (CT) has proved to be an excellent method for demonstrating the normal adrenal glands[47,63] and pathologic conditions of adrenal glands.[18,27,28] High spatial resolution is achieved with CT, and thin sections ranging from 1.5 to 5 mm can be performed to differentiate normal glands from those involved with multinodular disease or small primary adrenal masses. Rapid CT scan times minimize motion artifacts, and calcifications are well-demonstrated. The inherent contrast difference between adrenal glands and the surrounding perirenal fat makes it possible in many cases to adequately image the adrenal glands without the use of intravenous (IV) contrast agents. Intravenous contrast enhancement is sometimes needed to differentiate adrenal

nodules from a pseudotumor because of adjacent unenhanced vascular structures.[7] The primary limitation of CT is its inability to differentiate causes of adrenal enlargement. With the exception of myelolipoma and adrenal cyst, adrenal lesions cannot be reliably differentiated based on CT morphology.[28,39]

Magnetic resonance imaging (MRI) has several capabilities that make it useful for adrenal imaging: (1) direct multiplanar imaging to differentiate adrenal masses from liver, retroperitoneal, or renal masses,[44] (2) improved tissue contrast and potential for characterization of adrenal lesions, (3) excellent depiction of flow void in vascular structures without the need for IV contrast enhancement, (4) decreased artifacts from surgical clips that produce image degradation on CT scans, and (5) lack of ionizing radiation. Disadvantages of MRI in comparison with CT include decreased spatial resolution, increased scan times with more artifacts related to respiratory motion, greater expense, and poor depiction of calcifications within masses.[20]

TECHNIQUE

MRI of the adrenal glands is performed using axial and coronal planes. Sagittal images are useful in differentiating masses of adrenal origin from hepatic and renal lesions.[44] Spin-echo (SE) imaging is most commonly performed using a body coil scanner. T1-weighted images (T1WI) (i.e., weighted toward the spin-lattice or longitudinal relaxation time [T1], and in this case with a repetition time [TR] of 300 to 800 msec and an echo time [TE] of less than 30 msec) provide the greatest detail and contrast and are best for demonstrating anatomy.[21] Dual echo T2-weighted images (T2WI) (i.e., weighted toward the spin-spin or transverse relaxation time [T2]; TR 2000-2500, TE 20/80-100) are used for characterization of the lesion but provide less anatomic detail because of decreased contrast between the adrenal glands and perirenal fat. Slice thickness is 5 to 10 mm with 2.5 to 5 mm interslice gap. Oral contrast agents may be used to opacify the stomach and jejunum and decrease the possibility of pseudotumor from unopacified bowel. This has proved important in CT scanning[5] but has not yet been verified with oral contrast agents for MRI.

Fast gradient echo (GE) imaging is also applied to adrenal mass characterization. Images are obtained during suspended respiration using T2-weighting (TR 60 msec, TE 30 msec, flip angle of 15° at 1.5 T). Dynamic perfusion studies using IV gadopentetate dimeglumine are feasible using these fast scan techniques and are useful in adrenal mass characterization.[40]

Surface coil imaging of the adrenal glands has the ad-vantage of increased signal-to-noise ratio and spatial resolution, but it limits the field of view and ability to compare signal intensities with other abdominal organs, such as the liver.[19,20,61]

ANATOMY

The adrenal glands are paired endocrine organs located within Gerota's fascia in the perirenal space. The right adrenal gland is superior to the upper pole of the right kidney and lies immediately posterior to the inferior vena cava and medial to the right lobe of the liver. In axial CT images (Fig. 16-1, *A*), the right adrenal gland has a linear or inverted V configuration. The left adrenal gland is antero-medial to the upper pole of the left kidney and is com-

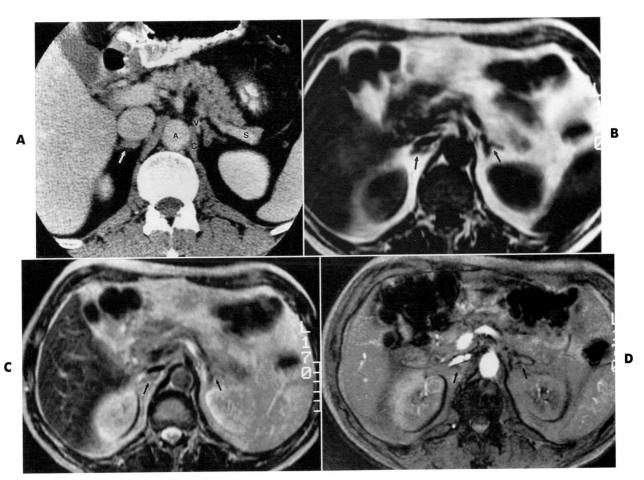

Fig. 16-1. Normal adrenal glands. **A,** CT scan. Left adrenal gland is shaped like an inverted Y, is surrounded by perinephric fat, and is located posterior to splenic vein *(s)* and lateral to aorta *(a)* and diaphragm crus *(c)*. Left inferior phrenic vein *(v)* is anteromedial to adrenal gland. Right adrenal gland is posterior to inferior vena cava *(arrow)*. **B,** T1-weighted MR (magnetic resonance) image (TR 600, TE 20). Signal intensity of adrenal glands *(arrows)* is similar to liver and greater than muscle and perinephric fat. Note signal void in adjacent vessels (inferior vena cava, splenic vein, and superior mesenteric artery). **C,** T2-weighted MR image (TR 2500, TE 80). Adrenal glands *(arrows)* are not as clearly delineated from perinephric fat in comparison with T1WI. **D,** GE image (TR 22, TE 13, flip angle 30°. Left adrenal gland is defined *(arrow)* but right adrenal gland cannot be seen. Vascular structures are well delineated.

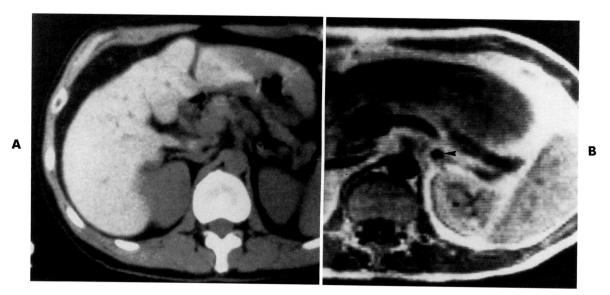

Fig. 16-2. Adrenal pseudomass caused by a varix. **A,** CT scan. Small ovoid mass *(v)* is on anterior aspect of left adrenal gland. **B,** T1-weighted MR image. Flow void in mass *(arrowhead)* indicates flowing blood in varix of left inferior phrenic vein. (From Brady TM, et al: *AJR* 145:301-304, 1985.)

monly triangular in shape but may appear as an inverted T, Y, or V on axial views. The normal adrenal gland is 2 to 4 cm in length and up to 1 cm in thickness.[47]

In a retrospective study of 100 normal patients undergoing MRI of the adrenal glands,[8] the left adrenal gland was demonstrated in 99 patients and was not seen in 1 patient because of scoliosis. The right adrenal gland was shown in 91 patients and was not seen in 8 patients because of the lack of retroperitoneal fat and in 1 patient because of hepatomegaly. On SE images, normal adrenal glands have homogeneous, low signal intensity, which is less than the signal intensity of adjacent fat and greater than the signal intensity of the crus of the diaphragm (Fig. 16-1, *B to D*). The adrenal glands are nearly isointense to the liver on T1WI and T2WI.[21] A difference in signal intensity between the cortex and medulla has been demonstrated in a small percentage of patients,[55] but this has not been confirmed by all investigators[8] and is not likely to have clinical significance.

Pseudotumors of the adrenal glands have been documented by CT scanning.[5] A pseudotumor can be produced by the bowel, including a fluid-filled gastric fundus or gastric diverticulum.[56] Prominent splenic lobulations, tortuous splenic vessels and varices of the left inferior phrenic vein, and masses arising in adjacent organs, such as the kidney or tail of the pancreas, may also mimic adrenal lesions on CT. Similar pitfalls may occur with MRI, although vascular abnormalities are less likely to be confused with nodules from flow phenomena demonstrated with MRI (Fig. 16-2).

HYPERFUNCTIONING LESIONS

The adrenal cortex and medulla have different embryonic origins and hormonal functions.[46] The cortex arises from mesodermal tissues of the urogenital ridge and contains three histologic layers: the zona glomerulosa, which produces mineralocorticoids, and the zona fasciculata and zona reticularis, which produce glucocorticoids and adrenal androgens. The adrenal medulla is of ectodermal origin and is derived from neural crest cells. These give rise to chromaffin cells (pheochromocytes), which produce epinephrine and norepinephrine, and autonomic ganglion cells.

Because the adrenal glands have many endocrine functions, adrenal disorders produce a variety of endocrine disturbances.[62] It is therefore practical to discuss adrenal diseases in terms of their clinical relevance as follows: diseases of adrenal hyperfunction affecting either the cortex or medulla, nonfunctional adrenal lesions, and diseases of adrenal hypofunction.

Cortical hyperfunction

Conn's syndrome. Primary hyperaldosteronism (or Conn's syndrome) results from mineralocorticoid excess. The predominant clinical findings include sodium and fluid retention and hypertension. Laboratory analysis reveals hypokalemia, elevated plasma aldosterone levels, and decreased plasma renin activity.[62] Of patients with Conn's syndrome, 75% to 80% have a benign, aldosterone-producing adenoma and are treated surgically.[27] Adrenal hyperplasia accounts for 20% to 25% of cases and is treated medically, since surgical therapy has limited benefit.[2,60] Excess aldosterone production by adrenal cortical carcinoma occurs rarely but is associated with profound hypokalemia and significant elevation in plasma aldosterone.[23]

Accurate diagnosis of aldosteronomas is essential for proper patient management. The technique for imaging the adrenal glands must be optimized using thin sections, because the tumors are usually small. In a study of 23 aldosterone-producing tumors, the average tumor diameter was 1.5 cm, with a range of 0.5 to 3.5 cm. CT scans performed with 4 mm sections detected 75% of the adenomas.[26] In a more recent study, the accuracy of CT for diagnosis of aldosteronoma was 86%.[33] On MRI, aldosteronomas are isointense or hyperintense to the liver on T2-weighted sequences.[54]

In Conn's syndrome caused by adrenal hyperplasia, the adrenal glands are frequently normal in appearance on imaging studies. The adrenal glands may contain bilateral nodules varying in size from 0.25 to 1 cm and occasionally up to 2 to 3 cm in diameter. Therefore, hyperplasia with a dominant nodule may be mistaken for a single adenoma, if image resolution is not adequate to allow detection of minimal nodularity in the contralateral gland (Fig. 16-3). In a study including four patients with hyperaldosteronism caused by nodular hyperplasia, MRI identified only the dominant nodule in three of four patients.[33] Because of

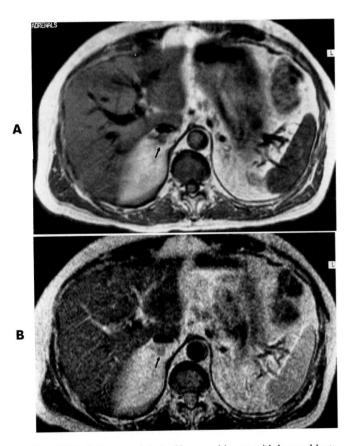

Fig. 16-3. Solitary nodule in 73-year-old man with hyperaldosteronism is caused by hyperplasia, based on adrenal vein samplings. **A,** T1-weighted MR image. Solitary nodule in right adrenal gland *(arrow)*, which is isointense with rest of the adrenal gland and liver. **B,** T2WI. Nodule *(arrow)* is isointense with normal adrenal glands and liver. This is the most common MR signal intensity pattern seen in adenomas. Differentiation of functional versus nonfunctional adenoma cannot be made on imaging studies.

its higher spatial resolution, CT is currently recommended over MRI for evaluating patients suspected of having Conn's syndrome. Alternative diagnostic procedures for primary hyperaldosteronism include selective adrenal vein sampling, which has a 96% accuracy rate,[26] and iodine-131 NP-59 scintigraphy.[8,33]

Cushing's syndrome. This syndrome results from glucocorticoid excess, and clinical manifestations include truncal obesity, hirsutism, abdominal striae, bruising, muscle wasting, osteoporosis, hypertension, and hypercortisolism.[62] Cushing's syndrome commonly results from exogenous glucocorticoid administration for treatment of medical problems. Endogeneous sources of glucocorticoid excess include cortisol-producing adrenal adenoma (20%), adrenal cortical carcinoma (10%), and adrenal cortical hypertension from excess adrenocorticotropic hormone (ACTH) production (70%).[18,62] The majority of patients with ACTH excess have Cushing's disease secondary to a hyperfunctioning pituitary adenoma. Ectopic sources account for approximately 10% of cases of excessive ACTH production and include oat cell carcinoma; bronchial carcinoid, ovarian, pancreatic, thymic, and thyroid tumors; and pheochromocytoma.[16] Petrosal sinus sampling for ACTH level is an accurate way to differentiate pituitary from ectopic ACTH production.[14]

Cortisol-producing adenomas are easily demonstrated with standard CT or MRI protocols. These tumors are usually greater than 2 cm in diameter and are surrounded by abundant retroperitoneal fat. When an adenoma is present, the remainder of the ipsilateral adrenal gland is usually not visualized, and the contralateral adrenal gland is normal or often atrophic.[14] The signal intensity of adenomas on MRI is variable. In a series of 30 adenomas evaluated at 0.35 T, 71% were isointense, 19% were hyperintense, and 10% were hypointense to the liver on T2WI (TR 2000, TE 40-50 or 100 msec).[54] Differentiation between non-functioning and functioning adenomas has not been possible based on MRI.[48] Rarely, adenomas are so hyperintense on T2WI, they are indistinguishable from metastatic disease or adrenal carcinoma (Fig. 16-4).[3]

Adrenal hyperplasia in Cushing's syndrome has a variable appearance.[18] The adrenal glands are normal in appearance in up to 50% of cases. Diffuse unilateral or bilateral enlargement and macronodular hyperplasia may also occur (Figure 16-5). When a dominant nodule is found and the contralateral gland is nodular, this most likely represents nodular cortical hyperplasia. Recognition of this prevents unnecessary adrenalectomy for a dominant nodule in patients with nodular hyperplasia. Petrosal sinus sampling for ACTH is then used to detect ACTH gradients that confirm a pituitary microadenoma that may not be visible on CT or MRI studies.[14]

A rare variant of Cushing's syndrome that occurs in children and young adults is known as primary pigmented nodular adrenocortical disease (PPNAD).[15] The clinical manifestations include short stature and profound osteo-

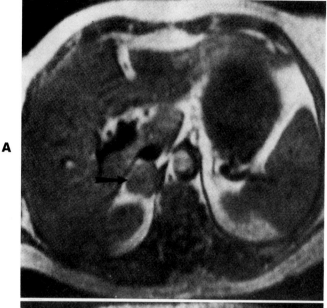

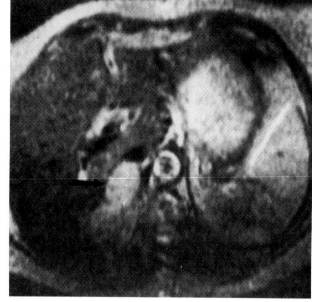

Fig. 16-4. Functioning adrenal adenoma mimics a malignant lesion. Pathologic analysis showed a cortical adenoma with multiple, small areas of hemorrhage. **A,** T1WI. Signal intensity of the mass *(arrow)* is equal to that of the liver. **B,** T2WI. Signal intensity of the mass *(arrow)* is significantly greater than that of the liver, which is usually characteristic of malignant lesions or pheochromocytomas. (From Baker ME et al: *AJR* 153:307-312, 1989.)

porosis. The adrenal glands contain multiple pigmented nodules of hyperplastic cells that produce atrophy of normal tissue between the nodules. With state-of-the-art CT and MRI techniques, multiple nodules ranging from 5 to 10 mm in size can be documented in these patients.[14] Treatment is bilateral adrenalectomy followed by hormonal replacement therapy. Accurate diagnosis of PPNAD

is important because of the association with the Carney complex, which includes calcified Sertoli cell tumors of the testes and cardiac and soft tissue myxomas.[15]

Carcinoma. Primary adrenal cortical carcinoma is a rare malignancy with an incidence of one to two per million persons.[18,57] Hormonal hyperfunction occurs in 50% of patients. Depending on the hormones produced, the patient may develop Cushing's syndrome, virilization, feminization, and rarely hyperaldosteronism. When the tumors are nonfunctioning, they remain clinically silent until their large size produces local mass effects or until metastatic disease develops. Metastatic disease may involve regional and paraaortic lymph nodes, the lungs, liver, or vascular invasion into the inferior vena cava.[57] Excision is performed by en bloc resection, but the prognosis is poor.

Radiologic examination shows adrenal carcinomas as large masses, greater than 5 cm and up to 22 cm in diameter with inhomogeneous enhancement and a low-density center, representing central necrosis.[28] Calcifications occur in 30% of the cases. MRI has been shown to be advantageous and superior to CT in determining the site of tumor origin, involvement of the liver, and invasion of the adrenal vein and inferior vena cava.[57] The signal characteristics reported for adrenal cortical carcinoma are similar to those seen with metastatic disease: lower signal intensity than the liver on T1WI, and higher intensity on T2WI (Fig. 16-6). Small carcinomas of less than 5 cm may be homogenous without necrosis and may simulate a benign adenoma.[28] Gadolinium-enhanced MRI can be used to differentiate thrombus from tumor thrombus invading the inferior vena cava.[22]

Medullary hyperfunction

Pheochromocytoma. Paragangliomas are rare neuroendocrine tumors that arise within the adrenal medulla or from paraganglionic tissue extending from the base of skull to the pelvis. Paraganglionic cells are classified as APUD (amine-precursor-uptake decarboxylation) cells and have vesicles containing catecholamines.[58] Paragangliomas that arise within the adrenal medulla (90%) are classified as pheochromocytomas. Pheochromocytomas are usually hormonally active and produce both norepinephrine and epinephrine. Extraadrenal paragangliomas arise from the sympathetic chain and retroperitoneal ganglia. They are less commonly hormonally active and secrete only norepinephrine. Parasympathetic paragangliomas, including branchiomeric (chemodectomas), visceral autonomic, and vagal paragangliomas are least likely to be hormonally active.[58]

The clinical symptoms and signs produced by hormonally active paragangliomas are due to excess catecholamine secretion. Symptomatic patients have sustained or paroxysmal hypertension and episodic attacks of anxiety, headache, visual blurring, sweating, and vasomotor changes caused by transient elevations in catecholamine

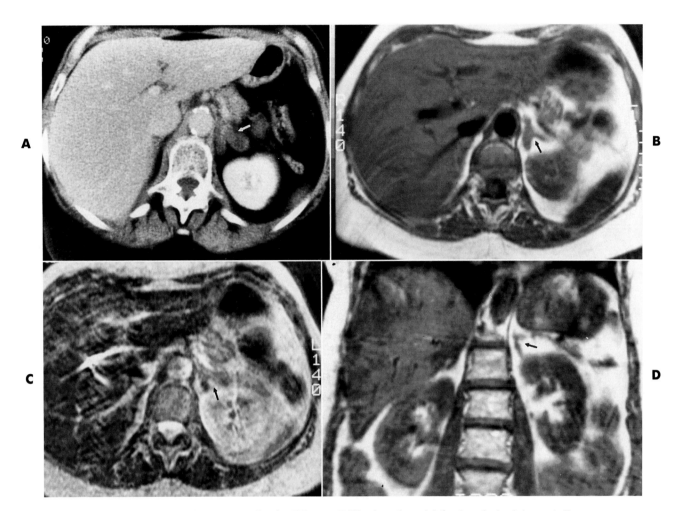

Fig. 16-5. Adrenal hyperplasia. **A,** CT scan. Diffusely enlarged left adrenal gland *(arrow).* **B,** T1WI. Enlarged left adrenal gland *(arrow)* has signal intensity equal to that of the liver. **C,** T2WI. Enlarged adrenal gland *(arrow)* is isointense with the liver. **D,** Coronal T1WI. Left adrenal gland *(arrow)* shows diffuse enlargement.

levels. Laboratory assessment reveals elevation of plasma and urinary catecholamines or their metabolites, including norepinephrine, vanillylmandelic acid (VMA), and metanephrine.

Extraadrenal paragangliomas are referred to as extraadrenal pheochromocytomas by many authors.[44,62] They occur along the sympathetic chain in paracaval or paraaortic regions, at the organ of Zuckerkandl near the aortic bifurcation, in the mediastinum, and in the wall of the urinary bladder. Pheochromocytoma has been termed a "10% tumor," because approximately 10% of pheochromocytomas are malignant, 10% are bilateral, and 10% are extraadrenal.[28] Bilateral tumors are more common in patients with multiple endocrine neoplasia syndromes, and 50% of these patients are asymptomatic. Syndromes associated with pheochromocytoma and extraadrenal paragangliomas include the following[62]:

1. Multiple endocrine neoplasia (MEN) syndrome, type IIa (Sipple's syndrome): pheochromocytoma, medullary carcinoma of the thyroid, and parathyroid hyperplasia
2. MEN syndrome, type IIb: pheochromocytoma, medullary carcinoma of the thyroid, mucocutaneous disorders (including mucosal neuromas), and marfanoid habitus
3. Neurofibromatosis
4. von Hippel–Lindau syndrome
5. Familial pheochromocytoma

Because pheochromocytomas of adrenal origin are generally greater than 3 cm in size at the time of diagnosis, they are readily diagnosed by CT or MRI. Larger tumors tend to be inhomogeneous, containing central necrosis or hemorrhage (Fig. 16-7).[24] Small pheochromocytomas can-

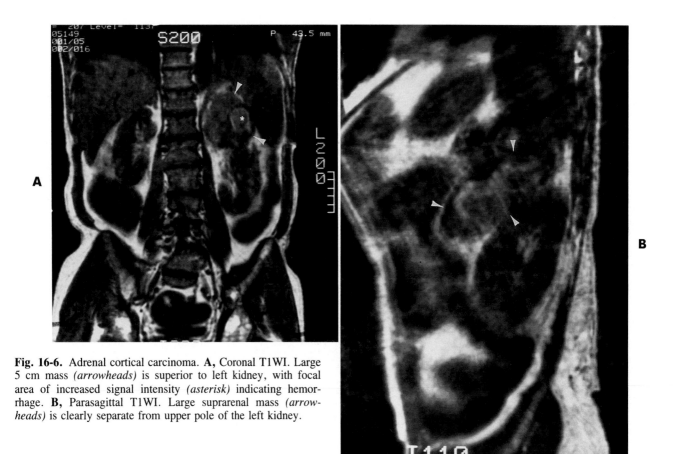

Fig. 16-6. Adrenal cortical carcinoma. **A,** Coronal T1WI. Large 5 cm mass *(arrowheads)* is superior to left kidney, with focal area of increased signal intensity *(asterisk)* indicating hemorrhage. **B,** Parasagittal T1WI. Large suprarenal mass *(arrowheads)* is clearly separate from upper pole of the left kidney.

not be differentiated from nonhyperfunctioning adenomas by CT; however, both pheochromocytomas and extraadrenal paragangliomas have distinctive signal characteristics on MRI because of a prolonged T1 and T2 within the tumor, showing low signal intensity on T1WI and very high signal intensity on the T2WI (Fig. 16-8).[44] Significant differences in the ratio of adrenal mass to liver signal intensity[24,52] and calculated T2 values[4] have been documented in pheochromocytomas in comparison with other adrenal masses. MRI has proved to be superior to CT in detection of extraadrenal tumors, particularly those located in a juxtacardiac location, in the wall of the urinary bladder or retroperitoneum near the inferior vena cava, or those located near surgical clips.[18] For recurrent or metastatic disease, iodine-131 metaiodobenzylguanidine (MIBG) scintigraphy is a useful method of initial evaluation and may be followed by scintigraphically directed MRI or CT scanning for anatomic information.[51] Some investigators suggest that MRI is the preferred method for initial evaluation of patients with suspected functioning paragangliomas.[58]

The other hyperfunctioning lesion of the adrenal medulla is the neuroblastoma, which occurs rarely in adults and is discussed in Chapter 18.

NONHYPERFUNCTIONING LESIONS

Adenoma. Nonhyperfunctioning adenomas of the adrenal glands are common incidental findings and are referred to as "incidentalomas."[28] In a series of 9866 consecutive autopsies, cortical adenomas greater than 3 mm in diameter were found in 2.9% of the patients.[10] If macroscopic and microscopic nodules found at autopsy are included, the incidence of adenoma is as high as 64.5%.[12] By CT examination, small nonhyperfunctioning adrenal masses are found in approximately 1% of patients.[30] Adenomas are more commonly seen with increasing age and in patients with hypertension and diabetes.[32]

Based on morphologic characteristics, benign adenomas cannot be differentiated from malignant masses by CT. However, a recent study showed a significant difference in the mean attenuation coefficient of 38 adenomas (-2.2 HU ± 16) in comparison with 28 malignant adrenal masses (28.9 HU ± 10.6).[41] The authors propose that a mass with CT attenuation values of less than 0 HU is a benign lesion. Masses with attenuation values of 1 to 10 HU are most likely benign but warrant close follow-up.

Many investigations have been conducted using MRI to characterize adrenal masses and differentiate adenomas from malignant lesions. At low and high magnetic field

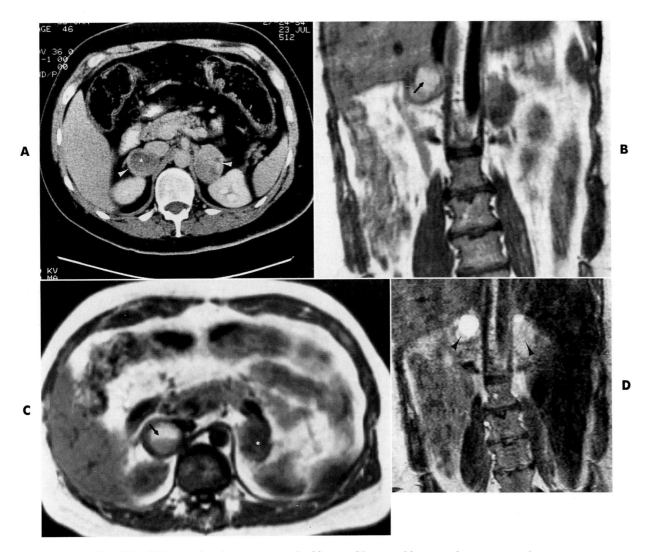

Fig. 16-7. Bilateral pheochromocytomas in 29-year-old man with mucosal neuroma syndrome (MEN 2B). **A,** CT scan. Bilateral adrenal masses *(arrows)* with soft tissue attenuation and region of decreased density *(asterisk)* within right adrenal mass. **B,** T1WI. Coronal image shows regions of high signal intensity *(arrow)* indicative of hemorrhage in the right adrenal mass. **C,** T1WI. Axial image shows hemorrhagic right adrenal mass with layering of blood products *(arrow)* and left adrenal mass *(asterisk)*. **D,** T2WI. Coronal image shows high signal intensity in adrenal masses bilaterally *(arrowheads),* with highest intensity in hemorrhagic portion of right adrenal pheochromocytoma.

strengths, most nonhyperfunctioning adenomas have low signal intensity similar to the liver on T1WI and T2WI (Fig. 16-9). In contrast, most metastases and adrenal carcinomas are typically hyperintense to the liver, and pheochromocytomas are extremely hyperintense on T2WI. Initial studies using adrenal mass to liver signal intensity ratios suggested that adenomas could be reliably differentiated from malignant lesions based on MR signal characteristics.[29,33] Further investigations have shown variability of signal characteristics in adenomas because of the presence of hemorrhage, necrosis, or calcifications, which

limit the ability of MRI to differentiate adenomas from malignant lesions. Using quantitative parameters and low-to-intermediate magnetic field strength (0.3 to 0.5 T), 21% to 31% of adrenal masses fall within an indeterminate range in which benign and malignant adrenal lesions cannot be differentiated.[27,53] This has proved true for adrenal mass to liver signal intensity ratios, adrenal mass to fat signal intensity ratios on T2WI, and mass to liver signal intensity ratios on T1WI.[9] Using high field-strength magnets (1.5 T) the adrenal mass to liver signal intensity ratios on T2WI have not differentiated adenomas from metastasis

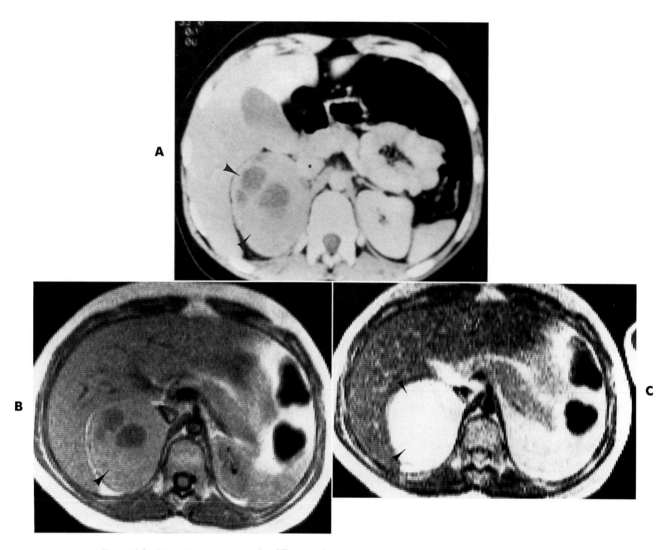

Fig. 16-8. Pheochromocytoma. **A,** CT scan. Large right adrenal mass *(arrowheads)* has hypodense regions, suggesting old hemorrhage or necrosis. Inferior vena cava *(asterisk)* is displaced anteriorly. **B,** T1-weighted MR image. Adrenal mass *(arrowhead)* has slightly higher signal intensity than adjacent liver and regions of low signal intensity corresponding to necrosis. **C,** T2WI. Homogeneously high signal intensity is seen within the right adrenal mass *(arrows)* and is characteristic of pheochromocytoma and extraadrenal paragangliomas.

or carcinomas. Instead, calculated T2 relaxation time has proved more useful in differentiating adrenal masses at 1.5 T.[4] Adrenal adenomas generally show calculated T2 values of less than 60 msec. Masses with calculated T2 values of greater than 60 msec are more commonly, but not always, malignant lesions. In one series, masses with T2 values of less than 60 msec included two hemorrhagic adrenal glands, two nonhyperfunctioning adenomas, six metastases, two pheochromocytomas, and one adrenal carcinoma.[38]

Fast GE imaging during suspended respiration is also used to characterize adrenal masses.[40] In a study of 38 masses, malignant tumors and pheochromocytomas had significantly higher signal intensities than benign adenomas on T2-weighted GE scans (TR 60 msec, TE 30 msec, flip angle 15°). Overlap between benign and malignant lesions occurred in 9 out of 38 cases. Using IV gadolinium injection and dynamic scanning (repeated single sections during and 1, 2, 3, 4, 5, 7, 9, 11, and 15 minutes after IV administration of 0.1 mmol/kg of gadopentetate dimeglumine), adenomas showed less enhancement and faster washout than metastases and pheochromocytomas. Use of dynamic scanning and gadolinium allowed 5 out of 9 equivocal cases to be correctly classified as adenomas, leaving 4 out of 9 in the equivocal range. Accuracy of characterizing adrenal masses was 31 out of 34 or 90%

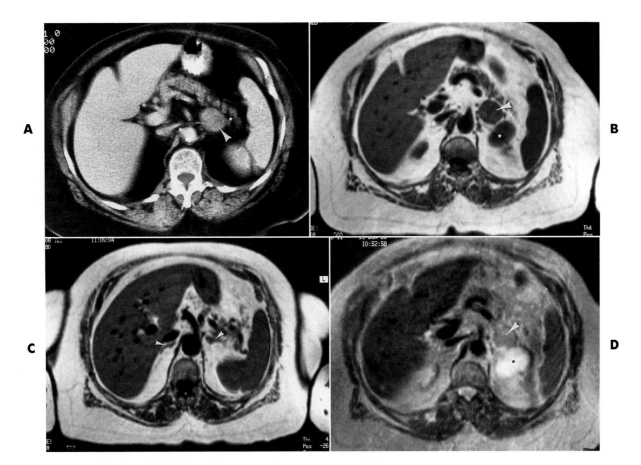

Fig. 16-9. Probable nonfunctioning adenoma in an elderly woman with no history of malignancy. **A,** CT scan. The 2.5 cm left adrenal mass *(arrowhead)* has homogeneous soft tissue density. Small projection from the lateral aspect may represent normal adrenal tissue *(asterisk)*. **B,** Axial T1WI. Adrenal mass *(arrowhead)* has homogeneous, low signal intensity. Renal cyst *(asterisk)* is seen posterior to adrenal gland. **C,** Axial T1WI. Right adrenal gland *(arrowhead)* and superior aspect of the left adrenal gland *(arrowhead)* are normal. **D,** T2-weighted MR image. Adrenal mass *(arrow)* has uniform signal intensity that is slightly greater than perinephric fat and greater than the liver. High signal intensity posteriorly *(asterisk)* is a left renal cyst.

when dynamic gadolinium perfusion studies were used.

In summary, adrenal adenomas can have a variable appearance by MRI. No imaging finding to date is pathognomonic for a nonfunctioning adrenal adenoma using standard MRI techniques.

Myelolipoma. Myelolipoma is an uncommon, benign neoplasm of the adrenal glands that contains fat and myeloid (bone marrow) elements. The mass may be primarily lipomatous or solid in appearance, with small foci of fat. Both CT and MRI demonstrate fat density or fat signal intensity within the tumor, which is highly suggestive of myelolipoma (Fig. 16-10).[18,44] Other retroperitoneal fat-containing tumors—including teratoma, lipoma, or liposarcoma—rarely involve the adrenal glands. In patients with known malignancy, adrenal masses containing only a small quantity of fat or peripherally located fat may represent metastasis with engulfment of surrounding perirenal fat.[31] Percutaneous biopsy may be considered in these cases, and aspiration of myeloid elements is confirmatory for myelolipoma.

Cysts. Cysts of the adrenal glands occur rarely, with a reported incidence of 0.06% in 14,000 autopsies.[59] Endothelial cysts are most common, comprising 45% of adrenal cysts, and are most often lymphangiomatous. Pseudocysts represent 39% of adrenal cysts and are the most common to be clinically diagnosed. They probably result from hemorrhage within the adrenal glands, have a fibrous wall with linear calcifications and internal septations, and contain reddish-brown fluid (Fig. 16-11). Epithelial cysts make up 9% of adrenal cysts and parasitic cysts account for 7%. Most of these are asymptomatic because of their small size.[34,36]

The MRI appearance of adrenal cysts depends on the content of the cyst. Most cysts are hypointense relative to

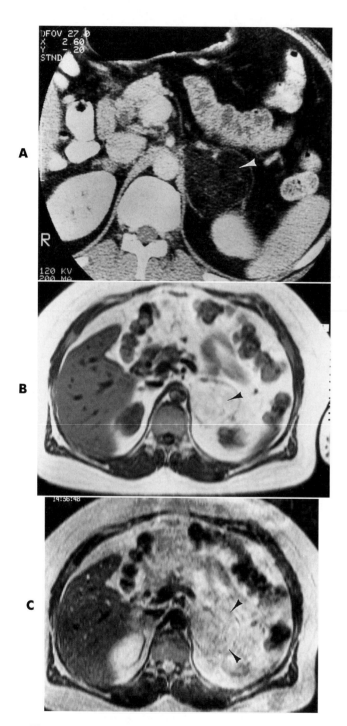

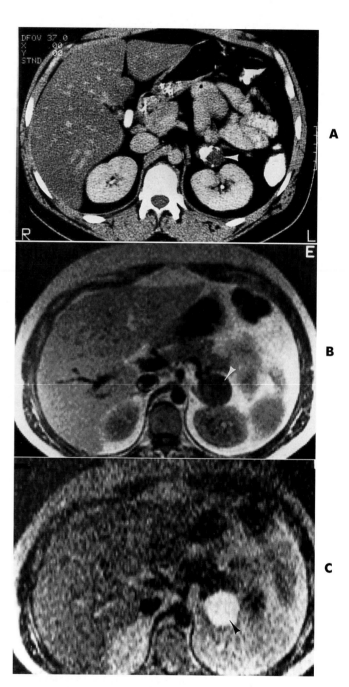

Fig. 16-10. Adrenal myelolipoma. **A,** CT scan. Large left adrenal mass *(arrowhead)* with fat density. **B,** T1-weighted MR image. Signal intensity within left adrenal mass *(arrowhead)* is nearly equal that of perinephric fat. **C,** T2WI. Myelolipoma *(arrowheads)* is defined by low intensity rim but is otherwise difficult to differentiate from perinephric fat.

Fig. 16-11. Hemorrhagic adrenal cyst, proven by surgical excision. **A,** CT scan. Left adrenal mass *(arrowhead)* is hypodense with peripheral calcifications. **B,** T1-weighted MR image. Round adrenal mass *(arrow head)* has low signal intensity. Rim calcifications are not visible. **C,** T2-weighted MR image. Adrenal mass *(arrowhead)* is homogeneous with high signal intensity.

the liver on T1WI and hyper-intense to the liver on T2WI. If hemorrhage is present, increased signal intensity may be present within the cyst on T1WI.

Metastasis. The adrenal glands are a common site of metastatic disease, representing the fourth most commonly involved organ after the lungs, liver, and bone.[39] In an autopsy study of 1000 patients with epithelial cancers, 27% had metastatic disease in the adrenal glands.[1] The primary tumors most often involved the lungs, breasts, thyroid glands, colon, and skin.[39] Although metastatic disease occurs commonly in patients with malignancies, an isolated adrenal mass in a cancer patient is still most likely to be benign. In a study of 25 patients with nonsmall bronchogenic carcinoma of the lung who underwent biopsy of solitary adrenal masses, 32% had metastasis and 68% had adenomas.[49] In another series, percutaneous biopsy of adrenal masses in patients with neoplasms showed adenomas in 43%.[35]

By CT imaging, adrenal metastases appear as rounded or oval soft tissue masses or diffuse enlargement of the adrenal glands. As discussed in the section on adrenal adenoma, MRI has been extensively evaluated as a means of discriminating between benign and malignant lesions. Most metastatic lesions have higher signal intensity than the liver on the T2WI. However, metastatic lesions arising from the lung, colon, and carcinoid tumors[28] and from lymphoma[4] have shown low signal intensity, simulating the appearance of a typical nonhyperfunctioning adenoma. Therefore, imaging criteria alone cannot accurately differentiate benign from malignant disease. If the diagnosis of metastatic disease to the adrenal glands will change therapy for a patient with a known malignancy, percutaneous biopsy of an adrenal mass is required to confirm the histologic diagnosis.

HYPOFUNCTIONING LESIONS

Clinical syndrome (Addison's disease). Chronic adrenocortical insufficiency is due to progressive destruction of the adrenal cortices. Clinical findings include weakness, fatigue, anorexia, increased skin pigmentation, and hypotension.[62] Laboratory assessment shows low levels of plasma cortisol and elevated levels of plasma ACTH. The most common cause of Addison's disease is idiopathic atrophy, which may have an autoimmune origin and is characterized on imaging studies by severe atrophy of the adrenal glands.[15,18,44]

Inflammatory diseases. Tuberculosis is the second most common cause of Addison's disease, accounting for one third of the cases. Histoplasmosis, blastomycosis, and fungal disease rarely involve the adrenal glands.[64] On imaging studies, adrenal glands involved with tuberculosis may be enlarged but of normal configuration, and in the late stages they are often calcified. Active involvement with tuberculosis may produce bilateral adrenal enlarge-

ment with high signal intensity on T2WI, mimicking malignant disease.[3]

Hemorrhage. Bilateral adrenal hemorrhage occurs in adults with coagulopathy caused by a bleeding disorder or anticoagulation or in association with stress from surgery, sepsis, trauma, or hypotension. CT of acute adrenal hemorrhage typically shows hyperdense adrenal masses, which become decreased in density with time, later forming pseudocysts with rim calcification. On MRI in the subacute phase, areas of high signal intensity are seen on T1WI that are caused by blood products, including methemoglobin (Fig. 16-12).[21] Adrenal hemorrhage in neonates is most often due to trauma and seldom results in adrenal insufficiency.

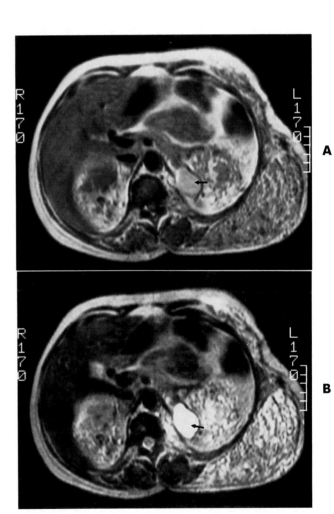

Fig. 16-12. Adrenal hemorrhage in patient with hemangioma. **A,** T1-weighted MR image. Left adrenal mass *(arrow)* has moderately high signal intensity indicative of blood products, predominantly methemoglobin. Note multiple vessels of the hemangioma involving the perinephric space, left subcutaneous tissues, and abdominal musculature. **B,** T2-weighted MR image. Uniform high signal intensity in the hemorrhagic left adrenal gland *(arrow).*

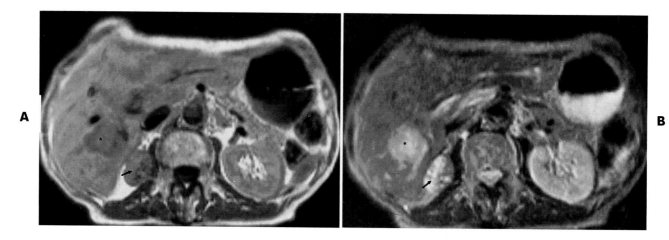

Fig. 16-13. Right adrenal mass in a patient with liver metastases from small cell carcinoma. Histologic diagnosis of right adrenal mass did not significantly alter the course of chemotherapy, and percutaneous biopsy was not performed. **A,** T1WI. Adrenal mass has *(arrow)* intermediate signal intensity with some inhomogeneity. Liver metastasis *(asterisk)* is well demonstrated. **B,** T2-weighted MR image. Adrenal mass *(arrow)* is inhomogeneous with areas of high signal intensity. Differential diagnosis includes adenoma with hemorrhage or necrosis, metastatic disease, or primary adrenal carcinoma. Liver metastasis is evident *(asterisk)*.

Metastasis. Metastatic disease is an uncommon cause of adrenal insufficiency because adrenal function can be maintained until greater than 90% of the glands are destroyed or replaced. Breast and lung cancer are the most common sites of tumor origin.[18] Non-Hodgkin lymphoma involves the adrenal glands in a small percentage of patients, occurring in 4% of 173 patients in one series, and may produce adrenal insufficiency when extensive and bilateral involvement occurs.[50]

RADIOGRAPHIC EVALUATION OF THE ASYMPTOMATIC ADRENAL MASS

The primary consideration in evaluating an adrenal mass is whether the patient has a known malignancy. In

Table 16-1. Summary: CT and MRI features of adrenal masses

Type of lesion	Morphology of lesion	CT	T1WI	T2WI
Nonfunctioning adenoma	< 3 cm, round or oval	Homogeneous, low density	Isointense with liver	Variable, predominantly isointense, but occasionally hyperintense or hypointense
Adenoma—Conn's syndrome	Small, mean of 1.5 cm, round or oval	Homogeneous, low density	Isointense with liver	Variable
Adenoma—Cushing's syndrome	>2 cm	Homogeneous, low density	Isointense	Variable
Adrenal cortical carcinoma	Large mass, 5-22 cm	Inhomogeneous, ± central necrosis, 30% calcified	Hypointense to liver	Hyperintense, ± region of necrosis
Pheochromocytoma	Usually >3 cm	Variable, cystic or solid mass, ± necrosis		Typically very hyperintense compared with liver, ± necrosis
Myelolipoma	Size variable	Fat density in tumor	Variable, with intensity of fat	Variable, with signal characteristic of fat within tumor
Metastasis	Size variable, often multiple other sites	Variable	Variable, most hypointense	Variable, most hyperintense to liver

the patient without an underlying neoplasm, the major differential diagnosis for an adrenal mass is nonhyperfunctioning adenoma and adrenal carcinoma.[28] Adenoma is common and adrenal carcinoma is rare. Conservative management of these patients is appropriate when the mass has benign features, including smooth contour, sharp margination, and a size of less than 3 cm. Some authors suggest that a mass less than 5 cm in diameter is also most likely benign.[11] Imaging follow-up is performed with serial CT or MRI scans obtained at 3 months, 6 months, and 1 year. If the mass is stable at 1 year, it can be considered benign.[45] Adrenal masses greater than 5 cm in diameter should be excised, because adrenal cortical carcinoma cannot be excluded based on percutaneous biopsy, and the possibility of carcinoma is increased in large lesions.[6]

In a patient with a known malignancy, an adrenal mass may represent a nonhyperfunctioning adenoma, metastasis, or adrenal carcinoma (Fig. 16-13). CT and MRI methods cannot definitively differentiate an adenoma from a malignant lesion. (See Table 16-1, summarizing CT and MRI features in adrenal masses.) Additional evaluation with NP-59 scintigraphy has proved useful in masses greater than 2 cm in diameter.[28] Magnetic resonance spectroscopy has shown promise in distinguishing adenomas from other lesions based on fat content and may prove clinically useful in the future.[42] However, the consensus based on literature to date is that a patient with an adrenal mass and a known malignancy should undergo percutaneous biopsy for definitive diagnosis, if the presence of metastatic disease will significantly alter therapy.[3,6,35,49] Before percutaneous biopsy, patients with hypertension or familial syndromes should be screened using laboratory tests to exclude pheochromocytoma, since biopsy of a pheochromocytoma may induce hypertensive crisis and death.[43] The risk of percutaneous adrenal biopsy is otherwise low, with complications including bleeding or pneumothorax. The benefit of a pathologic diagnosis of an adrenal mass in the cancer patient outweighs the risks of percutaneous biopsy when the diagnosis will alter therapy.

REFERENCES

1. Abrams HL, Spiro R, Goldstein N: Metastases in carcinoma: analysis of 1000 autopsied cases, *Cancer* 3:74-85, Jan 1950.
2. Auda SP, Brennan MF, Gill JR: Evolution of the surgical management of primary aldosteronism, *Ann Surg* 191:1-7, 1980.
3. Baker ME, Spritzer C, Blinder R, et al : Benign adrenal lesions mimicking malignancy on MR imaging: report of two cases, *Radiology* 163:669-671, 1987.
4. Baker ME, Blinder R, Spritzer C, et al: MR evaluation of adrenal masses at 1.5 T, *AJR* 153:307-312, 1989.
5. Berliner L, Bosniak MA, Megibow A: Adrenal pseudotumors on computed tomography, *J Comput Assist Tomogr* 6(2):281-285, 1982.
6. Bernardino ME: Management of the asymptomatic patient with a unilateral adrenal mass, *Radiology* 166:121-123, 1988.
7. Brady TM, Gross BH, Glazer GM, et al: Adrenal pseudomasses due to varices: angiographic-CT-MRI-pathologic correlations, *AJR* 145:301-304, 1985.
8. Chang A, Glazer HS, Lee JKT, et al: Adrenal gland: MR imaging, *Radiology* 163:123-128, 1987.
9. Chezmar JL, Robbins SM, Nelson RC, et al: Adrenal masses: characterization with T1-weighted MR imaging, *Radiology* 166:357-359, 1988.
10. Commons RR, Callaway CP: Adenomas of the adrenal cortex, *Arch Intern Med* 81:37-41, 1948.
11. Copeland PM: The incidentally discovered adrenal mass, *Ann Intern Med* 98:940-945, l983.
12. Dobbie JW: Adrenocortical nodular hyperplasia: the aging adrenal, *J Pathol* 99(1):1-18, 1969.
13. Doppman JL, Gill JR, Nienhuis AW, et al: CT findings in Addison disease, *J Comput Assist Tomogr* 6:757-761, l982.
14. Doppman JL, Miller DL, Dwyer AJ, et al: Macronodular adrenal hyperplasia in Cushing disease, *Radiology* 166:347-352, l988.
15. Doppman JL, Travis WD, Nieman L, et al: Cushing syndrome due to primary pigmented nodular adrenocortical disease: findings at CT and MR imaging, *Radiology* 172:415-420, 1989.
16. Doppman JL, Nieman L, Miller DL, et al: Ectopic adrenocorticotropic hormone syndrome: localization studies in 28 patients, *Radiology* 172:115-124, 1989.
17. Dunnick NR: CT and MRI of adrenal lesions, *Urol Radiol* 10:12-16, 1988.
18. Dunnick NR: Adrenal imaging: current status, *AJR* 154:927-936, 1990.
19. Edelman RR, McFarland E, Stark DD, et al: Surface coil MR imaging of the abdominal viscera. Part I. Theory, technique, and initial results, *Radiology* 157:425-430, 1985.
20. Egglin TK, Hahn PF, Stark DD: MRI of the adrenal glands, *Semin Roentgenol* 23(4):280-287, 1988.
21. Falke THM, te Strake L, Sandler MP, et al: Magnetic resonance imaging of the adrenal glands, *Radiographics* 7(2):343-370, 1987.
22. Falke THM, Peetoom JJ, de Ross A, et al: Gadolinium-DTPA enhanced MR imaging of intravenous extension of adrenocortical carcinoma, *J Comput Assist Tomogr* 12(2):331-334, 1988.
23. Farge D, Chatellier G, Pagny J, et al: Isolated clinical syndrome of primary aldosteronism in four patients with adrenocortical carcinoma, *Am J Med* 83:635-640, 1987.
24. Fink IJ, Reinig JW, Dwyer AJ, et al: MR imaging of pheochromocytomas, *J Comput Assist Tomogr* 9(3):454-458, 1985.
25. Francis IR, Smid A, Gross MD, et al: Adrenal masses in oncologic patients: functional and morphologic evaluation, *Radiology* 166:353-356, 1988.
26. Geisinger MA, Zelch MG, Bravo EL, et al: Primary hyperaldosteronism: comparison of CT, adrenal venography, and venous sampling, *AJR* 141:299-302, 1983.
27. Glazer GM: MR imaging of the liver, kidneys, and adrenal glands, *Radiology* 166:303-312, 1988.
28. Glazer GM, Francis IR, Quint LE: Progress in clinical radiology: imaging of the adrenal glands, *Invest Radiol* 23:3-11, 1988.
29. Glazer GM, Woolsey EJ, Borrello J, et al: Adrenal tissue characterization using MR imaging, *Radiology* 158:73-79, 1986.
30. Glazer HS, Weyman PJ, Sagel SS, et al: Nonfunctioning adrenal masses: incidental discovery on computed tomography, *AJR* 139:81-85, 1982.
31. Green KM, Brantly PN, Thompson WR: Adenocarcinoma metastatic to the adrenal gland simulating myelolipoma: CT evaluation, *J Comput Assist Tomogr* 9(4):820-821, 1985.
32. Hedeland H, Ostberg G, Hokfelt B, et al: On the prevalance of adrenocortical adenomas in an autopsy material in relation to hypertension and diabetes, *Acta Med Scand* 184:211-214, l968.
33. Ikeda DM, Francis IR, Glazer GM, et al: The detection of adrenal tumors and hyperplasia in patients with primary aldosteronism: comparison of scintigraphy, CT, and MR imaging, *AJR* 153:301-306, 1989.

34. Johnson CD, Baker ME, Dunnick NR: CT demonstration of an adrenal pseudocyst, *J Comput Assist Tomogr* 9(4):817-819, 1985.

35. Katz RL, Shirkhoda A: Diagnostic approach to incidental adrenal nodules in the cancer patient: results of a clinical, radiologic, and fine needle aspiration study, *Cancer* 55:1995-2000, 1985.

36. Kearney GP, Mahoney EM, Maher E, et al: Functioning and nonfunctioning cysts of the adrenal cortex and medulla, *Am J Surg* 134:363-368, 1977.

37. Kenney PJ, Stanley RJ: Calcified adrenal masses, *Urol Radiol* 9:9-15, 1987.

38. Kier R, McCarthy S: MR characterization of adrenal masses: field strength and pulse sequence considerations, *Radiology* 171:671-674, 1989.

39. Korobkin M: Overview of adrenal imaging/adrenal CT, *Urol Radiol* 11:221-226, 1989.

40. Krestin BP, Steinbrich W, Friedmann G: Adrenal masses: evaluation with fast gradient-echo MR imaging and Gd-DTPA-enhanced dynamic studies, *Radiology* 171:675-680, 1989.

41. Lee MJ, Hahn PF, Papanicolau N, et al: Benign and malignant adrenal masses: CT distinction with attenuation coefficients, size and observer analysis, *Radiology* 179:415-418, 1991.

42. Leroy-Willig A, Bittoun J, Luton JP, et al: In vivo MR spectroscopic imaging of the adrenal glands: distinction between adenomas and carcinomas larger than 15 mm based on lipid content, *AJR* 153:771-773, 1989.

43. McCorkell SJ, Niles NL: Fine-needle aspiration of catecholamine-producing adrenal masses: a possibly fatal mistake, *AJR* 145:113-114, 1985.

44. Mezrich R, Banner MP, Pollack HM: Magnetic resonance imaging of the adrenal glands, *Urol Radiol* 8:127-138, 1986.

45. Mitnick JS, Bosniak MA, Megibow AJ, et al: Non-functioning adrenal adenomas discovered incidentally on computed tomography, *Radiology* 148:495-499, 1983.

46. Mitty HA: Embryology, anatomy, and anomalies of the adrenal gland, *Semin Roentgenol,* 43(4):271-279, 1988.

47. Montagne J, Kressel HY, Korobkin M, et al: Computed tomography of the normal adrenal glands, *AJR* 130:963-966, 1978.

48. Moulton JS, Moulton JS: CT of the adrenal glands, *Semin Roentgenol* 43(4):288-303, 1988.

49. Oliver TW Jr, Bernardino ME, Miller JI, et al: Isolated adrenal masses in nonsmall-cell bronchogenic carcinoma, *Radiology* 153:217-218, 1984.

50. Paling MR, Williamson BRJ: Adrenal involvement in non-Hodgkin lymphoma, *AJR* 141:303-305, 1983.

51. Quint LE, Glazer GM, Francis IR, et al: Pheochromocytoma and paraganglioma: comparison of MR imaging with CT and I-131 MIBG scintigraphy, *Radiology* 165:89-93, 1987.

52. Reinig JW, Doppman JL, Dwyer AJ, et al: Adrenal masses differentiated by MR, *Radiology* 158:81-84, 1986.

53. Reinig JW, Doppman JL, Dwyer AJ, et al: MRI of indeterminate adrenal masses, *AJR* 147:493-496, 1986.

54. Remer EM, Weinfeld RM, Glazer GM, et al: Hyperfunctioning and nonhyperfunctioning benign adrenal cortical lesions: characterization and comparison with MR imaging, *Radiology* 171:681-685, 1989.

55. Schultz CL, Haaga JR, Fletcher BD, et al: Magnetic resonance imaging of the adrenal glands: a comparison with computed tomography, *AJR* 143:1235-1240, 1984.

56. Silverman PM: Gastric diverticulum mimicking adrenal mass: CT demonstration, *J Comput Assist Tomogr* 10(4):709-711, 1986.

57. Smith SM, Patel SK, Turner DA, et al: Magnetic resonance imaging of adrenal cortical carcinoma, *Urol Radiol* 11:1-6, 1989.

58. van Gils APG, Falke THM, van Erkel AR, et al: MR imaging and MIBG scintigraphy of pheochromocytomas and extraadrenal functioning paragangliomas, *Radiographics* 11:37-57, 1991.

59. Wahl HR: Adrenal cysts, *Am J Pathol* 27:798, 1951.

60. Weinberger MH, Grim CE, Hollifield JW, et al: Primary aldosteronism: diagnosis, localization and treatment, *Ann Intern Med* 90:386-395, 1979.

61. White EM, Edelman RR, Stark DD, et al: Surface coil MR imaging of abdominal viscera. Part II. The adrenal glands, *Radiology* 157:431-436, 1985.

62. Williams TC: Functional disorders of the adrenal glands: an overview, *Semin Roentgenol* 43(4):304-313, 1988.

63. Wilms G, Baert A, Marchal G, et al: Computed tomography of the normal adrenal glands: correlative study with autopsy specimens, *J Comput Assist Tomogr* 3:467-469, 1979.

64. Wilson, Muchmore HG, Tisdal RG, et al: Histoplasmosis of the adrenal glands studied by CT, *Radiology* 150:779-783, 1984.

Chapter 17

KIDNEY

Juri V. Kaude
Gladys M. Torres

A variety of well-established imaging modalities are routinely used for evaluating renal diseases. In recent years, magnetic resonance imaging (MRI) has emerged as a new imaging modality for the genitourinary (GU) tract. Compared with ultrasound (US) and computed tomography (CT) of the kidneys, MRI at first advanced slowly. Early clinical investigators encountered difficulty in overcoming motion artifacts, inferior spatial resolution, and high cost.

Since the first reports on MRI of the human kidney,[94,109] significant developments in technology have broadened the clinical applications of MRI in evaluating the GU tract. The ability to control motion artifacts by increased imaging speed, availability of an effective oral contrast agent for opacification of the bowel, and magnetic resonance angiography (MRA) are among the factors which have improved magnetic resonance (MR) image quality. The use of gadopentetate dimeglumine expands the indications for renal MRI. Renal function can be assessed and renal tumors can be better demarcated with a dynamic examination.* Gadopentetate dimeglumine (as well as other metal chelates and superparamagnetic iron oxide[30,71]) is freely filtered by the kidney; its excretion reflects the glomerular filtration rate and tubular absorption of water.

Examination cost and time still constrain the utilization of MRI. Nevertheless, MRI has become an important tool for staging renal malignancies and for detecting certain other pathologic processes.

TECHNIQUES

We use a technique for scanning the abdomen that requires supine position. Abdominal compression and a respiratory compensation belt are used. Every patient

---

*References 8, 9, 13, 14, 23, 46, 51, 69, 82, 105, 107.

receives 2 to 3 cups of barium sulfate suspension. For better delineation of the gastrointestinal (GI) tract and reduction of high intensity artifacts of peristaltic motion, one cup of barium sulfate is given at each of the following times before scanning; 60 minutes, 30 minutes, and 5 minutes.[62]

The fundamental MRI technique for renal evaluation is the spin-echo (SE) sequence. The kidneys are localized and examined with T1-weighted (i.e., weighted to the spin-lattice or longitudinal relaxation time) SE sequence using a pulse repetition time (TR) of 500 to 700 msec and a time to echo (TE) of 15 to 20 msec in the transaxial and coronal planes. T2-weighted images (i.e., weighted to the spin-spin or transverse relaxation time) are performed using a TR of 2000 to 2500 msec and a TE of 20 to 80 msec.

If the possibility of a pathologic condition involving the vessels exists, gradient-echo images are performed to enhance flow imaging. Single breath-hold sequences of 9 to 12 seconds duration are used to control respiratory motion artifacts. Multiple overlapping 10 mm axial scans cover the entire area of interest, as do single-section gradient reversal echo (GRE) scans, using a TR of 22 msec, a TE of 13 msec, and a flip angle of 30 degrees.

MRA also is used to evaluate abdominal vasculature. Two-dimensional time of flight angiography obtains a series of GRE images within a single breath-holding period (less than 15 seconds).

For evaluating the inferior vena cava (IVC), renal veins, and renal arteries, coronal views are done using a TR of 30 msec, a TE of 8 msec, and a flip angle of 30 degrees. Single-level dynamic GRE is used in conjunction with gadopentetate dimeglumine to obtain both anatomic and functional information.

Finally, fat suppression techniques[90] based on selective chemical-shift suppression imaging, especially with the use of contrast material, may be useful in diagnosing and characterizing small renal lesions.[11]

MORPHOLOGY OF NORMAL KIDNEYS

The difference in water content of the cortex and medulla of the kidney provides good contrast between renal parenchymal compartments by MRI without intravenous contrast administration. For this reason and freedom from the risk and cost of iodine contrast, MRI has major advantages over CT.

On T1-weighted images (T1WI), the cortical tissue is of higher signal intensity than that of the medulla (Fig. 17-1, A). Renal sinus fat is differentiated well by its high signal intensity, whereas the renal pelvis and calices, if distended, are well-outlined by the low signal intensity of

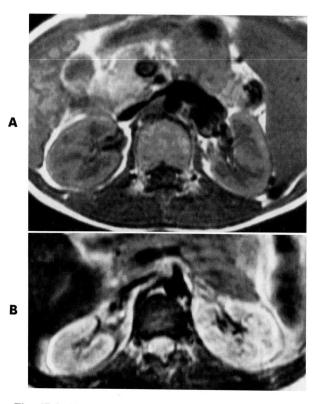

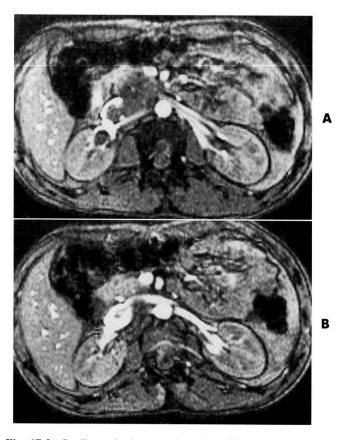

Fig. 17-1. Normal kidneys. **A,** T1-weighted image. Note good demarcation of cortex (higher signal intensity) and pyramids of medulla (lower signal intensity). **B,** T2-weighted image of normal kidneys.

Fig. 17-2. Gradient echo images of renal arteries and veins (TR 22 msec, TE 13 sec, flip angle of 30 degrees).

urine. Renal arteries and veins are frequently shown best on gradient echo images (Fig. 17-2).

On T2-weighted images (T2WI) the corticomedullary boundaries are less well-differentiated (Fig. 17-1, *B*). The same is true for renal imaging following gadopentetate dimeglumine administration, unless rapid scanning sequences are used. Thus renal MRI must always include T1WI for optimal anatomic depiction.

CONGENITAL DISEASE
Polycystic kidneys

Of the congenital renal abnormalities, adult polycystic kidney disease is most frequently encountered (Fig. 17-3). Some polycystic kidneys are detected incidentally, with the patient not yet having developed renal failure. Other patients with polycystic kidneys are usually examined in adulthood or in the advanced stage of the disease.

The cysts in the polycystic kidneys may have variable signal intensities, depending on whether they are uncomplicated simple, hemorrhagic, or infected cysts (Fig. 17-3).* Calcifications are frequently present in adult polycystic kidney disease and can be identified as foci of signal voids.

Other congenital abnormalities

Infantile polycystic kidneys or other congenital abnormalities are rarely imaged by MR. One report in the literature describes prenatal diagnosis of renal agenesis by MRI.[18] Occasionally, congenital hydronephrosis is encountered in adulthood, usually secondary to partial uretero-pelvic obstruction. Extrarenal pelvis should be considered as a normal variant. A horseshoe kidney may also be found in patients referred for MRI.[64]

INFLAMMATORY DISEASE

In acute glomerulonephritis or acute bacterial nephritis, corticomedullary differentiation in the usually enlarged and edematous kidney is difficult or impossible.[64,72,109] In acute tubular necrosis, Leung et al.[64] found the medulla to be swollen and the corticomedullary boundary less well-demarcated than in the normal kidney.

In hemorrhagic fever with uremia syndrome—a viral, rodent-transmitted disease—corticomedullary demarcation is preserved. The signal intensity of the outer medulla is decreased on T2WI because of medullary hemorrhages.[55] In hemosiderosis the cortical T2 relaxation time is shortened by the susceptibility effect of iron deposition, resulting in good corticomedullary demarcation.[72]

In paroxysmal nocturnal hemoglobinuria, the signal intensities between the cortex and medulla are reversed.[75] The cortical signal is lower than that of the medulla because of the paramagnetic effect of iron being deposited mainly in the proximal tubular cells of the cortex.[15]

*References 4, 34, 38, 48, 57, 64, 65, 101.

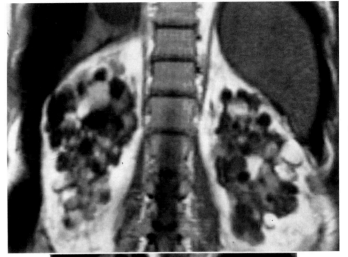

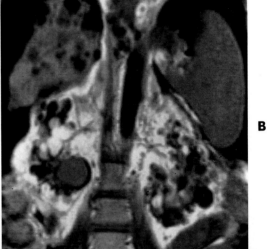

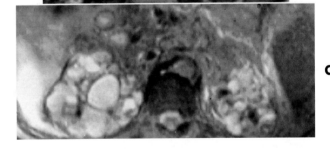

Fig. 17-3. Polycystic kidneys. **A,** Coronal T1-weighted image. Multiple cysts of varying signal intensity (low signal intensity for clear fluid; high signal intensity for hemorrhages) in both kidneys. **B,** Coronal T1-weighted image. Multiple simple cysts are also in the liver. **C,** Axial T2-weighted image of the same patient.

In sickle cell disease, a similar decrease of signal intensity in the cortex, in particular on T2WI, has been reported.[60] The decrease of signal intensity is thought to be caused by iron deposition in the cortex, reflecting an iron metabolism abnormality in sickle cell disease.

Acute focal disease

In an acute focal disease such as an abscess in its different stages of development, the diseased area produces lower or mixed signal intensity on T1WI (Fig. 17-4, *A*) and higher signal intensity than normal parenchyma on T2WI (Fig. 17-4, *B*).[31,101] Specific MR diagnosis of abscess versus focal lesions of other etiology is not possible, since renal neoplasm may cause similar signal intensity changes.

Chronic disease

Either in chronic pyelonephritis or glomerulonephritis, the kidneys are usually small, and the corticomedullary boundaries are blurred or entirely absent (Fig. 17-5).[38,64] Renal sinus fat is abundant,[38] and the remaining renal parenchyma may have low signal intensity (Fig. 17-5).[64] Focal scarring may be demonstrable in chronic pyelonephritis as decreased intensity on T1 and T2 sequences.

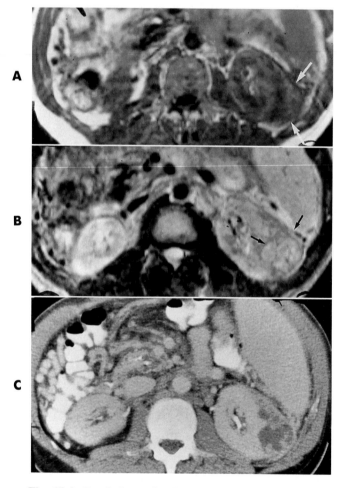

Fig. 17-4. Renal abscess in 40-year-old male with diabetes. **A,** T1-weighted image. **B,** T2-weighted image. Mass in the lateral aspect of the left kidney demonstrates mixed signal intensity *(arrows)*. On T2WI, signal intensity is increased. **C,** CT scan for comparison shows irregular areas of low attenuation within the mass.

Xanthogranulomatous pyelonephritis

This inflammatory disease frequently is manifested as a mass lesion associated with obstructive stone disease. The inflammatory mass demonstrates mixed signal intensity, and it may simulate a neoplasm (Fig. 17-6).[25,48,67] The diagnosis is aided by the signal void caused by renal calculus. The disease process may extend beyond the renal capsule and infiltrate the perirenal space and adjacent organs.[25,61]

HYDRONEPHROSIS

The diagnosis of hydronephrosis is readily made by MRI of the dilated collecting system in both axial or coronal projections, preferably on T1WI (Figs. 17-7 and 17-12).* According to Marotti et al.,[72] in acute obstruction the corticomedullary demarcation is preserved, whereas in chronic hydronephrosis the demarcation is absent. Using dynamic gadopentetate dimeglumine in acute obstruction, cortical enhancement is similar to a normal kidney, but medullary enhancement is higher.[91] In chronic obstruction, cortical enhancement is lower than in the normal kidney and the tubular phase is prolonged.[91] Kikinis et al.,[53] using gradient-echo imaging, also describes increased signal intensity in the medulla following contrast enhancement of the hydronephrotic kidney.

TRAUMA AND HEMORRHAGE

Few institutions have MRI available for emergency evaluation of abdominal trauma patients. Monitoring of vital signs and magnet safety issues concerning life-support devices are limiting factors. In addition the clinical status of the patient may not always permit the use of the scanning times of several minutes necessary for routine spin echo imaging. Therefore, most patients with renal trauma examined with MRI have suffered an iatrogenic trauma from either diagnostic or therapeutic procedures. They are patients who have had renal biopsy or nephrostomy (penetrating trauma) or have been treated with extracorporeal

*References 38, 48, 49, 64, 68, 72, 91.

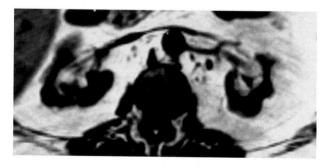

Fig. 17-5. Chronic pyelonephritis is shown by T1-weighted image. Both kidneys are small and severely scarred. Signal intensity is reduced, and fat is abundant in renal sinus.

shock wave lithotripsy (ESWL) therapy for renal stone disease (blunt trauma). Loss of corticomedullary demarcation is a frequent finding in patients who have undergone ESWL and is attributed to renal edema.[6,48,50,52] In experimental studies, Neuerburg et al.[76] were unable to prove that the loss of corticomedullary demarcation was caused by edema but found the explanation plausible.

Fresh renal or perirenal hemorrhage on T1WI is either isointense with renal cortex or has mixed signal intensity (Figs. 17-8 and 17-9). A subcapsular hemorrhage is well-outlined against the parenchyma and is surrounded by the renal capsule (Fig. 17-10).[48,50,52,101] In experimental studies, fresh subcapsular hemorrhage had increased signal intensity on T2WI.[78] However, fresh perirenal hemorrhage in kidney transplants after biopsy has been reported to have low signal intensity, both on T1WI and T2WI.[73] The signal intensity of blood depends on the timing of examination, the presence of intact or lysed red cells, and the oxidation state of hemoglobin in various parts of the hemorrhage. Intensity generally increases with the age of the hemorrhage, when clotting or organization has occurred (Fig. 17-10).[48,50,52,73] With resolution or liquefaction of the hemorrhage, the signal intensity decreases relative to the acute stage of bleeding because of the accumulation of hemosiderin.

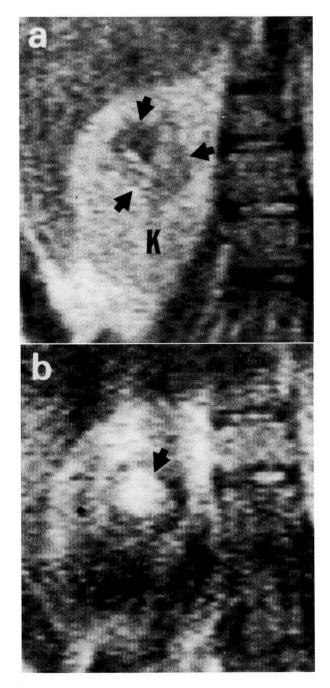

Fig. 17-6. Xanthogranulomatous pyelonephritis. **A,** T2-weighted image. Mass lesion of mixed but generally lower signal intensity than renal parenchyma *(arrows).* **B,** T2-weighted image, delayed echo sequence. Signal intensity in lesion is much higher *(arrow).* No stone obstructing the collecting system was present in this case. (From Kaude JV, Kinard RE: In Löhr E, Leder L-D, eds: *Renal and adrenal tumors,* ed 2, Berlin, 1987, Springer-Verlag.)

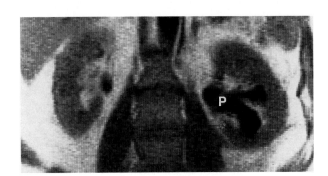

Fig. 17-7. Hydronephrosis of left kidney is shown by T1-weighted image. Dilated kidney pelvis has low signal intensity *(P).* Right kidney is normal.

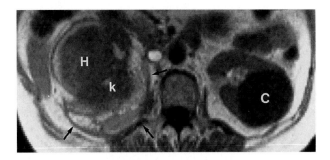

Fig. 17-8. Large perirenal hemorrhage 18 days after biopsy is shown by T1-weighted image. Kidney *(K)* is squeezed between the well-defined hematoma *(H)* anteriorly and a more diffuse hemorrhage posteriorly *(arrows).* Large cyst *(C)* is in the left kidney.

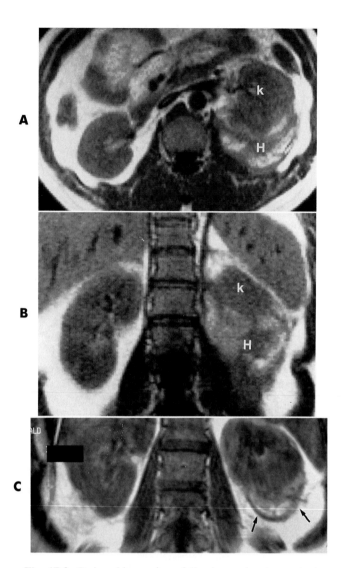

Fig. 17-9. Perirenal hemorrhage following nephrostomy. **A,** Axial T1-weighted image. **B,** Coronal T1-weighted image. Left kidney *(K)* is pushed anteriorly and cranially by a large perirenal-retroperitoneal hemorrhage of mixed echogenicity *(H)*. **C,** Follow-up scan 6 years later shows some remaining scarring around lower pole of left kidney *(arrows)*.

ATRAUMATIC VASCULAR DISEASES
Arteriovenous fistulas and aneurysms

Renal vascular abnormalities include congenital or spontaneous arteriovenous fistulas and renal artery aneurysms. Smaller vascular lesions may be occult on MRI but can be detected by angiography (Fig. 17-11, *B*) or noninvasively and easily with (color) Doppler ultrasound (Fig. 17-11, *C*). Larger lesions may be very impressive on MRI (Fig. 17-11, *A*). Differential diagnosis includes hemorrhagic masses or cysts.

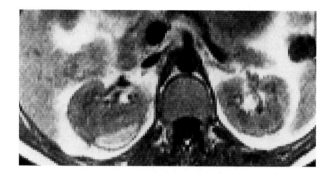

Fig. 17-10. Six-week-old subcapsular hemorrhage of right kidney (after ESWL for renal stones) is shown by T1-weighted image. Signal intensity is high in well-defined hemorrhage in the posterior aspect of the right kidney. Hemorrhage was resolved 6 months later with minimal residual scarring. (From Kaude et al: *AJR* 145:305-313, 1985.)

Ischemia

The results of early experimental investigations of renal ischemia were somewhat controversial. Although London et al.[68] did not observe any change of the T1 relaxation time in the ischemic kidney, Slutsky et al.[93] and Yuasa and Kundel[111] observed a prolongation of the T1 relaxation time. Their observations have been confirmed clinically.[43,77]

Renal vein thrombosis

In experimental renal vein thrombosis, Uhlenbrock et al.[103] have observed increased T2 relaxation times in the cortex and reduced T2 relaxation times in the medulla, and they believe that MRI is a sensitive test for evaluation of renal vein thrombosis.

Patients with renal vein thrombosis who are referred for MRI are usually cancer patients. The diagnosis and appearance of tumor thrombi is discussed in this chapter under "Malignant Neoplasms."

PERIRENAL DISEASE
Retroperitoneal fibrosis

This disease, first described by Albarran in 1905, is discussed in detail in Chapter 15. There are rare individuals in whom the disease is primary or involves only the perirenal space. In such a patient examined with MRI, bilateral perirenal masses encapsulated the kidneys and obstructed the renal pelves (Fig. 17-12, *A*).[106] The masses were of low signal intensity on T2WI, indicating that fibrous tissue was the main component of the perirenal disease process (Fig. 17-12, *B*).

Perirenal hemorrhage

Perirenal hemorrhage (see Figs. 17-8 and 17-9) is usually associated with trauma to the kidney (see "Trauma

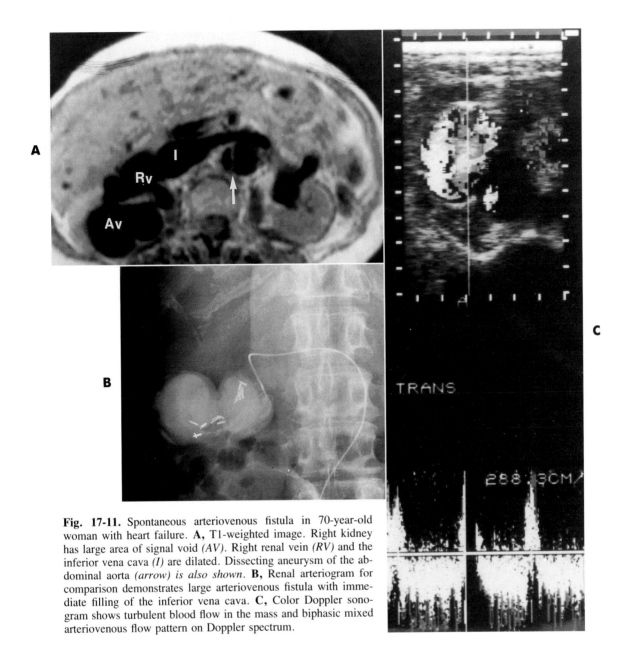

Fig. 17-11. Spontaneous arteriovenous fistula in 70-year-old woman with heart failure. **A,** T1-weighted image. Right kidney has large area of signal void *(AV)*. Right renal vein *(RV)* and the inferior vena cava *(I)* are dilated. Dissecting aneurysm of the abdominal aorta *(arrow) is also shown.* **B,** Renal arteriogram for comparison demonstrates large arteriovenous fistula with immediate filling of the inferior vena cava. **C,** Color Doppler sonogram shows turbulent blood flow in the mass and biphasic mixed arteriovenous flow pattern on Doppler spectrum.

and Hemorrhage" in this chapter). However, hypervascular renal tumors may also produce perirenal hemorrhage following vessel rupture.

Perirenal abscess

Perirenal abscesses are frequently associated with acute renal infections (Fig. 17-4).[31] They may represent infected hematomas.

MRI OF RENAL PHYSIOLOGY AND PATHOPHYSIOLOGY

The availability of MR contrast agents (gadopentetate dimeglumine) and rapid imaging sequences has permitted

the use of MRI as a renal function test. Both renal perfusion[8,9,30,82] and glomerular filtration rate[14] can be determined. The investigation by Choyke et al.[14] on glomerular filtration rate indicates that MRI is accurate for most clinical purposes. Its advantages over radionuclide studies are patient convenience and shorter examination time.

BENIGN MASSES
Cysts

Cysts are the most frequent renal mass lesions and are often detected incidentally, particularly in the elderly population.

Simple. On MRI, simple cysts are well defined and

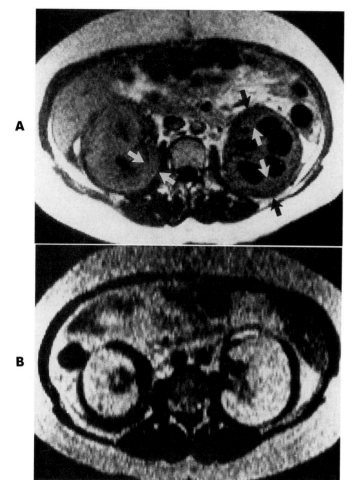

have low signal intensity (clear fluid) on T1WI (see Figs. 17-8; 17-13; 17-15, *A;* and 17-21, *A*). On T2WI, their signal intensity is high (Figs. 17-15, *B;* 17-18, *A;* and 17-21, *B*). With these characteristics the diagnosis of simple cysts is not difficult.* The smallest cysts detectable with state-of-the-art equipment have a diameter of approximately 0.5 to 1 cm.

Complicated. These cysts lack one or more of the characteristics of simple cysts. They may have irregular borders (inflammatory reaction) or wall calcifications. They may be septated, hemorrhagic, or contain a high concentration of protein or milk of calcium. Any of these aberrations results in changes of signal intensities or cyst outlines. Differential diagnosis versus a cystic or necrotic neoplasm may be difficult or impossible. Thin septa in the cysts may not be demonstrated by MRI.

Hemorrhagic cysts or cysts containing a high concentration of proteinaceous material demonstrate a variable degree of increased signal intensity on T1WI. In hemorrhagic cysts, intensity depends on the amount and age of the blood products (Figs. 17-3 and 17-14).[34,39,48,70,101]

Milk of calcium in the cyst is visualized as a signal void because of the calcium content (Fig. 17-15).[56] The configuration of the signal void changes when the patient changes position. Signal void caused by wall calcifications

*References 4, 39, 48, 57, 67, 70, 94.

Fig. 17-12. Perirenal retroperitoneal fibrosis in 35-year-old female with deteriorating renal function and with history of pancreatitis and pancreatic pseudocyst. **A,** T1-weighted image. Band of tissue *(arrows),* poorly demarcated from thinned renal parenchyma, results in bilateral hydronephritis. **B,** T2-weighted image. Abnormal (fibrous) tissue has low signal intensity. (From Yancey JM, Kaude JV: *J Comput Assist Tomogr* 12:335-337, 1988.)

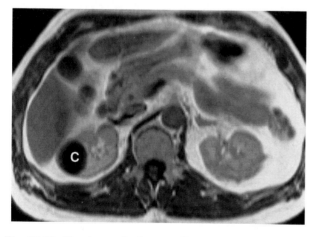

Fig. 17-13. Simple cyst is shown on T1-weighted image. Signal intensity in the simple cyst *(C)* (clear fluid) is very low.

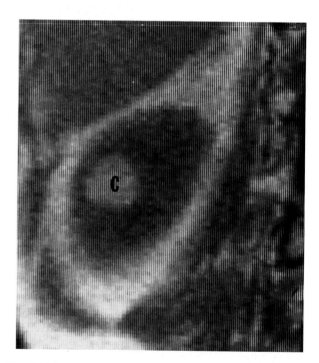

Fig. 17-14. Hemorrhagic cyst *(C),* shown by T1-weighted image, has high homogeneous signal intensity. (From Kaude JV, Kinard RE: In Löhr E, Leder L-D, eds: *Renal and adrenal tumors,* ed 2, Berlin, 1987, Springer-Verlag.)

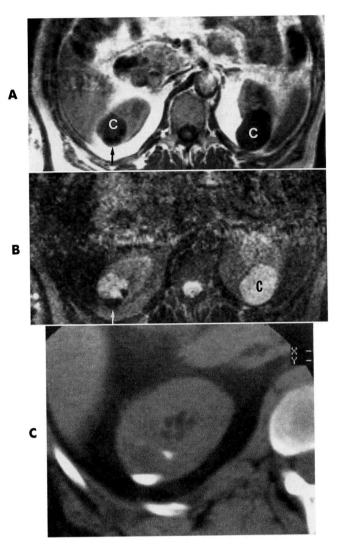

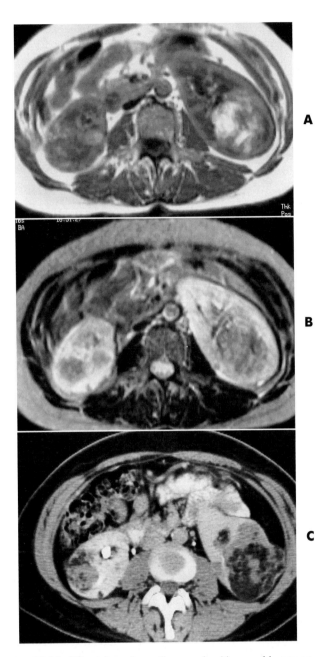

Fig. 17-15. Milk of calcium in renal cyst. **A,** T1-weighted image. Signal void *(arrow)* is in posterior aspect of the cyst in right kidney. Simple cyst *(C)* is in left kidney. **B,** T2-weighted image. Delineation of signal void area against fluid of high signal intensity is much better. **C,** CT scan for comparison shows calcium-fluid level in the cyst. (From Kinard RE et al: *J Comput Assist Tomogr* 10:1057-1059, 1986.)

Fig. 17-16. Bilateral angiomyolipomas in 44-year-old woman with left flank pain. **A,** T1-weighted image. Bilateral renal masses with high intensity signal equal to that of fat are demonstrated and best shown in tumor in the left kidney. **B,** T2-weighted image. Bilateral tumors have same intermediate signal intensity as subcutaneous fat. **C,** CT scan for comparison shows low attenuation areas (fat) in both tumors.

is not position-dependent.[19] True pathologic signal voids must be distinguished from chemical shift artifacts (see Chapter 2).

Multilocular cystic nephroma

Multilocular cystic nephromas are uncommon benign neoplasms.[3] The cystic components of these masses (cystic dysplasia) may have varying intensity, depending on the composition of the fluid, which may be clear or hemorrhagic or may have high protein content.[20] In the case reported by Kim et al.,[54] the cysts had low signal intensity on T1WI and high signal intensity on T2WI. The capsule

and the septa of multilocular cystic nephromas can be clearly delineated.

Angiomyolipoma

Angiomyolipomas are benign neoplasms, either focal or diffuse (as found in patients with tuberous sclerosis). Their signal intensity varies with the degree of fat content within the lesion.[23,48,67,100] Usually they contain a considerable amount of fat, resulting in high signal intensity on T1WI (Fig. 17-16). Only one case reported in the literature describes an angiomyolipoma that could not be differentiated from renal cell carcinoma, perhaps because of technical limitations.[17]

Fibrolipomatosis and lipomas

Renal sinus fibrolipomatosis is characterized by excessive proliferation of renal sinus fat. Affected patients frequently have a history of repeated or chronic ureteral obstruction, chronic infection, or central loss of parenchyma. The condition may be associated with renal parenchymal disease, including renal transplant rejection.[47] Renal sinus fat proliferation may resemble a mass lesion; however, the signal intensity of renal sinus fibrolipomatosis does not differ from that of normal peripelvic fat (Fig. 17-17).[38,48]

Fibroma

Small renal fibromas are common, but clinically significant fibromas in the kidney are rare. Because the signal intensity of renal fibroma is low both on T1WI and T2WI, typical for collagenous hypocellular tumors, differentiation of fibroma against malignant neoplasms is possible.[16]

Other benign neoplasms

Leung et al.[64] describe a sclerosing leiomyoma examined by MRI. Such a tumor is difficult to differentiate from a malignant neoplasm.

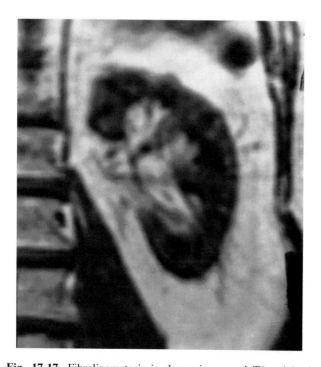

Fig. 17-17. Fibrolipomatosis is shown in coronal T1-weighted image of left kidney. Renal sinus fat is abundant.

POTENTIALLY MALIGNANT NEOPLASMS
Oncocytoma

First described in the parotid gland, oncocytomas are interesting neoplasms.[32] They are composed of eosinophilic cells, are frequently clinically asymptomatic, and are discovered incidentally. They can cause problems in differential diagnosis from renal cell carcinomas. Oncocytomas may be multifocal or bilateral.[74]

Oncocytomas were for a long time regarded as benign neoplasms, but increased evidence now indicates that they may contain foci of malignant cells and perhaps should be classified as low-grade renal malignancies.[66,83,85,110]

Only a few cases of oncocytoma have been examined with MRI. Oncocytomas are generally of homogeneous, intermediate signal intensity. The central scar, often present in larger oncocytomas, is expected to have low signal intensity on T2WI. However, in one reported case the scar had high signal intensity, apparently because of high water content.[86] Occasionally an oncocytoma may simulate a renal cell carcinoma with central necrosis and hemorrhage, resulting in mixed signal intensity.[95] Calcifications in oncocytoma may be present as demonstrated by signal voids on MR images. After administration of gadopentetate dimeglumine, oncocytoma may demonstrate intense, homogeneous enhancement.[23] As reported recently, a cystic oncocytoma is rare.[79]

The signal intensity of one oncocytoma the authors examined was homogeneous and intermediate on T1WI. The tumor had a high signal intensity on T2WI, suggesting fluid or a malignant neoplasm (Fig. 17-18, *A*). Histologic examination revealed that the tumor was an oncocytoma containing only a few small foci of atypical cells.

Adenomas

Some adenomas are not clearly distinguished from renal cell carcinoma by histologic examinations. The conventional wisdom is that adenomas larger than 3 cm in diameter must be considered malignant. However, adenomas less than 2 cm in size have been reported to metastasize, whereas larger ones do not necessarily spread.[63]

On MRI, adenomas are reported to be isointense with renal parenchyma on T1WI. The signal intensity is high on T2WI. A central scar, which may be present, has low signal intensity.[70]

MALIGNANT NEOPLASMS
Renal cell carcinoma

Statistics show that every year 18,000 Americans are diagnosed as having renal cell carcinoma and that 9000 die every year from this tumor.[10] Therefore, when MRI became available, considerable efforts were made to provide early diagnosis and preoperative staging of the disease.

MRI probably does not offer any advantages over CT in diagnosing the primary tumor. On the contrary, small tumors that are isointense with renal parenchyma may be

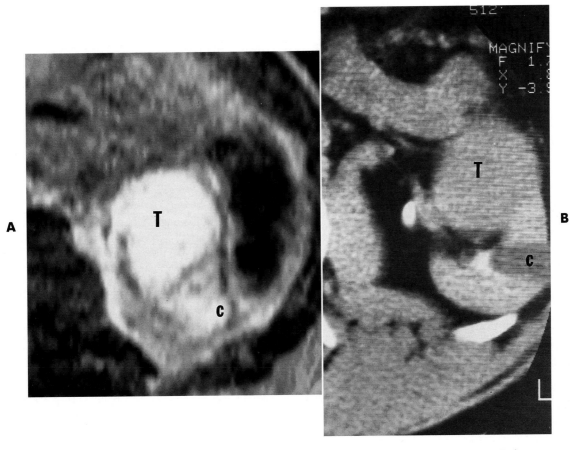

Fig. 17-18. Oncocytoma. **A,** Axial T2-weighted image. High signal intensity in tumor *(T)* is equal to that of cyst *(C)*. On T1-weighted image (not shown), tumor is isointense with renal parenchyma. **B,** CT scan for comparison shows better delineation of tumor *(T)* and cyst *(C)*, with different attenuations than on MR images.

better delineated by CT.[48] The inherent advantages of MRI over CT are imaging without iodinated contrast agent and examination in different projections.

In one tertiary care center with highly qualified clinical faculty for treatment of complicated urinary tract malignancies, MRI is usually performed only when CT or other studies performed there or outside the institution leave some doubt about the nature or extension of a renal neoplasm. Mainly MRI is used for staging renal cell carcinoma, particularly for vascular assessment, therefore obviating the need for renal angiography. With very few exceptions, angiography is performed only in conjunction with preoperative tumor embolization.

The signal intensity of primary renal adenocarcinoma is variable.[39,48,64,84,92] On T1WI the signal intensity is frequently lower than that of the cortex of a normal kidney (Figs. 17-19 and 17-23, *A*). Hemorrhagic or necrotic carcinomas have mixed signal intensities and may have areas of high signal intensity on T1WI and T2WI (Fig. 17-20). Some tumors have low signal intensity.[98,101] In a case reported by Sussman, Glickstein, and Krzymouski,[98] this

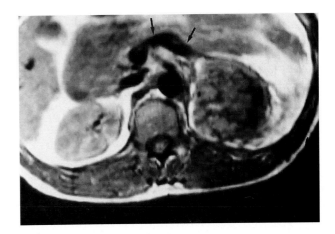

Fig. 17-19. Renal cell carcinoma, as shown by T1-weighted image has low, mixed signal intensity with areas of signal void (vessels in richly vascularized tumor). Renal vein *(arrows)* is open.

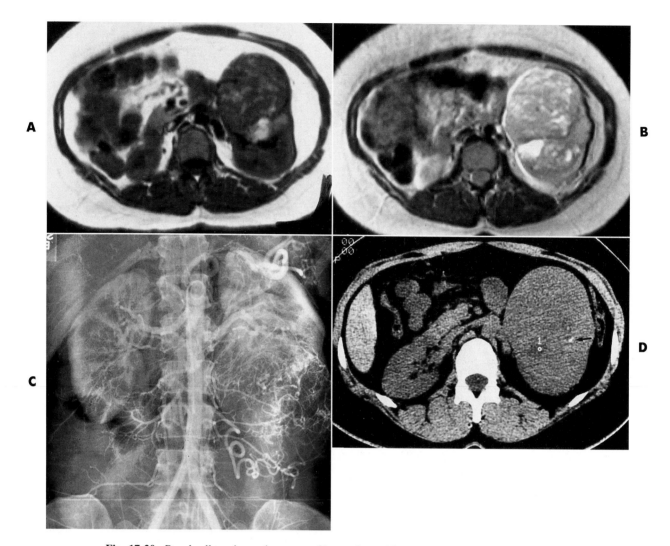

Fig. 17-20. Renal cell carcinoma has areas of hemorrhage, identified by high signal intensity with all echo sequences. **A,** T1-weighted image. **B,** T2-weighted image. **C,** Angiography for comparison. **D,** Non-contrast-enhanced CT of same tumor. One low attenuation area *(marker)* is demonstrated. Small tumor calcifications *(arrow)* are present but not identifiable (as signal void) on MR images.

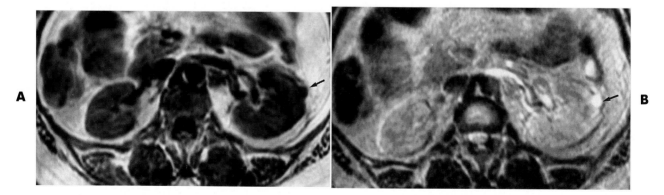

Fig. 17-21. Renal cell carcinoma of left kidney isointense with renal parenchyma. **A,** T1-weighted image. **B,** T2-weighted image. Tumor cannot be outlined against renal parenchyma. However, left kidney is greatly enlarged, and corticomedullary boundary is ill defined. Small cyst is present in periphery of the left kidney *(arrow)*.

was attributed to iron contents in the tumor, almost resulting in a signal void. Other authors report tumors of high signal intensity.[12,33,88] Renal cell carcinomas may be isointense with renal parenchyma and may be distinguishable only by contour changes or renal enlargement (Fig. 17-21).[10,48] They may escape detection when they are in-

trarenal without causing any mass effect. The size of the smallest detectable renal cell carcinoma by MRI is around 2 cm,[26,48,57] but Mallek et al.[69] reported a tumor measuring only 1 cm in size. This small carcinoma was best demonstrated on T2WI.

Gadopentetate dimeglumine administration enhances

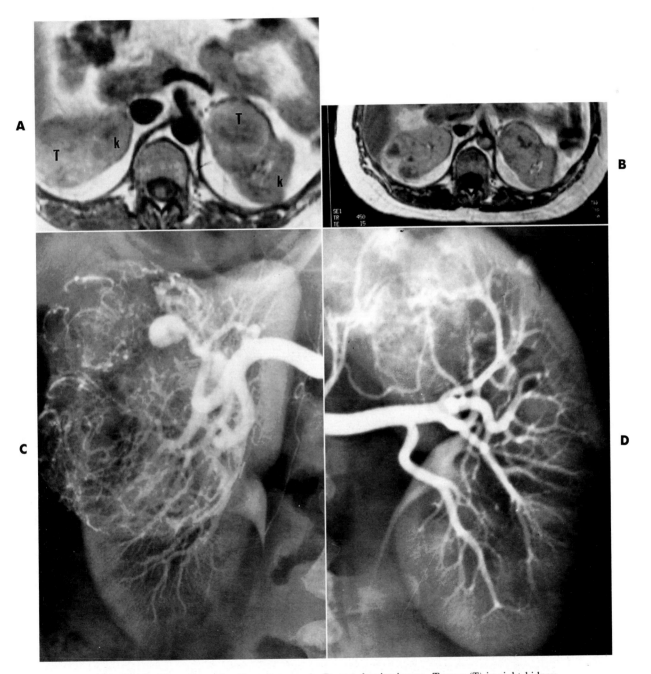

Fig. 17-22. Bilateral renal cell carcinoma. **A,** Proton density image. Tumor *(T)* in right kidney *(K)* is approximately isodense with renal cortex. Tumor in left kidney has rim of higher intensity signal than that of renal parenchyma. Center of the tumor has low signal intensity. **B,** T1-weighted image following administration of gadopentetate dimeglumine shows tumors are enhanced except for well-delineated necrotic areas. **C,** Angiogram of right side for comparison. **D,** Angiogram of left side for comparison. Both tumors are highly vascularized.

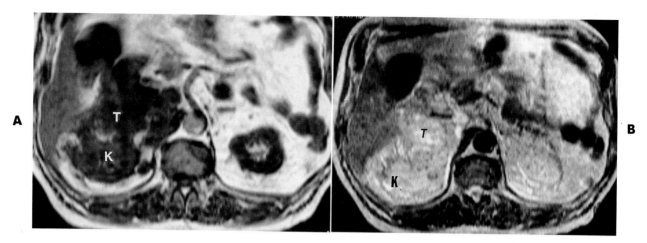

Fig. 17-23. Extracapsular extension of renal cell carcinoma of the right kidney *(T)*. *K,* Kidney. **A,** T1-weighted image. Tumor has low signal intensity. **B,** T2-weighted image. Tumor with its higher signal intensity is better delineated against bowel.

Fig. 17-24. Adrenal metastasis from renal cell carcinoma after right nephrectomy. **A,** Coronal T1-weighted image. Adrenal tumor *(t)* invades inferior vena cava *(i)*. *a,* Aorta. **B,** Angiogram of inferior vena cava for comparison demonstrates tumor invasion. *t,* tumor. (From Kaude JV, Kinard RE: In Löhr E, Leder L-D, eds: *Renal and adrenal tumors*, ed 2, Berlin, 1987, Springer-Verlag.)

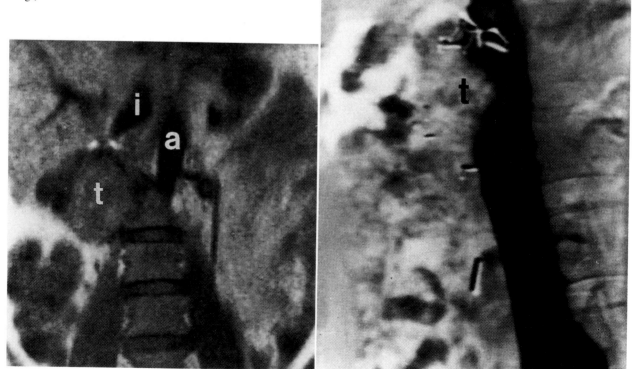

small tumor detection, as demonstrated in experimental investigations and in clinical reports.[51,58,59,64,107] The dosage of gadopentetate dimeglumine should be 0.1 mmol/kg of body weight. The best tumor enhancement and differentiation from normal parenchyma is obtained about 10 to 15 minutes after intravenous administration of gadopentetate dimeglumine.[107] Images must be obtained with short TE and TR times (T1WI,) because T2WI do not permit tumor delineation after gadopentetate dimeglumine. Necrotic areas show no contrast enhancement (Fig. 17-22, *B*).[59,107] Gradient echo image can also be used after gadolinium-

DTPA injection to observe pattern of enhancement by renal cell carcinomas.

Extrarenal spread of renal cell carcinoma is well-demonstrated by MRI (Fig. 17-23). Coronal or sagittal scans may be useful in determining or excluding invasion of adjacent organs or the IVC by a renal neoplasm (Figs. 17-24, *A;* 17-25; 17-28, *B;* and 17-31).

Vascular invasion of the renal vein, IVC, or right atrium is one of the most important indications for MRI of patients with renal neoplasms (Figs. 17-25 and 17-28).[21,35,36,48] Using both axial and coronal scans, MRI

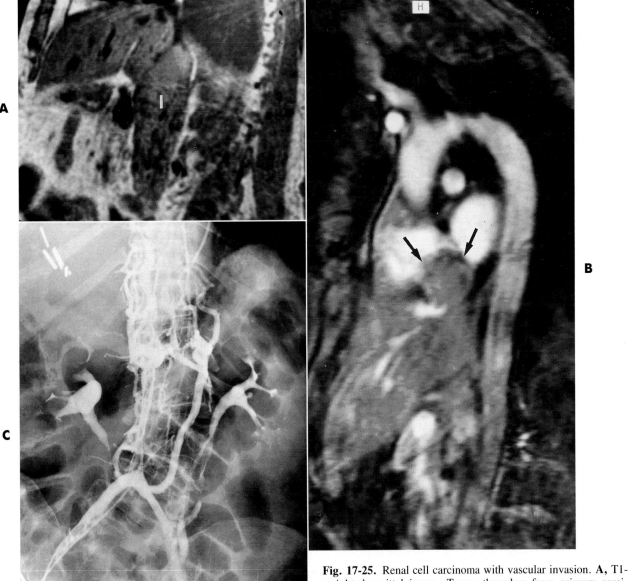

Fig. 17-25. Renal cell carcinoma with vascular invasion. **A,** T1-weighted sagittal image. Tumor thrombus from primary carcinoma of the right kidney fills the distended inferior vena cava *(I).* **B,** Gradient echo sagittal image shows extension of tumor into the right atrium *(arrows).* **C,** Cavogram for comparison. Inferior vena cava is totally obstructed with extensive collateral venous channels.

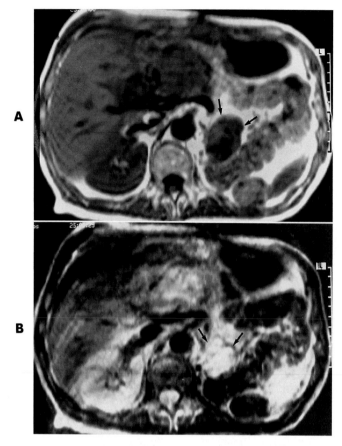

Fig. 17-26. Metastatic renal cell carcinoma in retroperitoneal lymph nodes after left nephrectomy. **A,** T1-weighted image demonstrates mixed signal intensities in tumor *(arrows).* **B,** T2-weighted image demonstrates high signal intensity in tumor *(arrows).*

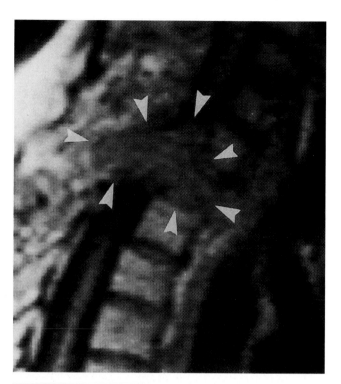

Fig. 17-27. Metastatic renal cell carcinoma in cervical spine *(arrows)* is shown by T1-weighted image. (From Kaude JV, Kinard RE: In Löhr E, Leder L-D, eds: *Renal and adrenal tumors,* ed 2, Berlin, 1987, Springer-Verlag.)

is capable of depicting venous invasion by the tumor without contrast administration. According to Horan et al.,[36] venacavography and MRI of the IVC are for practical purposes equal in detecting tumor thrombi. Amendola et al.[1] report a 95% negative predictive value and 100% positive predictive value of MRI for evaluation of the IVC for tumor thrombus without using contrast.

Nodal (Fig. 17-26) and distant metastases of renal carcinoma (Fig. 17-27)[29,48,81] or recurrent tumors (see Fig. 17-24) are detected well with MRI. That metastatic lesions of renal cell carcinoma may have the same T1 and T2 relaxation times as the primary tumor is noteworthy.[81]

Robson's classification of renal cell carcinoma is commonly used for staging purposes (Table 17-1). In the literature a 74% to 96% correlation between pathologic-histologic and MR staging of renal cell carcinoma has been reported.* In one recent investigation, 80% of the carcinomas were correctly staged with MRI.[1] Fein et al.[24] found that MRI was not reliable in differentiating stage I from

*References 1, 2, 4, 24, 40, 42, 87, 89, 102.

stage II disease. According to Patel, Stack, and Turner,[80] CT and MRI are comparable for stages I, II, IIB, and IV, but MRI has a higher accuracy than CT in staging IIIA and IVA carcinomas. Overall, several authors agree that MRI is more reliable than CT for staging purposes.[24,102] With the advent of fat suppression techniques, increases in accuracy, particularly for stages I and II, are expected.

Wilms' tumor

This childhood malignancy, which may be bilateral, appears on MRI frequently as a homogeneous tumor with

Table 17-1. Robson's classification of renal cell carcinoma for staging

Stage	Extent
I	Tumor confined to the kidney
II	Tumor spread to perinephric fat but within Gerota's fascia
IIIA	Tumor spread to the renal vein or inferior vena cava
IIIB	Tumor spread to local lymph nodes
IIIC	Tumor spread to local veins and lymph nodes
IVA	Tumors spread to adjacent organs (including adrenal glands)
IVB	Distant metastases

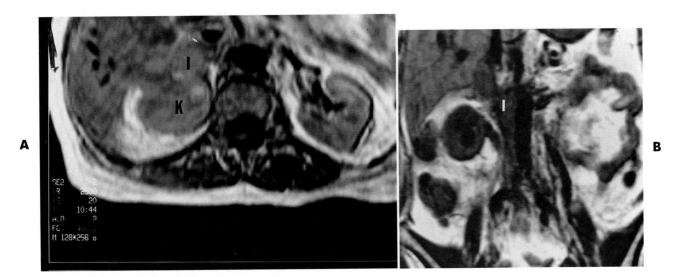

Fig. 17-28. Transitional cell carcinoma with venous tumor thrombi. **A,** Proton density axial image. Tumor infiltrated right kidney *(K)* and extended into inferior vena cava *(I)*. **B,** T1-weighted coronal image. Tumor thrombus is in inferior vena cava.

low or intermediate signal intensity on T1WI and with high signal intensity on T2WI.[7,19,45] Tumors with central necrosis have also been reported,[67] as has tumor extension into the renal veins and IVC.[28] There is additional discussion of this entity in Chapter 18.

Transitional cell carcinoma

Transitional cell carcinoma is the second most frequent renal malignancy in adulthood. To depict a small primary tumor that does not cause any obstruction of the collecting system is difficult, if not impossible, by MRI. In the early days of our MR operations (1984), even a 2 cm size tumor in a nondilated renal pelvis was missed. With hydronephrosis a tumor is well depicted as a solid mass against the urine-filled renal pelvis.

Larger, infiltrating transitional cell carcinomas are readily detectable with MRI; however, they are indistinguishable from other renal neoplasms. They even occasionally extend into the renal vein and IVC (Fig. 17-28).

Lymphoma and leukemia

Renal lymphoma may be diffuse or may be manifested as a focal mass lesion. MRI demonstrates a focal renal lymphoma as any other neoplasm, not permitting histologic differentiation. Diffuse lymphomatous or leukemic infiltration of the kidney results in enlargement of the kidney and indistinctness or in loss of corticomedullary demarcation (Fig. 17-29).[19,48,67,72]

Other malignancies

Many other malignant neoplasms of the kidney exist, but their occurrence is rare.[63] We have examined one patient with recurrent leiomyosarcoma of the kidney. MRI

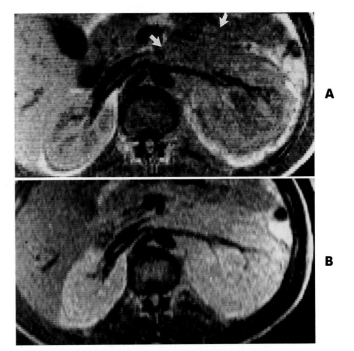

Fig. 17-29. Renal lymphoma (T-cell) in diffusely enlarged left kidney. **A,** T1-weighted image. **B,** T2-weighted image. Corticomedullary boundary is ill-defined. Extrarenal tumor has extended *(arrows)*. Both renal arteries and the right renal vein are well demonstrated. (From Kaude JV, Kinard RE: In Löhr E, Leder L-D, eds: *Renal and adrenal tumors,* ed 2, Berlin, 1987, Springer-Verlag.)

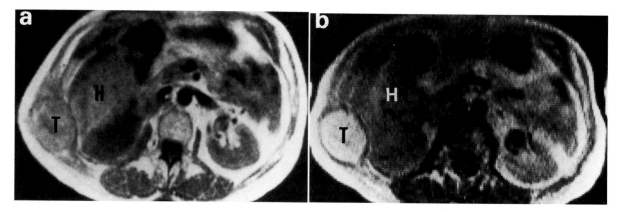

Fig. 17-30. Recurrent leiomyosarcoma after right nephrectomy. **A,** T1-weighted image. **B,** T2-weighted image. Tumor in soft tissues *(T)* is probably an implant secondary to surgery. Note extrinsic compression of liver *(H)*. (From Kaude JV, Kinard RE: In Löhr E, Leder L-D, eds: *Renal and adrenal tumors,* ed 2, Berlin, 1987, Springer-Verlag.)

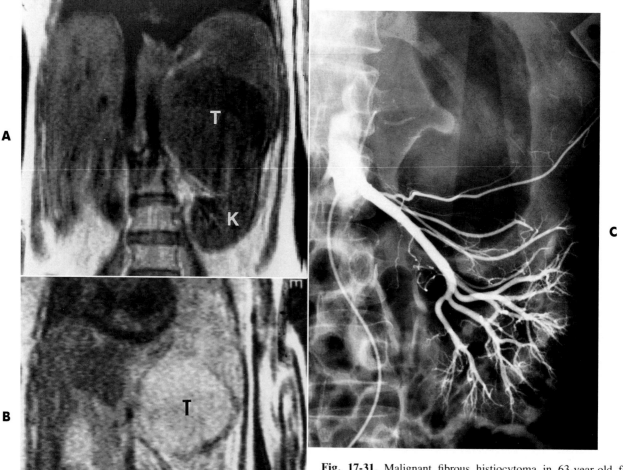

Fig. 17-31. Malignant fibrous histiocytoma in 63-year-old female. **A,** Coronal T1-weighted image. Large mass of intermediate signal intensity *(T)* involves upper pole of the left kidney *(K)*. Spleen is not invaded. **B,** T2-weighted image. Tumor is isointense with kidney. **C,** Angiography for comparison. Mass is hypovascular. (From Kaude JV, Kinard RE: In Löhr E, Leder L-D, eds: *Renal and adrenal tumors,* ed 2, Berlin, 1987, Springer-Verlag.)

demonstrated a tumor in the soft tissues (probably implant) after nephrectomy (Fig. 17-30).

In another patient with a large neoplasm involving the kidney, no specific tissue diagnosis could be determined from MRI (Fig. 17-31). The tumor was poorly vascularized as shown by angiography. On histologic examination the tumor was proved to be a malignant fibrous histiocytoma.

Metastatic neoplasms

Metastatic carcinomas are indistinguishable from primary neoplasms of the kidney (Figs. 17-32 and 17-33). Metastasis from a bronchial carcinoid demonstrated low signal intensity on T1WI and enhancement following gadolinium-DTPA administration (Fig. 17-33, *A*).

RENAL TRANSPLANTS

A renal transplant was first imaged with MR by Young et al.[109] in 1982. Generally, as in any normal kidney, in a normally functioning renal transplant the corticomedullary boundary is well defined on T1WI (Fig. 17-34). In earlier publications, reduced or absent corticomedullary demarcation was reported in acute or chronic rejection,[27,37,67] whereas in acute tubular necrosis the presence of corti-

comedullary demarcation was variable.[27] In experimental studies these observations were confirmed, with the exception of acute tubular necrosis, in which the corticomedullary demarcation was found not to be substantially altered compared with normally functioning kidney transplants.[87] Hricak et al.[41] reported a 98% accuracy for MRI in diagnosing renal transplant rejection. However, in histologically well-correlated studies by several other authors, it has been found that the blurring or loss of corticomedul-

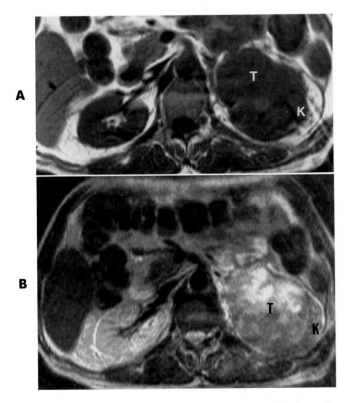

Fig. 17-32. Metastatic squamous cell carcinoma of the lung. Tumor *(T)* is not distinguishable from any of the primary renal neoplasms. **A,** T1-weighted image. Tumor *(T)* is isointense with remaining renal parenchyma. **B,** T2-weighted image. Tumor is better delineated and now demonstrates higher signal intensity than that of the kidney *(K)*.

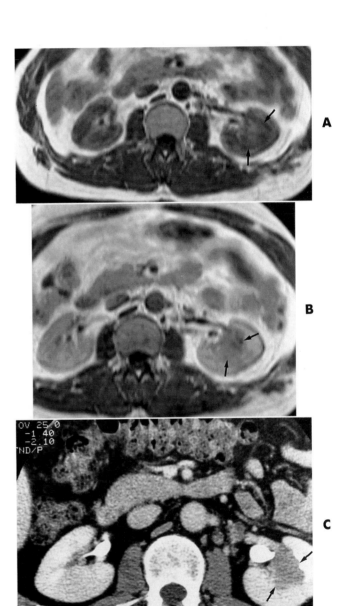

Fig. 17-33. Metastasis from bronchial carcinoid. **A,** T1-weighted image following gadopentetate dimeglumine. Enhanced tumor in renal hilum *(arrows)* is isointense with renal cortex but is well delineated. **B,** T2-weighted image. Tumor intensity *(arrows)* is slightly lower than that of parenchyma. **C,** Contrast-enhanced CT scan for comparison.

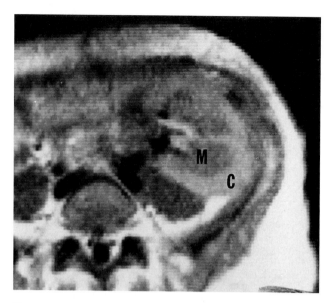

Fig. 17-34. Normal kidney transplant in left iliac fossa is shown by axial T1-weighted image. Note good demarcation between cortex *(C)*, which has higher signal intensity, and medulla *(M)*, which has lower signal intensity.

lary demarcation may be a rather sensitive indicator for renal transplant dysfunction (Figs. 17-35 and 17-36), but its specificity in regard to different parenchymal causes of transplant failure is low.* Corticomedullary demarcation also may be lost in cases of infarction and ischemia.[43] On the other hand the cortico-medullary boundary is preserved in some cases of rejection,[5,73] acute tubular necrosis,[40] or cyclosporin toxicity.[99]

Yap et al.[108] reported a sensitivity of no higher than 64% for MRI in detecting acute rejection. This agrees with the experiences of Winsett et al.[104] who regard MRI as not sufficiently accurate for investigation of renal transplant disease. They report considerable overlap of findings with only 60% sensitivity and specificity.

Ureteral obstruction resulting in hydro-nephrosis[37] or perirenal fluid collections such as lymphocele, perirenal hemorrhage,[37,73] or abscesses[37] are easily demonstrated by MRI. However, MRI is not the most cost-effective method

*References 5, 22, 44, 96, 97, 99, 104.

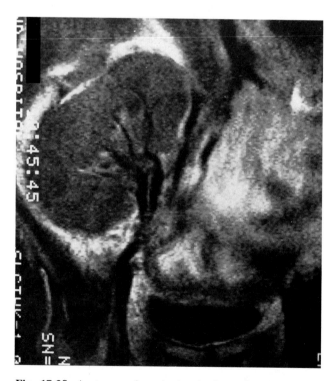

Fig. 17-35. Acute vascular rejection is shown by T1-weighted image. Note homogeneous, intermediate signal intensity with loss of corticomedullary demarcation. (From Dunbar KR et al: *Am J Kidney Dis* 12:200-207, 1988.)

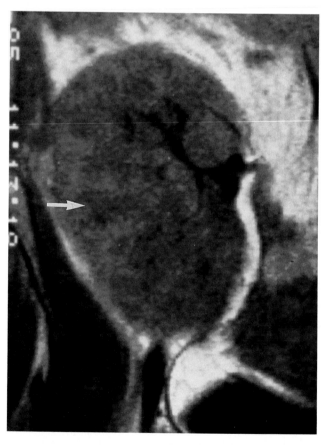

Fig. 17-36. Acute cellular rejection is shown by T1-weighted image. Only a few poorly delineated areas of lower signal intensity (pyramids of medulla) are present *(arrow)*. Otherwise, corticomedullary demarcation is lost. Intrarenal vessels are compressed. (From Dunbar KR et al: *Am J Kidney Dis* 12:200-207, 1988.)

and should not be used as the primary imaging modality for these purposes.

SUMMARY

After 10 years of experimental and clinical experience with MRI, certain conclusions can be drawn for indications and usefulness of MRI in evaluating renal disease. For practical purposes one should always consider the cost-effectiveness and availability of MRI. The usual question is this: "Can MRI offer additional and more useful information than CT?" Although with state-of-the-art equipment the sensitivity for disease detection with MRI is approximately equal to CT, in some cases MRI may be more specific than CT (for example, detection of hemorrhage in cysts).

A second advantage of MRI over CT is the ability to examine the patient in any desired projection, which is particularly useful in delineating tumor from surrounding organs (kidney, liver) or for evaluating tumor thrombi in the venous system.

A third advantage of MRI is good anatomic depiction without iodinated contrast agent administration.

A final advantage of MRI is the avoidance of ionizing radiation.

Disadvantages of MRI in evaluating renal disease are (1) relatively high cost, (2) prolonged examination time (approximately 45 to 60 minutes per study), and (3) unavailability or impracticality for emergency evaluations. However, these disadvantages may be overcome with more advanced technology using fast scanning sequences.

In spite of all accumulated experience and advances in technology, MRI cannot be expected to differentiate among various renal neoplasms. In many cases, even distinction between malignant and benign masses is not possible. On the other hand, MRI may become the imaging modality of choice for evaluation of renal function, vascular abnormalities, and hemorrhagic lesions.

REFERENCES

1. Amendola MA et al: Staging of renal carcinoma using magnetic resonance imaging at 1.5 Tesla, *Cancer* 66:40-44, 1990.
2. Auberton E et al: Etude comparative IRM-TDM du bilan d'extension des cancers du rein de l'adulte, *J Radiol* 70:327-336, 1989.
3. Banner MP, Pollack HM, Chatten J, et al: Multilocular renal cysts: radiologic-pathologic correlation, *AJR* 136:239-247, 1981.
4. Baumgartner BR, Chezmar JL: Magnetic resonance imaging of the kidneys and adrenal glands, *Semin Ultrasound CT MR* 10:43-62, 1989.
5. Baumgartner BR, Nelson RC, Ball TI, et al: MR imaging of renal transplants, *AJR* 147:949-953, 1986.
6. Baumgartner BR, Dickey KW, Ambrose SS, et al: Kidney changes after extra-corporeal shock wave lithotripsy: appearance on MR imaging, *Radiology* 163:531-534, 1987.
7. Belt TG, Cohen MD, Smith JA, et al: MRI of Wilms' tumor: promise as the primary imaging modality, *AJR* 146:955-961, 1986.
8. Carvlin MJ, Arger PH, Kundel HL, et al: Acute tubular necrosis:

use of gadolinium-DTPA and fast MR imaging to evaluate renal function in rabbit, *J Comput Assist Tomogr* 11:488-495, 1987.
9. Carvlin MJ, Arger PH, Kundel HL, et al: Use of Gd-DTPA and fast gradient-echo and spin-echo MR imaging to demonstrate renal function in the rabbit, *Radiology* 170:705-711, 1989.
10. Choyke PL: MR imaging of renal cell carcinoma, *Radiology* 169:572-573, 1988.
11. Choyke PL: MR imaging of the kidneys and retroperitoneum. In *MR Imaging Syllabus,* Chicago, 1991, Radiological Society of North America, pp 165-173.
12. Choyke PL, Kressel HY, Pollack HM, et al: Focal renal masses: magnetic resonance imaging, *Radiology* 152:471-477, 1984.
13. Choyke PL, Frank JA, Girton ME, et al: Dynamic Gd-DTPA enhanced MR imaging of the kidney: experimental results, *Radiology* 170:713-720, 1989.
14. Choyke PL, Frank JA, Austin HA, et al: Determination of glomerular filtration rate with gadolinium clearance, *Radiology* 177(P): 110, 1990.
15. Clark DA et al: The kidneys in paroxysmal nocturnal hemoglobinuria, *Blood* 59:83-89, 1981.
16. Comier P, Patel SK, Turner DA, et al: MR imaging findings in renal medullary fibroma, *AJR* 153:83-84, 1989.
17. Cranidis A et al: Is magnetic resonance imaging insufficient in diagnosing preoperatively renal angiomyolipoma? *Urol Int* 44:316-318, 1989.
18. De Cleyn K et al: MRI in the prenatal diagnosis of bilateral renal agenesis, *Fortschr Roentgenstr* 150:104-105, 1989.
19. Demas B, Thurnher S, Hricak H: The kidney, adrenal gland and retroperitoneum. In Higgins CB, Hricak H, eds: *Magnetic resonance imaging of the body,* New York, 1987, Raven Press.
20. Dikengil A, Benson M, Sanders L, et al: MRI of multilocular cystic nephroma, *Urol Radiol* 10:95-99, 1988.
21. DiStefano D et al: Cancer du rein: bilan de'extension veineuse en imagerie par résonance magnétique, *Ann Urol* 24:122-126, 1990.
22. Dunbar KR et al: Loss of cortico-medullary demarcation on magnetic resonance imaging: an index of biopsy-proven acute renal transplant dysfunction, *Am J Kidney Dis* 12:200-207, 1988.
23. Eilenberg SS, Lee JKT, Brown JJ, et al: Renal masses: evaluation with gradient-echo Gd-DTPA-enhanced dynamic MR imaging, *Radiology* 176:333-338, 1990.
24. Fein AB, Lee JKT, Balte DM, et al: Diagnosis and staging of renal cell carcinoma: a comparison of MR imaging and CT, *AJR* 148:749-753, 1987.
25. Feldberg MAM, Driessen LP, Witkamp TD, et al: Xanthogranulomatous pyelo-nephritis: comparison of extent using computed tomography and magnetic resonance imaging in one case, *Urol Radiol* 10:92-94, 1988.
26. Fritzsche PJ: Current state of MRI in renal mass diagnosis and staging of RCC, *Urol Radiol* 11:210-214, 1989.
27. Geisinger MA, Risius B, Jordan, ML, et al: Magnetic resonance imaging of renal transplants, *AJR* 143:1229-1234, 1984.
28. Gibson JM, Hall-Craggs MA, Dicks-Mireaux C, et al: Intracardiac extension of Wilms' tumor: demonstration by magnetic resonance, *Br J Radiol* 63:568-569, 1990.
29. Gindea AJ et al: Unusual cardiac metastasis in hypernephroma: the complementary role of echocardiography and magnetic resonance imaging, *Am Heart J* 116:1359-1361, 1988.
30. Granier N, Trilland H, Louail C, et al: Evaluation of renal perfusion with turbo FLASH MR imaging and superparamagnetic iron oxide particles, *Radiology* 177(P):167, 1990.
31. Hamlin DJ et al: Magnetic resonance imaging of renal abscess in an experimental model, *Acta Radiol Diagn* 26:315-319, 1985.
32. Hamperl HP: Beiträge zur normalen und pathologischen Histologie menschlicher Speicheldrüsen, *Z Mikrosk Anat Forsch* 27:1-55, 1931.

33. Herman SD et al: Magnetic resonance imaging of papillary renal carcinoma, *Urol Radiol* 7:168-171, 1985.

34. Hilpert PL, Friedman AC, Radecki PD, et al: MRI of hemorrhagic renal cysts in polycystic kidney disease, *AJR* 146:1167-1172, 1986.

35. Hockley NM et al: Use of magnetic resonance imaging to determine surgical approach to renal cell carcinoma with vena caval extension, *Urology* 36:55-65, 1990.

36. Horan JJ et al: The detection of renal carcinoma extension into the renal vein and inferior vena cava: a prospective comparison of vena cavography and magnetic resonance imaging, *J Urol* 142:943-948, 1989.

37. Hricak H, Terrier F, Demas B: Renal allografts: evaluation by MR imaging, *Radiology* 159:435-441, 1986.

38. Hricak H, Crooks L, Sheldon P, et al: Nuclear magnetic imaging of the kidney, *Radiology* 146:425-432, 1983.

39. Hricak H, Williams RD, Moon KL, et al: Nuclear magnetic resonance imaging of the kidney: renal masses, *Radiology* 147:765-772, 1983.

40. Hricak H, Demas BE, Williams RD, et al: Magnetic resonance imaging in the diagnosis and staging of renal and perirenal neoplasms, *Radiology* 154:709-715, 1985.

41. Hricak H, Terrier F, Marotti M, et al: Posttransplant renal rejection: comparison of quantitative scintigraphy: US and MR imaging, *Radiology* 162:685-688, 1987.

42. Hricak H, Thoeni RF, Carroll PR, et al: Detection and staging of renal neoplasms: a reassessment of MR imaging, *Radiology* 166:643-649, 1988.

43. Ishikawa I et al: Magnetic resonance imaging in renal infarction and ischemia, *Nephron* 51:99-102, 1989.

44. Jennerholm S, Backman U, Bohman S-O, et al: Magnetic resonance imaging of the transplanted kidney: correlation to function and histopathology, *Acta Radiol* 31:499-503, 1990.

45. Kangarloo H et al: Magnetic resonance imaging of Wilms' tumor, *Urology* 28:203-207, 1986.

46. Katzberg RW, Sahler LG, Duda SW, et al: Renal handling and physiologic effects of the paramagnetic contrast medium Gd-DTPA, *Invest Radiol* 25:714-719, 1990.

47. Kaude J, Fuller TJ, Soong J: Fibrolipomatosis of the transplanted kidney, *Fortschr Roentgenstr* 130:300-302, 1979.

48. Kaude JV, Kinard RE: Magnetic resonance imaging of renal mass lesions. In Löhr E, Leder L-D, eds: *Renal and adrenal tumors,* ed 2, Berlin, 1987, Springer-Verlag, pp 115-131.

49. Kaude JV et al: Imaging of unilateral hydronephrosis in an experimental animal model: with special reference to magnetic resonance, *Acta Radiol Diagn* 25:501-506, 1984.

50. Kaude JV, Williams CM, Millner MR, et al: Renal morphology and function immediately after extracorporeal shock wave lithotripsy, *AJR* 145:305-313, 1985.

51. Kaude JV et al: Improvement of MRI diagnosis of renal carcinoma by gadolinium-DTPA: an experimental study in rabbits. Fifth Annual Meeting, Society of Magnetic Resonance in Medicine, Montreal, 1986, *Book of Abstracts,* pp 275-276.

52. Kaude JV et al: Magnetic resonance imaging of the kidney after ESWL. In Gravenstein JS, Peter K, eds: *Extracorporeal shockwave lithotripsy for renal stone disease: technical and clinical aspects,* Boston, 1986, Butterworths, pp 125-139.

53. Kikinis R, von Schulthess GK, Jager P, et al: Normal and hydronephrotic kidney: evaluation of renal function with contrast enhanced MR imaging, *Radiology* 165:837-842, 1987.

54. Kim SH, Choi BI, Han MC, et al: Multilocular cystic nephroma: MR findings, *AJR* 153:1317, 1989.

55. Kim SH, Sim S, Lee JS, et al: Hemorrhagic fever with renal syndrome: MR imaging of the kidney, *Radiology* 175:823-825, 1990.

56. Kinard RE, Orrison WW, Brogdon BG, et al: MR imaging of milk of calcium renal cyst, *J Comput Assist Tomogr* 10:1057-1059, 1986.

57. Kulkarni MV, Shaff MI, Sandler MP, et al: Evaluation of renal masses by MR imaging, *J Comput Assist Tomogr* 8:861-865, 1984.

58. Laniado M, Fiegler W, Claussen C, et al: Gd-DTPA in imaging of renal tumors, *Radiology* 157(P):276, 1985.

59. Laniado M et al: Dynamic MRI of renal tumors with fast imaging sequences and intravenous gadolinium-DTPA. Fifth Annual Meeting, Society of Magnetic Resonance in Medicine, Montreal, 1986, *Book of Abstracts,* pp 1541-1542.

60. Lande IM, Glazer GM, Sarnaik S, et al: Sickle cell nephropathy: MR imaging, *Radiology* 158:379-393, 1986.

61. Langareil P et al: Pyélonéphrite xanthogranulomateuse avec proliferation graisseuse de la loge rénale, *J Radiol* 70:295-297, 1989.

62. Langmo LS, Ros PR, Torres GM, et al: Barium MR imaging for pelvic disease, *Radiology* 177(P):357, 1990.

63. Leder L-D, Richter HJ: Pathology of renal and adrenal neoplasms. In Löhr E, Leder L-D, eds: *Renal and adrenal tumors,* ed 2, Berlin, 1987, Springer-Verlag, pp 1-68.

64. Leung AW-L, Bydder GM, Steiner RE, et al: Magnetic resonance imaging of the kidneys, *AJR* 143:1215-1227, 1984.

65. Levine E, Grantham JJ: Perinephric hemorrhage in autosomal dominant polycystic kidney disease: CT and MR findings, *J Comput Assist Tomogr* 11:108-111, 1987.

66. Lieber MM, Tomera KM, Farron GM: Renal oncocytoma, *J Urol* 125:481-485, 1981.

67. LiPuma JP: Magnetic resonance imaging of the kidney, *Radiol Clin North Am* 22:925-941, 1984.

68. London DA, Davis PL, Williams RD, et al: Nuclear magnetic resonance imaging of induced renal lesions, *Radiology* 148:167-172, 1983.

69. Mallek R et al: Contrast MRI in multiple endocrine neoplasia type I (MEN) associated with renal cell carcinoma, *Eur J Radiol* 10:105-108, 1990.

70. Marotti M, Hricak H, Fritzsche P, et al: Complex and simple renal cysts: comparative evaluation with MR imaging, *Radiology* 162:679-684, 1987.

71. Marotti M et al: Metal chelates as urographic contrast agents for magnetic resonance imaging, *Fortschr Roentgenstr* 146:89-93, 1987.

72. Marotti M, Hricak H, Terrier F, et al: MRI in renal disease, *Magn Reson Med* 5:160-172, 1987.

73. Mitchell DG, Roza AM, Spritzer CE, et al: Acute renal allograft rejection: difficulty in diagnosis of histologically mild cases by MR imaging, *J Comput Assist Tomogr* 11:655-683, 1987.

74. Mooring FJ, Kaude JV, Wajsman Z: Bilateral renal oncocytomas, *J Med Imaging* 3:27-30, 1989.

75. Mulopulos GP, Turner DA, Schwartz MM, et al: MRI of the kidneys in paroxysmal nocturnal hemoglobinuria, *AJR* 146:51-52, 1986.

76. Neuerburg JM, Daus HJ, Recker F, et al: Effects of lithotripsy on rat kidney: evaluation with MR imaging, histology, and electron microscopy, *J Comput Assist Tomogr* 13:82-89, 1989.

77. Newhouse JH, Markisz JA, Kazam E: Magnetic resonance imaging of the kidneys, *Cardiovasc Intervent Radiol* 8:351-366, 1986.

78. Paajanen H, Schmiedl U, Aho HJ, et al: Magnetic resonance imaging of experimental renal hemorrhage, *Invest Radiol* 22:792-798, 1987.

79. Palmer WE, Chew FS: Renal oncocytoma, *AJR* 156:1144, 1991.

80. Patel SK, Stack CM, Turner DA: Magnetic resonance imaging in staging renal cell carcinoma, *Radiographics* 7:703-728, 1987.

81. Pettersson H et al: Magnetic resonance imaging and tissue characterization of a renal cell carcinoma and its osseous metastases, *Acta Radiol Diagn* 26:193-196, 1985.

82. Price PR, Pickens DR, Lorenz CH, et al: Gd-DTPA kinetics in an excised kidney model with use of snapshot FLASH MR imaging, *Radiology* 177(P):110, 1990.

83. Psihramis KE et al: Further evidence that renal oncocytoma has malignant potential, *J Urol* 139:585-587, 1988.

84. Quint LE, Glazer GM, Chenevert TL, et al: In vivo and in vitro MR imaging of renal tumors: histopathologic correlation and pulse sequence optimization, *Radiology* 169:359-362, 1988.

85. Rainwater LM, Farrow GM, Lieber MM: Flow cytometry of renal oncocytoma: common occurrence of deoxyribonucleic acid polyploidy and aneuploidy, *J Urol* 135:1167-1171, 1986.

86. Remark PR et al: Magnetic resonance imaging of renal oncocytoma, *Urology* 31:176-179, 1988.

87. Rholl KS, Lee JKT, Ling D, et al: Acute renal rejection versus acute tubular necrosis in a canine model: MR evaluation, *Radiology* 160:113-117, 1986.

88. Rofsky NM, Bosniak MA, Weinrep JC, et al: Giant renal cell carcinoma: CT and MR chacteristics, *J Comput Assist Tomogr* 13:1078-1080, 1989.

89. Schmidt HC, Tscholakoff D, Hricak H, et al: MR image contrast and relaxation times of solid tumors in the chest, abdomen and pelvis, *J Comput Assist Tomogr* 9:738-748, 1985.

90. Semelka RC et al: Improved MR imaging in the upper abdomen with fat saturation imaging technique, *Radiology* 173(P):388, 1989.

91. Semelka RC, Hricak H, Tomei E, et al: Obstructive nephropathy: evaluation with dynamic Gd-DTPA-enhanced MR imaging, *Radiology* 175:797-803, 1990.

92. Singer J, McClennan BL: The diagnosis, staging, and follow-up of carcinomas of the kidney, bladder and prostate: the role of cross-sectional imaging, *Semin Ultrasound CT MR* 10:481-487, 1989.

93. Slutsky RA et al: In vitro magnetic resonance relaxation times of the ischemic and reperfused rabbit kidney, *J Nucl Med* 25:38-41, 1984.

94. Smith FW et al: Renal cyst or tumor? differentiation by whole body nuclear magnetic resonance imaging, *Diagn Imaging* 50:61-65, 1981.

95. Sohn HK, Kim SY, Seo HS: MR imaging of a renal oncocytoma, *J Comput Assist Tomogr* 11:1085-1087, 1987.

96. Steinberg HV, Nelson RC, Murphy FB, et al: Renal allograft rejection: evaluation by Doppler US and MR imaging, *Radiology* 162:337-342, 1987.

97. Stendel A et al: MR-Tomographie nach Nierentransplantation, *Fortschr Roentgenstr* 147:514-520, 1987.

98. Sussman SK, Glickstein MF, Krzymovski GA: Hypointense renal cell carcinoma: MR imaging with pathologic correlation, *Radiology* 177:495-497, 1990.

99. te Strake L, Schultze Kool LJ, Paul LC, et al: Magnetic resonance imaging of renal transplants: its value in the differentiation of acute rejection and cyclosporin A nephrotoxicity, *Clin Radiol* 39:220-228, 1988.

100. Uhlenbrock D, Fischer C, Beyer HK: Angiomyolipoma of the kidney: comparison between magnetic resonance imaging, computed tomography and ultrasonography for diagnosis, *Acta Radiol* 29:523-526, 1988.

101. Uhlenbrock D, Schörner W, Sahlen S: Differential-diagnose fokaler Nierenerkrankungen mit der Kernspintomographie, *Fortschr Rontgenstr* 149:76-83, 1988.

102. Uhlenbrock D et al: Kernspintomographie und Computertomographie des malignen Hypernephroms, *Fortschr Rontgenstr* 146:664-674, 1987.

103. Uhlenbrock D et al: Kernspintomographische Untersuchungen bei experimenteller Nierenvenen-ligatur, *Fortschr Rontgenstr* 147:68-75, 1987.

104. Winsett MZ, Amparo EG, Fawcett HO, et al: Renal transplant dysfunction: MR evaluation, *AJR* 150:319-323, 1988.

105. Wolfgang S et al: Gd-DTPA enhances uses for MR imaging of body, *Diagn Imaging* 3:114-119, 1990.

106. Yancey JM, Kaude JV: Diagnosis of perirenal fibrosis by MR imaging, *J Comput Assist Tomogr* 12:335-337, 1988.

107. Yancey JM, Ackerman N, Kande JV, et al: Gadolinium-DTPA enhancement of VX-2 carcinoma of the rabbit kidney on T1-weighted magnetic resonance images, *Acta Radiol Diagn* 28:479-482, 1987.

108. Yap HK et al: Acute renal allograft rejection: comparative value of ultrasound venous magnetic resonance imaging, *Transplantation* 43:249-252, 1987.

109. Young IR, Bailes DR, Buol M, et al: Initial clinical evaluation of whole body NMR tomograph, *J Comput Assist Tomogr* 6:1-18, 1982.

110. Young RH, Dunn J, Dickersin R: An unusual oncocytic renal tumor with sarcomatoid foci and osteogenic differentiation, *Arch Pathol Lab Med* 112:937-939, 1988.

111. Yuasa Y, Kundel HL: Magnetic resonance imaging following unilateral occlusion of the renal circulation in rabbits, *Radiology* 154:151-156, 1985.

Chapter 18

PEDIATRIC ABDOMINAL AND PELVIC MRI

Paula J. Keslar

The disease processes in the pediatric population are quite different from those of the adult population. Ultrasonography (US) is often used as the initial imaging study on children since it is portable and the abdominal organs are imaged well. Pediatric patients also have little perivisceral fat, which can make computed tomography (CT) and magnetic resonance imaging (MRI) studies difficult to interpret. However, US exams can be limited by overlying bowel gas, which is not a problem with CT scanning or MRI. CT and MRI are being used more frequently in the abdominal evaluation of children.

The abdominal organs can be visualized well by MRI; however, clarity varies with each patient. Motion degradation is decreasing as faster scanning times are obtained.

The liver has the shortest T1 (spin-lattice or longitudinal) and T2 (spin-spin or transverse) relaxation times; relaxation times increase for the pancreas, spleen, renal cortex, and renal medulla in that order. In general, long T1 relaxation times result in low signal intensity on T1-weighted images, and long T2 relaxation times have high signal intensity on T2-weighted images (Fig. 18-1).

LIVER

Imaging studies determine the location and type of an abdominal mass for planning before resection, and they evaluate obstructive jaundice, vascular anatomy, and congenital anomalies before liver transplantation.

Although CT is the examination of choice for the evaluation of trauma, MRI has the advantage of multiplanar scanning, and vessels are imaged well without the use of intravenous contrast agents. In addition, no ionizing radiation is used. Sedation is required for either exam in patients less than 5 to 6 years of age.

The normal liver has greater signal intensity than the spleen on T1-weighted images and lower intensity than the spleen on T2-weighted images. The intrahepatic vessels are visualized well; however, nondilated bile ducts are not visualized. The gallbladder is visualized well, but its appearance depends on the fasting state of the patient, because bile becomes more concentrated with the removal of of water. Fresh bile has long T1 relaxation times and has

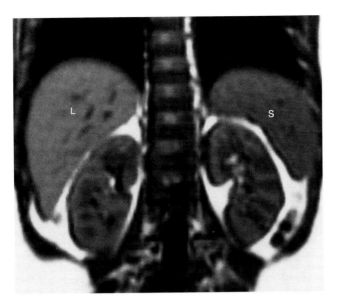

Fig. 18-1. Normal liver, spleen, and kidneys (coronal image; TR 500/TE 20 [repetition time of 500 msec; echo time of 20 msec]). Liver has higher signal intensity compared with the spleen. Note corticomedullary differentiation in the kidneys. *L,* Liver; *S,* spleen.

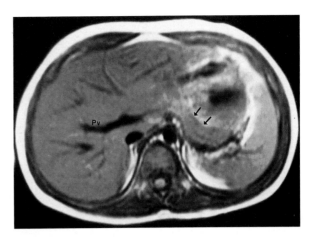

Fig. 18-2. Normal liver, spleen, and pancreas (axial image; TR 2000/TE 30). Portal veins, inferior vena cava, and aorta are well visualized. Pancreas has signal intensity similar to that of the spleen *(arrows). PV,* Portal vein.

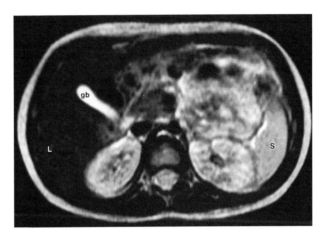

Fig. 18-3. Normal liver, spleen, kidneys, and gallbladder (axial image; TR 2000/TE 90). Liver has low signal intensity compared with the spleen. Gallbladder has high signal intensity. *L,* Liver; *S,* spleen; *gb,* gallbladder.

low signal intensity on T1-weighted images. Concentrated bile has short T1 relaxation times and high signal intensity on T1- and T2-weighted images (Figs. 18-2 and 18-3).[11]

Congenital anomalies

Biliary atresia. Most anomalies of the gallbladder and biliary tree are rare. The gallbladder may be congenitally absent or duplicated.

Biliary atresia is a disease process with progressive obliteration of the extrahepatic biliary ducts. Biliary atresia and neonatal hepatitis are the most common causes of prolonged neonatal conjugated hyperbilirubinemia. Neonatal hepatitis, which is treated medically, must be differentiated from biliary atresia, which requires surgical treatment.

US and the technetium-99m-disopropyl-iminodiacetic acid (DISIDA) scan are performed to evaluate neonatal jaundice. US can exclude other causes of obstructive jaundice, such as choledochal cyst. In biliary atresia the gallbladder is frequently small or absent, but occasionally it is normal. The DISIDA scan of a patient primed with phenobarbital shows hepatocellular dysfunction with excretion into the bowel in neonatal hepatitis. In biliary atresia, hepatocyte clearance is relatively well-preserved, but no bowel excretion occurs. A biopsy is often required for confirmation of the diagnosis.

Biliary atresia is treated with the Kasai procedure (portoenterostomy) or liver transplantation. The Kasai procedure is most successful if it is performed before 3 months of age. Complications include cholangitis, portal hyperten-

sion, and malabsorption of fat and fat soluble vitamins.[27] Liver transplantation is curative.

Approximately 10% to 15% of patients with biliary atresia have anomalies of the polysplenia syndrome (interrupted inferior vena cava, preduodenal portal vein, intestinal malrotation, and bilateral bilobed lungs) that are not associated with congenital heart anomalies.[24] The incidence of choledochal cyst is also slightly increased. Although MRI plays no role in the diagnosis of biliary atresia, it demonstrates the anomalies associated with polysplenia syndrome and is used for evaluation before liver transplantation.

Choledochal cyst. Choledochal cysts are focal areas of dilation of the biliary tree and are classified by the location of the dilated segment. Dilation of the common bile duct

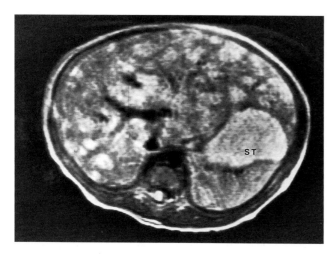

Fig. 18-4. Hepatic hemangioendothelioma is demonstrated by axial MRI (TR 1500/TE 56) of 1-month-old boy. Note diffuse involvement of liver with high signal intensity lesions. *ST,* Stomach. (From Boechat MI, Kangarloo H, Ortega J et al: *Radiology* 169:727-732, 1988.)

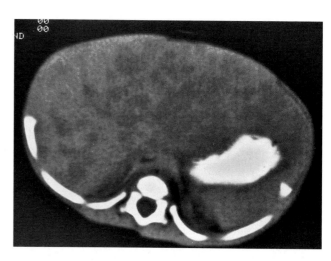

Fig. 18-5. Non-contrast-enhanced CT corresponding to Fig. 18-4. Multiple low-density lesions are present throughout the liver. (From Boechat MI, Kangarloo H, Ortega J et al: *Radiology* 169:727-732, 1988.)

(type 1) is most common; diverticulum of the common bile duct (type 2), choledochocele (type 3), multiple cysts of the intrahepatic and extrahepatic ducts (type 4A), and multiple cysts of the extrahepatic duct (type 4B or Caroli's disease) are the other types.[27] The etiology is thought to be a more proximally located pancreaticobiliary junction that permits reflux of pancreatic secretions into the bile duct. Clinical findings include abdominal pain, jaundice, and an abdominal mass.

Imaging studies reveal a mass in the right upper abdomen. The DISIDA scan confirms its connection to the biliary tree. The MRI signal intensity within the cyst is the same as that of bile in the gallbladder on all pulse sequences.[2]

Treatment is complete excision, because the incidence of developing biliary carcinoma is 2.5% to 4.7%.

Tumors

Infantile hemangioendothelioma. This liver tumor is usually diagnosed in early infancy, most often in the first 6 months. Patients with hemangioendotheliomas have hepatomegaly and congestive heart failure if arteriovenous shunting is extensive.[3]

CT studies show well-defined, low density lesions with early peripheral enhancement after intravenous contrast agent injection. MRI demonstrates low signal intensity lesions on T1-weighted images (Figs. 18-4 to 18-6). Large hemangioendotheliomas may have an heterogeneous appearance caused by areas of thrombosis and fibrosis. This makes them difficult to distinguish from other liver tumors.[6] The hepatic artery is often enlarged as well.

Treatment depends on the clinical status of the patient.

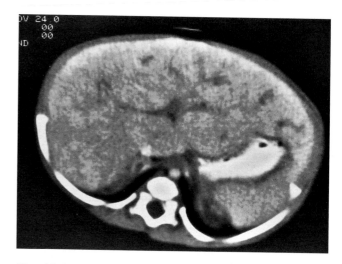

Fig. 18-6. Contrast-enhanced CT corresponding to Fig. 18-4. Note marked enhancement of the hemangioendothelioma. (From Boechat MI, Kangarloo H, Ortega J et al: *Radiology* 169:727-732, 1988.)

Many require no treatment at all. Most hemangioendotheliomas spontaneously resolve within the first year of life, but hepatic artery embolization or surgery may be required if medical therapeutic measures fail or in cases of rupture.[22]

Mesenchymal hamartoma. Mesenchymal hamartoma is a rare cystic, benign mass that contains gelatinous serous fluid within cystic spaces, with a matrix of bile ducts and mesenchymal tissue. These lesions are more often found in

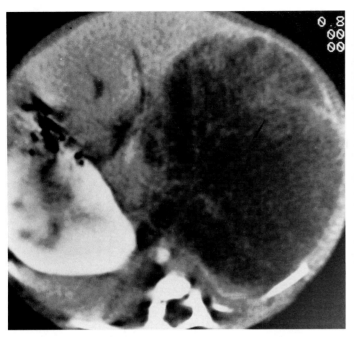

Fig. 18-7. Contrast-enhanced CT of mesenchymal hamartoma. Large, low attenuation lesion occupies most of right lobe of the liver and contains a few internal septations.

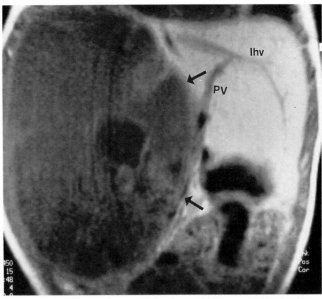

Fig. 18-8. MRI of mesenchymal hamartoma (coronal image; TR 450/TE 15) in 14-month-old boy with abdominal mass. Huge cystic lesion *(arrows)* occupies entire right hepatic lobe and contains loculated fluid of signal intensities different from main cystic mass. Main portal vein *(PV)* is displaced to the left. *lhv,* Left hepatic vein.

males than in females. Patients younger than 2 years of age may present with an asymptomatic abdominal mass.

CT examination demonstrates a large, nonenhancing low density mass with internal septations, most frequently in the right lobe of the liver. The septations may enhance (Fig. 18-7).[35] MRI shows a well-defined lesion with low signal intensity on T1-weighted images and high signal intensity on T2-weighted images (Figs. 18-8 and 18-9). This is consistent with the cystic nature of the lesion.

Hepatoblastoma and hepatocellular carcinoma. Malignant liver tumors are the third most frequent pediatric abdominal neoplasm. Hepatoblastoma is more common than hepatocellular carcinoma and is rarely seen after 4 years of age. Hepatoblastoma has a better prognosis than hepatocellular carcinoma. Incidence of hepatoblastoma is increased in patients with hemihypertrophy and Beckwith-Wiedemann syndrome. Hepatocellular carcinoma is uncommon before 5 years of age and is more frequently seen between 12 and 15 years of age. An increased incidence is seen in children with chronic liver disease, especially in tyrosinemia.[7] The patient usually has abdominal pain and discomfort. Less than half the children have resectable lesions at presentation.

CT and MRI easily identify liver lesions. Calcification, which is best seen by CT, is present 25% to 50% of the time. It appears as fine stippled or coarse chunks of calcium. The lesion has low attenuation on CT and enhances after bolus intravenous (IV) contrast agent injection. Areas

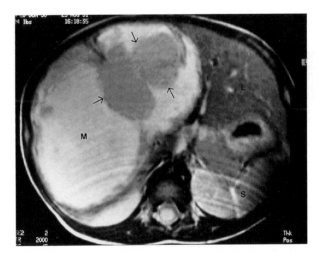

Fig. 18-9. T2-weighted axial image (TR 2000/TE 45) corresponding to Fig. 18-8. Large mass *(M),* with fairly homogeneous high signal intensity, reflects cystic nature of lesion. Loculated fluid of differing intensity is within lesion *(arrows). L,* Liver; *S,* spleen.

of necrosis and hemorrhage do not enhance. On MRI the mass generally has low signal intensity on T1-weighted images and higher signal intensity on T2-weighted images compared with the normal liver. Calcification is not visualized well by MRI (Figs. 18-10 to 18-12). For evaluation

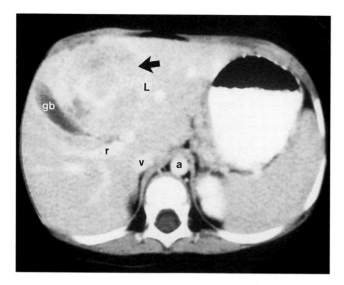

Fig. 18-10. Hepatoblastoma in an 18-month-old boy who had an abdominal mass. Contrast-enhanced CT shows enhanced mass in the liver *(arrow)*. *gb,* Gallbladder; *L,* liver; *r,* right portal vein branch; *v,* inferior vena cava; *a,* aorta. (From Cohen MD, Edwards MK, eds: *Magnetic resonance imaging in children,* St. Louis, 1990, Mosby–Year Book.)

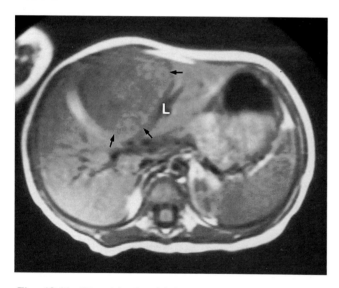

Fig. 18-11. T1-weighted axial image (TR 550/TE 26) corresponding to Fig. 18-10. Lesion *(arrows)* has slightly lower signal intensity compared with normal liver. *L,* Liver. (From Cohen MD, Edwards MK, eds: *Magnetic resonance imaging of children,* St. Louis, 1990, Mosby–Year Book.)

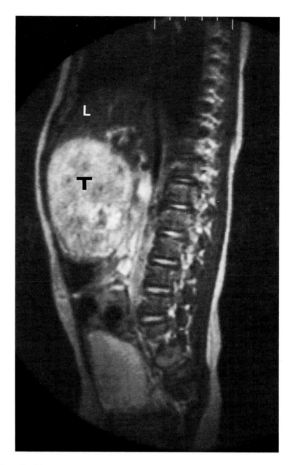

Fig. 18-12. T2-weighted sagittal image (TR 2000/TE 80) corresponding to Fig. 18-10. Tumor *(T)* has an inhomogeneous appearance and has higher signal intensity compared with normal liver *(L)*. (From Cohen MD, Edwards MK, eds: *Magnetic resonance imaging of children,* St. Louis, 1990, Mosby–Year Book.)

of resectability, MRI demonstrates vascular anatomy better than CT. It is also better in detecting neoplastic recurrence.[13] The most common metastatic site of primary liver tumors in children is the lungs, which are better evaluated by CT.

Metastases and lymphoma

The most common tumors that metastasize to the liver are Wilms' tumor, neuroblastoma, and lymphoma. In-volvement may be focal or diffuse. Infants with stage IV-S neuroblastoma often have diffuse liver involvement. However, the prognosis is good because of the frequent spontaneous regression of the disease.

Most metastases have a high signal intensity on T2-weighted images and variable signal intensity on T1-weighted images. The appearance is nonspecific because most pathologic conditions have increased T1 and T2 relaxation times compared with the normal liver.

Diffuse diseases

Hemosiderosis. This iron storage disease is seen in patients undergoing continual blood transfusions for hemolytic anemias and chronic renal failure. Hemosiderin, which contains iron in the ferric state, accumulates in the reticuloendothelial system. This decreases both T1 and T2 relaxation times because of the paramagnetic effect of the iron on adjacent hydrogen nuclei.[8] However, the overall effect is low signal intensity in the liver on both T1- and T2-weighted images (Fig. 18-13). Although MRI is sensi-

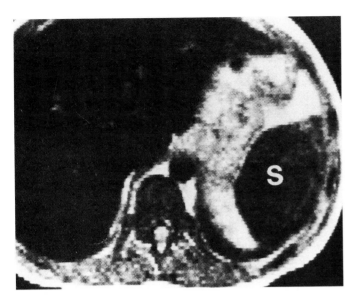

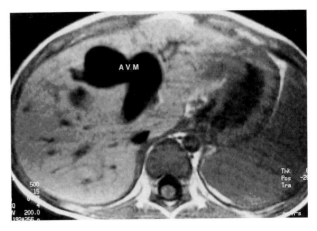

Fig. 18-14. Huge arteriovenous malformation in an 18-month-old girl with hepatosplenomegaly (axial image; TR 500/TE 15). Large dumbbell-shaped structure within liver has flow void. Arteriovenous malformation *(AVM)* has connections to hepatic artery and portal vein.

Fig. 18-13. Sickle cell anemia with hemosiderosis (axial image; TR 2000/TE 28). Liver and spleen *(S)* have low signal intensities because of shortened T1 and T2 relaxation times from deposited hemosiderin. (From Cohen MD, Edwards MK, eds: *Magnetic resonance imaging of children,* St. Louis, 1990, Mosby–Year Book.)

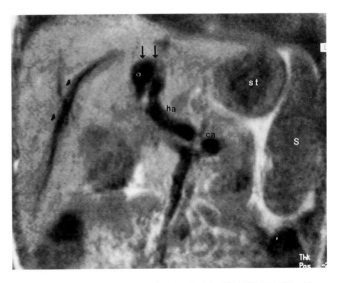

Fig. 18-15. Coronal view of Fig. 18-14 (TR 450/TE 15). Enlarged hepatic artery *(ha)* is supplying arteriovenous malformation *(arrows)*. Note enlarged celiac axis *(ca)*. *Arrowheads,* hepatic vein; *st,* Stomach; *S,* spleen.

tive in detecting iron overload, it only qualitatively estimates the amount of iron deposited in tissues.[23,34]

Portal hypertension and portal vein thrombosis. The most common cause of portal hypertension in children is idiopathic extrahepatic portal vein thrombosis, which often occurs during the neonatal period and is associated with umbilical venous catheterization. Intrahepatic causes include biliary atresia and metabolic disorders. In a child with extrahepatic portal vein obstruction, the most common manifestation is gastrointestinal bleeding from esophageal varices. Cavernous transformation of the portal vein represents the development of collateral vessels.

MRI features of portal vein thrombosis include (1) the signal involving the entire width of the portal vein lumen in which the signal intensity of the portal vein exceeds that of the liver on the T2-weighted image and flow void being present in hepatic veins and (2) complete nonvisualization of the portal vein and major branches in images that show a flow void in portal collaterals and hepatic veins.[31]

Arterial abnormalities. Congenital arteriovenous malformations (AVMs) of the liver are rare. An arteriovenous fistula may develop in the liver after trauma. An AVM was found in a 2½-year-old girl who had hepatomegaly and an abdominal thrill. She had no history of trauma or umbilical venous catheterization. An MRI examination demonstrated a large dumbbell-shaped lesion with flow void. An enlarged hepatic artery and portal vein were also present (Figs. 18-14 and 18-15). An angiogram showed that the right and left hepatic arteries fed the fistula, with drainage through the portal vein.

Transplantation

The preoperative evaluation of liver transplantation candidates requires assessment of the portal vein and inferior vena cava (IVC). Imaging studies also evaluate the extent of liver disease and the presence of hepatic tumors, varices, and ascites.

Biliary atresia is the most common reason for liver transplantation in children, of whom approximately 10% to 15% have some of the associations of polysplenia syndrome. MRI has been shown to be more sensitive than US in detecting these abnormalities.[5] The minimal portal vein diameter required to perform liver transplantation is 3 mm.

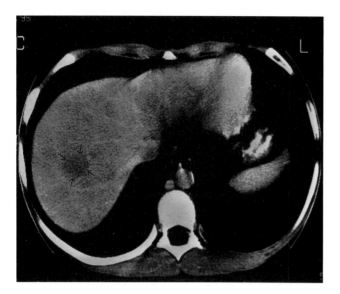

Fig. 18-16. Hepatocellular carcinoma in cirrhotic liver. Evaluation in a 10-year-old girl before liver transplant demonstrated several lesions within the liver. Contrast-enhanced CT shows non-enhancing lesion *(arrows)*.

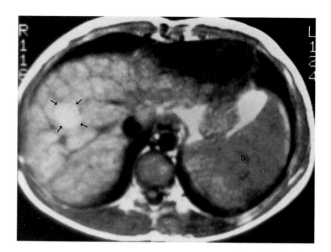

Fig. 18-17. Axial MRI in same patient as in Fig. 18-16 (TR 300/TE 20). Nodular appearance of cirrhotic liver is more apparent on MRI. Hyperintense lesion *(arrows)* is noted. Hepatocellular carcinoma was found within the liver at the time of transplantation. *S,* Spleen.

However, grafts can be placed from the confluence of the portal and splenic veins, if the main portal vein is too small or in cases of portal vein thromboses.[38] Patients with end-stage liver disease also have an increased incidence of hepatocellular carcinoma, which can be detected before transplantation. This finding is not a contraindication for transplantation (Figs. 18-16 to 18-18). That MRI should be the pretransplantation imaging technique of choice in children with end-stage liver disease has been suggested.[5] The authors, however, continue to use US as the main preoperative study and MRI for difficult cases.

PANCREAS

Pancreatic tumors and acute pancreatitis are uncommon in childhood. In general the CT examination of pancreatitis is reserved for those thought to have complications. Since a pancreatic tumor often presents in pediatric cases as a palpable mass, imaging studies are useful in the initial evaluation.

US is often the initial imaging procedure because it does not utilize ionizing radiation. Pediatric patients have little retroperitoneal fat, which often makes it difficult to delineate the pancreas from surrounding bowel. With a good oral contrast examination, the pancreas is well-defined by CT. Visualization of the pancreas is variable with MRI, however.

Tumor

Although pancreatic tumors are rare in the pediatric population, benign and malignant epithelial tumors and those with and without endocrine function may occur. Patients with von Hippel-Lindau syndrome have an increased

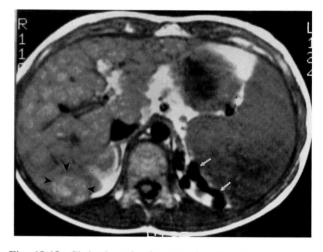

Fig. 18-18. Cirrhosis and splenomegaly with collateral vessels. Axial MRI (TR 300/TE 20) in same patient as in Fig. 18-16 demonstrates cirrhotic liver with lesion *(arrowhead),* splenomegaly, and collateral vessels *(arrows).*

incidence of developing pancreatic carcinomas and cysts.[30] To date, no reports based on MRI of pancreatic tumors in the pediatric population have been made.

Diffuse disease

Most patients with cystic fibrosis have severe pancreatic insufficiency and steatorrhea. This is caused by obstruction of the small ducts of the pancreas by viscous secretions, which results in atrophy of the acinar tissue and fatty and fibrous degeneration. Although extensive pancreatic changes occur, pancreatitis is relatively rare because very little residual tissue maintains pancreatic function.

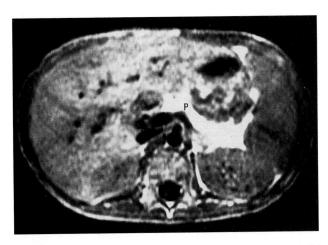

Fig. 18-19. Fatty replacement of pancreatic insufficiency. Axial T1-weighted image (TR 300/TE 20) shows hyperintense pancreas *(p).* (From Murayama S, Robinson AE, Mulvihill DM et al: *Pediatr Radiol* 20:536-539, 1990).

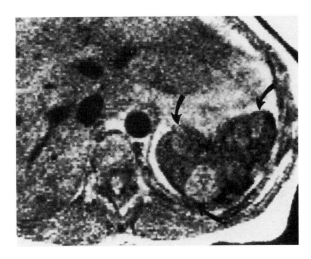

Fig. 18-20. Sickle-cell anemia with secondary splenic infarction. Axial T2-weighted image (TR 2000/TE 28) shows multiple hyperintense splenic lesions *(arrows)* consistent with multiple infarcts. (From Cohen MD, Edwards MK, eds: *Magnetic resonance imaging of children,* St. Louis, 1990, Mosby–Year Book.)

MRI of the pancreas in cystic fibrosis has been reported. A hyperintense pancreas on T1-weighted images is consistent with fatty replacement associated with pancreatic insufficiency (Fig. 18-19).[33] The potential for routine clinical application of MRI to cystic fibrosis is not known at this time.

SPLEEN

Imaging studies are used to evaluate the presence or absence of the spleen. MRI is used to detect possible abscess formation in cases of sepsis, and it is used to evaluate for a possible mass in the left upper quadrant, splenomegaly, and acute trauma.

CT and MRI demonstrate the spleen equally well. MRI has the added advantage of multiplanar imaging. MRI plays little role, however, in the evaluation of the acutely traumatized patient.

Infection

Splenic abscesses demonstrate prolonged T1 and T2 relaxation times. An abscess is seen as a poorly or well-defined lesion of low signal intensity on T1-weighted images and of high signal intensity on T2-weighted images. Air fluid levels may also be present. (See Chapter 13)

Infarction

Splenic infarction may be a complication of sickle-cell anemia or splenomegaly with vascular compromise. The appearance on MRI is variable, depending on whether the spleen is normal or is involved with hemosiderosis before infarction. In an otherwise normal spleen, infarction may be difficult to detect. In patients with hemosiderosis, areas of infarction have increased signal intensity on T2-weighted images compared with the low signal intensity of the spleen (Fig. 18-20).[1]

Sickle cell anemia

Hemosiderosis occurs in patients with sickle-cell anemia because of the iron deposited from repeated blood transfusions. Low signal intensity is present on T1- and T2-weighted images in the liver and spleen. The spleen may also undergo infarction (Figs. 18-13 and 18-20).

ADRENAL GLANDS

The most useful role of MRI is the evaluation of neuroblastoma. MRI is also helpful for screening patients with family history of pheochromocytoma, von Hippel-Lindau syndrome, and multiple endocrine neoplasms. Adrenal hemorrhage is primarily imaged in the neonatal period, with US being the preferred technique because of its portability.

MRI has been shown to accurately evaluate neuroblastoma for the extent of tumor, metastases, resectability, and response to therapy.[16] It demonstrates vessel encasement by tumor without the use of intravenous contrast agents and demonstrates intraspinal extension.

Hemorrhage

Normal adrenal tissue has an intermediate signal intensity that is slightly less than that of the liver and renal cortex on T1-weighted images and that is lower than the surrounding fat on heavily weighted T2 images. The cortex and medulla cannot be distinguished by MRI.

The adrenal gland is quite large at birth and decreases in size within a few weeks. Trauma, coagulation abnormalities, or abrupt venous pressure changes may cause this vascular organ to bleed in the neonatal period. Adrenal hemorrhage is also associated with renal vein thrombosis. In clinically apparent cases, the hemorrhage is from the

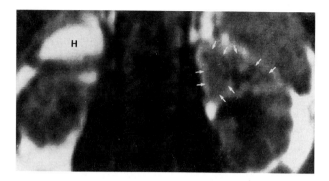

Fig. 18-21. Right adrenal gland hemorrhaging in a 6-day-old newborn. Coronal T1-weighted image (TR 500/TE 35) demonstrates enlarged right adrenal gland, with hyperintense focus in central and lower portions of the gland. This is consistent with hemorrhaging *(h)*. Upper pole pyramids of the left kidney are indicated with arrows. (From Brill PW, Jagannath A, Winchester P et al: *Radiology* 170:95-98, 1989).

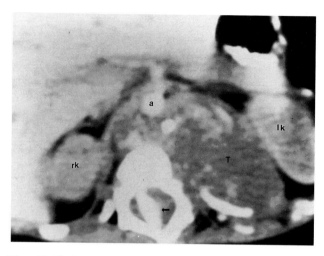

Fig. 18-22. Neuroblastoma in 3-month-old girl. Contrast-enhanced CT exam demonstrates nonenhancing tumor *(T)* with calcification. Aorta *(a)* is displaced anteriorly by tumor. Tumor also extends into spinal canal *(arrow)*. *rk,* Right kidney; *lk,* left kidney.

right side in 70% of the cases and is bilateral in 5% to 10% of the cases.

The diagnosis of adrenal hemorrhage is made with US. The US appearance may be similar to that of neuroblastoma; however, adrenal hemorrhage is more common than neuroblastoma in the neonatal period. The US diagnosis is confirmed over time with resolution of the hematoma. The MRI appearance is characterized by a hyperintense signal on T1- and T2-weighted images (Fig. 18-21).[9] Neuroblastoma usually has a medium-level signal. The kidneys, renal vein, and IVC can also be evaluated. A hemorrhagic neuroblastoma may not be differentiable from an adrenal hemorrhage.[6]

Tumors

Neuroblastoma. Neuroblastoma is one of the most common solid tumors in children and may be present at birth. Approximately 60% of neuroblastomas are found in the abdomen, with over 60% of these arising in the adrenal medulla. Most occur before the age of 8. Neuroblastoma originates from neural crest cells and can be found anywhere along the sympathetic ganglion chain. It tends to metastasize early to the bone marrow, skeleton, liver, lymph nodes, or skin. Approximately 15% of patients have intraspinal extension of neuroblastoma. Prognosis depends on the age of the patient when the tumor is discovered and the stage of disease. Infants have a better prognosis than older patients. Stage IV-S (special)—which occurs in infants with a small adrenal primary tumor, liver, skin, or bone marrow involvement—has an excellent prognosis. Frequently the tumor undergoes spontaneous regression. Skeletal metastases in bone cortex exclude a patient from stage IV-S.

CT examination demonstrates an irregular, low density pararenal lesion if the neuroblastoma is present in the adrenal gland. Calcifications are frequently present, and dystrophic calcification occurs with treatment. Retroperitoneal lymphadenopathy is often present with encasement and anterior displacement of the aorta and IVC (Fig. 18-22). MRI identifies the site of origin of the tumor, vascular involvement, bone marrow and dural metastases, and intraspinal extension of the tumor. The coronal view is quite useful for differentiating adrenal tumor from the kidney. Compared with the liver and renal cortex, neuroblastoma has decreased signal intensity on T1-weighted images and slightly increased signal intensity on T2-weighted images. The blood vessels are evaluated without the use of intravenous contrast agent. Calcification is poorly evaluated with MRI and appears as an area of signal void (Figs. 18-23 to 18-25).[16,19]

Pheochromocytoma. Pheochromocytomas arise from chromaffin cells of the sympathetic nervous system. They are rare in children, with less than 5% of pheochromocytomas being found in the pediatric age group. An increased incidence is found in patients with multiple endocrine adenomatosis (MEA type 2), von Hippel–Lindau syndrome, and neurofibromatosis. Children usually have sustained hypertension.[14]

Pheochromocytomas are usually greater than 2 cm in diameter when they are discovered. The CT appearance is nonspecific. The lesion may contain low density areas that represent necrosis or hemorrhage. Rim enhancement may be present, and calcifications are rare. The appearance on MRI is usually low signal intensity on T1-weighted images and hyperintensity compared with the liver on T2-weighted images.[18]

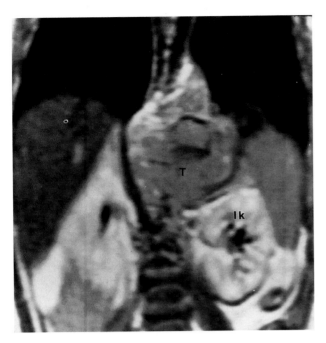

Fig. 18-23. Coronal T1-weighted image (TR 550/TE 20) of same patient as in Fig. 18-22. Heterogeneous tumor mass *(T)* is visualized well, with extension into spinal canal and displacement of IVC. *lk,* Left kidney.

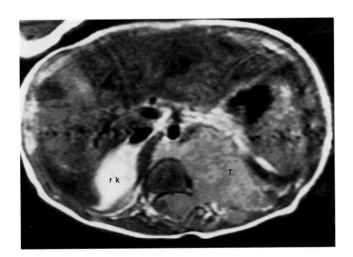

Fig. 18-24. Axial T2-weighted (TR 550/TE 20), gadolinium-enhanced image of same patient as in Fig. 18-22. Left neuroblastoma *(T)* is visualized well, with extension into spinal canal *(arrows)*. Aorta is displaced from the spine. Note enhancement of the right kidney *(rk)* after administration of gadolinium.

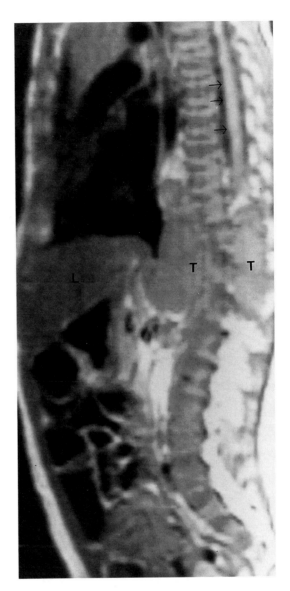

Fig. 18-25. Neuroblastoma and its extension into the spinal canal is visualized well in this sagittal plane image (TR 600/TE 20). *Arrows,* Spinal cord; *L,* liver.

KIDNEYS

The indications for imaging the kidneys include evaluation of urinary tract infections, mass lesion, hematuria, trauma, and renal failure and to define anatomy.

The screening procedure for the evaluation of pediatric renal disease is ultrasound. High frequency transducers are

used because of the small size of the patient, and this allows excellent visualization of the kidneys. CT or MRI are used for additional information. Since the field of view in ultrasound is limited by the shape of the US beam, large renal lesions are best evaluated by CT or MRI. Bowel gas may also obscure the kidneys on ultrasound images. Nuclear medicine scans, MRI, or CT are used to evaluate for ectopic location of the kidneys. CT is best for evaluation of trauma. Renal calcifications are best visualized with nonenhanced CT or US.

The appearance of the kidney on MRI varies with age. Renal pyramids are more prominent in infants and young children. The signal intensity from hilar adipose tissue increases with age. Little increased hilar signal is noted before 10 years of age. The corticomedullary differentiation is best visualized on T1-weighted images in the coronal plane, which give the best overall view of the kidneys. On T1-weighted images the cortex has a higher signal intensity than the renal medulla. Less differentiation between cortex and medulla is noted on T2-weighted images. The urine within the pelvocalyceal system has low signal intensity on T1-weighted images (see Fig. 18-1).[15]

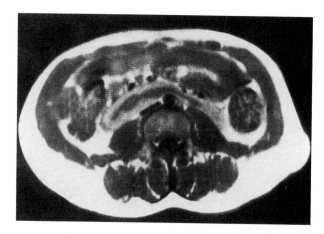

Fig. 18-26. Horseshoe kidney. Axial image (TR 500/TR 28) demonstrates fusion of lower poles of the kidneys across the midline. (From Cohen MD, Edwards MK, eds: *Magnetic resonance imaging of children*, St. Louis, 1990, Mosby–Year Book.)

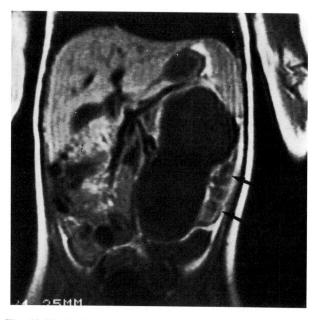

Fig. 18-27. Duplex renal collecting system with an infected, obstructed upper pole collecting system. Coronal T1-weighted image (TR 500/TE 28) shows low intensity fluid-filled upper pole collecting system displacing lower pole of the kidney laterally and inferiorly *(arrows)*. (From Cohen MD, Edwards MK, eds: *Magnetic resonance imaging of children*, St. Louis, 1990, Mosby–Year Book.)

Congenital anomalies

The kidney may be located in an ectopic position in the pelvis, or less commonly, in the intrathoracic region. Nuclear medicine studies or cross-sectional imaging (CT or MRI) are preferred methods to define ectopic location versus renal agenesis. In renal agenesis the ipsilateral adrenal gland is present. Associated anomalies of the uterus and vagina may also be present.

Fusion anomalies are better defined by MRI than by CT. Coronal images best demonstrate crossed-fused ectopia. Axial images best demonstrate horseshoe kidneys (Fig. 18-26).

Hydronephrosis

Hydronephrosis and multicystic dysplastic kidney are the most common causes of a renal mass in the neonate. Hydronephrosis may be caused by obstruction at the ureteropelvic junction or ureterovesical junction. Posterior urethral valves and ureterocele may also cause hydronephrosis. Other reasons for hydronephrosis include vesicoureteral reflux, primary megacalyces, prune-belly syndrome, and sepsis.[40] US is usually used to evaluate hydronephrosis, with little added information being obtained from MRI.

In duplex kidneys the upper pole ureter inserts in an ectopic location, medial and caudal to the normal insertion. The condition is commonly associated with an ureterocele. This obstructs the upper pole collecting system. Reflux is usually noted in the lower pole ureter, however, the ureterocele may also obstruct the lower pole ureter or cause bladder outlet obstruction (Figs. 18-27 and 18-28).

Renal cystic disease

Multicystic dysplastic kidney. The most common renal cystic disease in the neonatal period is multicystic dysplastic kidney. It is thought to be caused by intrauterine

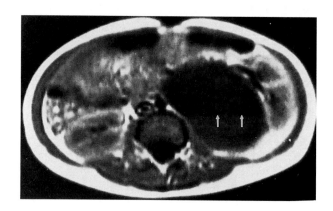

Fig. 18-28. Axial image (TR 500/TE 28) corresponding to Fig. 18-27 demonstrates fluid-fluid level *(arrows)* within infected upper pole collecting system. (From Cohen MD, Edwards MK, eds: *Magnetic resonance imaging of children*, St. Louis, 1990, Mosby–Year Book.)

ureteral obstruction. The two types are the classic type, which consists of multiple cysts of varying size with no functional renal tissue, and the hydronephrotic form, which has one dominant, central cyst with smaller peripheral cysts. The renal artery is hypoplastic or atretic. The diagnosis can be made by US, but a nuclear medicine renal scan may help confirm it by demonstrating absence of blood flow to the involved kidney. To distinguish multicystic dysplastic kidney from ureteropelvic junction obstruction may be difficult; however, the cysts do not communicate in multicystic dysplastic kidney. Magnetic resonance (MR) images demonstrate multiple cysts with a small amount of dysplastic tissue. Bilateral multicystic dysplastic kidney is incompatible with life. The contralateral kidney may be abnormal. The abnormal kidney is usually not removed unless it is very large, because the cysts regress over time.[17]

Autosomal recessive polycystic kidney disease (RPKD). This disease is also known as infantile polycystic disease. RPKD is rare, with a wide spectrum of clinical manifestations and pathologic conditions. Hepatic and renal involvement are present, and the severity of the disease tends to vary inversely with liver disease. However, severe renal disease may coexist with liver disease.[21] The pathologic defect is dilation of the collecting tubules. Clinical detection is most frequently by the palpation of large kidneys on physical examination. Patients often have hypertension. The prognosis depends on the severity of renal disease but tends overall to be poorer than that of the autosomal dominant type.

US demonstrates large kidneys that are echogenic. MRI also demonstrates large kidneys with cysts and may detect the presence of hemorrhage (Figs. 18-29 and 18-30).

Autosomal dominant polycystic kidney disease (DPKD). This disease involves dilation of tubules throughout the nephron. Cysts may also develop in the liver, pancreas, spleen, thyroid gland, ovary, and seminal vesicles. Although DPKD may occur in childhood, typically it is detected in young adulthood. It may be detected during family studies performed after a parent or relative is diagnosed with DPKD. Patients frequently have hematuria. The kidneys may be normal at birth, or one kidney may have a simple cyst. Eventually both kidneys enlarge and contain many cysts that increase in size with age. MRI demonstrates large kidneys with multiple cysts, some of which contain blood.

Syndromes associated with cysts. Many syndromes—such as Meckel syndrome, Zellweger cerebrohepatorenal syndrome, Jeune's syndrome, Ivemark syndrome, von Hippel–Lindau syndrome, and tuberous sclerosis—are associated with cysts. Multiple angiomyolipomas are also present in tuberous sclerosis.[21]

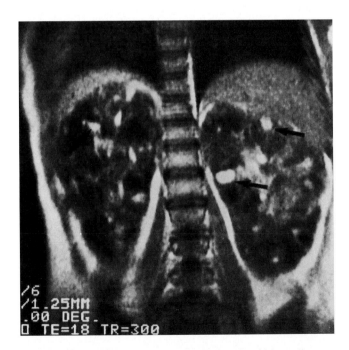

Fig. 18-29. Juvenile onset autosomal recessive kidney disease. Coronal T1-weighted image (TR 300/TE 18) shows that both kidneys are enlarged. Multiple low signal intensity cysts are present, some of which contain high signal intensity areas *(arrows)*. This is consistent with hemorrhage within cysts. (From Cohen MD, Edwards MK, eds: *Magnetic resonance imaging of children,* St. Louis, 1990, Mosby–Year Book.)

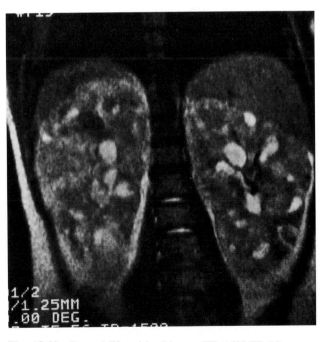

Fig. 18-30. Coronal T2-weighted image (TR 1500/TE 56) corresponding to Fig. 18-29. Both hemorrhagic and nonhemorrhagic cysts have high signal intensity. (From Cohen MD, Edwards MK, eds: *Magnetic resonance imaging of children,* St. Louis, 1990, Mosby–Year Book.)

Vascular abnormalities

Renal vein thrombosis. Renal vein thrombosis is common in the neonatal period. It is associated with infants of diabetic mothers, severe dehydration, poor renal perfusion and a high hematocrit; clot may extend into the IVC. MRI demonstrates enlargement of the kidney and thrombus in the renal vein and IVC.[9]

Sickle-cell nephropathy. Sickle cell nephropathy includes hyposthenuria, hematuria, nephrotic syndrome, renal tubular acidosis, hyperuricemia, and progressive renal insufficiency. MR findings have been reported in sickle-cell anemia patients and include a decreased cortical signal intensity compared with medullary signal intensity on T1- and T2-weighted images. This finding is not thought to be caused by cortical hemosiderin deposition, because the phenomenon has not been observed in other patients with iron overload.[29]

Tumors

Nephroblastomatosis. Nephroblastomatosis represents a complex pathologic condition in which primitive renal tissue (metanephric blastema) is found within the periphery of the kidney. It is classified into two main types, multifocal and diffuse, and is seen mainly before the age of 4 months. Lesions are rarely present beyond infancy and presumably regress with time. On CT the kidneys are large, with nonenhancing cortical areas. In the multifocal type the kidneys may be normal in size. The process is bilateral. Nephroblastomatosis is thought to be a precursor to Wilms' tumor.[20]

Wilms' tumor. Wilms' tumor is the most common malignant renal tumor in children, occuring in heritable and sporadic forms. Most children are diagnosed with Wilms' tumor between the ages of 1 to 5 years, with a mean of 3 years. The tumor occurs as an asymptomatic abdominal mass and is associated with aniridia, hemihypertrophy, and Beckwith-Wiedemann syndrome. Wilms' tumor metastasizes to the local lymph nodes, liver, and lungs. Extension into the renal vein or IVC may occur.[28]

MRI is an excellent technique to image Wilms' tumor. The tumor signal intensity is consistent, with prolonged T1 and T2 relaxation times. Areas of necrosis or hemorrhage are often seen with Wilms' tumor, and therefore the signal intensity is variable. The organ of origin is visualized well in the coronal plane. Although MRI detects liver metastases, CT is better for detecting lung metastases. MRI detects IVC involvement without the use of intravenous contrast agents, which is important for surgical planning (Figs. 18-31 and 18-32).[4,26]

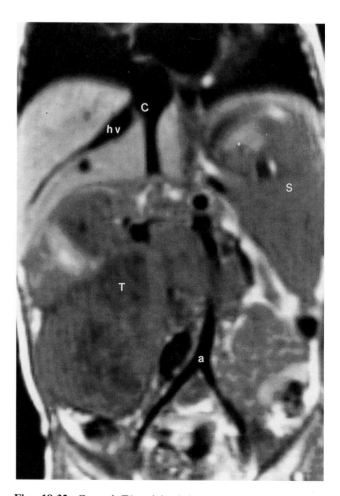

Fig. 18-32. Coronal T1-weighted image (TR 524/TE 15) of same patient as in Fig. 18-31. Extensive renal tumor *(T)* displaces aorta to the left and occludes IVC *(C)*. *hv,* Hepatic vein; *S,* spleen.

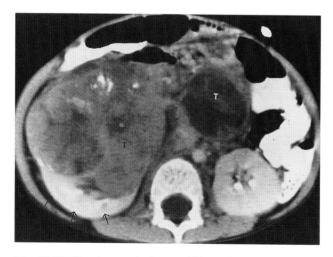

Fig. 18-31. Renal tumor in 5-year-old boy with abdominal mass is thought to represent large Wilms' tumor. Pathologic diagnosis was mesothelioma. Contrast-enhanced CT shows large heterogenous tumor *(T)* with calcifications arising from right kidney *(arrows)*. Tumor is also outside the kidney in left abdomen.

UTERUS AND OVARIES

Imaging of the pelvic organs is performed for the evaluation of ambiguous genitalia, congenital anomalies, primary amenorrhea, and pelvic masses.

CT is usually not used to evaluate the female pelvis, except in cases of pelvic masses. US is usually the initial imaging study. MRI is being used more frequently. The uterus and cervix are evaluated best in the sagittal plane, but the vagina and ovaries are visualized best in the axial plane. The coronal and oblique coronal planes along the long axis of the uterus are also useful. MRI has excellent soft tissue contrast, which is helpful for visualizing the pelvic organs.

Congenital anomalies

The appearance of the uterus, cervix, and vagina depends on the age of the patient and hormonal status. During the neonatal period, under maternal hormonal influence, the uterine body is longer than the cervix. On T2-weighted MRI the endometrial lining has high signal intensity with medium myometrial signal. The low signal junctional line found in the postpubertal uterus is also present. After the loss of maternal hormonal stimulation, the uterine body and cervix are approximately equal in length. Poor endometrial-myometrial differentiation is also present. At puberty the MRI findings are those of the adult uterus. Because of their small size the ovaries are often difficult to identify. They are best identified by location, which is normally adjacent to the internal iliac vessels. Ovaries have low to medium signal intensity on T1-weighted images and high signal intensity on T2-weighted images. They may be difficult to distinguish from adjacent bowel loops or fat.[12,25]

Ambiguous genitalia. Ultrasound is often the initial imaging study in cases of ambiguous genitalia. However, MRI can be helpful in difficult cases. The presence or absence of the uterus, cervix, vagina, ovaries, or testes must be determined. A true hermaphrodite has both ovarian and testicular tissue. A uterus may be present but may be hypoplastic. A female pseudohermaphrodite has ovaries and a uterus, but masculinization of the external genitalia is present. A male pseudohermaphrodite has testes, but the external genitalia are not fully masculinized.

Uterine malformations. The fallopian tubes, uterus, cervix, and the proximal vagina develop from the paired müllerian ducts. The distal two thirds of the vagina develops from the urogenital sinus.

Failure of fusion may result in the following malformations:

1. Uterus didelphys—Total failure of fusion, producing two vaginas, two cervixes and two uterine bodies
2. Uterus bicornis bicollis—Partial fusion producing one vagina, two cervixes and two uterine bodies

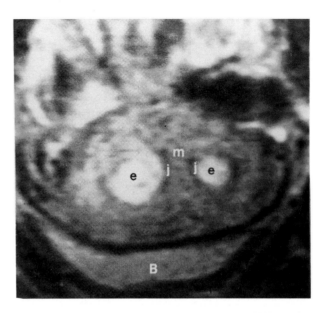

Fig. 18-33. Bicornate uterus (coronal image; TR 2000/TE 80). Two separate endometrial canals (high signal intensity), each with its own low signal intensity junctional zone, are separated by myometrium. *e,* Endometrium; *j,* junctional zone; *m,* myometrium; *b,* bladder. (From Mintz MC, Thickman DI, Gussman D et al: *AJR* 148:287-290, 1987.)

3. Uterus bicornis unicollis—Partial fusion producing one vagina, one cervix, and two uterine bodies[10]

Arrested development of the mullerian ducts results in uterine aplasia or atresia, but this is uncommon. Incomplete resorption of the sagittal septum results in uterus septus. MRI can differentiate between bicornate uterus and uterus septus in postpubertal females. The axial T2-weighted image demonstrates a medium signal intensity strip of myometrium that separates two low signal junctional zones in a bicornate uterus (Fig. 18-33).[32]

Müllerian duct anomalies are associated with renal anomalies such as renal agenesis or malposition of the kidney.

Hydrometrocolpos. Hydrometrocolpos is the accumulation of secretions and blood in the uterus and vagina. It is caused by obstruction of the vagina (or cervix, in which case it causes hydrometra) from an intact hymen, vaginal membrane, or vaginal atresia and may be accompanied by congenital anomalies such as imperforate anus. Hydrometrocolpos is manifested as an abdominal mass in infancy.[37] A dilated vagina and uterus are visualized best in the sagittal plane. If they are filled with blood, the fluid is seen as high signal intensity on T1- and T2-weighted images (Fig. 18-34). Treatment is by vaginoplasty.

Ovarian tumors

Ovarian tumors occur at any age; however, most occur around puberty. Patients may present with pelvic or ab-

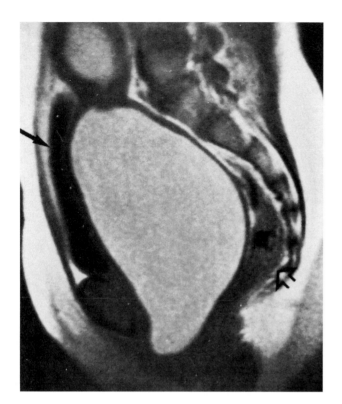

Fig. 18-34. Hematometrocolpos in 12-year-old girl. Sagittal midline T1-weighted image (TR 500/TE 28) demonstrates high signal intensity fluid (blood) in uterus. Compressed bladder *(solid arrow)* and rectum *(open arrow)* are also visualized. (From Dietrich RB, Kangarloo H: *Radiology* 163:367-372, 1987.)

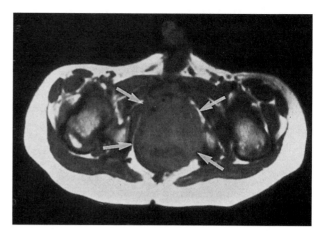

Fig. 18-35. Pelvic rhabdomyosarcoma in 2-year-old boy (axial image; TR 800/TE 26). Large mass lesion *(arrows)*, with signal intensity similar to muscle, occupies most of the pelvic cavity. (From Cohen MD, Edwards MK, eds: *Magnetic resonance imaging of children*, St. Louis, 1990, Mosby – Year Book.)

dominal masses because of the small size of the pelvis. Pain may be caused by hemorrhage into the mass, torsion, or rupture. Functional cysts are the most common cause of an ovarian mass in the neonate or adolescent. In the neonate, cyst development is thought to be caused by maternal hormonal stimulation. Most are of follicular origin and are easily diagnosed by ultrasound.

Of the primary ovarian neoplasms found in children, 60% are of germ cell origin. The most common of these is the teratoma. Most are benign, with malignant changes noted in 10%. Teratomas contain elements from all three germ cell layers. On MRI, signal intensity similar to that of fat on T1- and T2-weighted images is found in most lesions. Internal debris within the lesion has an intermediate signal intensity. Calcification, which is obvious on plain films or CT, is often missed on MRI.[41] Other germ cell tumors found in children include dysgerminoma and embryonal carcinoma. Granulosa-theca cell tumor is the most common ovarian tumor of stromal origin. Epithelial tumors, serous cystadenoma being the most common type, are rare before puberty.[39]

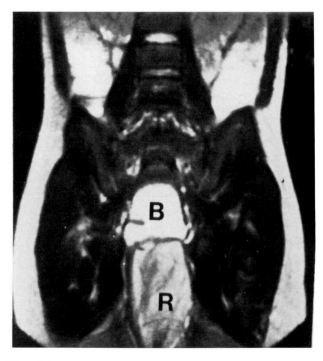

Fig. 18-36. Coronal image (TR 2000/TE 80) corresponding to Fig. 18-35. Tumor *(R)* demonstrates increased signal intensity, which is less intense than that of urine in the bladder *(B)*. (From Cohen MD, Edwards MK, eds: *Magnetic resonance imaging of children*, St. Louis, 1990, Mosby – Year Book.)

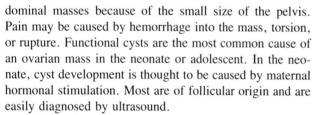

PELVIS
Rhabdomyosarcoma

Rhabdomyosarcoma is the most common soft tissue sarcoma in childhood. The neck and pelvis are the sites most frequently involved, but in the pelvis the bladder trigone, prostate gland, vagina, and uterus are most frequently involved. The tumor is usually fixed to the pelvic wall and is not evident as an abdominal mass, as are other ovarian neoplasms. The multiplanar imaging ability of MRI is helpful in evaluating the bladder base and pelvic walls. Rhabdomyosarcoma produces medium signal intensity on T1-weighted images and high signal intensity on T2-weighted images (Figs. 18-35 and 18-36).[12]

Sacrococcygeal teratoma

Although sacrococcygeal teratoma is the most common neoplasm in the neonate, it is uncommon. The tumor arises from the coccyx and has internal and external com-

ponents. Ninety percent of the teratomas found at birth are benign. Most are obvious because of the large external component. The majority of tumors found after the neonatal period are malignant. A predominantly cystic tumor is usually benign. The cystic component of the lesion has low signal intensity on T1-weighted images and high signal intensity on T2-weighted images. Teratomas often contain calcifications that may be missed on MRI; however, MRI is useful for characterizing the tissue types in the teratoma to determine the extent of the depth of the mass and to detect the presence of intraspinal involvement.

Anal atresia

The preoperative evaluation of perirectal anatomy in patients with anal atresia is important to determine the degree of the anal atresia and to demonstrate the size and position of the levator sling and associated fistulas. Patients with incontinence after surgery may have a malpositioned rectum.

CT and MRI demonstrate the perirectal anatomy, but MRI has the advantages of imaging in three planes and using no ionizing radiation for the inital and follow-up studies, and only T1-weighted images are required.

The internal anal sphincter is composed of the inner circular layer of smooth muscle of the bowel wall. The exter-

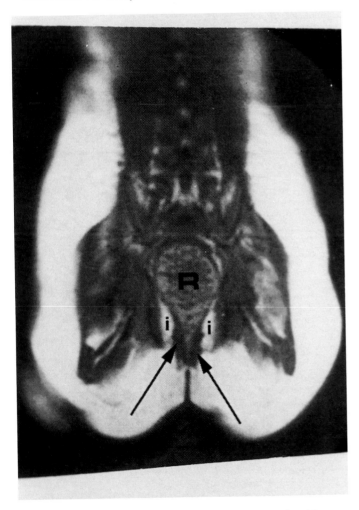

Fig. 18-37. Low anal atresia with normal external sphincter muscles (coronal image; TR 800/TE 26). Rectum *(R)* is easily identified between external sphincter muscles *(arrows)*. Note ischiorectal fossae *(i)* filled with fat. (From Cohen MD, Edwards MK, eds: *Magnetic resonance imaging of children,* St. Louis, 1990, Mosby–Year Book.)

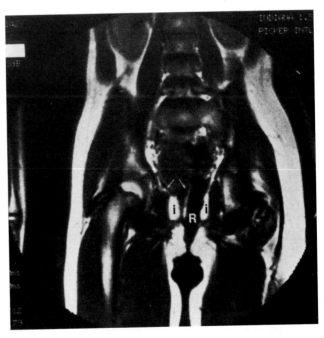

Fig. 18-38. Repaired anal atresia with malpositioned rectum. Coronal T1-wieghted image (TR 800/TE 30) shows rectum *(R)* to the left of midline. Fibers of the levator ani muscle appear as low intensity oblique bands *(arrows)*. Rectum is lateral to the left levator ani muscle. Ischiorectal fossae *(i)* are demarcated by fat. Rectum passes through fat of the left ischiorectal fossa. (From Cohen MD, Edwards MK, eds: *Magnetic resonance imaging of children,* St. Louis, 1990, Mosby–Year Book.)

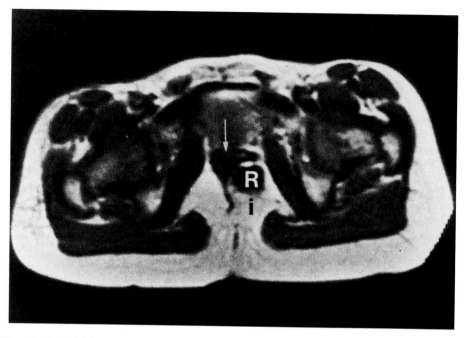

Fig. 18-39. Axial image corresponding to Fig. 18-38. Malpositioned rectum *(R)* lies within the fat of the ischiorectal fossa *(i)* but is outside of the levator sling complex *(arrow)*. (From Cohen MD, Edwards MK, eds: *Magnetic resonance imaging of children,* St. Louis, 1990, Mosby–Year Book.)

nal anal sphincter is composed of striated muscle and fibers of the levator ani muscle that blend with the deep external sphincter. Anal atresia is classified as high, intermediate, and low. In high atresia the colon terminates as a blind pouch above the level of the levator muscles. In intermediate atresia the lumen stops at the levator ani muscle. In low atresia the anus is patent through the levator ani muscle, with a superficial covering at the skin margins.

On CT or MRI the transverse plane through the ischial rami and ischial tuberosity is at the level of the external anal sphincter. The coronal plane through the rectum demonstrates the anal canal between the fat-filled ischiorectal fossa. The muscle of the external sphincter is just medial to the ischiorectal fossa and has the signal intensity of muscle (Fig. 18-37). The obturator internus muscle is just lateral to the ischiorectal fossa.[36]

Low atresias are treated by anoplasty or fistula dilation. High lesions require a colostomy with definitive surgery at a later date. Postoperative imaging may demonstrate a malpositioned rectum (Figs. 18-38 and 18-39).[41]

REFERENCES

1. Adler DD, Glazer GM, Aisen AM: MRI of the spleen: normal appearance and findings in sickle-cell anemia, *AJR* 147:843-845, 1986.
2. Alexander MC, Haaga JR: MR imaging of a choledochal cyst, *J Comput Assist Tomogr* 9:357-359, 1985.
3. Becker JM, Heitler MS: Hepatic hemangioendotheliomas in infancy, *Surg Gynec Obstet* 168:189-198, 1989.
4. Belt TG, Cohen MD, Smith JA et al: MRI of Wilms' tumor: promise as the primary imaging method, *AJR* 146:955-961, 1986.
5. Bisset GS, Strife JL, Balistreri WF: Evaluation of children for liver transplantation: value of MR imaging and sonography, *AJR* 155:351-356, 1990.
6. Boechat MI, Kangarloo H: MR imaging of the abdomen in children, *AJR* 152:1245-1250, 1989.
7. Boechat MI, Kangarloo H, Gilsanz V: Hepatic masses in children, *Semin Roentgenol* 23:185-193, 1988.
8. Brasch RC: Methods of contrast enhancement for NMR imaging and potential applications, *Radiology* 147:781-788, 1983.
9. Brill PW, Jagannath A, Winchester P et al: Adrenal hemorrhage and renal vein thrombosis in the newborn: MR imaging, *Radiology* 170:95-98, 1989.
10. Callen PW: Ultrasonography in obstetrics and gynecology, Philadelphia, 1988, WB Saunders, pp 393-411.
11. Cohen MD: MRI of the gastrointestinal and musculoskeletal systems in children, *Appl Radiol* 16:50-53, 1987.
12. Cohen MD, Edwards MK, eds: Magnetic resonance imaging of children, St. Louis, 1990, Mosby-Year Book, pp 611-893.
13. Dachman AH, Pakter RL, Ros PR et al: Hepatoblastoma: radiologic-pathologic correlation in 50 cases, *Radiology* 164:15-19, 1987.
14. Daneman A: Adrenal neoplasms in children, *Semin Roentgenol* 23:205-215, 1988.
15. Dietrich RB, Kangarloo H: Kidneys in infants and children: evaluation with MR, *Radiology* 159:215-221, 1986.
16. Dietrich RB, Kangarloo H, Lenarsky C et al: Neuroblastoma: the role of MRI imaging, *AJR* 148:942-987, 1987.
17. Donaldson JS, Shkolnik A: Pediatric renal masses, *Semin Roentgenol* 23:194-204, 1988.
18. Egglin TK, Hahn PF, Stark DD: MRI of the adrenal glands, *Semin Roentgenol* 23:280-287, 1988.
19. Fletcher BD, Kopiwoda SY, Strandjord SE et al: Abdominal neuroblastoma: magnetic resonance imaging and tissue characterization, *Radiology* 155:699-703, 1985.
20. Franken EA, Yiu-Chiu V, Smith WL et al: Nephroblastomatosis:

clinicopathologic significance and imaging characteristics, *AJR* 138:950-952, 1982.

21. Gagnadoux MF, Habib R, Levy M et al: Cystic renal diseases in children, *Adv Nephrol* 18:33-57, 1989.

22. Guzzetta PC, Randolph JG: Pediatric hepatic surgery, *Surg Clin North Am* 69:251-257, 1989.

23. Hernandez RJ, Sarnaik SA, Lande I et al: MR evaluation of liver iron overload, *J Comput Assist Tomogr* 12:91-94, 1988.

24. Hernanz-Schulman M, Ambrosino MM, Genieser NB et al: Current evaluation of the patient with abnormal visceroatrial situs, *AJR* 154:797-802, 1990.

25. Hricak H: MRI of the female pelvis: a review, *AJR* 146:1115-1122, 1986.

26. Kangarloo H, Dietrich RB, Ehrlich RM et al: Magnetic resonance imaging of Wilms tumor, *Urology* 28:203-207, 1986.

27. Karrer FM, Hall RJ, Stewart BA et al: Congenital biliary tract disease, *Surg Clin North Am* 70:1403-1419, 1990.

28. Kobrinsky NL, Talgoy M, Shuckett B et al: Wilms' tumor, *Pediatr Ann* 17:238-250, 1988.

29. Lande IM, Glazer GM, Sarnaik S et al: Sickle-cell nephropathy: MR imaging, *Radiology* 158:379-383, 1986.

30. Levine E, Collins DL, Horton WA et al: Screening of the abdomen in von Hippel-Lindau disease, *AJR* 139:505-510, 1982.

31. Levy HM, Newhouse JH: MR imaging of portal vein thrombosis, *AJR* 151:283-286, 1988.

32. Mintz MC, Thickman DI, Gussman D et al: MR evaluation of uterine anomalies, *AJR* 148:287-290, 1987.

33. Murayama S, Robinson AE, Mulvihill DM et al: MR imaging of pancreas in cystic fibrosis, *Pediatr Radiol* 20:536-539, 1990.

34. Querfeld U, Dietrich R, Taira RK et al: Magnetic resonance imaging of iron overload in children treated with peritoneal dialysis, *Nephron* 50:220-224, 1988.

35. Ros PR, Goodman ZD, Ishak KG et al: Mesenchymal hamartoma of the liver: radiologic-pathologic correlation, *Radiology* 158:619-624, 1986.

36. Sachs TM, Applebaum H, Touran T et al: Use of MRI in evaluation of anorectal anomalies, *J Pediatr Surg* 25:817-821, 1990.

37. Solvis TL, Sty JR, Haller JO: Imaging of the pediatric urinary tract, Philadelphia, 1989, WB Saunders, pp 237-240.

38. Starzl TE, Demetris AJ: Liver transplantation: a 31-year perspective (part I). *Curr Probl Surg* 27:55-116, 1990.

39. Sty JR, Wells RG: Other abdominal and pelvic masses in children, *Semin Roentgenol* 23:216-231, 1988.

40. Teele RL, Share JC: The abdominal mass in the neonate, *Semin Roentgenol* 23:175-184, 1988.

41. Togashi K, Nishimura K, Itoh K et al: Ovarian cystic teratoma: MR imaging, *Radiology* 162:669-673, 1987.

Part III

PELVIS

Chapter 19

OVERVIEW OF PELVIC MAGNETIC RESONANCE IMAGING

Gladys M. Torres

Luis H. Ros Mendoza

Magnetic resonance imaging (MRI) has become an important imaging modality for studying the male and female pelvis. Its freedom from ionizing radiation and noninvasive nature, coupled with multiplanar imaging capability, excellent contrast resolution, and visualization of the vessels, make it an ideal imaging modality for evaluating the pelvis. MRI is considered a primary tool for staging pelvic malignancies and a problem solving technique in evaluating certain pathologic conditions. In general the advantages, disadvantages, contraindications, and general indications of MRI of the pelvis and upper abdomen are similar. In this chapter the criteria for MRI that apply to the pelvic region and its pathologic conditions are discussed.

INDICATIONS

MRI is indicated for evaluation of a number of pathologic conditions of the pelvis (Table 19-1). A major role is the evaluation of local tumor spread, as in the pelvis, in which the major organs normally are well-delineated from one another or are surrounded by fat.[1]

In the female pelvis, MRI is helpful for evaluation of pregnant and young patients who have obstetric and gynecologic conditions. Since a full bladder is not a pre-requisite for MRI, patients with equivocal ultrasound (US) find-

ings can be examined with MRI.[20] MRI is used to evaluate benign diseases of the pelvis and to delineate developmental uterine anomalies. Pelvic MRI also is useful for the diagnosis and localization of uterine leiomyomas and for differentiating leiomyomas from adenomyosis.[30,43,44,46] These findings are helpful in determining appropriate management for some patients. MRI is also valuable in the study of adnexal masses and polycystic ovarian diseases.

T1-weighted images (T1WI) characterize fatty and hemorrhagic lesions, including teratomas, endometriomas, and hemorrhagic cysts.[3,42,47] The multiplanar imaging (sagittal and coronal) capability of MRI helps to accurately determine the origin of large pelvic masses that extend into the abdomen. MRI is valuable for staging cervical and endometrial carcinomas because it demonstrates tumor location, size, depth of myometrial or cervical penetration, and extension to surrounding tissues. MRI is an adjunct to clinical staging in selected patients with gynecologic malignancies.[23,26]

The major role of MRI of the male pelvis is the staging of prostatic carcinoma, for which its accuracy ranges from 70% to 90%.[12-14] With MRI it is possible to evaluate invasion of the periprostatic fat, obstruction of the periprostatic venous plexus, and involvement of the seminal vesicles. Using endorectal coils, fat suppression and other techniques that allow better anatomical detail, the accuracy of MRI is expected to approach 80% to 90%.[36]

MRI is also useful for evaluating testicular pathologic conditions. It has been proved to be a sensitive study for the localization of undescended testes.[15,16,25] Its lack of ionizing radiation and multiplanar imaging capabilities are

Table 19-1. Indications

Female pelvis	Male pelvis	Others
Developmental uterine anomalies	Prostate carcinoma staging	Bladder carcinoma staging
Diagnosis and localization of leiomyomas	Undescended testes	Rectal carcinoma staging and detection of local recurrence
Diagnosis of adenomyosis	Testicular tumors	
Gynecologic tumor staging	Extratesticular pathologic conditions	
Characterization of adnexal masses		
Localization of pelvic masses in cases of indeterminate ultrasound findings		

the principal advantages for evaluating these patients.

In evaluating testicular masses MRI differentiates normal testicular parenchyma from a testicular mass and intratesticular from extratesticular masses. The size, margins, and extension of tumors are well-demonstrated with MRI. Testicular tumors are usually inhomogeneous masses with lower signal intensity than the normal testicle.[4,19,20]

Benign processes also are evaluated with MRI. T2-weighted images (T2WI) of testicular inflammatory disease show testicular enlargement with decreased signal intensity.[4] The ability of MRI to show the tunica albuginea makes it suitable for evaluating acute scrotal trauma. In cases of testicular torsion, MRI characteristically shows absent or diminished vascular flow to the affected side and sometimes shows the twisted stalk.[22]

Other extratesticular conditions, such as spermatoceles, varicoceles, hydroceles, and epididymal abnormalities, are easily identified by MRI.[4] The signal intensity of the normal epididymis is isointense or hypointense to the normal testis. On T2WI the epididymis becomes hypointense. In cases of epididymitis the signal intensity increases, particularly on T2WI.[45]

MRI is also used for staging neoplasms of the bladder.[2,7,9,34] The normally high signal intensity of perivesical fat provides a favorable background against which extravesicular tumor extention is readily demonstrated. MRI has the advantage of determining the depth of bladder wall invasion and delineating the seminal vesicles and prostate gland for evaluation of tumor extension. MRI is also helpful in the pathologic evaluation of tumors, including analysis of tumor size and site and pattern of tumor growth. The ability of MRI to differentiate tumors with deep muscle invasion from tumors without muscle invasion helps the surgeon choose between segmental and radical cystectomy.

In the evaluation of rectal neoplasms the role of MRI is limited. Initial series were disappointing, with a reported staging accuracy of 59% in a study done by Hodgman, MacCarthy, and Wolff.[19] Guinet et al.[17] report that MRI correlates with surgical staging in 73% of cases and has a 40% sensitivity for metastatic lymph nodes. A recent study by DeLange et al.[12] showed more encouraging results in the determination of the local extent of rectal carcinoma,

particularly in patients who have not received radiation therapy or surgery. However, in the evaluation of lymphadenopathy, there is no improvement in detection compared with prior MRI studies.

MRI and computed tomography (CT) are used extensively to determine the presence or absence of recurrent colorectal carcinoma.[8,27,35] Both methods have proved to be helpful in detecting recurrence in patients who are asymptomatic or in whom carcinoembryonic antigens are normal. MRI also is useful for detecting presacral masses. Early studies reported that MRI helps differentiate tumor recurrence from fibrosis based on the signal intensity. However, more recent studies have found that whereas it is helpful in detecting masses after surgery, MRI has relatively low specificity. MRI cannot separate benign from malignant tissue on the basis of signal intensity, particularly in tumors that have desmoplastic reaction or in patients who have received radiation therapy and have inflammatory changes.

CONTRAINDICATIONS

The contraindications described in Chapter 8 apply also to pelvic MRI but are not reported in this chapter.

In recent years MRI has been used as an alternate imaging modality for evaluating pregnant patients who have indeterminate US examinations. Although MRI is thought to be free from causing adverse effects to the fetus, at present no large, controlled study documents this.[37,38] The potentially adverse effects of exposure to radiofrequency fields, static magnetic fields, and pulsed gradient magnetic fields must be considered. Because of these factors, MRI must not be performed unnecessarily during the first gestational trimester, in which organogenesis takes place. Until further studies are done, during this period of organogenesis, MRI should be performed only in patients with precise clinical indications and in whom this study offers a definite advantage over other imaging modalities known not to be harmful to the fetus.[11]

ADVANTAGES

Of all the advantages described in Chapter 8, those most pertinent to the pelvis are summarized here. The high signal intensity of fat in all pulsing sequences

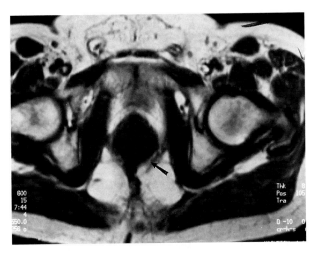

Fig. 19-1. Axial T1-weighted image of pelvis shows clear delineation of the prostate gland *(arrow)*, surrounded by hyperintense periprostatic fat.

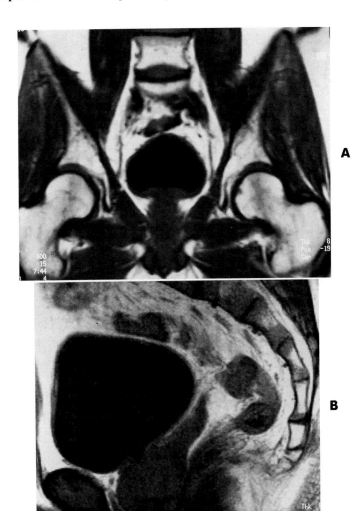

Fig. 19-2. A, Coronal T1-weighted image of pelvis shows good delineation of the normal pelvic anatomy because of its excellent soft tissue contrast of fat, muscles, and fluid within the bladder. **B,** Sagittal T1-weighted image demonstrates relationship between the bladder, prostate gland (posterior to bladder), and rectum.

provides natural contrast for the delineation of the rectum and other pelvic organs (Fig. 19-1).[29] The multiplanar imaging capability and wide field of view of MRI make it an ideal imaging modality for survey examination of normal anatomy and for detection and local staging of neoplasms (Fig. 19-2). In these cases, MRI helps localize space-occupying lesions, determine tumor volume, and delineate tumor extension to adjacent structure—factors that are important in treatment planning, follow-up, and estimating the prognosis of the patient.[39] In MRI of the pelvis, physiologic motion is less of a problem than in the upper abdomen.

MRI versus CT

The major advantage of MRI over CT is its superior soft tissue contrast resolution and its freedom from image degradation from beam hardening by the osseous structures in the pelvis, factors that limit the value of CT for staging neoplasms. MRI is more accurate for defining the soft tissue extent of malignant diseases and for demonstrating the invasion of adjacent structures by neoplasm.[1]

MRI differentiates vascular structures from lymphadenopathy without intravenous contrast agents. Soft tissue characterization is possible in some cases because of the different relaxation times of tissues on appropriate pulse sequences. This property is helpful for tumor detection and for differentiating tumor recurrence from postsurgical fibrosis.[31]

MRI is used as the imaging modality for follow-up patients after pelvic surgery (radical cystectomy and radical retroperitoneal lymph node dissection). These patients frequently have metallic clips that create artifacts on CT scans but produce no significant adverse effects in MRI (Fig. 19-3).

In the female pelvis, MRI demonstrates the morpho-

logic changes produced in the genital tract as a response to the different hormonal stimuli during the normal menstrual cycle.[13,18,31] It delineates the normal anatomy of the genital tract, a characteristic useful in evaluating tumor depth extension.[32,33] The absence of ionizing radiation is a major advantage in obstetric examinations.[40]

MRI versus US

In MRI, soft tissue contrast resolution depends on multiple physical parameters. Contrast resolution in ultrasound is based on differences in acoustic impedance. The advantage of MRI over US in pelvic imaging is based primarily on the delineation of the structures of the lateral pelvic walls, sensitive detection of lymphadenopathy, and freedom from artifacts caused by skeletal structures. MRI does not require an acoustic window to the pelvic organs; there-

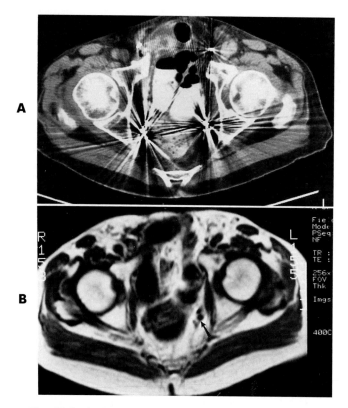

Fig. 19-3. A, Axial CT of pelvis shows degradation of the image caused by streak artifacts from surgical clips. **B,** Axial T1-weighted image of same area shows no significant evidence of artifacts. Round signal void *(arrow)* in left pelvis represents a clip.

fore, a full bladder is not needed. Technically, MRI is less operator-dependent and the quality of the image is not affected by the patient's position, body habitus, bowel gas, or a gravid uterus (in the case of pregnant patients). In certain cases, contact with the ultrasound transducer exacerbates patients' symptomatology (as in testicular disease). MRI is an alternative technique for evaluating these patients. Compared to transvaginal US, MRI is more comfortable to the patient. MRI also has a wider field of view than either endorectal or transvaginal US, making it more accurate for staging neoplastic disease.[30]

DISADVANTAGES

The disadvantages of MRI of the pelvis compared with CT or US are similar to those of MRI of the upper abdomen. The first disadvantage of MRI is cost. It is an expensive study compared with the other imaging modalities, and for this reason it is not as widely available as US and CT. The second disadvantage is time. The patient must lie motionless in the bore of the magnet for a period of 45 to 60 minutes. The third disadvantage of MRI is that it cannot be performed on all patients. Patients who are claustrophobic or morbidly obese and those who have pacemakers, metallic foreign bodies, intraocular foreign

bodies, or cerebral aneurysm clips are not candidates for MRI. A fourth disadvantage of MRI is its relatively low specificity.[28]

REFERENCES

1. Aisen A: Body MR imaging and the local staging of neoplasms, *Radiology* 176:617-619, 1990.
2. Amendola MA, Glazer GM, Grossman HB, et al: Staging of bladder carcinoma: MRI-CT-surgical correlation, *AJR* 146:1179-1183, 1986.
3. Arrive L, Hricak H, Martin MC: Pelvic endometriosis: MR imaging, *Radiology* 171:687-692, 1989.
4. Baker LL, Halek PC, Burkhard TK, et al: MR imaging of the scrotum: pathologic conditions, *Radiology* 163:93-98, 1987.
5. Bezzi M, Kressel HY, Allen KS, et al: Prostatic carcinoma: staging with MR imaging at 1.5 T, *Radiology* 169:339-346, 1988.
6. Biondetti PR, Lee JKT, Ling D, et al: Clinical stage B prostate carcinoma: staging with MR imaging, *Radiology* 162:325-329, 1987.
7. Bryan PJ, Butler HE, Li Puma JP, et al: CT and MR imaging in staging bladder neoplasms, *J Comput Assist Tomogr* 11(1):96-101, 1987.
8. Butch RJ, Stark DD, Wittenberg J, et al: Staging rectal cancer by MR and CT, *AJR* 146:1155-1160, 1986.
9. Buy JN, Moss AA, Guinet C, et al: MR staging of bladder carcinoma: correlation with pathologic findings, *Radiology* 169:695-700, 1988.
10. Chang YCF, Hricak H, Thurnher S, et al: Vagina: evaluation with MR imaging. II. Neoplasms, *Radiology* 169:175-179, 1988.
11. Consensus conference magnetic resonance imaging, *JAMA* 259(14):2132-2138, 1988.
12. DeLange EE, Fechner RE, Edge SB, et al: Preoperative staging of rectal carcinoma with MR imaging: surgical and histopathologic correlation, *Radiology* 176:623-628, 1990.
13. Demas BE, Hricak H, Jaffe RB: Uterine MR imaging: effects of hormonal stimulation, *Radiology* 159:123-126, 1986.
14. Ebner F, Kressel HY, Mintz MC, et al: Tumor recurrence versus fibrosis in the female pelvis: differentiation with MR imaging at 1.5 T, *Radiology* 166:333-340, 1988.
15. Friedland GW, Chang P: The role of imaging in the management of the impalpable undescended testis, *AJR* 151:1107-1111, 1988.
16. Fritzsche PJ, Hricak H, Kogan BA, et al: Undescended testis: value of MR imaging, *Radiology* 164:169-173, 1987.
17. Guinet C, Buy JN, Sezeur A, et al: Preoperative assessment of the extent of rectal carcinoma: correlation of MR, surgical and histopathologic findings, *J Comput Assist Tomogr* 12:209-214, 1988.
18. Haynor DR, Mack LA, Soules MR, et al: Changing appearance of the normal uterus during the menstrual cycle: MR studies, *Radiology* 161:459-462, 1986.
19. Hodgman CG, MacCarty RL, Wolff BG: Preoperative staging of rectal carcinoma by computed tomography and 0.15 T magnetic resonance imaging: preliminary report, *Dis Colon Rectum* 29:446-450, 1986.
20. Hricak H, Chang YCF, Thurnher S: Vagina: evaluation with MR imaging. I. Normal anatomy and congenital anomalies, *Radiology* 169:169-174, 1988.
21. Hricak H, Stern JL, Fisher MR, et al: Endometrial carcinoma staging by MR imaging, *Radiology* 162:297-305, 1987.
22. Hricak H, Doomes GC, Jeffrey RB Jr, et al: Prostatic carcinoma: staging by clinical assessment, CT, and MR imaging, *Radiology* 162:331-336, 1987.
23. Hricak H, Lacey CG, Sandles LG, et al: Invasive cervical carcinoma: comparison of MR imaging and surgical findings, *Radiology* 166:623-631, 1988.
24. Johnson JO, Mattrey RF, Phillipson J, et al: Differentiation of seminomatous from nonseminomatous testicular tumors with MR imaging, *AJR* 154:539-543, 1990.

25. Kier R, McCarthy S, Rosenfield AT, et al: Nonpalpable testes in young boys: evaluation with MR imaging, *Radiology* 169:429-433, 1988.

26. Kim SH, Choi BI, Lee HP, et al: Uterine cervical carcinoma: comparison of CT and MR findings, *Radiology* 175:45-51, 1990.

27. Krestin GP, Steinbrich W, Friedmann G: Recurrent rectal cancer: diagnosis with MR imaging versus CT, *Radiology* 168:307-311, 1988.

28. Ling D, Lee JKT, Heiken JP, et al: Prostatic carcinoma and benign prostatic hyperplasia: inability of MR imaging to distinguish between the two diseases, *Radiology* 158:103-107, 1985.

29. LiPuma JP, Bryan PJ: Magnetic resonance imaging of the genitourinary tract. In Kressel HY, ed: *Magnetic resonance annual, 1985,* New York, 1985, Raven Press.

30. Mark AS, Hricak H, Heinrichs LW, et al: Adenomyosis and leiomyoma: differential diagnosis with MR imaging, *Radiology* 163:527-529, 1987.

31. McCarthy S, Tanber C, Gore J: Female pelvic anatomy: MR assessment of variations during the menstrual cycle and with use of oral contraceptives, *Radiology* 160:119-123, 1986.

32. McCarthy SM, Filly RA, Stark DD, et al: Obstetrical magnetic resonance imaging: fetal anatomy, *Radiology* 154:427-432, 1985.

33. McCarthy SM, Stark DD, Filly RA, et al: Obstetrical magnetic resonance imaging: maternal anatomy, *Radiology* 154:421-425, 1985.

34. Neuerburg JM, Bohndorf K, Sohn M, et al: Urinary bladder neoplasms: evaluation with contrast-enhanced MR imaging, *Radiology* 172:739-743, 1989.

35. Rafto SE, Amendola MA, Gefter WB: MR imaging of recurrent colorectal carcinoma versus fibrosis, *J Comput Assist Tomogr* 12(3):521-523, 1988.

36. Schnall MD, Linkinski RE, Pollack HM, et al: Prostate: MR imaging with an endorectal surface coil, *Radiology* 172:570-574, 1989.

37. Shellock FG, Crues JV: MRI: potential adverse effects and safety considerations, *MRI Decisions* 2:25-30, 1988.

38. Shellock FG: Biological effects of MRI, *Diagn Imaging* 9:96-101, 1987.

39. Special NIH consensus report. II. Clinical indications for MRI and comparison and other diagnostic modalities, *MRI Decisions* 2:14-16, 1988.

40. Stark DD, McCarthy SM, Filly RA, et al: Pelvimetry by magnetic resonance imaging, *AJR* 144:947-950, 1985.

41. Thurnher, Hricak H, Carroll PR, et al: Imaging the testis: comparison between MR imaging and US. *Radiology* 167:631-636, 1988.

42. Togashi K, Nishimura K, Itoh K, et al: Ovarian cystic teratomas: MR imaging, *Radiology* 162:669-673, 1987.

43. Togashi K, Nishimura K, Itoh K, et al: Adenomyosis: diagnosis with MR imaging, *Radiology* 166:111-114, 1988.

44. Togashi K, Ozasa H, Konishi I, et al: Enlarged uterus: differentiation between adenomyosis and leiomyomas with MR imaging, *Radiology* 171:531-534, 1989.

45. Trambert MA, Mattrey RF, Levine D, et al: Subacute scrotal pain: evaluation of torsion versus epididymitis with MR imaging, *Radiology* 175:53-56, 1990.

46. Weinreb JC, Barkoff ND, Megibow A, et al: The value of MR imaging in distinguishing leiomyomas from other pelvic masses when sonography is indeterminate, *AJR* 154:295-299, 1990.

47. Zawin M, McCarthy S, Scoutt LM, et al: Endometriosis: appearance and detection at MR imaging, *Radiology* 171:693-696, 1989.

Chapter 20

ANATOMY OF THE PELVIS

Barry B. Kraus

Magnetic resonance imaging (MRI) provides details of pathologic conditions or anatomic variation within the pelvis. Unlike images of the upper abdomen, images of the the pelvis do not suffer significant degradation from respiratory motion artifacts. This allows the operator to decrease the number of signals averaged without greatly reducing image quality. The scan time saved is used to improve spatial resolution by increasing the matrix from 128 to 192 or 256 phase-encoding steps for T1-weighted acquisitions (i.e., weighted to the spin-lattice or longitudinal relaxation time [T1]). Of course, time constraints usually limit matrix size to 128 for T2-weighted scans (i.e., weighted to the spin-spin or transverse relaxation time [T2]) with long repetition times (TR). However, newly developed pulse sequences that employ multiple phase steps per TR may allow for larger matrices (512×512, for example) with little increase in time.

To recognize pathologic conditions and anatomic variations in the pelvis, one must have a knowledge of normal pelvic anatomy. Computed tomography (CT) provides excellent spatial resolution in the transverse plane. Although it cannot yet equal the resolution of CT, MRI provides superior contrast between normal and pathologic tissue.

Both the male and female pelvises can be subdivided into groups of structures for the purpose of anatomic discussion. Each consists of the urinary tract, reproductive tract, gastrointestinal (GI) tract, vascular system, nervous system, supporting structures (muscles, bones, joints), and various tissue planes, spaces, and ligaments.

What follows is a description and atlas of anatomy and signal characteristics of normal pelvic structures and comments regarding planes for optimal imaging of the structures.

URINARY TRACT

The pelvic portion of the urinary tract consists of the distal ureters, bladder, and urethra. The kidneys and proximal ureters normally reside within the upper abdomen and a description of them may be found in Chapter 9.

Ureters

The ureter, a small, tubular structure anterior to the psoas muscle in the lower abdomen, crosses the pelvic inlet anterior to the bifurcation of the common iliac artery. It then passes inferiorly and slightly posteriorly in front of the internal iliac artery to the level of the ischial spine. Distal to this, the ureter passes anteriorly and medially to reach the posterosuperior portion of the bladder. Each ureter is crossed by the gonadal vessels and the colic vessels. The right ureter is also crossed by the ileocolic vessels.[5] Transverse images generally display the ureter and its anatomic and pathologic relations best. However, in the case of a mass near the ureters, coronal images best reveal the degree of ureteral displacement.

Bladder

The urinary bladder lies anteriorly in the pelvis behind the anterior abdominal wall; medial to the obturator internus muscles, femoral vessels, and iliac vessels; anterior to the uterus and vagina (females) or seminal vesicles and rectum (males); inferior to the uterus and ovaries (females) and bowel loops; and superior to the prostate (males) and pubic bone (Figs. 20-1 to 20-7).[5]

Patients should be evaluated with a distended bladder to assess the vesical wall, which has a low signal intensity on T1-weighted sequences. The signal intensity of the bladder decreases somewhat on T2-weighted images (T2WI).[9,13,23] The perivesical fat emits high intensity signal on both T1-weighted images (T1WI) and T2WI, and urine emits low intensity signal on T1WI and high intensity signal on T2WI.[13,16,23] On T2WI the bladder wall is therefore seen as an area of low signal intensity of uniform thickness surrounded by urine and fat of higher signal intensity.[10] Because of the low signal intensity of urine, the inner margin of the bladder wall cannot be distinguished on T1WI.

Key to Figs. 20-1 to 20-11. *a,* Deep dorsal vein of penis; *b,* spermatic cord (including pampiniform plexus, vas deferens); *c,* crus of penis; *d,* cavernous urethra; *e,* bulb of penis; *f,* anal canal; *g,* external anal sphincter; *h,* ischial tuberosity; *i,* ischiorectal fossa; *j,* Buck's fascia; *k,* pectineus muscle; *l,* adductor brevis muscle; *m,* obturator externus muscle; *n,* rectus femoris muscle; *o,* sartorius muscle; *p,* lesser trochanter of femur; *q,* semimembranosus muscle; *r,* gluteus maximus muscle; *s,* long head of biceps femoris muscle; *t,* inferior gluteal vessels; *u,* iliopsoas muscle; *u*,* iliacus muscle; *u**,* psoas muscle; *v,* great saphenous vein; *w,* femoral artery; *x,* femoral vein; *y,* lateral femoral circumflex vessels; *z,* sciatic nerve; *A,* pubic symphysis; *A',* pubic bone; *B,* adductor longus muscle; *C,* obturator internus muscle; *D,* urethra; *E,* vagina; *F,* levator ani muscle; *G,* vaginal venous plexus; *H,* internal pudendal vessel; *J,* tensor fascia lata muscle; *K,* urinary bladder; *L,* head of femur; *M,* greater trochanter; *N,* rectum; *P,* ischium; *Q,* superior pubic ramus; *R,* vesicovaginal venous plexus; *S,* obturator vessels; *T,* gemellus muscles; *U,* ilium; *V,* cervical mucus and mucosa; *W,* rectus abdominus muscle; *X,* coccyx; *Y,* coccygeus muscle; *Z,* gluteus minimus muscle; *aa,* gluteus medius muscle; *bb,* uterovaginal venous plexus; *cc,* ileum; *dd,* inferior epigastric vessel; *ee,* external iliac artery and vein; *ff,* femoral nerve; *gg,* uterus; *gg*,* endometrium; *hh,* rectouterine space; *jj,* sacrum; *kk,* neural foramen; *ll,* bifurcation of common iliac vein; *mm,* internal iliac artery; *nn,* external iliac artery; *oo,* multifidus muscle; *pp,* sacrospinalis muscle; *qq,* oblique abdominal muscles; *rr,* descending colon; *ss,* transversus abdominus muscle; *tt,* common iliac artery; *uu,* inferior vena cava; *vv,* common iliac vein; *ww,* lumbar plexus of nerves; *xx,* linea alba; *yy,* L5 vertebral body; *zz,* spinal canal; *AA,* L4 vertebral body; *BB,* intervertebral disk; *DD,* piriformis muscle; *EE,* cecum; *FF,* ascending colon; *GG,* jejunum; *HH,* vastus intermedius muscle; *JJ,* vastus lateralis muscle; *KK,* vastus medialis muscle; *LL,* ovary; *MM,* seminal vesicle; *NN,* aorta; *PP,* prostate; *QQ,* retropubic space of Retzius; *RR,* sigmoid colon; *SS,* corpus cavernosum.

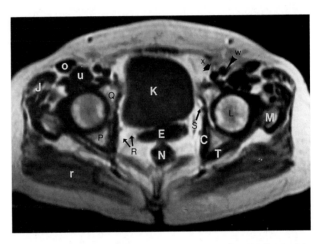

Fig. 20-1. Hip joints (female). Transverse T1-weighted spin-echo image through pelvis at level of the hip joints.

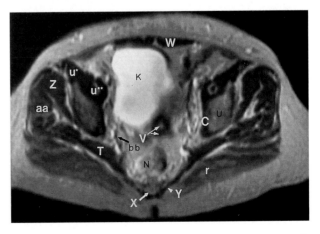

Fig. 20-2. Midpelvis (postmenopausal female). Transverse T2-weighted spin echo image through midpelvis, 2 cm superior to hip joint. Note distended bladder and small uterine corpus. Compare with Fig. 20-32.

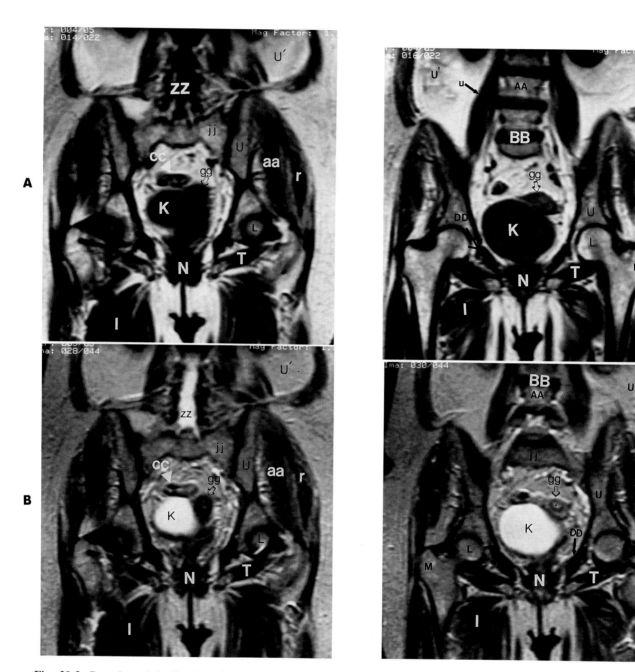

Fig. 20-3. Posterior pelvis (female). Coronal T1-weighted **(A)** and T2-weighted **(B)** spin-echo images through posterior pelvis at level of the spinal canal.

Fig. 20-4. Midpelvis (female). Coronal T1-weighted **(A)** and T2-weighted **(B)** spin-echo images through pelvis, approximately 1 cm anterior to spinal canal.

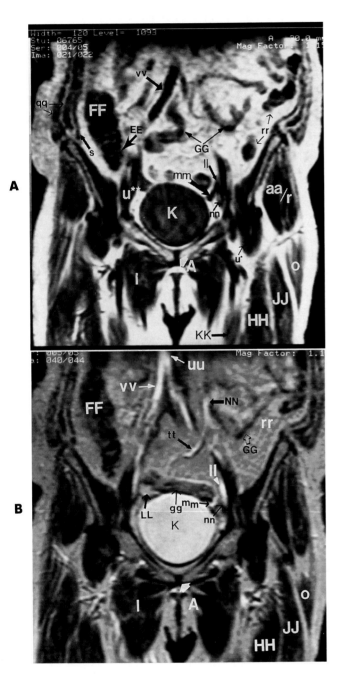

Fig. 20-5. Anterior pelvis (female). Coronal T1-weighted **(A)** and T2-weighted **(B)** spin-echo images through pubic symphysis.

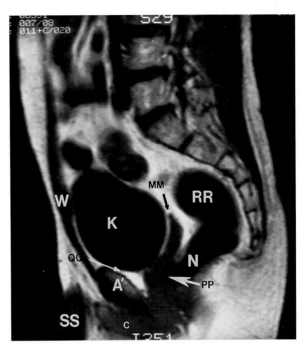

Fig. 20-6. Midpelvis (male). Sagittal T1-weighted spin-echo image through midline of the pelvis.

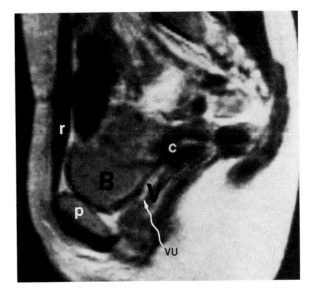

Fig. 20-7. Midpelvis (female). Sagittal T2-weighted (2000/60, or a TR of 2000 ms to a TE [echo time] of 60 msec) spin-echo image through midline of the pelvis. *B,* Urinary bladder; *C,* cervix; *P,* pubic bone; *R,* rectus abdominus muscle; *V,* vagina, *VU,* vesicouterine space. Note that high signal intensity cervical mucus can be distinguished from lower signal intensity cervical stroma. (From Hricak H et al: *AJR* 146:1115-1122, 1986.)

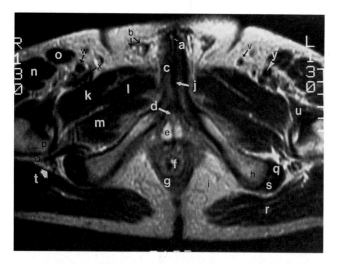

Fig. 20-8. Transverse T2-weighted spin-echo image through base of the penis.

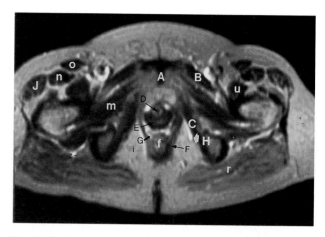

Fig. 20-9. Transverse T2-weighted spin-echo image through pelvic floor of a female.

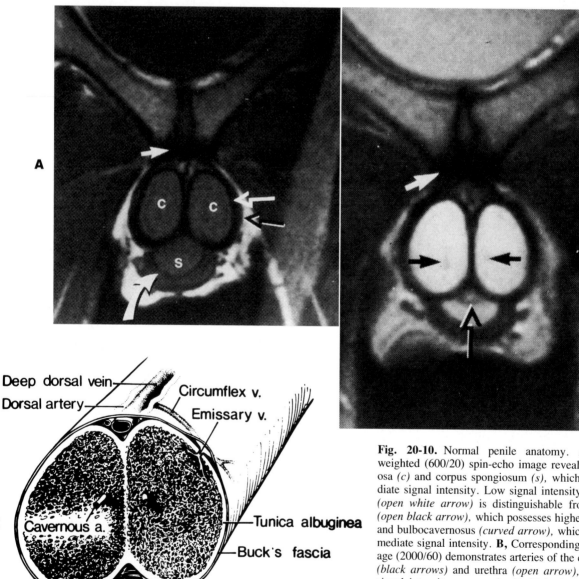

Deep dorsal vein
Dorsal artery
Circumflex v.
Emissary v.

Cavernous a.
Tunica albuginea
Buck's fascia

Urethral a.
Urethra

Fig. 20-10. Normal penile anatomy. **A,** Coronal T1-weighted (600/20) spin-echo image reveals corpora cavernosa *(c)* and corpus spongiosum *(s),* which possess intermediate signal intensity. Low signal intensity tunica albuginea *(open white arrow)* is distinguishable from Buck's fascia *(open black arrow),* which possesses higher signal intensity, and bulbocavernosus *(curved arrow),* which possesses intermediate signal intensity. **B,** Corresponding T2-weighted image (2000/60) demonstrates arteries of the corpora cavernosa *(black arrows)* and urethra *(open arrow),* which have low signal intensity compared with high signal intensity of the corpora. Suspensory ligament of the penis *(solid white arrow* in **A** and **B**) is between Buck's fascia and the pubis. **C,** Diagram of penis in cross section. (From Hricak H, Chang YCF, Thurnher S: *Radiology* 169:683-690, 1988.)

Transverse images show most pathologic conditions of the bladder well. However, for suspected lesions in the dome or base of the bladder, coronal and sagittal images should be obtained.

Urethra

The urethra appears as a thin-walled, collapsed structure originating from the bladder. In males it courses through the prostate gland and urogenital diaphragm, and after passing inferior to the pubic symphysis, it courses through the corpus spongiosum of the penis to terminate at the external urethral orifice (Figs. 20-8 to 20-18). In females, the urethra originates from the bladder, passes through the urogenital diaphragm, and terminates just superior to the vagina. Along its distal course, it runs close to the anterior vaginal wall.[5] The urethra emits low intensity signal on T1WI and high intensity signal on T2WI.[19,20] This signal intensity is usually lower than that of urine in the bladder on T2WI. It is currently thought that the signal intensity derives from the copious vascularity of the urethral mucosa.[19]

The tortuous superoinferior course of the urethra often makes imaging in the transverse plane suboptimal. However, since the urethra lies in the midline, sagittal imaging often demonstrates it well.

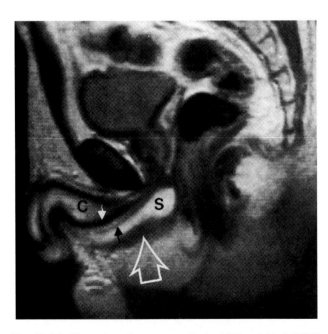

Fig. 20-11. Normal penile anatomy. Sagittal T2-weighted (2000/60) spin-echo image shows bulb of the penis *(S),* urethra *(black arrow)* penetrating roof of the bulb and curving to center of the corpus spongiosum, and bulbocavernosus *(open arrow).* Transverse septum *(white arrow)* separates corpus cavernosum *(C)* from corpus spongiosum. (From Hricak H et al: *Radiology* 169:683-690, 1988.)

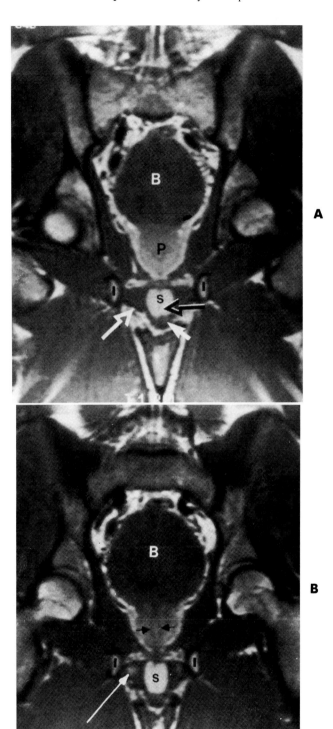

Fig. 20-12. Base of penis. **A,** Coronal proton-density–weighted image (2000/20) through base of penis shows corpus spongiosum *(s)* with low signal intensity septum *(open black arrow),* bulbocavernosus *(solid arrow),* ischium *(I),* ischiocavernosus *(open white arrow),* prostate gland *(P),* and bladder *(B).* **B,** Similar image taken 5 mm anterior to **A** shows intraprostatic urethra *(black arrows)* extending into penile bulb *(s),* proximal crura of the corpora cavernosa *(white arrow),* ischium *(I),* and bladder *(B).* (From Hricak H et al: *Radiology* 169:683-690, 1988.)

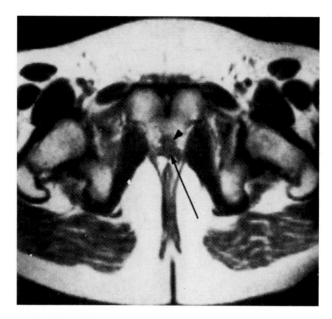

Fig. 20-13. Premenarchal vagina in 9-year-old girl. Transverse T2-weighted (2000/60) spin-echo image reveals small vagina *(long arrow),* which contains thin central area of mucus and low signal intensity vaginal wall. Arrowhead denotes urethra. (From Hricak H, Chang YCF, Thurnher S: *Radiology* 169:169-174, 1988.)

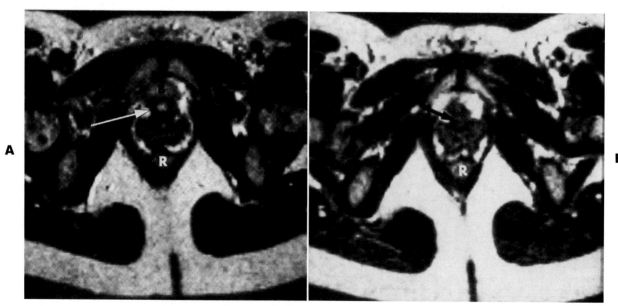

Fig. 20-14. Vagina in 28-year-old woman. **A,** Transverse T2-weighted (2000/80) spin-echo image through middle third of the vagina. *B,* Bladder; *arrow,* bladder neck; *R,* rectum. **B,** Image with same qualifications through lower third of the vagina, which lies between the urethra *(arrow)* and rectum *(R).* (From Hricak H, Chang YCF, Thurnher S: *Radiology* 169:169-174, 1988.)

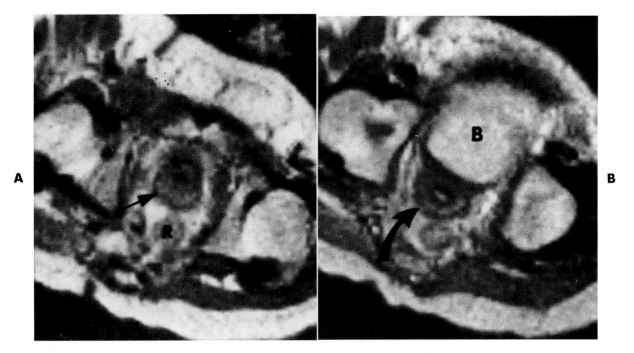

Fig. 20-15. Vagina in 1-month-old infant. **A,** Transverse T2-weighted (2000/80) spin-echo image through lower third of the vagina *(arrow)*. *Arrowhead,* Urethra; *R,* rectum. **B,** Image through uterine corpus *(arrow)*. Appearance of the vagina and uterus is similar to that during reproductive age. This results from the influence of maternal hormones in utero. (From Hricak H, Chang YCF, Thurnher S: *Radiology* 169:169-174, 1988.)

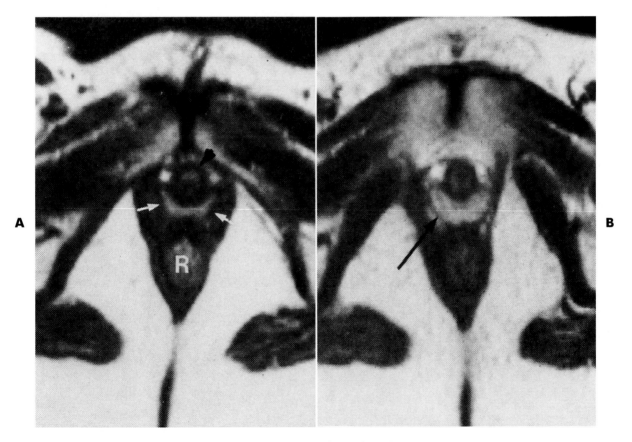

Fig. 20-16. Vaginal changes during menstrual cycle are shown by transverse T2-weighted (2000/60) spin-echo images through lower third of the vagina: **A,** Proliferative phase. **B,** midsecretory phase. Low signal intensity wall (**A,** *white arrows*) and high signal intensity central area of mucus and epithelium are present during early proliferative phase. In secretory phase, vaginal wall possesses medium intensity signal (**B,** *black arrow*), and mucus part of the vagina increases in thickness. *Arrowhead,* Urethra; *R,* rectum. (From Hricak H, Chang YCF, Thurnher S: *Radiology* 169:169-174, 1988.)

Fig. 20-17. Vagina in pregnant woman (32 weeks gestation). Transverse T2-weighted (2000/60) spin-echo image. Vagina *(V)* possesses intermediate signal intensity. Vaginal wall blends with central mucosa and perivaginal tissue. *Arrow,* Urethra; *R,* rectum. (From Hricak H, Chang YCF, Thurnher S: *Radiology* 169:169-174, 1988.)

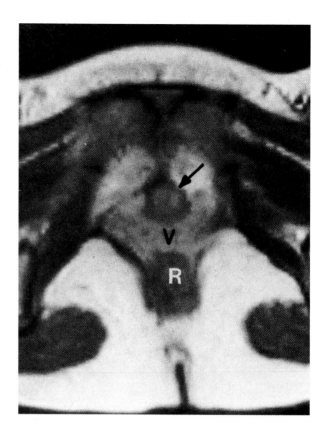

Fig. 20-18. Postmenopausal vagina. Transverse T2-weighted (2000/60) spin-echo images obtained in 65-year-old not taking estrogen replacement **(A)** and 65-year-old on estrogen replacement therapy **(B)**. **A,** Vagina *(solid arrow)* possesses low signal intensity and central mucus is not seen. **B,** Vagina *(solid arrow)* possesses low signal intensity and central mucus is not seen. Vagina *(curved arrow)* looks similar to that of a woman of reproductive age. *Open arrow,* Urethra; *R,* rectum. (From Hricak H, Chang YCF, Thurnher S: *Radiology* 169:169-174, 1988.)

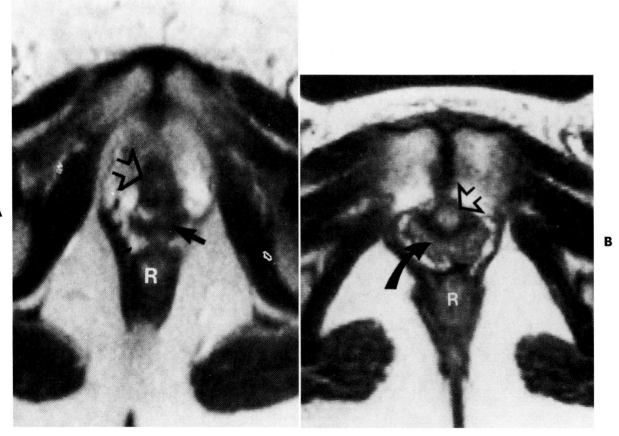

MALE REPRODUCTIVE TRACT

The male reproductive tract comprises the prostate, seminal vesicles, vas deferens, testes, erectile tissue, and epididymis and spermatic cord. With appropriate patient preparation and coil selection, all of these structures can be imaged with MRI.

The prostate, seminal vesicles, and distal vas deferens lie within the pelvis and are usually imaged with the body coil. However, the scrotum and its contents lie beyond the pelvic cavity and are relatively mobile. Because of this, it is important to immobilize these structures for diagnostic imaging. One can position the patient supine and place a folded towel under the scrotum to maintain it in a longitudinal plane.[1,11,21,27] Alternatively, one can have the patient squeeze his thighs together and rest the scrotum on them. The former method is usually more comfortable for the patient.

The scrotum contains relatively small structures for which high spatial resolution is needed. With body coil imaging, however, the increased resolution carries with it a reduction in signal-to-noise ratio (SNR). Fortunately, because the scrotum lies outside the pelvis, surface coils can be used to obtain a high SNR, making high-resolution scans possible.[1,27]

Prostate gland

The prostate gland lies inferior to the neck of the bladder, superior to the urogenital diaphragm, posterior to the retropubic space (or Retzius' space), anterior to the rectum, and medial to the levator ani muscles. A portion of the urethra traverses the prostate gland.[5] The prostate gland contains three zones of tissue: the peripheral zone, central zone, and transition zone (Figs. 20-19 to 20-24). Differentiation of these zones depends on magnetic field strength and the type of pulsing sequence used. At lower field strengths (0.35 T) the prostate emits a uniformly intermediate signal on T1WI, and the three zones are indistinct.* However, at higher field strengths (1.5 T) T1WI may allow for differentiation of zonal anatomy.[19] T2WI at any field strength reveal the zonal anatomy well. The peripheral zone shows higher signal intensity than either the central or transition zone.† This may be attributed to a prolonged T2 within the peripheral zone from fluid and secretions and a shortened T2 in the central zone from compact smooth muscle fibers.[11,19,21,26]

One may consistently differentiate the peripheral and central zones in younger patients. However, separation of the zones is less dependable in older patients because of changes in the prostate tissue that occur with age.[10,13,19] T2WI also allow for differentiation of the peripheral zone and the levator ani muscle. Regardless of the field strength or spin echo (SE) pulsing sequence used, differentiation

*References 10, 11, 13, 16, 22, 23.
†References 10, 11, 13, 19, 21, 22, 23.

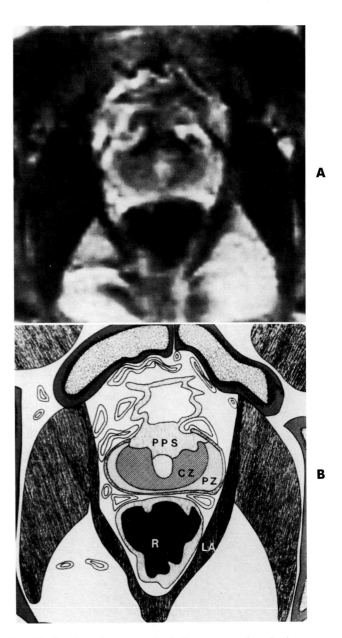

Fig. 20-19. Normal prostate gland. Transverse spin echo image (1500/80) **(A)** and accompanying diagram **(B),** 1 cm superior to verumontanum in 30-year-old. Smooth muscle of the periprostatic sphincter *(PPS)* blends with base of the bladder. *CZ,* Central zone of prostate; *PZ,* peripheral zone of prostate; *R,* rectum; *LA,* levator ani muscle. (From Koslin DB et al: *Invest Radiol* 22:947-953, 1987.)

between the central and transitional zones is currently not possible.

The various zones of the prostate are best imaged in the coronal plane (Fig. 20-22). The relation of the prostate to the rectum is best seen in the midsagittal plane (Fig. 20-23). The relationship of the prostate gland to the bladder may be imaged either in the coronal or sagittal plane. However, imaging of the relationship between the urethra

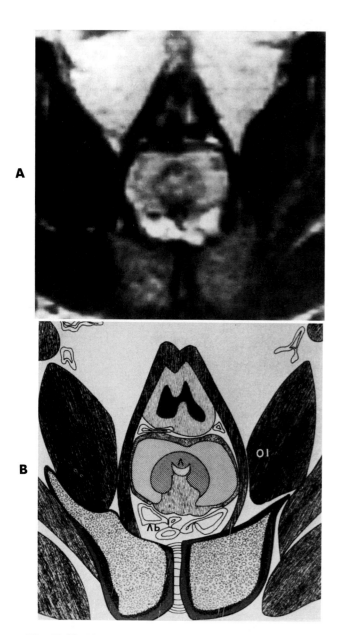

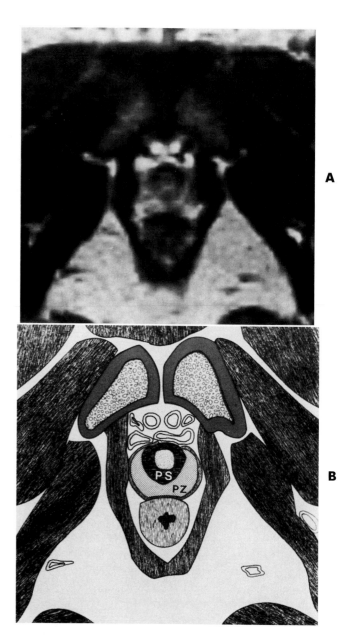

Fig. 20-20. Normal prostate gland. Transverse spin-echo image (1500/80) **(A)** and accompanying diagram **(B)** at level of the verumontanum in 30-year-old. Urethra and periurethral stroma are seen as an area of high signal intensity anterior to the veru-montanum *(V)*. Note thick posterior capsule. *OI,* Obturator internus muscle; *VP,* periprostatic venous plexus. (From Koslin DB et al: *Invest Radiol* 22:947-953, 1987.)

Fig. 20-21. Normal prostate gland. Transverse spin-echo image (1500/80) **(A)** and accompanying diagram **(B),** 1 cm inferior to verumontanum in 30-year-old. Prostate gland is smaller, and striated muscle of the prostatic sphincter appears as low-intensity ring. Also note absence of central zone tissue at this level. *PS,* Prostatic sphincter; *PZ,* peripheral zone. (From Koslin DB et al: *Invest Radiol* 22:947-953, 1987).

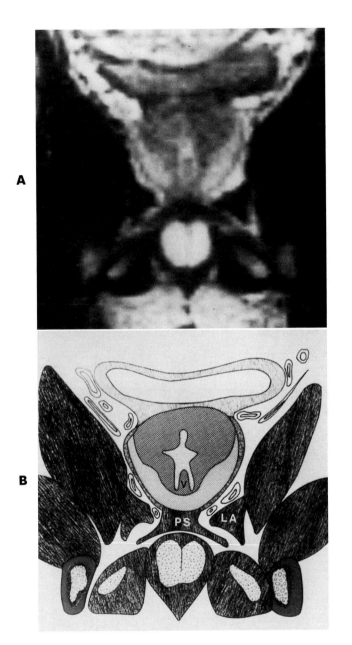

Fig. 20-22. Normal prostate gland. Coronal spin-echo image (1500/80) **(A)** and accompanying diagram **(B)** through the verumontanum *(V)*. *PS,* Prostatic sphincter; *LA,* levator ani muscle. (From Koslin DB et al: *Invest Radiol* 22:947-953, 1987).

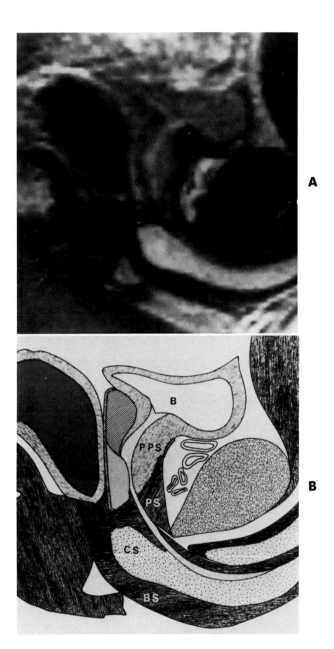

Fig. 20-23. Normal prostate gland. Midsagittal spin-echo image **(A)** and accompanying diagram **(B)** of the prostate. Urethra passes through prostate gland at 45-degree angle. A paucity of glandular tissue is in the midline. Sphincter muscle comprises the majority of tissue anterior to the urethra. Note that smooth muscle of the bladder wall and periprostatic sphincter blend with lower intensity striated muscle of the prostatic sphincter. *B,* Bladder; *R,* rectum; *PPS,* periprostatic sphincter; *PS,* prostatic sphincter; *CS,* corpus spongiosum; *BS,* bulbospongiosus muscle. (From Koslin DB: *Invest Radiol* 22:947-953, 1987).

and zonal anatomy is best in the transverse plane (see Figs. 20-19 to 20-21).[4,11,16,19]

The periprostatic venous plexus is recognizable as a round, tubular structure of low signal intensity on the first echo of a dual echo T2-weighted acquisition (Figs. 20-20 to 20-24). The plexus may emit high intensity signals on the second echo because of even echo rephasing.[11,13,19,22] The prostatic capsule cannot be consistently visualized by

MRI.[10,13,19,21,23] However, the posterior fascial covering of the prostate gland, Denonvillier's fascia, is visible as a line of low signal intensity between the peripheral zone of prostate gland and the anterior wall of the rectum (Figs. 20-18, 20-20, and 20-24).[13,23]

Seminal vesicles

The seminal vesicles form a V-shaped structure lying on the base of the bladder (see Figs. 20-6, 20-24, and 20-25). They are posterior and inferior to the bladder, superior to the prostate gland, anterior to the rectum, lateral to the ductus deferens and terminal part of the ureters, and me-

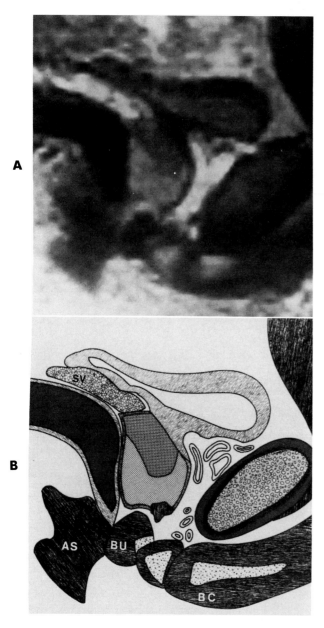

Fig. 20-24. Normal prostate gland. Parasagittal spin-echo image (1500/80) **(A)** and accompanying diagram **(B),** 1 cm from midline. High intensity signal from seminal vesicle results from its fluid content. Central zone and peripheral zone of the prostate gland are visualized well. *SV,* Seminal vesicle; *BU,* bulbourethral gland; *AS,* anal sphincter; *BC,* bulbocavernosus muscle. (From Koslin DB et al: *Invest Radiol* 22:947-953, 1987).

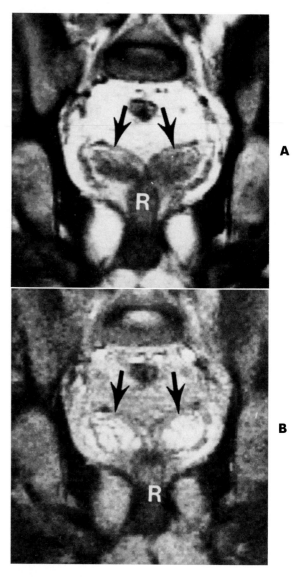

Fig. 20-25. Normal seminal vesicles. Coronal spin-echo images reveal seminal vesicles *(arrows)* and rectum *(R).* **A,** Proton-density image (2100/30) shows seminal vesicles possess intermediate signal intensity. **B,** T2-weighted image (2100/90) shows that they possess high signal intensity. (From Lee JKT, Rholl KS: *AJR* 147:732-736, 1986.)

dial to the levator ani muscle. The seminal vesicles are surrounded by fat in their retroperitoneal position.[5]

The signal intensity of the seminal vesicles varies with the pulsing sequence. On T1WI they exhibit medium signal intensity. On T2WI they exhibit higher signal intensity, often blending with the signal from surrounding fat.[11,16,23] This variation is presumably secondary to fluid secretions. The seminal vesicles are best seen either in the transverse or coronal plane.

Vas deferens

The vas deferens travels a winding path from its origin in the epididymis through the inguinal canal as part of the spermatic cord, turning medially and crossing anterior to the iliac vessels to enter the pelvis. In its course along the lateral pelvic wall, the vas deferens crosses the umbilical artery, the obturator nerves and vessels, the vessels of the bladder, and the ureter. Near the level of the ischiadic spine, it turns medially to loop over the superior pole of the seminal vesicle, the structure with which it joins to form the ejaculatory duct.[5]

The vas deferens emits medium intensity signal on T1WI. With images weighted more heavily to T2, its signal intensity increases.[16] Because of its circuitous course,

the vas deferens cannot be imaged completely in any one plane. The portion of the vas deferens within the spermatic cord can be imaged quite well in the coronal or transverse plane.

Spermatic cord

The spermatic cord runs from the testis through the scrotum and inguinal canal (Figs. 20-8, 20-22, 20-26, and 20-27). Its signal intensity is mixed, owing to its components. MRI often distinguishes the vas deferens from the internal spermatic vessels by the differences in signal intensity. As stated before, the vas deferens emits medium intensity signal on T1WI, which increase with longer TR and TE (echo time) sequences. The internal spermatic vessels emit low signal intensity on T1- and T2-weighted images because of flowing blood. Coronal and transverse planes are generally most beneficial for imaging the structures of the spermatic cord.

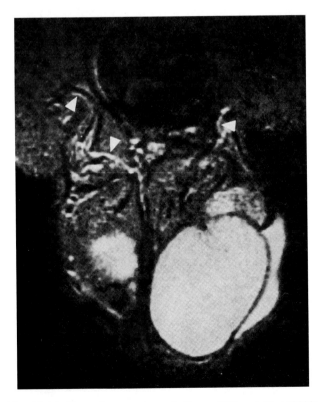

Fig. 20-26. Normal spermatic cord. Coronal T2-weighted (2000/70) spin-echo image shows spermatic cord in inguinal canal. Areas of high signal intensity represent vascular structures. Note phase shift artifact from blood flow (*arrowheads*). (From Baker LL et al: *Radiology* 163:89-92, 1987.)

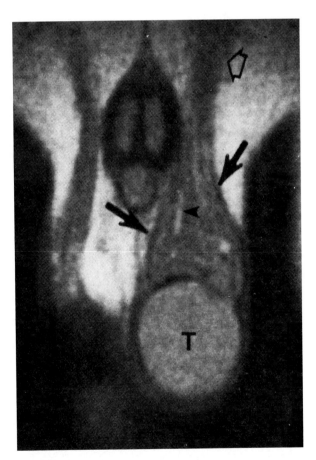

Fig. 20-27. Normal pampiniform plexus. Coronal T1-weighted (600/35) spin-echo image shows striated appearance of the pampiniform plexus of veins (*arrows*). High-intensity area (*arrowhead*) within plexus likely indicates slow blood flow. Also seen are spermatic cord (*open arrow*) and testis (*T*). (From Rholl KS et al: *Radiology* 163:99-103, 1987.)

Scrotum, testes, and epididymides

The testes normally reside within the scrotum (Figs. 20-28 and 20-30). They are surrounded by a dense layer of fascia, the tunica albuginea (Figs. 20-28, 20-29). The epididymis lies on the posterior aspect of the testis, with the epididymal head situated superiorly (Figs. 20-28 and 20-30). The tail of the epididymis continues as the proximal part of the vas deferens, which then passes to the pelvis through the spermatic cord.

The testis normally exhibits a signal intensity lower than that of fat on T1WI and a higher signal intensity (comparable to fat) on T2WI.[28] The tunica albuginea, composed of fibrous tissue, and the tunica vaginalis, which adheres to the tunica albuginea, emit low intensity signals on most pulse sequences. The mediastinum testis, arising from the tunica albuginea, appears as a 1 to 3 cm area of low signal intensity on T2WI.[1,3,11,21,27]

On T1WI the epididymis exhibits a mixed signal intensity, similar to or somewhat lower than that of the testis. With increased T2-weighting the epididymis has a signal intensity lower than that of the testis.[1,27]

The scrotal sac comprises an area of low signal intensity outlined by high intensity subcutaneous fat. Within this tissue the dartos muscle appears as a thin layer of moderate signal intensity (Fig. 20-29).[1]

In general, transverse and coronal images show the scrotal contents best. The transverse plane reveals the relationship between the testis and the epididymis, whereas the coronal plane reveals the testis and spermatic cord (Fig. 20-31). The sagittal plane shows the testis and epididymis, the tunica albuginea, and the layers within the scrotal wall, including the dartos muscle.[1,11]

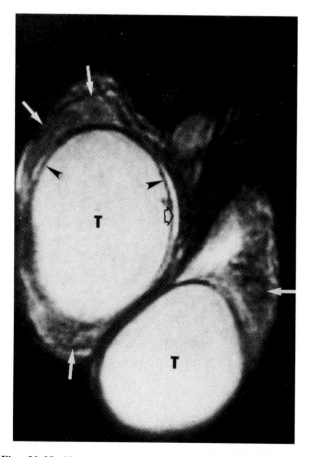

Fig. 20-28. Normal scrotum. Coronal T2-weighted (2000/70) spin-echo image shows testes *(T)*, epididymis *(white arrows)*, and tunica albuginea *(arrowheads)*. A small amount of fluid is present *(open arrow)*. (From Baker LL et al: *Radiology* 163:89-92, 1987.)

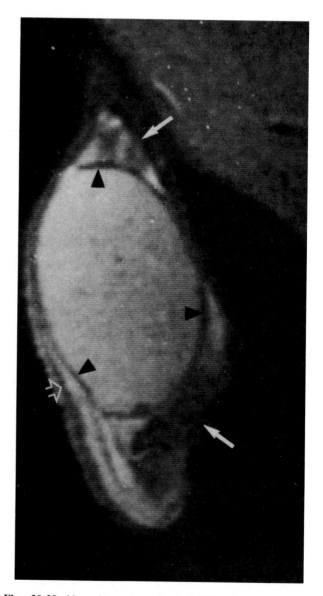

Fig. 20-29. Normal scrotum. Sagittal T2-weighted (2000/70) spin-echo image shows tunica albuginea *(arrowheads)*, head and tail of the epididymis *(arrows)*, and layers of the scrotal wall, including dartos muscle *(open arrow)*. (From Baker LL et al: *Radiology* 163:89-92, 1987.)

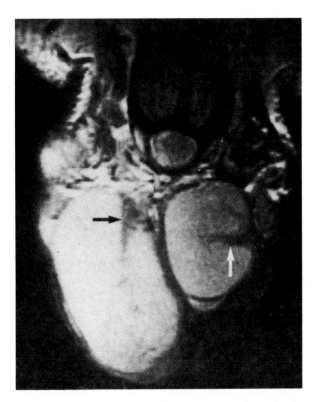

Fig. 20-30. Normal testes. Coronal proton-density weighted (2000/25) spin-echo image shows mediastinum testis *(arrows)* in long and short axes. Right testis possesses higher signal than left testis because of its more central position relative to the surface coil. (From Baker LL et al: *Radiology* 163:89-92, 1987.)

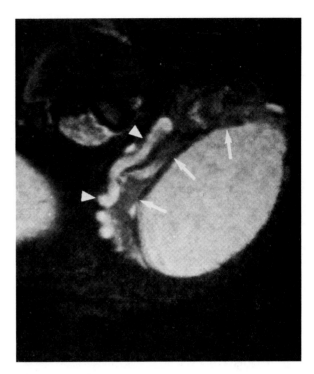

Fig. 20-31. Normal epididymis. Coronal T2-weighted spin-echo image shows entire left epididymis *(arrows)*. Note vas deferens *(arrowheads),* which possesses signal intensity similar to that of the testis. (From Baker LL et al: *Radiology* 163:89-92, 1987.)

Penis and erectile tissue

The penis contains several structures visible with MRI (Figs. 20-6 and 20-8). The erectile tissue consists of the corpus spongiosum and the two corpora cavernosa (Figs. 20-10 to 20-12 and 20-32). The corpus spongiosum originates within the superficial space of the perineum as the bulb of the penis and continues ventrally into the body of the penis to terminate as the glans. Within the corpus spongiosum lies the penile urethra. The corpora cavernosa originate from the ischia as the crura of the penis and continue dorsally and laterally into the body of the penis. The three corpora are invested in fascia and are separated from each other by septa.[5] The corpora exhibit medium signal intensity on T1WI and high signal intensity on T2WI (Fig. 20-32). Their appearances vary with the amount of blood in each at a given time. Buck's fascia is seen as a line of low signal intensity surrounding the corpora.[20]

The penis is best imaged in the midsagittal plane, which shows the course of the urethra and corpora through the penis. The transverse plane (a plane through the penis that shows its contents in cross section) reveals the anatomic relationship between the corpora, their surrounding fascia, and the urethra. A true coronal plane through the base of

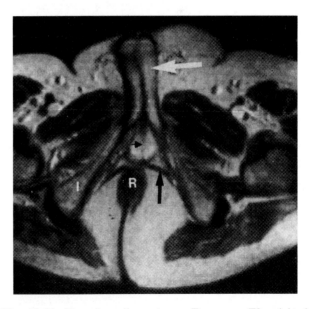

Fig. 20-32. Normal penile anatomy. Transverse T2-weighted (2000/60) spin-echo image reveals septum in the posterior penile bulb *(arrowhead)* as area of low signal intensity. Corpus cavernosum *(white arrow)* possesses high signal intensity and superficial transverse perineal muscle *(black arrow)* possesses low signal intensity. *R,* Rectum; *I,* ischium. (From Hricak H et al: *Radiology* 169:683-690, 1988.)

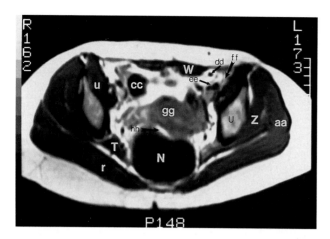

Fig. 20-33. Midpelvis (female). Transverse T1-weighted spin-echo image through midpelvis, 2 cm superior to hip joint. Non-distended bladder is below imaging plane. Note uterine fundus in this female of child bearing age. Compare with Fig. 20-2.

the penis reveals its structures in cross section and is useful to examine their relationship to surrounding pelvic anatomy.[20]

FEMALE REPRODUCTIVE TRACT

The female reproductive tract comprises the ovaries, fallopian tubes, uterus, cervix, vagina, and labia. MRI depicts all of these structures well, except for the ovaries, which are difficult to visualize. Unlike imaging of the male reproductive tract, special patient preparation and coil selection is not necessary.

Uterus

The uterus lies within the pelvis between the bladder and rectum (Figs. 20-3, 20-4 and 20-5, *B*). It usually bends anteriorly to overhang the bladder and form a right angle with the vaginal canal. The uterus lies posterior to the bladder, anterior to the rectouterine pouch and rectum, inferior to the ileum, superior to the vagina, and medial to the fallopian tubes and uterine ligaments.[5]

The signal intensity and morphology of the uterus varies with pulsing sequence, zonal anatomy, and menstrual cycle. On T1WI the uterus appears homogeneous with low to intermediate signal intensity, and the three tissue layers cannot be distinguished (Fig. 20-33).

T2WI provide contrast between the endometrium and

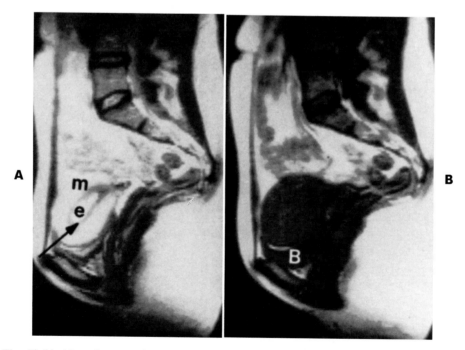

Fig. 20-34. Normal uterus of woman of reproductive age. Sagittal T2-weighted (2000/60) **(A)** and T1-weighted (500/30) **(B)** images through the uterus. Uterine corpus is seen above dome of empty urinary bladder *(B)*. Myometrium *(M)* is clearly differentiated from endometrium *(E)* on T2-weighted image. Arrow in **A** shows junctional zone. Zonal anatomy is obscured on T1-weighted image. (From Hricak H: *AJR* 146:1115-1122, 1986.)

myometrium (Figs. 20-34 and 20-35). Within the corpus the endometrium and myometrium possess high signal intensities and are separated by a junctional zone of low signal intensity (Fig. 20-34). This zone is thought by some to represent mainly venous structures within the inner third of the myometrium and to others to represent lower water content in this part of the uterus.[6,18,24,25] The appearance of the corpus depends on hormonal stimulation and thus changes with the menstrual cycle. The endometrium changes in width, being thickest in the midsecretory phase and thinnest just after menses. Also, the total uterine volume increases during the secretory phase.[12-14] The myometrium possesses a higher signal intensity on T2WI during the secretory phase. These two tissue layers are still distinguishable with the junctional zone interposed, regardless of the phase of the menstrual cycle.

Oral contraceptive pills change the appearance of the uterus (Fig. 20-35). The distinction between the endometrium and myometrium becomes poor, the junctional zone is not always seen, and the endometrium becomes noticeably atrophic.[14] Uteruses of premenarchal and postmenarchal women also differ in appearance from the uteruses of menstruating women. These patients have small uterine corpora and atrophic endometrium (Fig. 20-36).[13,14] The uteruses of postmenarchal women who take estrogen have an appearance similar to those of menstruating women.[14]

Cervix

Like the uterus the cervix has anatomical zones that can be imaged with MRI. T1WI display the cervix as a structure of homogeneous intermediate signal intensity. T2WI reveal two distinct zones: a central zone of high signal intensity representing cervical epithelium and mucus (Figs. 20-2, 20-7, 20-35, and 20-36)[17,24] and a more peripheral zone encircling the central zone and emitting low intensity signals. The latter area represents the fibrous cervical stroma.[17] In some women the peripheral zone contains two areas of distinct signal intensity.[24] In addition to the low-intensity area, a layer of tissue with moderate signal intensity may be seen even more peripherally.

The cervix is imaged optimally in the sagittal and transverse planes.

Vagina

The vagina is divided into two anatomic parts. The upper two thirds lies above the level of the bladder base and is of müllerian duct origin. The lower one third lies below the level of the bladder base and is of urogenital sinus origin.

On T1WI the vagina appears as a line of low signal intensity between the bladder and rectum (see Fig. 20-1). Because the vagina is under hormonal influence, its appearance on T2WI depends on the stage of the menstrual

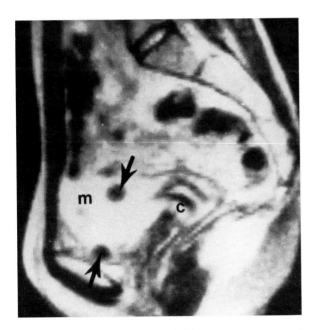

Fig. 20-35. Uterus of woman of reproductive age who is taking oral contraceptives. Sagittal T2-weighted (2000/56) image shows that uterine corpus is globular. Myometrium *(M)* possesses high signal intensity and differentiating between it and endometrium is not possible. Two small leiomyomas are present *(arrows)*. Normal cervix *(C)*, with a distinct stroma and central mucus, is visible. (From Hricak H: *AJR* 146:1115-1122, 1986.)

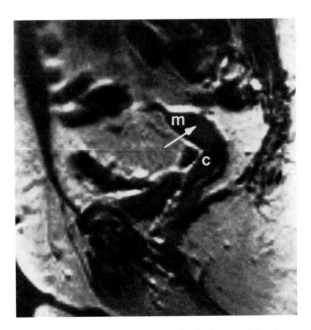

Fig. 20-36. Postmenopausal uterus. Sagittal T2-weighted image (2000/40) reveals that length of the uterine corpus is similar to length of the cervix *(C)*. It is difficult to distinguish the myometrium *(M)* from the endometrium *(arrow)*. Myometrium possesses lower signal intensity than myometrium of woman of reproductive age. This volunteer was 10 years past menopause. (From Hricak H: *AJR* 146:1115-1122, 1986.)

cycle and on other factors, such as the woman being pregnant, premenarchal, or postmenopausal or using oral contraceptives).[2,14,15] These factors generally influence the vaginal mucosa in a manner similar to their affect on the uterus.

Generally, T2WI display the vagina as a mucus-containing area of high signal intensity surrounded by an area of low signal intensity, representing the vaginal wall (Figs. 20-7, 20-9, 20-14, and 20-37).[14] High intensity signal from surrounding pelvic fat delineate the outer margin of the wall. During the early proliferative phase of the menstrual cycle, the vagina appears on T2WI as described previously. During the late proliferative phase, the vaginal wall possesses higher signal intensity and the central, mucus-containing area thickens and possesses even higher signal intensity. During the midsecretory phase the vaginal wall possesses moderate to high signal intensity, and the central area is even thicker and more intense (Fig. 20-16). During this phase, one also sees a high intensity rim around the vaginal wall on the second, even echo on T2WI. This area represents slow flowing blood in congested perivaginal vessels.[15]

T2WI of the vagina in premenarchal girls show the vaginal wall with low signal intensity and the thin central area with low signal intensity (Fig. 20-13). However, in children less than 1 month old, the vagina looks similar to that of women of reproductive age (Fig. 20-15). Images of the vagina of a postmenopausal woman show the wall as a low intensity area and the central area as quite thin (Fig. 20-18). If these women take exogenous estrogens, the vagina appears similar to that of a woman of reproductive age. Transverse and sagittal images are essential when evaluating the vagina. Coronal scans also show the vagina but are not as advantageous.[15]

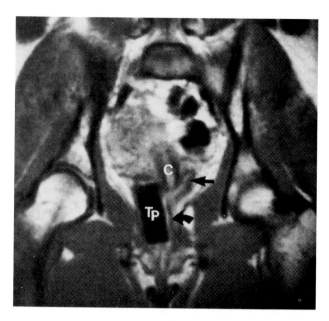

Fig. 20-37. Proton-density (2000/30) spin echo coronal image of vagina at 0.35 T shows tampon *(Tp)* in place. Left fornix *(straight arrow)*, left vaginal wall *(curved arrow)*, and cervix *(C)* are visible. (From Hricak H, Chang YCF, Thurnher S: *Radiology* 169:169-174, 1988.)

Adnexa

The normal ovaries and fallopian tubes may be difficult to visualize with MRI. On T1WI, the ovaries emit low to moderate intensity signals similar to those of fluid-filled bowel loops. They emit higher intensity signal on T2WI, often appearing hyperintense relative to the surrounding fat, but often appearing isointense (Fig. 20-38).[13] The ad-

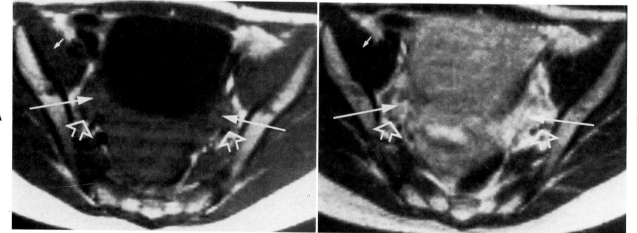

Fig. 20-38. Normal ovaries. Transverse images through the adnexa. **A,** T1-weighted (500/28) spin-echo image demonstrates ovaries *(long arrows)*, which possess low signal intensity similar to that of striated muscle *(small arrow)*. **B,** T2-weighted (2000/56) spin-echo image shows ovaries with high signal intensity, approaching the signal intensity of fat. *Open arrows,* Ovarian vessels. (From Dooms GC, Hricak H, Tscholakoff D: *Radiology* 158:639-646, 1986.)

nexa are often seen in relation to their surrounding structures, the ovarian and obturator vessels.

In women of reproductive age, the ovaries often are visible with thin, contiguous slices obtained in either the transverse or coronal plane. Unlike imaging of the uterus, the sagittal plane does not demonstrate the ovaries well. The ovaries are even more difficult to visualize in postmenopausal women, owing to their involution. In a study using an 0.35 T system, investigators identified normal ovaries in 87% of women of reproductive age but in only 47% of post-menopausal women.[7] MRI is quite helpful in identifying the adnexal origin of pelvic lesions, however. In the same study, investigators correctly identified the adnexal origin of 100% of the lesions imaged.

STRUCTURES OF THE PELVIS
Bowel

The distal small bowel, cecum, much of the colon, and rectum are seen routinely on MR (magnetic resonance) images of the pelvis (Fig. 20-5). The differentiation between these structures is based on location and morphology, not on differences in signal characteristics. All emit variable signal intensities depending on their luminal content. The bowel wall emits low intensity signals on both T1- and T2-weighted images. The outer aspect of the wall is seen in contrast to the surrounding pelvic fat. However, the inner aspect of the wall cannot be seen unless the lumen contains material of relatively higher signal intensity, such as fluid, or lower signal intensity, such as an agent with negative contrast effects. In addition the thickness of the bowel wall is inconsistent and depends on the amount of distension from luminal content. Barium preparations may be used to distend the upper and lower GI tract.

Coronal and transverse planes display parts of the GI tract well. Unfortunately, even in the pelvis the images may be degraded by motion artifact. Although respiratory motion artifacts do not play a role, blurring from peristalsis does. In the future, some type of peristalsis-reducing contrast agent may will be advantageous.

Musculature

The pelvis contains several groups of muscles, all of which normally emit low intensity signals on T1- and T2-weighted images. These include the muscles of the lower abdominal wall, lower back, iliopsoas complex, and pelvic floor and hip muscles that originate in the pelvis (Figs. 20-1, 20-6, 20-8, 20-9, 20-32, 20-39, and 20-40). Individual muscles often are distinguishable from surrounding musculature by the different signal intensities from fascial planes. However, muscle groups are best recognized by their location, not their signal intensity.

Bones and joints

Although MRI of the pelvis is usually not done primarily to evaluate bones and joints, these are seen routinely (Figs. 20-1, 20-6, 20-8, 20-9, 20-32, 20-39, and 20-40). Generally, cortical bone is shown as an area of low signal intensity on all sequences. Fat-containing medullary bone possesses higher signal intensity on T1- and T2-weighted images. Knowledge of normal marrow signal intensities is essential, because many disease processes may invade the marrow and produce variable signal intensities. Joint spaces contain small amounts of synovial fluid, which emits moderate intensity signals on T1WI and high intensity signals on T2WI, relative to cartilage or cortical bone.

Bones that should be examined on images of the pelvis include the ilium, ischium, pubis, sacrum, coccyx, lumbar vertebrae, and femur. Joints that should be examined include the intervertebral joints, pubic symphysis, sacroiliac joints, and hip joints. As with the evaluation of pelvic muscles, bones and joints of the pelvis are best recognized by their location, not their signal intensity.

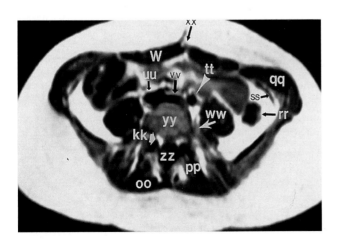

Fig. 20-39. Upper pelvis. Transverse T1-weighted spin echo image through upper pelvis. Note confluence of the common iliac veins at this level.

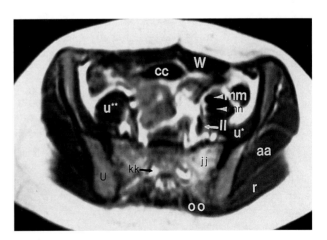

Fig. 20-40. Sacroiliac joint. Transverse T1-weighted spin echo image through pelvis at the sacroiliac joint. Note iliac vessels and their branches.

Vessels

The pelvis contains many blood vessels and nerves. Vessels that can be specifically evaluated with MRI include the aorta, inferior vena cava (IVC), azygous system, and iliac vessels and the gonadal, pudendal, rectal, and femoral vessels (Figs. 20-1, 20-6, 20-8, 20-9, 20-32, 20-39, and 20-40).

All of these vessels possess the same signal characteristics, which depend on the rate of blood flow. The aorta is seen as a large tubular structure just to the left of the spine (Fig. 20-5, *B*). Like the other vessels, it possesses low signal intensity on SE images and higher signal intensity on gradient-echo (GE) images. Presaturation pulses help create a more uniform low intensity signal on SE, and gradient moment nulling (flow compensation) helps create a more uniform, high intensity signal on GE (see Chapter 7). Transverse images usually provide sufficient information to evaluate the aorta. However, coronal images often give a better view of medial or lateral deviation.

The IVC is similar in appearance to the aorta but lies to the right of the spine (Figs. 20-5, *B*, and 20-39). The smaller azygous vein is seen just posterior to the IVC. The hemiazygous vein is seen on the left side of the spine, originating at the level of the renal vein.

The iliac arteries arise at the bifurcation of the aorta at the level of the fourth lumbar vertebra (Fig. 20-39). Each artery passes inferiorly and laterally for a short distance and then divides into an internal and an external branch. The right common iliac artery crosses anterior to the IVC and is anterior to the right common iliac vein. The left common iliac artery is slightly lateral to its corresponding vein. Branches of the inferior mesenteric artery to the rectum pass anterior to the left common iliac artery.

The external iliac arteries arise at the level of the lumbosacral joint, just anterior to the sacroiliac joint (Figs. 20-5 and 20-40). They pass inferiorly and slightly laterally just anterior to the psoas muscle. Each artery lies anterior to its paired vein at its origin but eventually becomes lateral to it. The sigmoid colon crosses the left external iliac artery. Other structures that cross the arteries are the ureters, ovarian vessels, vas deferens and ligamentum teres uteri. The artery terminates as the femoral artery as it crosses the inguinal ligament.

The internal iliac arteries course inferiorly from their origin, posterior to the ureter and anterior to the corresponding internal iliac vein, and terminate in anterior and posterior divisions (Figs. 20-5 and 20-40).

The iliac veins roughly parallel their corresponding arteries (Figs. 20-5, 20-40). The common iliac veins originate from the junction of the external and internal iliac veins on each side of the pelvis. The right vein courses almost directly superior, whereas the left vein crosses anterior to the vertebral column to join and form the IVC at the level of the fifth lumbar vertebra.

The rectum derives its blood supply from various sources. The superior rectal (hemorrhoidal) artery arises from the inferior mesenteric artery and supplies blood to the upper two thirds of the rectum before its branches anastomose with the inferior rectal artery at the level of the anal columns. The middle rectal artery arises from the internal iliac artery and supplies blood to the muscular layer of the lower third of the rectum. The inferior rectal artery arises from the internal pudendal artery and supplies blood to the lower end of the anal canal and the perianal area.

The rectal veins parallel the rectal arteries in their course through the pelvis. That the rectal veins provide an important site for anastomosis of venous drainage is apparent from their different sites of termination. This allows the rectal veins to be used frequently as sites for collateral blood flow.

The pair of testicular arteries arise from the anterior surface of the aorta, inferior to the origin of the renal arteries. Each passes inferiorly and laterally to the deep inguinal ring and becomes part of the spermatic cord. Each artery passes through the inguinal canal and descends anteriorly to the vas deferens to reach the upper end of the testis.

The right testicular artery initially lies anterior to the aorta; it then crosses anterior to the IVC and the ureter to reach the psoas major muscle. It lies within the retroperitoneum and is crossed anteriorly by the third part of the duodenum, the colic vessels, the root of the mesentery, and the cecum and appendix. The left testicular artery passes to the left, anterior to the ureter and sympathetic trunk on the psoas muscle, and crosses the external iliac vessels to reach the inguinal canal.

The ovarian arteries travel along the same course as the testicular arteries down to the rim of the pelvis. Beyond this, each courses medially, anterior to the external iliac artery, to enter the pelvic cavity and the broad ligament.

The testicular and ovarian veins arise from the pampiniform plexus of veins and follow the course of their corresponding arteries proximally to the internal inguinal ring, past which they diverge from their arteries. The left vein drains into the left renal vein, whereas the right vein drains directly into the IVC.

Occasionally, branches of the internal iliac vessels are seen with MRI. The internal pudendal artery, for example, arises from the anterior division of the internal iliac artery and courses inferiorly and posteriorly along the obturator internus muscle (Fig. 20-9). It exits the pelvis through the greater ischiadic foramen.

Nerves

Nerves lying within the pelvis generally originate from three sources: the lumbar plexus, sacral plexus, and -sympathetic chain. The lumbar plexus consists of segments of nerves from the first four lumbar levels of the spinal cord (Fig. 20-39). The plexus itself lies mostly outside the pelvis, but its branches course through the pelvis. Notable nerves are the ilioinguinal nerve, which passes through the inguinal canal to terminate as a cutaneous nerve of the external genitalia; the femoral nerve, which innervates the psoas and iliacus muscles before passing distally to terminate in the thigh; the obturator nerve, which courses on the medial side of the psoas major muscle and along the lateral wall of the pelvis, passes through the obturator foramen, and innervates the lower limb; and the genitofemoral nerve, which passes through the anterior surface of the psoas major muscle and divides into branches that course either through the inguinal canal (genital branch) or into the thigh (femoral branch).

The sacral plexus derives from the first through fourth sacral nerves but receives contributions from the fourth and fifth lumbar nerves and fifth sacral nerve. Most branches of the sacral plexus terminate in the lower limb. However, some course through the pelvis to end in the perineum. The pudendal nerve arises from the sacral plexus, courses through the pelvis with the internal pudendal artery, and exits the pelvis through the greater ischiadic foramen. It passes within the pudendal canal on the obturator internus muscle and lateral wall of the ischiorectal fossa. It innervates the external anal sphincter, levator ani muscle, and muscles of the urogenital triangle and provides cutaneous innervation to the external genitalia.

The autonomic nervous system innervates the viscera of the abdomen and pelvis. It is divided into craniosacral and thoracolumbar segments. The former provides parasympathetic innervation and the latter sympathetic innervation. The sacral portion of the autonomic nervous system arises from the second through fourth sacral segments, which form the pelvic nerve. Branches of this nerve are generally not visualized well with MRI.

Lymph nodes

As with other areas of the body, the lymph nodes of the pelvis are named for the structures near which they lie. In the pelvis, these groups of nodes include the common iliac, external iliac, internal iliac, obturator, sacral, and inguinal nodes. The common iliac, external iliac, and internal iliac nodes are found near the arteries bearing the same names. The obturator nodes lie near the obturator internus muscle. The sacral nodes lie in the anterior concavity of the sacrum. The inguinal nodes lie near the inguinal ligament and are comprised of deep and superficial groups.

Studies comparing MRI to CT in the evaluation of pelvic adenopathy have shown that CT, because of its superior spatial resolution, may be better than MRI in assessing normal-sized (less than 10 mm) nodes. However, MRI appears to be better than CT in assessing abnormally large (greater than 13 to 15 mm) nodes because of the superior contrast resolution, allowing for clear demonstration of nodes from surrounding tissue, especially fat and blood vessels.[8]

Miscellaneous pelvic structures

The ischiorectal fossa forms a large wedge-shaped area on each side of the anus and rectum (Figs. 20-8 and 20-9). Its boundaries are anteriorly, the transverse muscles of the perineum; posteriorly, the gluteus maximus muscle and sacrotuberous ligament; laterally, the obturator internus muscle; and medially, the levator ani and external anal sphincter muscles. This space contains mostly fat, but several important structures pass through it. They include the inferior rectal arteries and nerves, the pudendal nerve, and the internal pudendal artery. Abscesses that form in the ischiorectal fossa can cross the midline since the two fat pads are continuous anterior and posterior to the anus.

The retropubic space (also called the prevesical space or Retzius' space) is bounded by the pubic symphysis anteriorly, the bladder (and in males the prostate gland) posteriorly, and the urogenital diaphragm inferiorly. The space contains fat and the puboprostatic ligaments. It is best seen in the sagittal plane (Fig. 20-6).

The paravesical space, as its name indicates, is found lateral to the urinary bladder and contains fat (Figs. 20-1 and 20-5).

The rectovesical space in males is the space between the urinary bladder and rectum (Fig. 20-6). In its superior portion lies the rectovesical pouch, the inferior reflection of the peritoneum.

The uterovesical space lies between the bladder and uterus and is a thin space consisting of a double reflection of peritoneum between the bladder and uterus (Fig. 20-7).

The rectouterine space in females lies between the uterus and the rectum and contains the rectouterine pouch (or Douglas' pouch) (Fig. 20-32). This pouch lies just posterior to the posterior vaginal fornix, a fortuitous relation for transvaginal culdocentesis.

Because of their symmetric location within the pelvis, all of the previously mentioned spaces are best imaged in the mid- and parasagittal planes. Transverse images are also useful, and both planes are usually necessary to fully evaluate pathologic conditions in this area.

MRI demonstrates fat planes within the pelvis quite well. Fat planes around the bladder, rectum, prostate gland, and cervix are especially important to visualize in cases of carcinomas of these structures, all of which tend to invade the surrounding fat.

In the female the broad ligament is seen between the uterus and the lateral wall of the pelvis. It consists of peritoneal reflections and contains the uterine tube and round ligament (ligamentum teres uteri). Transverse and coronal images best display these relations.

SUMMARY

MR of the pelvis is rapidly emerging as a useful imaging modality. The relative lack of artifacts from physiologic motion allows the operator to obtain high resolution images without a significant loss in SNR. This can be achieved in reasonable scan times by using a high matrix (256 × 256) and low number of averages.[1,2]

More than any other region of the body (except perhaps the central nervous system), the symmetry of pelvic structures about the midline allows for excellent imaging in the sagittal plane. As elsewhere, adequate imaging of the pelvis also requires imaging in the transverse plane.

Visceral organs such as the urinary bladder, prostate gland, seminal vesicles, testes, uterus, cervix, vagina, and rectum are evaluated quite well. MRI of these and other pelvic structures cannot yet achieve the spatial resolution of CT. However, MRI provides superior tissue contrast resolution and allows for imaging in multiple planes. For this reason MRI appears to be competitive with, if not better than, CT in many instances.

REFERENCES

1. Baker LL, Hajek PC, Burkhard TK, et al: MR imaging of the scrotum: normal anatomy, *Radiology* 163:89-92, 1987.
2. Baumgartner BR, Nelson RC: MRI delineates anatomy of female pelvic organs, *Diagn Imaging* (December) 68-72, 1989.
3. Bryan PJ, Butler HE, LiPuma JP: Magnetic resonance imaging of the pelvis, *Radiol Clin North Am* 22(4):897-915, 1984.
4. Bryan PJ, Butler HE, Lipuma JP, et al: Magnetic resonance imaging of the prostate, *AJR* 146:543-548, 1986.
5. Crafts RC: *A textbook of human anatomy,* ed 2, New York, 1979, John Wiley & Sons.
6. Demas BE, Hricak H, Jaffe RB, et al: Uterine MR imaging: effects of hormonal stimulation, *Radiology* 159:123-126, 1986.
7. Dooms GC, Hricak H, Tscholakoff D: Adnexal structures: MR imaging, *Radiology* 158:639-646, 1986.
8. Dooms GC, Hricak H, Crooks LE, et al: Magnetic resonance imaging of the lymph nodes: comparison with CT, *Radiology* 153:719-728, 1984.
9. Fisher MR, Hricak H, Crooks LE: Urinary bladder MR imaging. I. Normal and benign conditions, *Radiology* 157:467-470, 1985.
10. Fishman-Javitt MC, Lovecchio JL, Stein HL: Imaging strategies for MRI of the pelvis, *Radiol Clin North Am* 26(3):633-649, 1988.
11. Fritzsche PJ, Smith D: MRI's role in male pelvis includes staging of tumors, *Diagn Imaging* (August) 113-117, 1988.
12. Haynor DR, Mack LA, Soules MR, et al: Changing appearance of the normal uterus during the menstrual cycle: MR studies, *Radiology* 161:459-462, 1986.
13. Heiken JP, Lee JKT: MR imaging of the pelvis, *Radiology* 166:11-16, 1988.
14. Hricak H: MRI of the female pelvis: a review, *AJR* 146:1115-1122, 1986.
15. Hricak H, Chang YCF, Thurnher S: Vagina: evaluation with MR imaging. I. Normal anatomy and congenital anomalies, *Radiology* 169:169-174, 1988.
16. Hricak H, Williams RD, Spring DB, et al: Anatomy and pathology of the male pelvis by magnetic resonance imaging, *AJR* 141:1101, 1983.
17. Hricak H, Alpers C, Crooks LE, et al: Magnetic resonance imaging of the female pelvis: initial experience, *AJR* 141:1119-1128, 1983.
18. Hricak H et al: Gynecologic masses; value of MRI, *Am J Obstet Gynecol* 153(1):31-37, 1985.
19. Hricak H, Dooms GC, McNeal JE, et al: MR imaging of the prostate gland: normal anatomy, *AJR* 148:51-58, 1987.
20. Hricak H, Marotti M, Gilbert TJ, et al: Normal penile anatomy and abnormal penile conditions: evaluation with MR imaging, *Radiology* 169:683-690, 1988.
21. Janus C, Martin A: MRI of the male pelvis: current applications, *Appl Radiol* pp 36-39, 1989.
22. Koslin DB, Kenney PJ, Koehler RE, et al: Magnetic resonance imaging of the internal anatomy of the prostate gland, *Invest Radiol* 22:947-953, 1987.
23. Lee JKT, Rholl KS: MRI of the bladder and prostate, *AJR* 147:732-736, 1986.
24. Lee JKT, Gersell PJ, Balte DM, et al: The uterus: in vitro MR anatomic correlation of normal and abnormal specimens, *Radiology* 157:175-179, 1985.
25. McCarthy S, Scott G, Majundar S, et al: Uterine junctional zone: MR study of water content and relaxation properties, *Radiology* 171:241-243, 1989.
26. McNeal JE et al: The prostate gland: morphology and pathobiology, *Monogr Urol* 4(1):5, 1983.
27. Rholl KS, Lee JKT, Ling D, et al: MR imaging of the scrotum with a high-resolution surface coil, *Radiology* 163:99-103, 1987.
28. Seidenwurm D, Smathers RL, Lo RK, et al: Testes and scrotum: MR imaging at 1.5 T, *Radiology* 164:393-398, 1987.

Chapter 21

FEMALE PELVIS

Cynthia L. Janus
David S. Mendelson

The role of magnetic resonance imaging (MRI) in the evaluation of the female pelvis is evolving. This technique must be assessed in the context of the currently established cross-sectional examinations, namely ultrasound (US) and computed tomography (CT). All three modalities must be judged on the quality of information they provide, the potential harm to the patient, the ease of the examination, and the cost of the procedure.

US in particular has proved to be an excellent modality for evaluating the female pelvis. It is safe even during pregnancy, is relatively inexpensive, and usually depicts uterine and adnexal anatomy well. Its limitations are the inability to demonstrate the deeper portions of the pelvis and to provide tissue characterization. US is thus of little value in the staging of gynecologic malignancies, since pelvic tumor extension cannot be accurately assessed.

CT provides an excellent anatomic depiction of the pelvic anatomy, including several nodal chains relevant to the staging of malignancies, and is currently the mainstay of nonsurgical staging. Interestingly, CT is generally regarded as inferior to sonography in evaluating the uterus and adnexal structures, for although they are identifiable on CT, little morphologic information is provided about these structures. Limitations in soft tissue contrast resolution and the restriction to the axial plane for imaging account in part for the lack of information CT provides regarding the uterus and adnexa. Clearly, the exposure to ionizing radiation is a negative feature of CT, particularly in premenopausal women, and has all but eliminated CT as a useful examination during pregnancy. Optimal CT of the abdomen and pelvis usually is accomplished with the administration of intravenous iodinated contrast agents. However, the associated morbidity and rare mortality associated with these agents is another disadvantage of this examination.

MRI has several features that make it attractive as a technique to evaluate the female pelvis. It competitively, if not superiorly, depicts all pelvic anatomy,[4,12,13,26,54] based on good-to-excellent spatial resolution, the capability of multiplanar imaging, and the fact that the pelvic organs have physical characteristics that result in good MRI contrast resolution. This last feature is exemplified by the demonstration of uterine zonal anatomy as it varies during the menstrual cycle.[11,13,20,25] These qualities are countered by a variety of current drawbacks, in particular, that motion degenerates MR (magnetic resonance) images. Sources of motion include respiration, peristalsis, vascular pulsation, and patient inability to remain still, all four of which can be handled to an extent. For the advantageous reasons given, one anticipates that MRI would be a good imaging technique for evaluation of the female pelvis. Its qualities seem to overlap those of both sonography and CT. MRI appears safe in general[37,53] and is used, although only to a limited degree, during pregnancy. The place of MRI alongside US and CT continues to be assessed by comparative studies. The following discussion reviews the current role of MRI in imaging the female pelvis.

TECHNIQUES

The ability to image in any plane is one of the attributes of MRI. This asset requires the intelligent prescription of an imaging protocol by the radiologist, so as to obtain the most useful information from the examination. Generally, T1- and T2-weighted axial images are obtained (that is, images weighted to the spin-lattice or longitudinal relaxation time [T1] or to the spin-spin or transverse relaxation time [T2]). Such images provide a good overview of the pelvic anatomy, demonstrating the gynecologic structures, as well as nodal chains, deep vessels, bladder, rectum, parametria, and pelvic sidewalls. These images aid in tumor staging and the T1- and T2-weighted images together provide some information regarding tissue characterization.

When evaluating a patient for potential uterine abnormalities, T2-weighted sagittal images are particularly useful (Fig. 21-1). The zonal anatomy of the uterus is best demonstrated on T2-weighted images (T2WI). Since the long axis of the uterus is craniocaudal, sagittal images provide an excellent perspective for viewing this organ. The relationship of uterine masses to the normal portions of the uterus and adjacent organs are assessed well in this plane.

Likewise, the examination can be tailored for evaluation of the ovaries by the addition of coronal images. Separation of the ovaries from bowel loops may be difficult on axial images alone, particularly if oral or rectal contrast agents are not used. T1-weighted coronal images may aid in allowing one to trace the course of the bowel and to help separate these structures from the ovaries (Fig. 21-2).

The fact that the radiologist can tailor the examination should be emphasized. Views other than those suggested above may be added to address questions that arise or are not answered from the routine examination.

Image thickness and spacing are in part determined by the inherent capability of any given machine. Generally, images of 1 cm thickness are obtained. Although many MR units require some gap between images, this should be minimized to maintain good image quality. Thinner sections may provide better anatomic detail when specific problems arise. One must remember that although decreasing section thickness may be desirable ideally, other image quality problems may arise (such as signal-to-noise ratio) that require adjustments in imaging parameters, usually lengthening examination time.

Although most pelvic imaging is performed with whole body coils, the use of surface coils may at times help ad-

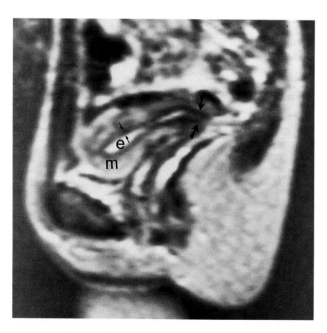

Fig. 21-1. Sagittal T2-weighted image of the uterus shows clear delineation of the normal zonal anatomy. Junctional zone is low signal intensity region between the endometrium and peripheral myometrium. Curved arrows point to the cervix. Junctional zone is between small straight arrows. *e*, Endometrium; *m*, myometrium.

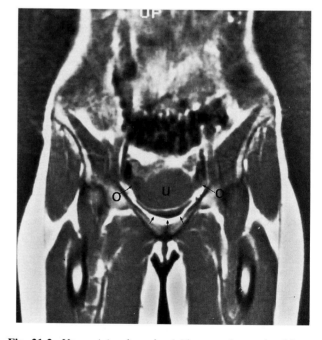

Fig. 21-2. Uterus *(u)* and ovaries *(o)* have moderate signal intensity on this T1-weighted coronal image. Urine-filled bladder (above *arrows*) has low signal intensity. High signal intensity fat surrounding pelvic structures provides good tissue contrast.

dress a specific problem. Again, the selection of such coils varies with the manufacturer. One should be aware of their availability and consider the use of such a coil when a specific problem arises. Usually the coils provide better spatial resolution over a limited anatomic region.

A variety of pharmaceuticals help in performing an MRI examination. If not contraindicated, glucagon (1 mg intramuscularly), minimizes peristalsis and improves image quality. When imaging a pregnant patient, some form of sedation that crosses the placenta can be used to diminish fetal motion and the associated artifacts. If distinguishing bowel from possible masses is a problem, oral or rectal contrast agents may be helpful.[29,35] Such contrast agents may be water, barium, or paramagnetic substances. Positive or negative contrast agents may be used, depending on the substance and whether T1-weighted images (T1WI) or T2WI are performed.

Respiratory gating is not routinely employed; however, in a patient with excessive abdominal wall motion, a significant improvement in image quality may result by the use of respiratory gating techniques.

ANATOMY

T2-weighted sagittal images provide an excellent depiction of uterine anatomy. The corpus and cervix can be identified, and the zonal anatomy of the uterus is demonstrated well, particularly in women of reproductive age. A central band of high signal intensity represents the endometrium. A peripheral zone of intermediate to high signal strength is characteristic of the myometrium. Separating these two zones is a third, low-intensity region, the junctional zone. This last zone is thought to correspond histologically to the inner third of myometrium (Fig. 21-1).[12,13]

The hormonal variations of the menstrual cycle result in characteristic changes in the uterine zones that are reflected in MR images (Fig. 21-3). The endometrial and junctional zones increase in width during the menstrual cycle, with the greatest proliferation in the periovulatory stage. Just before the onset of menses, the intensity of the endometrial zone may abruptly diminish. This is secondary to the presence of blood clots. The lack of hormonal influence in premenarchal girls and postmenopausal women is manifested by an extremely thin endometrial signal, 2 mm or less in width; an indistinct or nonexistent junctional zone; and a slight diminution of the myometrial signal intensity. In postmenopausal women receiving exogenous estrogen, the zonal anatomy is maintained, similar to that of a woman of reproductive age. The use of oral contraceptives may result in endometrial atrophy.[25]

The uterus is identifiable on T1WI, but its zonal anatomy is not (Fig. 21-4). The uterus has a homogeneous intermediate signal intensity and is featureless. Axial T1WI

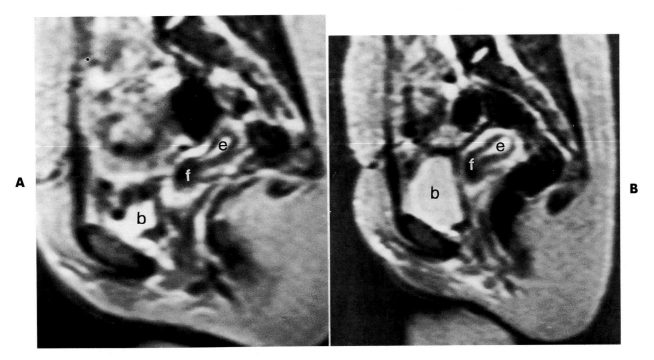

Fig. 21-3. A, T2-weighted image shows zonal anatomy in retroverted uterus on day 6 of the menstrual cycle in woman of reproductive age. Area of low signal intensity in the lower uterine segment represents a fibroid. *e,* Endometrium; *b,* urinary bladder; *f,* fibroid. **B,** On day 12 of the cycle, endometrium has increased in thickness. Note that demonstration of zonal anatomy is not dependent on the degree of bladder distension. *e,* Endometrium; *b,* urinary bladder; *f,* fibroid.

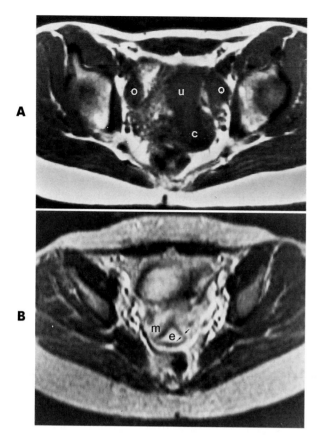

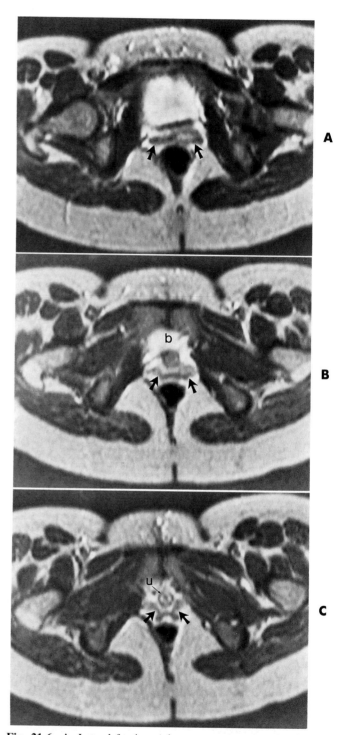

Fig. 21-4. A, Uterus *(u)*, cervix *(c)*, and ovaries *(o)* are identified on this axial T1-weighted image but appear featureless. **B,** Axial T2-weighted image of the uterus in another patient shows zonal anatomy. Junctional zone is between arrows. *e,* Endometrium; *m,* myometrium.

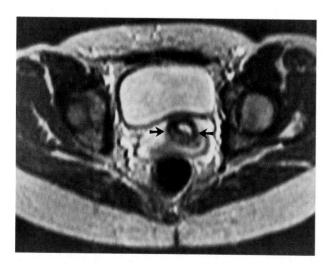

Fig. 21-5. Cervix (between *arrows*) is represented on axial T2-weighted image by high signal intensity of the endocervical glands, mucous centrally, and surrounding low signal intensity fibrous stroma. Pericervical tissues generally have high signal intensity with T2 weighting.

Fig. 21-6. A, Lateral fornices *(above arrows)* mark upper third of the vagina. Vaginal wall has low signal intensity, and vaginal contents have high signal intensity on T2-weighted sequences. **B,** Middle third of the vagina *(above arrows)* is found at level of the bladder base *(b)*. **C,** Urethra *(u)* is seen anterior to the lower third of the vagina *(arrows)*.

serve to demonstrate the relationship of the uterus to adjacent organs and better demonstrate the other anatomic features of the pelvis. The sagittal T2WI also provide an excellent portrayal of bladder or rectal involvement by uterine pathologic conditions.

The cervix is also well-demonstrated on the T2-weighted sagittal view (see Fig. 21-1). Its appearance is less influenced by hormones and appears the same in pre- and postmenopausal women. Centrally, the endocervical glands and mucus produce a band of high signal intensity, surrounded by the low intensity band of fibrous cervical stroma (Fig. 21-5). The pericervical tissues have intermediate signal strength on T1WI and become variably brighter on T2WI.

The normal vaginal anatomy is readily identified on transverse images. Again, the T2WI provide the best demarcation. The upper third of the vagina is identified by the lateral fornices (Fig. 21-6, *A*). The base of the bladder serves as the landmark for the middle third (Fig. 21-6, *B*), with the urethra as a landmark for the lower third (Fig. 21-6, *C*). The vaginal walls have relatively low signal intensity, surrounding a bright central region of high signal intensity that represents mucus. Once again, hormonal variation alters this basic appearance. The central bright band of mucus is thin in both premenarchal girls and postmenopausal women not receiving estrogen supplements. In women of reproductive age the central band generally has greater prominence. With the onset of the secretory phase of the menstrual cycle, this central region thickens, representing an increase in the amount of mucus and enlargement of the epithelium. With changes in the epithelium and vascular congestion at this time, the wall appears brighter to the extent that it becomes difficult to distinguish the wall from the mucus in many patients. Pregnancy, especially during the second and third trimesters, duplicates this latter appearance, with the interface between the thickened vaginal wall and central mucus being blurred. The vagina of postmenopausal women receiving estrogen therapy has an MR appearance similar to that of women of reproductive age during the proliferative phase of their cycles, hence the bright central band surrounded by the low signal intensity of the vaginal walls.

Multiplanar imaging again is valuable in that the sagittal view offers an excellent depiction of the relationship of the vagina to the bladder, cervix, and rectum. The origin and spread of pathologic conditions through these juxtaposed organs and spaces is better demonstrated in several planes.

The ovaries are identifiable on axial and coronal images in women of reproductive age. They may be difficult to identify in premenarchal girls or postmenopausal women. The ovaries have low to intermediate signal strength on T1WI and are difficult to separate from adjacent bowel loops (see Figs. 21-2 and 21-4, *A*). On T2WI the ovaries become bright, compounding the problem of delineating

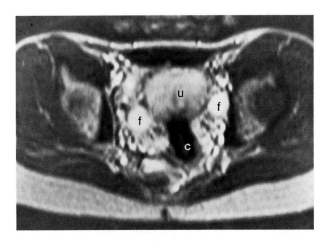

Fig. 21-7. Developing preovulatory follicles *(f)* are seen as high signal intensity structures on T2-weighted axial image. *u,* Uterus; *c,* cervix.

these structures, because they may blend with adjacent fat or unopacified bowel. The combination of axial and coronal images aids in resolving this problem. On T2WI, individual follicles are identifiable (Fig. 21-7), and changes in follicular size can be followed.

MRI also provides reliable pelvimetry data.[34,48] Pertinent pelvic distances and angles that aid the obstetrician in planning delivery can be accurately assessed. These include the anteroposterior pelvic inlet diameter, the interspinal distance, and intertuberal distance. Clearly, this method of obtaining pelvimetry measurements is advantageous in that no ionizing radiation is involved.

Utilizing MRI, the safety and appearance of intrauterine devices (IUD) have been assessed. Several such devices have been suspended in magnetic fields without demonstrating any deflection,[24,39] nor have any heating effects been noted. At least those evaluated would appear safe to image with MRI.

Two of the more common devices, the Copper-7 and Lippes Loop, are identifiable as regions of signal void.[24] One should remember that these structures are viewed in cross section, often oblique to the major axes of the device. Thus the regions of signal void may not resemble the gross structure of the IUD. The signal void of the IUD must be distinguished from that of blood vessels and surgical clips. The latter usually demonstrate some local artifacts, whereas the IUDs mentioned previously do not. MRI may prove useful in confirming the presence and location of the so-called missing IUD, in which the thread has migrated into the uterine cavity.

CONGENITAL ANOMALIES

Congenital abnormalities are evaluated well by MRI, particularly with axial images.* Because the major anoma-

*References 5, 8, 15, 22, 43, 47.

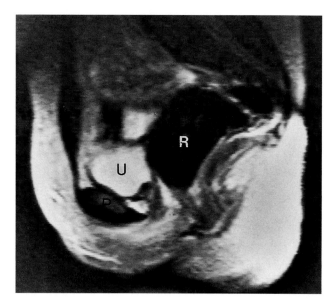

Fig. 21-8. Absence of the uterus and cervix is depicted on a sagittal T2-weighted image. Vaginal atresia is also present in this 13-year-old girl. *U,* Urinary bladder; *R,* rectum; *P,* symphysis pubis.

lies are characterized by absence of the vagina or uterus or improper fusion of their embryologic müellerian ducts anlage, the major function of imaging is full delineation of these organs. This may be difficult on sonography, hysterosalpingography, or CT. In a young patient in whom may be a clinically suspected abnormality, MRI affords an accurate means of fully delineating the female reproductive organs without exposing the patient to ionizing radiation. For example, a newly discovered mass during pregnancy may be identified as a duplication.[22] First, the presence or absence of the uterus and vagina must be established (Fig. 21-8). Patients with hematocolpos or hematometra have primary amenorrhea. These are characterized by the distension of the vagina or uterus by fluid of intermediate to high signal intensity on T1WI and high signal intensity on T2WI. The characterization of the fluid is secondary to the blood in it.

A variety of fusion abnormalities exist. In a bicornate uterus, myometrial tissue forms a wall between two endometrial cavities. The MRI characterization of this tissue is the same as that for the rest of the myometrium. This must be distinguished from septate uteri, in which fibrous bands traverse the endometrial cavity, dividing it. Such fibrous bands have low signal intensity on both T1WI and T2WI. Thus, the two conditions and their variants are distinguishable by tissue characterization. Such differentiation has therapeutic significance. Patients with these abnormalities have a spectrum of obstetric difficulties.

CERVICAL INCOMPETENCE

Cervical incompetence is a condition that results in spontaneous abortion in the second or early third trimester.

Hysterosalpingography and US have proved unreliable in assessing the nonpregnant female suspected of having this problem. US has also proved to have limitations for evaluating pregnant women, and physical examination during pregnancy remains the major means of diagnosis, prompting cerclage. In a study of cervical incompetence, Hricak et al.[19] developed a set of MRI criteria for the diagnosis of cervical incompetence that may prove useful in evaluating women with a history of spontaneous abortions or of exposure to diethylstilbestrol during pregnancy.

BENIGN UTERINE LESIONS
Leiomyoma

The most common uterine tumor is the benign leiomyoma, which occurs in 20% to 30% of women of reproductive age. For infertility, recurrent spontaneous abortion, uterine bleeding, or planning myomectomy, the location, number, and size of the leiomyomas is important.[9,51,56] Sonography, the current mainstay for evaluating patients with such conditions, has several known pitfalls. MRI may be a valuable adjunct examination or may be used alone to provide an accurate assessment of the tumors. The location of the tumors can be accurately categorized as subserosal, intramural, or submucosal.

The uncomplicated fibroid has a characteristic low signal intensity on T1WI and T2WI (see Fig. 21-3). Degenerating fibroids (hyaline, myxomatous, or fatty) create a diagnostic problem for MR. The intensity of these lesions is variable, with particularly high signal intensity on T2WI. The characteristics of these lesions are dependent on their constituents and the presence of hemorrhage. Unfortunately, their MRI characterization overlaps that of malignant neoplasms, and hence the two may not be distinguishable (Fig. 21-9).

MRI is competitive with, if not superior to, sonography in assessing leiomyomas.[51,56] In one study, MR demonstrated leiomyomas located in the lateral and posterior portions of the pelvis better than did sonography.[56] MRI is useful if a pelvic mass does not meet the sonographic criteria of a leiomyoma. If the mass also fails to meet the MRI criteria of a simple leiomyoma, the likelihood that it is a malignant neoplasm is substantial.[51]

Adenomyosis

Adenomyosis is a poorly defined clinical condition that has variable manifestations, including pain, menorrhagia, and an enlarged uterus. The histologic definition is the presence of basalis-type endometrial glands and stroma deep within a hypertrophic myometrium. Several MR findings may be noted. In diffuse adenomyosis the uterus is often enlarged. The low signal intensity band of the junctional zone on T2WI is thickened.[44] This condition also occurs focally and is referred to as an adenomyoma. The appearance of adenomyosis on T2WI may be confused with that of a leiomyoma, because both have low signal intensity. Unlike the leiomyoma, which is well-marginated

of this hormone include extrauterine germ cell tumors and other forms of neoplasia. Thus it is important to establish whether the uterus is indeed the site of the primary tumor. Sonography has been the modality of choice in this regard. CT, notoriously poor for uterine evaluation, is utilized primarily to stage a patient once a tumor has been identified. Such staging usually includes the lungs, entire abdomen and pelvis, and often the brain, all being known sites of metastases.

MRI has proved to be a useful tool for evaluating GTN.[16,27] T2WI demonstrate a high signal intensity mass. The hypervascularity of this mass is distinguishable from the prominent low signal intensity serpiginous structures traversing the tumor and adjacent pelvic structures. This combination of features results in a bubbly appearance of the tumor. The normal zonal anatomy of the uterus is distorted or lost (Fig. 21-10, A and B). The intensity of the tumor on T1WI is similar to that of normal myometrium, making the tumor difficult to detect. However, the presence of prominent vessels may be evident on these images, as well as focal areas of high signal intensity representing hemorrhage (Fig. 21-10, C).

Given the excellent sensitivity of MRI for demonstrating GTN, it is especially useful for evaluating deep myometrial invasion without manifestation on the endometrial surface. Curettage specimens of GTN are negative and not helpful, if not misleading. Associated changes include prominent adnexal theca lutein cysts that are easily identified on MR studies. Invasion of local structures is also well delineated.

Fortunately, successful chemotherapeutic regimens have been developed for GTN. MRI provides an excellent means of confirming tumor regression in the uterus. Conversely, in the rare patient in whom HCG levels remain elevated, MR serves to depict residua within the uterus. At this time, MRI cannot be regarded as a replacement for CT in staging, because the high incidence of pulmonary metastases in these patients necessitates CT scanning and also because MRI is expensive. However, MRI should be considered for staging the abdomen and pelvis in patients in whom iodinated contrast agents are contraindicated.

Cervical carcinoma

Carcinoma of the cervix is one of the most common malignancies of women. The features of the primary tumor are fairly typical,* one being a high signal intensity mass on T2WI that is easily distinguishable from the normal low signal intensity wall of the cervix (Fig. 21-11). These changes are nonspecific, and benign conditions, including nabothian cysts and inflammation, may mimic them. MRI should not be considered a screening modality.

The clinical and radiologic staging (Table 21-1) of the patient are important for determining therapy.[36,50,52] The

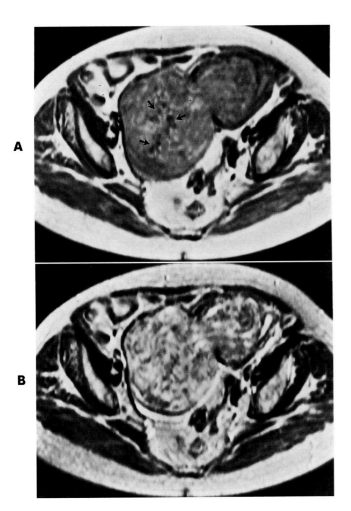

Fig. 21-9. A, Fibroids that are complicated by degeneration or hemorrhage have mixed signal intensity pattern. Axial T1-weighted image shows small areas of signal void that correspond to calcifications *(straight arrows)*. Small areas of high signal intensity represent either fat or hemorrhage. **B,** Axial T2-weighted image through fibroids shows heterogeneous pattern of signal intensity with generalized high signal intensity. This appearance overlaps that of malignant uterine tumors.

and often has a pseudocapsule, a distinguishing feature of the adenomyoma is its interdigitation with the adjacent myometrium and poorly defined margins. On T1WI, adenomyosis blends with normal myometrium.

MALIGNANT UTERINE NEOPLASMS
Gestational trophoblastic neoplasia

The term gestational trophoblastic neoplasia (GTN) refers to three entities that represent a spectrum of benign to malignant neoplasms. The hydatidiform mole is benign, whereas a chorioadenoma is a locally invasive mole. Choriocarcinoma is a malignant process that metastasizes to other organs. Elevated levels of human chorionic gonadotropin (HCG) provide a sensitive means of serologically detecting the presence of choriocarcinoma. Other sources

*References 1, 14, 18, 23, 40, 41, 45, 49.

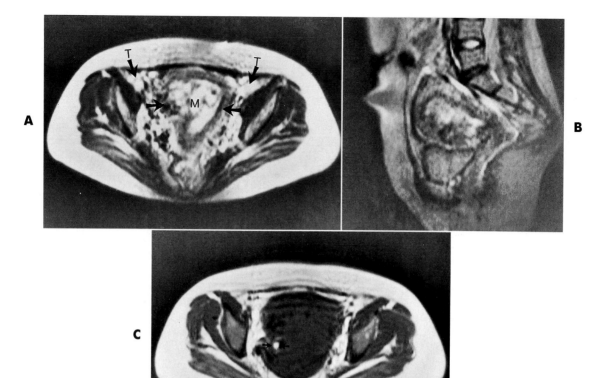

Fig. 21-10. A, T2-weighted axial image of patient with an invasive mole *(M)* demonstrates predominantly high signal intensity tumor filling the uterine cavity *(arrows* point to uterus). Tumor has bubbly or vesicular-like appearance. Low signal intensity areas represent enlarged vessels in the tumor and adjacent pelvic structures. Theca lutein cysts *(T)* are present bilaterally. **B,** Sagittal T2-weighted image shows extension of the tumor into the myometrium and loss of the normal zonal architecture. **C,** Focal area of hemorrhage in the tumor *(between arrows)* is region of high signal intensity on T1-weighted image.

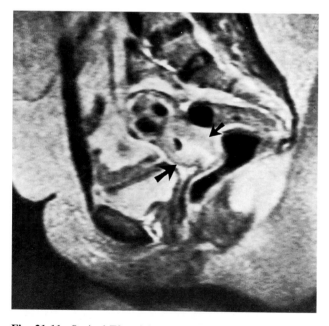

Fig. 21-11. Sagittal T2-weighted image reveals enlargement and abnormal high signal intensity of the cervical region in this patient with cervical carcinoma *(between arrows)*. Focal areas of low signal intensity in the myometrium represent fibroids.

Table 21-1. International Federation of Gynecology and Obstetrics (FIGO) classification in staging cervical carcinoma

Staging	Criteria
0	Carcinoma in situ
I	Carcinoma confined to the cervix (extension to the corpus disregarded)
IA	Microinvasive (preclinical invasive carcinoma)
IB	All other cases of Stage I
II	Carcinoma extends beyond cervix but not to pelvic sidewall or lower third of vagina
IIA	No parametrial involvement
IIB	Parametrial involvement
III	Extension to pelvic sidewalls or lower third of vagina, or ureteral obstruction
IIIA	No extension to pelvic sidewall
IIIB	Extension to pelvic sidewall or ureteral obstruction
IV	Extension beyond the true pelvis or invasion of the mucosa of bladder or rectum
IVA	Spread to adjacent organs
IVB	Spread to distant organs

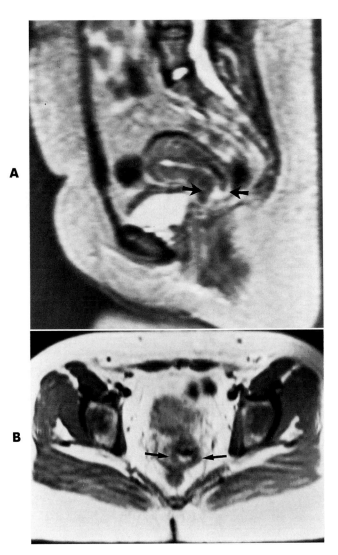

Fig. 21-12. A, Area of high signal intensity is seen in the cervical region *(between arrows)* on T2-weighted sagittal image in patient with early stage cervical carcinoma. **B,** Low signal intensity ring *(arrows)* of the cervix is intact, and parametria are not involved.

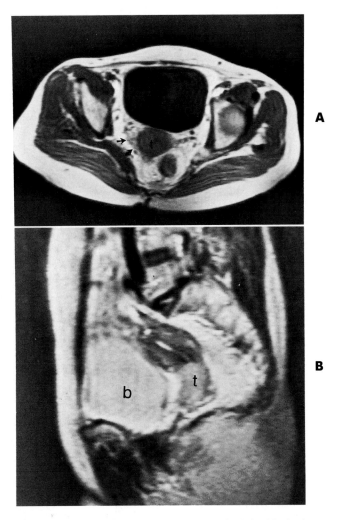

Fig. 21-13. A, Parametrial involvement of the left side is depicted as irregular area of low signal intensity in the paracervical fat on axial T1-weighted view *(arrows)*. *t,* Cervical tumor. **B,** This patient had bulky cervical tumor, which has high signal intensity on T2-weighted sagittal view. *t,* Cervical tumor; *b,* urinary bladder.

lower stages may be treated with surgery or radiation therapy (Fig. 21-12), but the higher stages require irradiation and occasionally chemotherapy. Paradoxically, the current forms of noninvasive staging are inaccurate, often resulting in surgery in a patient with an unresectable tumor.

It is most important to determine whether the vagina (Stage IIA) or pericervical-parametrial tissues (Stage IIB) are involved (Figs. 21-13 and 21-14). Although sagittal T2WI identify the tumor and demonstrate involvement of the uterine corpus and vagina, the axial T1WI and T2WI accurately portray the parametrial tissues. Irregularity of the lateral cervical interface with the parametria and pericervical tissues has proved a highly accurate sign of invasion of these structures.

Several recent studies support this assessment of MRI.[1,18,23,40,45] In a study performed by Togashi et al.,[45] MRI had a 95% accuracy in demonstrating invasive disease (Stage IB or higher), with an 89% accuracy in evaluation of the parametria. The overall staging accuracy in this study was 76%. In a study by Hricak et al.,[18] overall staging accuracy was 81%. All evaluations negative for bladder, rectal, and pelvic sidewall involvement were accurate. There were false positives with positive predictive values of 75% for the pelvic sidewall and 67% for the bladder (Figs. 21-15 and 21-16). Accuracy was high for the two important areas influencing treatment: 93% for evaluation of high vaginal disease and 88% for the evaluation of the parametrial region. Tumor location was accu-

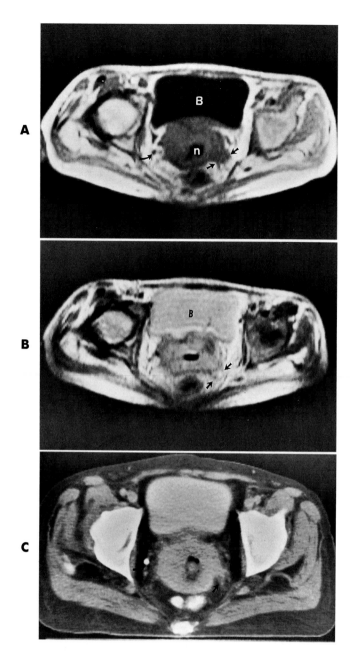

A,

B,

C,

Fig. 21-14. A, Parametrial tumor extension into left side *(arrows)* is represented as nodular soft tissue mass on axial T1-weighted image. Area of low signal intensity within the large cervical tumor represents necrosis *(n).* Curved arrow points to right urter. *B,* Urinary bladder. **B,** Cervical and parametrial tumors increase in signal intensity with T2 weighting. *B,* Urinary bladder. **C,** CT scan corresponding to **B** shows bulky necrotic cervical tumor and parametrial extension on left side *(arrows).* Ureter *(curved arrow)* is easily identified on this contrast-enhanced scan.

rately defined in 91% of the patients and size correctly judged to within 0.5 cm in 70% of the patients. In a study of Stage IB patients, Angel et al.[1] found that MRI proved more accurate in predicting size and extension of the tumor than clinical examination. Kim et al.[23] found that

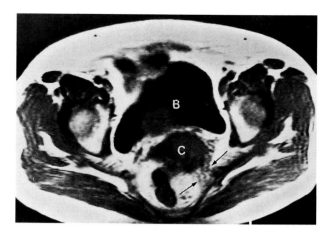

Fig. 21-15. Extension of cervical carcinoma to the left pelvic sidewall *(arrows)* is shown on axial T1-weighted image of patient with stage IIIB cervical carcinoma. *B,* Urinary bladder; *C,* cervical tumor.

MRI with an accuracy of 83% compared favorably to CT with an accuracy of 63% and to clinical staging with an accuracy of 70%. The most recent study by Sironi et al.[40] confirmed the results of Kim et al., demonstrating an overall accuracy of 88% in staging parametrial involvement in patients with disease clinically confined to the cervix. In this regard, sensitivity was 100% with a specificity of 80%.

Certainly, these data suggest that MRI represents an advance in the staging of patients. As the spatial resolution of this technique improves, one can expect the role of MR to increase, since staging has therapeutic implications.

Endometrial carcinoma

Endometrial carcinoma is a common gynecologic tumor in which appropriate staging (Table 21-2) determines whether a patient receives surgical therapy (early stages) or radiation therapy (more advanced disease). Patients with clinical Stage I disease that is confined to the uterus benefit from surgical resection. Unfortunately, a significant number of clinical Stage I patients are found to have more advanced disease, particularly lymph node metastases, at the time of surgery. If the patients were more thoroughly evaluated in advance, they would have been put on radiation therapy protocol.

Limited, small tumors have variable appearance on MR images.[7,17] The normal high signal intensity endometrium seen on T2WI may become heterogeneous or may appear with a low signal intensity region (Fig. 21-17). On T1WI the endometrium may appear normal or become bright. All these changes are nonspecific, and at times no abnormalities may be detected. Some changes are secondary to hem-

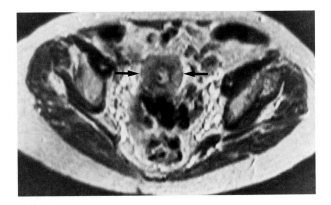

Fig. 21-17. Axial T2-weighted image at level of the uterine fundus (between *arrows*) in patient with biopsy-proven endometrial carcinoma shows heterogeneous signal intensity in the endometrial region. This appearance, however, is nonspecific and does not necessarily indicate a tumor.

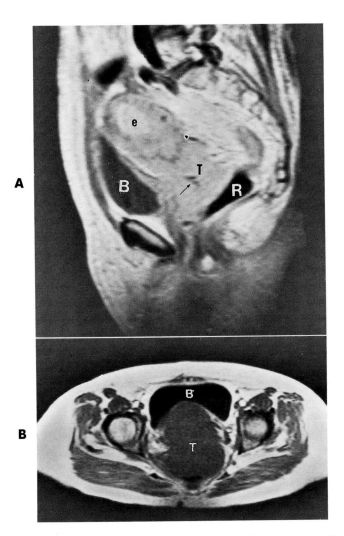

Fig. 21-16. A, Sagittal proton-density image shows patient with advanced cervical carcinoma. Cervical tumor *(T)* is large and bulky and contains area of necrosis *(arrow)*. There is associated obstruction of the endometrial cavity *(e)*. Tumor extends to and was found to involve walls of the urinary bladder *(B)* and rectum *(R)*. **B,** Involvement of the parametria and right pelvic sidewall is seen on axial T1-weighted image in this patient. *B,* Urinary bladder; *T,* cervical tumor.

Table 21-2. International Federation of Gynecology and Obstetrics (FIGO) Surgical Staging of Endometrical Carcinoma

Staging	Criteria
O	Carcinoma in situ
I	Tumor confined to corpus
IA	Tumor limited to endometrium
IB	Invasion of less than half of the myometrial width
IC	Invasion of more than half of the endometrial width
II	Tumor invades cervix but does not extend beyond uterus
IIA	Endocervical glandular involvement only
IIB	Cervical stromal invasion
III	Tumor extends beyond the uterus and adnexa, but not outside the true pelvis
IIIA	Tumor invades serosa and adnexa, peritoneal cystology
IIIB	Vaginal metastases
IIIC	Pelvic or paraaortic lymph nodes
IVA	Tumor invades mucosa of bladder or bowel
IVB	Distant metastasis including intraabdominal or inguinal lymph nodes

orrhage. Thus for early stages of disease, MR has limited value.

The major current niche of MRI is in detecting bulkier Stage I disease and distinguishing it from higher stages, hence nonsurgical cases. The direct identification of extrauterine disease is not only important, but definition of myometrial invasion is also valuable. The incidence of metastases is much greater if myometrial invasion is deep. Detection of such invasion might thus alter patient management. To date, the task of distinguishing Stage I from Stage II disease has not been accurately accomplished without surgery. The early literature suggests that MR has a great contribution to make in this regard.[14]

Interruption of the junctional zone is evidence of superficial myometrial invasion (Fig. 21-18). When this zone is absent, as in postmenopausal women, irregularity of the endometrial-myometrial interface may also indicate superficial myometrial invasion. Extension of the region of abnormal signal intensity across greater than one half the thickness of the myometrium is regarded as evidence of deep myometrial invasion (Fig. 21-19). In a study of 51 patients, 45 with histologic confirmation, Hricak et al.[17] showed MR to have an overall accuracy of 72% regarding

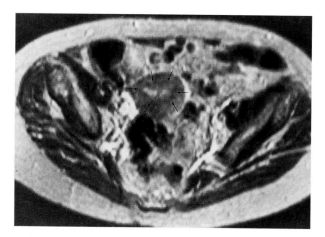

Fig. 21-18. Indistinctness of the junctional zone *(arrows)* on axial T2-weighted image reflects superficial myometrial invasion in patient with endometrial carcinoma.

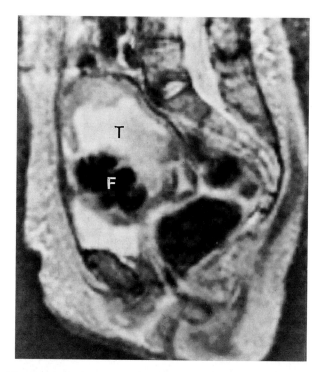

Fig. 21-19. In patient with endometrial carcinoma *(T)* and deep myometrial invasion, tumor is large area of heterogeneous, high signal intensity. Fibroid *(f)*, located anteriorly, maintains low signal intensity on this sagittal T2-weighted image.

staging. The technique was 82% accurate in evaluating the depth of myometrial invasion. Chen, Rumancik, and Spiegel[7] evaluated 50 clinical Stage I patients. Staging was advanced in 18% of the patients by MR imaging. Deep myometrial invasion was accurately predicted in 94% of the patients.

Leiomyosarcoma

This primary tumor of the myometrium has an MR presentation indistinguishable from endometrial carcinoma with myometrial invasion. The tumor is bright on T2WI and may destroy the normal zonal anatomy.[21,38] A complicated benign leiomyoma may mimic this appearance as well. The major attribute of MR is an accurate depiction of the local extent of the tumor.

VAGINAL AND VULVAL TUMORS

Primary carcinoma of the vagina is rare and is identified as a region of increased signal intensity on T2WI. However, it is indistinguishable from inflammatory lesions of the vagina, as well as metastatic disease, particularly from adjacent pelvic organs. MR is useful for staging the local extension of a primary neoplasm once it is identified. In an overall study of all vaginal neoplasms, including primary and metastatic tumors, MRI had an accuracy of 92%.[6] Another promising use of MR is the identification of vaginal tumor recurrence and differentiation of such recurrence from fibrosis. Preliminary data suggest that fibrosis has low signal intensity on T2WI, whereas a tumor is bright.

Tumors of the vulva, including carcinomas and sarcomas, can be delineated on MRI, and the location and degree of extension into adjacent pelvic structures can be assessed[21] (Fig. 21-20).

ENDOMETRIOSIS

Endometriosis is a common condition, usually affecting women in their third and fourth decades of life.[2,55,57]

Functioning endometrial tissue is found outside the uterus, most often in the pelvis. The ovaries are the most common site of involvement, but any organ may be involved. The clinical presentation is quite variable. Endometriosis may be responsible for pelvic pain or infertility, and it may also be an incidental finding at laparotomy or laparoscopy in asymptomatic women. Once diagnosed, patients may respond to hormonal manipulation, although surgical resection may be required at times.

Currently, laparoscopy is necessary to establish a diagnosis. US and CT are not sufficiently sensitive or specific in evaluating patients suspected of having this disease. The MR characteristics of endometriosis have been described.[2,30,33,55,57] The T1 and T2 characteristics of endometriosis demonstrate a wide spectrum, with virtually all combinations of T1 and T2 signals. The presence of hemorrhage and hence the presence of hemoglobin in its various oxidative states is thought to account for the variety of signal intensities.

Like CT and sonography, in two series of patients, MR proved to have limited sensitivity and specificity in identifying endometriosis.[2,55] Zawin et al.[55] demonstrated a sensitivity of 71% and specificity of 82%, whereas Arrive, Hricak, and Martin[2] demonstrated a sensitivity of 64% and specificity of 60%. Both groups of authors concluded that MR should not be used currently as the primary means of evaluating patients suspected of having endometriosis. In a subsequent study, Zawin et al.[57] did find MR useful for

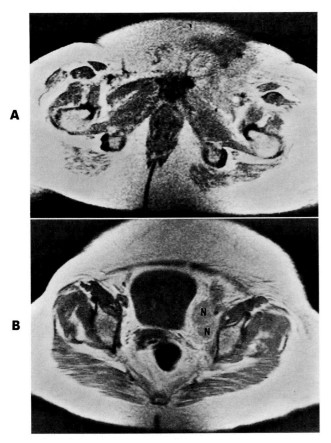

Fig. 21-20. **A,** An irregular and ill-defined area of abnormal signal intensity represents infiltrative tumor and soft tissue edema and extends into subcutaneous fat and pelvic musculature in patient with carcinoma of the vulva. **B,** Lymphadenopathy *(N)* is present along left pelvic sidewall in this patient. Signal intensity of the tumor-replaced lymph node is less than that of fat but greater than that of muscle on this proton-density image. *B,* Urinary bladder.

following patients who had endometriosis and who were subsequently placed on hormonal therapy. These authors recognized that they were only following gross disease and that neither their baseline nor follow-up examinations were accurate portrayals of smaller lesions and fibrosis. However, the response of gross disease may prove to be an adequate indicator of overall response.

OVARIAN LESIONS
Benign

As discussed in the anatomy and technique section, the normal ovaries are delineated with a combination of axial and coronal images. Simple follicular cysts are easily identified. The fluid of such cysts has long T1 and T2 relaxation times, resulting in low signal intensity on T1WI and high signal intensity on T2WI.

All other ovarian cysts, benign or malignant, have a less specific appearance.[31,42] Hemorrhagic cysts, chocolate cysts, and endometriomas have somewhat variable appear-

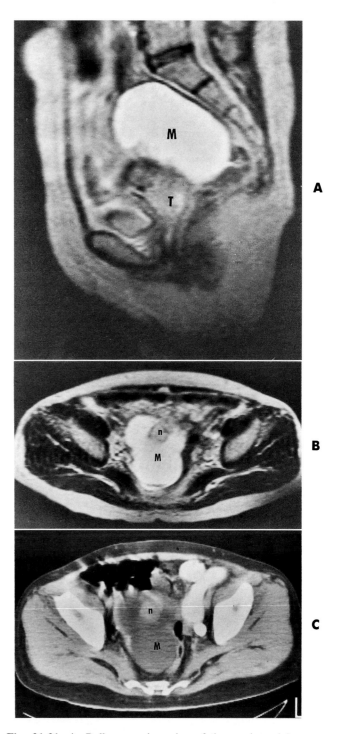

Fig. 21-21. **A,** Bulky mass in region of the cervix and lower uterine segment in this patient is cervical carcinoma *(T).* Large mass *(M)* is also present posterior to the uterus, is largely cystic, and demonstrates high signal intensity on T2-weighted sagittal scan. **B,** On this T2-weighted axial image, solid nodule *(n)* is seen projecting into the otherwise cystic mass *(M),* which is an ovarian carcinoma. **C,** Image corresponding to **B** at level of the ovarian tumor *(M)* from CT examination shows solid nodule *(n)* anteriorly. Extensive areas of low attenuation throughout the remainder of the mass represent the fluid component. Benign and malignant tumors often overlap in appearance on MRI and CT examinations.

ances, depending on the amount of blood products and protein present. Frequently, these cysts have high signal intensities on T1WI and signal intensities similar to that of fat on T2WI. Dermoid cysts also have a variable appearance, not reflecting the contents of any particular tumor.[42] Cystic fat has a characterization similar to the fat elsewhere, but cystic calcification produces a signal void. It is important to recognize that lesions other than the simple cysts previously described may be difficult to distinguish from solid malignant neoplasms. Benign and malignant lesions may have foci of hemorrhage, which contribute to this overlap in appearance.

Ovarian carcinoma

MR is capable of demonstrating ovarian carcinoma,[14,28,32]; however, although a mass can be identified, the findings are nonspecific. The signal characteristics of the mass are dependent on the tumor architecture, which is often complex (Fig. 21-21). On T1WI, cystic and solid

components have low signal intensity and intermediate signal intensity, respectively. On T2WI the cystic regions become bright, but the solid elements tend to maintain intermediate signal strength. Often, signals reflecting hemorrhage are characterized by brightness on T1WI and T2WI. With the great overlap of these findings with benign entities, MR cannot specifically aid in the diagnosis of ovarian

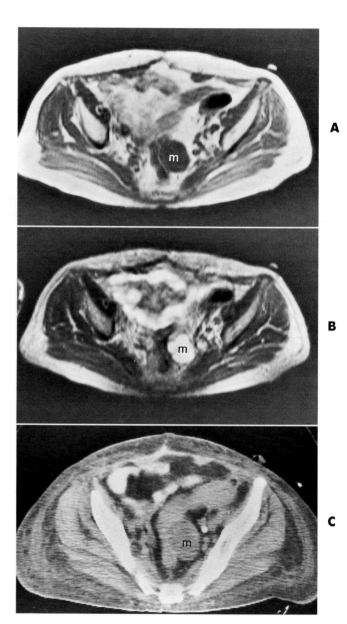

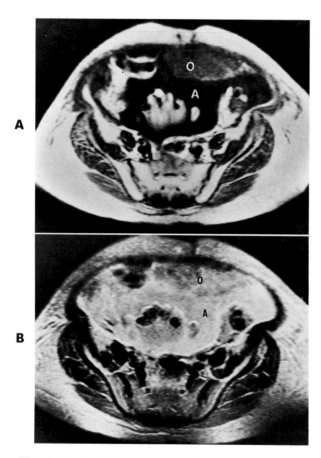

Fig. 21-22. A, Extensive ascites *(A)* are in this patient with ovarian carcinoma. This is represented by extensive areas of low signal intensity surrounding bowel loops. Large mass of moderate signal intensity anteriorly represents omental cake of tumor *(O)* on this T1-weighted image. **B,** On T2-weighted axial image, ascites *(A)* and omental tumor *(O)* increase in signal intensity and are less well-delineated from each other.

Fig. 21-23. A, Mass *(m)* is seen adjacent to bowel loop in patient who has undergone radical hysterectomy for cervical carcinoma. Mass has moderate signal intensity on T1-weighted image and represents recurrent spread of the tumor and associated microscopic invasion of the bowel wall. **B,** On T2-weighted axial image corresponding to **A,** tumor has high signal intensity. **C,** CT scan also shows tumor mass *(m)* and its close relationship to adjacent bowel.

carcinoma, unless metastatic involvement is identified (Fig. 21-22).

Large studies to determine the accuracy of MRI for staging ovarian carcinoma have not been performed to date. For the moment, CT remains the mainstay for such staging. MRI should be regarded as an adjunct for addressing specific problems as they arise.

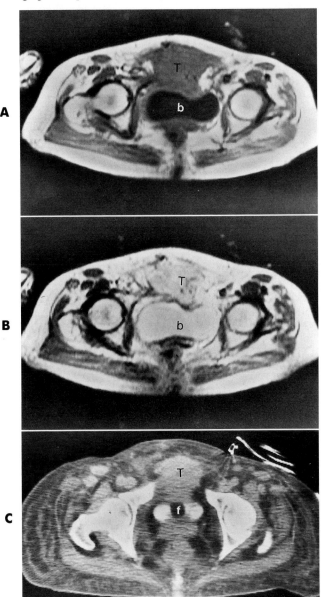

Fig. 21-24. A, Same patient as shown in Fig. 21-22 also had involvement of the lower abdominal wall and urinary bladder *(b)* by recurrent tumor *(T)*. Extent of the mass is well demonstrated on T1-weighted scan. **B,** Tumor *(T)* increases in signal intensity on T2-weighted image, and its borders are less distinct. Areas of active inflammation or acute radiation change may also show high signal intensity on T2-weighted views. *b,* Urinary bladder. **C,** CT scan shows tumor recurrence *(T)* anterior to the opacified, contracted bladder. On CT scan, areas of active inflammation or active tumor are more difficult to differentiate from scar tissue. *f,* Foley catheter balloon.

RADIATION CHANGES

MRI studies of changes in the pelvis induced by radiation have been performed.[3,46] Specifically, the overall signal intensity of the myometrium on T2WI may diminish after high doses of radiation have been given.

Perhaps more importantly, the presence of residual or recurrent tumor has been reliably detected after radiation therapy in patients with cervical carcinoma.[10,46] Neoplastic masses maintain intermediate to high signal intensity on T2WI (Figs. 21-23 and 21-24). Early fibrosis (1 to 6 months of growth) may mimic this appearance, probably secondary to edema or inflammation. Mature fibrosis (greater than 12 months of age) usually demonstrates low signal intensity on T2WI, enabling differentiation from tumor.

SUMMARY

MRI has an expanding role in the evaluation of gynecologic disorders. Clearly this modality, with multiplanar imaging and new forms of soft tissue contrast resolution (T1 and T2) successfully demonstrates normal pelvic anatomy and pathologic conditions. Cost and duration of the examination are currently limiting factors. Sonography remains the first-line modality for the initial evaluation of suspected pathologic conditions. CT is used for specific indications, usually the staging of pelvic malignancies, often with extrapelvic metastases being the focus of the examination. MR often provides supplemental information to the studies. MR may be performed and tailored to address issues that arise from the preliminary studies. On occasion US or CT may provide ambiguous results for technical reasons, and MR may provide the information being sought.

To recognize that MR is a technology merely in its adolescence, if not infancy, is exciting. Technical and pharmaceutic developments are occurring at a rapid pace. Newer and shorter imaging protocols, improved spatial resolution, and spectroscopy are developments that promise faster and more accurate examinations, with the hope of specific tissue characterization. As the number of studies assessing different imaging protocols and the accuracy of MR in the evaluation of pelvic pathologic conditions increases, MRI is likely to have growing importance and to assume a first-line role in many situations.

REFERENCES

1. Angel C et al: Magnetic resonance imaging and pathologic correlation in stage IB cervix cancers, *Gynecol Oncol* 2:357-365, 1987.
2. Arrive L, Hricak H, Martin MC: Pelvic endometriosis: MR imaging, *Radiology* 171:687-692, 1989.
3. Arrive L, Chang YCF, Hricak H, et al: Radiation-induced uterine changes: MR imaging, *Radiology* 170:55-58, 1989.
4. Bies JR, Ellis JH, Kopecky KK, et al: Assessment of primary gynecologic malignancies: comparison of 0.15 T resistive MRI with CT, *AJR* 43:1249-1257, 1984.
5. Carrington BM, Hricak H, Nuruddin RN, et al: Müellerian duct anomalies: MR imaging evaluation, *Radiology* 176:715-720, 1990.

6. Chang YCF, Hricak H, Nhurnher S, et al: Vagina: evaluation with MR imaging. II. Neoplasms, *Radiology* 169:175-179, 1988.

7. Chen SS, Rumancik WM, Spiegel G: Magnetic resonance imaging in stage I endometrial carcinoma, *Obstet Gynecol* 75:274-277, 1990.

8. Dietrich RB, Kangerloo H: Pelvic abnormalities in children: assessment with MRI imaging, *Radiology* 163:367-372, 1987.

9. Dudiak CM, Turne DA, Patel SK, et al: Uterine leiomyomas in the infertile patient: preoperative localization with MR imaging versus US and hysterosalpingography, *Radiology* 167:627-630, 1988.

10. Ebner F, Kressel HY, Mintz MC, et al: Tumor recurrence versus fibrosis in the female pelvis: differentiation with MR imaging at 1.5 T, *Radiology* 166:333-340, 1988.

11. Haynor DR, Mack LA, Soules MR, et al: Changing appearance of the normal uterus during the menstrual cycle: MR studies, *Radiology* 161:459-462, 1986.

12. Heiken JP, Lee JKT: MR imaging of the pelvis, *Radiology* 166:11-16, 1988.

13. Hricak H: MRI of the female pelvis: a review, *AJR* 1115-1122, 1986.

14. Hricak H: Carcinoma of the female reproductive organs: value of cross-sectional imaging, *Cancer* 67:1209-1218, 1991.

15. Hricak H, Chang YCF, Thurnher S: Vagina: evaluation with MR imaging. I. Normal anatomy and congenital anomalies, *Radiology* 169:169-174, 1988.

16. Hricak H, Demas BE, Braga CA, et al: Gestational trophoblastic neoplasm of the uterus: MR assessment, *Radiology* 161:11-16, 1986.

17. Hricak H, Stern JL, Fisher MR, et al: Endometrial carcinoma staging by MR imaging, *Radiology* 162:297-305, 1987.

18. Hricak H, Lacey CG, Sandles LG, et al: Invasive cervical carcinoma: comparison of MR imaging and surgical findings, *Radiology* 166:623-631, 1988.

19. Hricak H, Chang YCF, Cann, CE, et al: Cervical incompetence: preliminary evaluation with MR imaging, *Radiology* 174:821-826, 1990.

20. Janus CL, Wiczyk HP, Laufer N: Magnetic resonance imaging of the menstrual cycle, *Magn Reson Imaging* 6(6):669-674, 1988.

21. Janus CL et al: Uterine leiomyosarcoma—magnetic resonance imaging, *Gynecol Oncol* 32:79-81, 1989.

22. Kelly JL III et al: Magnetic resonance imaging to diagnose a müellerian anomaly during pregnancy, *Obstet Gynecol* 75:521, 1990.

23. Kim SH, Choi BI, Lee HP, et al: Uterine cervical carcinoma: comparison of CT and MR findings, *Radiology* 175:45-51, 1990.

24. Mark AS, Hricak H: Intrauterine contraceptive devices: MR imaging, *Radiology* 162:311-314, 1987.

25. McCarthy S, Tauber C, Gore J: Female pelvic anatomy: MR assessment of variations during the menstrual cycle with use of oral contraceptives, *Radiology* 160:119-123, 1986.

26. Mintz MC, Thickman DG, Gussman D, et al: MR evaluation of uterine anomalies, *AJR* 148:287-290, 1987.

27. Mirich DR et al: Metastatic adnexal trophoblastic neoplasm: contribution of MR imaging, *J Comput Assist Tomogr* 12(6):1061-1067, 1988.

28. Mitchell DG, Mintz MC, Spritzer CE, et al: Adnexal masses: MR imaging observations at 1.5 T, with US and CT correlation, *Radiology* 162:319-324, 1987.

29. Niemi P, Katevuo K, Kormano M, et al: Superparamagnetic particles as gastrointestinal contrast agent in magnetic resonance imaging of lower abdomen, *Acta Radiol* 31:409-411, 1990.

30. Nishimura K, Togashi K, Itoh K, et al: Endometrial cysts of the ovary: MR imaging, *Radiology* 162:315-324, 1987.

31. Nyberg DA, Porter BA, Olds MO, et al: MR imaging of hemorrhagic adnexal masses, *J Comput Assist Tomogr* 11(4):664-669, 1987.

32. Perkins AC et al: A protective evaluation of OC125 and magnetic resonance imaging in patients with ovarian carcinoma, *Eur J Nucl Med* 16:311-316, 1987.

33. Posniak HV, Keshavarzian A, Jabamoni R: Diaphragmatic endometriosis: CT and MR findings, *Gastrointest Radiol* 15:349-351, 1990.

34. Powell MC et al: Magnetic resonance imaging (MRI) in obstetrics. I. Maternal anatomy, *Br J Obstet Gynaecol* 95:31-37, 1988.

35. Rinck PA, Smerik O, Nilsen G, et al: Oral magnetic particles in MR imaging of the abdomen and pelvis, *Radiology* 178:775-779, 1991.

36. Rubens D, Thornbury JR, Angel C, et al: Stage IB cervical carcinoma: comparison of clinical, MR and pathologic staging, *AJR* 150:135-138, 1988.

37. Schwartz JL, Crooks LE: NMR imaging produces no observable mutations or cytotoxicity in mammalian cells, *Radiology* 139:583-585, 1983.

38. Shapeero LG, Hricak H: Mixed müellerian sarcomas of the uterus: MR imaging findings, *AJR* 153:317-319, 1989.

39. Shellock F: MR imaging of metallic implants and materials, a complication of the literature, *AJR* 151:811-814, 1988.

40. Sironi S, Belloni C, Taccagni GL, et al: Carcinoma of the cervix: value of MR imaging in detecting parametrial involvement, *AJR* 156:753-756, 1991.

41. Togashi K, Nishimura K, Itoh K, et al: Uterine cervical cancer: assessment with high-field MR imaging, *Radiology* 160:431-435, 1986.

42. Togashi K, Nishimura K, Itoh K, et al: Ovarian cystic teratomas: MR imaging, *Radiology* 162:669-673, 1987.

43. Togashi K, Nishimura K, Itoh K, et al: Vaginal agenesis: classification by MR imaging, *Radiology* 162:675-677, 1987.

44. Togashi K, Nishimura K, Itoh K, et al: Adenomyosis: diagnosis with MR imaging, *Radiology* 166:111-114, 1988.

45. Togashi K, Nishimura K, Sagoh T, et al: Carcinoma of the cervix: staging with MR imaging, *Radiology* 171:245-251, 1989.

46. Sugimura K, Carrington BM, Quivey JM, et al: Postirradiation changes in the pelvis: assessment with MR imaging, *Radiology* 175:805-813, 1990.

47. Vainright JR, Fulp CJ, Schiebler ML: MR imaging of vaginal agenesis with hematocolpos, *J Comput Assist Tomogr* 12(5):891-893, 1988.

48. Van Loon AJ et al: Pelvimetry by magnetic resonance imaging in breech presentation, *Am J Obstet Gynecol* 163:1256-1260, 1990.

49. Waggenspack GA, Amparo EG, Hannigan EV: MR imaging of uterine cervical carcinoma, *J Comput Assist Tomogr* 12(3):409-414, 1988.

50. Walsh JW, Vick CW: Staging of female genital tract cancer. In Walsh JW, ed: *Computed tomography of the pelvis,* New York, 1985, Churchill Livingstone.

51. Weinreb JC, Barkoff ND, Megibow A, et al: The value of MR imaging in distinguishing leiomyomas from other solid pelvic masses when sonography is indeterminate, *AJR* 154:295-299, 1990.

52. Whitley NO, Brenner DE, Francis A, et al: Computed tomographic evaluation of carcinoma of the cervix, *Radiology* 142:439-446, 1982.

53. Wolff S, Crooks LE, Brown P, et al: Tests for DNA and chromosomal damage induced by nuclear magnetic resonance imaging, *Radiology* 136:707-710, 1980.

54. Worthington JL, Balte DM, Lee JKT, et al: Uterine neoplasms: MR imaging, *Radiology* 159:725-730, 1986.

55. Zawin M, McCarthy S, Scoutt LM, et al: Endometriosis: appearance and detection at MR imaging, *Radiology* 171:693-696, 1989.

56. Zawin M et al: High-field MRI and US evaluation of the pelvis in women with leiomyomas, *Magn Reson Imaging* 8:371-376, 1990.

57. Zawin M, McCarthy S, Scoutt LM, et al: Monitoring therapy with a gonadotropin releasing hormone analog: utility of MR imaging, *Radiology* 175:503-506, 1990.

OBSTETRICS

Lisa M. Langmo
Pablo R. Ros

Sonography is currently the primary imaging modality used in obstetrics. It is inexpensive, widely available, and safe. Magnetic resonance imaging (MRI) has recently been advocated for obstetric indications, especially when sonography is limited by technical factors. MRI is noninvasive, does not use ionizing radiation, and provides images in multiple planes. For these reasons, it is preferable to radiography or computed tomography (CT).

In contrast to sonography, MRI allows simultaneous imaging of the entire maternal pelvis and is not limited by interference from maternal skeletal, fatty, or gas-containing structures. MRI is not dependent on the presence of an acoustic window for imaging deep pelvic structures. Oligohydramnios, which is detrimental to sonography, is ac-

tually an advantage for MRI in that fetal movement is restricted. MRI is usually performed in the third trimester, when fetal movement is restricted by the diminished amount of amniotic fluid, and when the limited field of view of the ultrasound transducer is most limited.

TECHNIQUE

Motion artifacts caused by fetal movement are one disadvantage of MRI. By the tenth week of gestational age, fetal movement may be identified using sonography. The movement becomes more vigorous and frequent and gradually progresses up to a short time before labor.[21] This may cause degradation of MRI images if long acquisition times are utilized. Although motion artifacts may decrease in the later stages of pregnancy, the use of short repetition time (TR) parameters reduces motion artifacts.

Several investigators have suggested various ways to reduce fetal movement. One is for the mother to refrain from eating several hours before imaging, since fetal movement may increase with glucose administration.[23,24] Some reports also claim that obstetric imaging should be performed in the morning because fetal movement is greater in the evenings.[25,26] Fetal immobilization is successfully performed using drugs such as pancuronium, vancuronium, and diazepam.[22,27]

The appropriate pulse sequences and planes for fetal imaging depend to a certain extent on the reasons for the study. Fetal anatomy and presentation are best displayed in the sagittal plane. Placental location and cervical anomalies are also best demonstrated in the sagittal plane.

T1-weighted images (T1WI; images weighted to the spin-lattice or longitudinal relaxation time [T1]) allow the advantage of greater contrast between the uterus and surrounding fat and between subcutaneous fetal adipose tissue and amniotic fluid. T2-weighted images (T2WI; images weighted to the spin-spin or transverse relation time [T2]) improve delineation of the brain and lungs, as well as the internal and external cervical os. T1WI are preferred for pelvimetry because of good delineation of bony and muscular structures. The relatively short acquisition times of T1WI also allow them to be obtained quickly in multiple planes.

FETAL ANATOMY
Central nervous system

Because of the high incidence of multiple anomalies in the fetus with ventriculomegaly, accurate delineation of intracranial pathologic conditions is imperative for obstetric and neurosurgical management.[1,2,4] Although cranial sonography is used for detection of ventriculomegaly, some investigators have reported that MRI has substantiated or significantly clarified the intracranial anomalies identified by US. Abnormalities such as aqueductal stenosis, Dandy-Walker syndrome, encephalocele (Fig. 22-1), hydranencephaly (Fig. 22-2), and porencephaly have been successfully imaged.[1]

In the adult, T1-weighted pulse sequences provide distinct contrast between white matter and gray matter.[3] In contrast, the fetal brain is homogeneous in signal intensity, demonstrating intermediate to low signal intensity on T1WI and higher signal intensity on T2WI. This is consistent with the high water content of the fetal brain: 90% in the 10- to 34-week-old fetus versus 72% in a child.[3] Myelination begins in midgestation and continues into the second decade. The greatest change occurs during the first postnatal year.[3,10,12] The extent of myelination determines the degree of contrast between gray and white matter. Since MRI displays the progression of myelination, it has potential for detecting delays or deficits in brain development. The ventricles, tentorium, falx, and calvarium have low signal intensity, as in the adult brain.

The signal characteristics of the spinal cord are similar to those of the brain. However, the fetal spine is usually visualized only in part. Therefore, spinal meningomyeloceles cannot be imaged reliably.[1,5]

Cardiovascular system

The heart is identifiable in almost all fetuses, but the image plane through the heart depends on fetal position.[5] Consistent assessment of the cardiac chambers is therefore unreliable. The fetal heart and major vessels appear dark on T1WI and T2WI because of the flow void phenomenon. The umbilical vessels and their insertion into the placenta also are well demonstrated by MRI.[3]

Pulmonary system

The fetal lungs are readily examined with MRI. Because of their high fluid content, fetal lungs have low signal intensity on T1WI and high signal intensity on T2WI (Fig. 22-3), reflecting their prolonged T1 and T2 relaxation times. Although the liver has similar low signal intensity on T1WI, the relaxation time of the liver is shorter in T2-weighted sequences. Thus the lower intensity of the liver allows differentiation from the lungs. The fetal lung is easily separable from the low intensity central vascular structures and the thoracic wall. Fetal lung maturation begins at approximately 24 weeks of gestation with the production of surfactant phospholipids.[3,4] As the concentration of surfactant increases, the MR (magnetic resonance) signal is altered because of shortening of the T1 and T2 relaxation times of pulmonary tissue. Currently, the most sensitive indicator of prenatal pulmonary maturity is the lecithin/sphingomyelin ratio of amniotic fluid. Determination of this ratio requires amniocentesis,[7] but this is difficult to perform in patients with severe oligohydramnios. In the future, MRI potentially could provide a noninvasive method of determining lung maturity.

Abdominal viscera

The fetal liver, which occupies much of the fetal abdomen, is easily identified (Fig. 22-4). Its signal intensity is homogeneous and intermediate. A signal change has been noted during the third trimester—most likely caused by

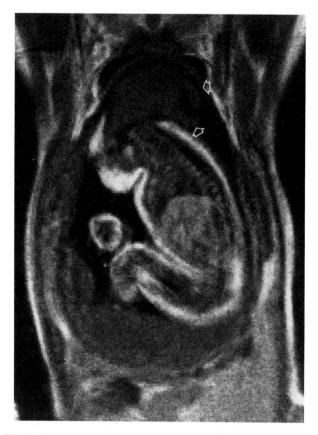

Fig. 22-1. Coronal magnetic resonance (MR) scan with TR of 700 msec and echo time (TE) of 15 msec. Large occipital encephalocele *(arrows)* is visualized just above vertebral column. (From Dinh DH, Wright RM, Hanigan WC: *Childs Nerv Syst* 6[4]:212-215, 1990.)

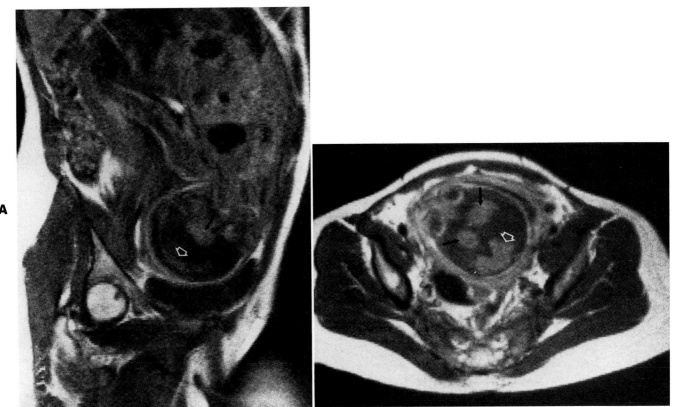

Fig. 22-2. A, Sagittal MR (TR 500/TE 70). Hydranencephaly is demonstrated with basal ganglia *(solid arrows)* and remnant of the parietal cortex *(hollow arrow).* **B,** Axial image at level of the orbits. (From Dinh DH, Wright RM, Hanigan WC: *Childs Nerv Syst* 6[4]:212-215, 1990.)

the change in glycogen composition and declining hemato-poietic function of the liver.[8] The portal and hepatic veins may also become visible.

The fetal kidneys may not be consistently visualized on a limited MRI survey. Bladder identification depends on the degree of its distention by urine, as well as on the plane of section. Urine has a low signal intensity on T1WI and high signal intensity on T2WI. As on sonography, patterns of persistent bladder distention and oligohydramnios (persistent posterior urethral valves), abnormal bladder position (extrophy), or persistent empty bladder (renal anomalies such as infantile polycystic disease) are important diagnostic signs.

Extremities

The musculoskeletal detail that is imaged during the third trimester depends on the amount of fetal motion during the scan time. Scan quality is therefore variable.[3,8] The bone marrow has moderate to high signal intensity, whereas cortical bone produces no signal. Muscle has low signal intensity (long T1, short T2), and fat has high signal intensity (short T1, intermediate T2). Fetal bone, muscle,

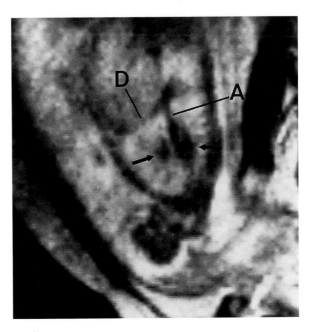

Fig. 22-3. Sagittal MR image (TR 2000/TE 56) gives oblique view of the lungs. Demonstrated are the pulmonary hilar vessels *(arrows),* aorta *(A),* and diaphragm *(D).* (From McCarthy SM et al: *Radiology* 154:427-432, 1985.)

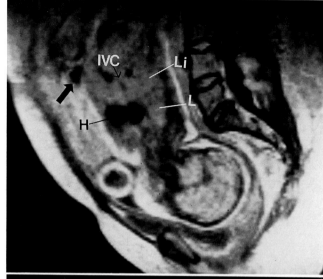

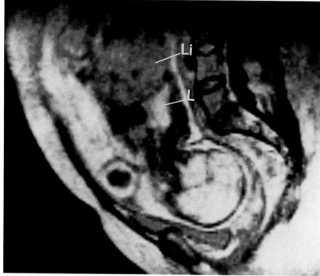

Fig. 22-4. A, MR image (TR 2000/TE 28) showing that fetal lungs *(L)* are intermediate intensity, as is liver *(Li)*. Also note heart *(H)*, inferior vena cava *(IVC)*, and umbilical cord *(arrow).* **B,** On second echo (TE 56), lungs greatly increase in intensity, clearly delineating thorax from liver. (From McCarthy SM et al: *Radiology* 154:427-432, 1985.)

and subcutaneous fat therefore have signal intensities similar to adult tissues. The central and subcutaneous fetal fat stores are easily imaged after 30 weeks of gestation. Measurement of fetal fat stores by MRI may be valuable in assessing intrauterine growth retardation (IUGR), but further work in this area is required.[3,5,8]

MATERNAL ANATOMY

The female pelvic anatomy is particularly well-demonstrated by MR.[9,10] The disadvantages of sonography are significant operator dependence, limitated depth of penetration of the beam, and relative inability to characterize tissues. CT is also limited because it uses ionizing radiation, is distorted by metallic clips, and needs iodinated contrast media. MRI is noninvasive, uses no ionizing radiation, has superb soft tissue contrast, is capable of multidirectional imaging, and demonstrates blood vessels without iodinated contrast agents.

Uterus and placenta

The appearance of the uterus depends on age-related hormonal stimuli. In premenarchal girls the normal uterus is seen as an ovoid structure under 5 cm in length. The cervix accounts for over half the total uterine length as viewed on sagittal MR images. The myometrium has low to medium signal intensity on a short TR sequence and higher signal intensity on a longer TR sequence. The myometrial signal intensity is lower in premenarchal females than in females of reproductive age.[11] The junctional zone, which is thought to be caused by vascular structures located within the inner third of the myometrium, is visible on T2WI but is indistinct.[9-11] Because of the small mass of the premenarchal uterus, the optimal imaging sections are 5 mm thick and contiguous. The MRI appearance of the corpus uteri is greatly influenced by hormone-induced secretory activity and tissue hypertrophy. In women of reproductive age, a T2-weighted sequence shows the high signal intensity endometrium separated from the medium signal intensity myometrium by the low signal intensity of the junctional zone. In the midsecretory phase, the endometrial width increases, and to a lesser extent the myometrial width increases. The signal intensity of the myometrium increases, reflecting its increase in T1 and T2 relaxation times (Fig. 22-5).[9,11]

Women of reproductive age who are taking oral contraceptives have noticeable atrophy of the endometrium, which may limit its visibility in some women. The junctional zone is not well-defined.[11]

In postmenopausal women not taking exogenous estrogen, the endometrium is atrophic and the corpus uteri is small. Thin, 5 mm contiguous sections are ideal for imaging in these patients. Routine 10 mm thick sections may be used in women of reproductive age.

In imaging of the placenta, some researchers have shown that iron and manganese produce dose-dependent decreases in T1 and T2 relaxation times that alter the signal intensity of the placenta.[12] This data suggest future opportunity for noninvasive measurement of transplacental pharmacokinetics, placental flow, and diagnosis of placenta previa and abdominal pregnancies using paramagnetic labels on endogenous substances.

Cervix

MRI is excellent in demonstrating cervical morphology and changes during pregnancy. Three layers can be de-

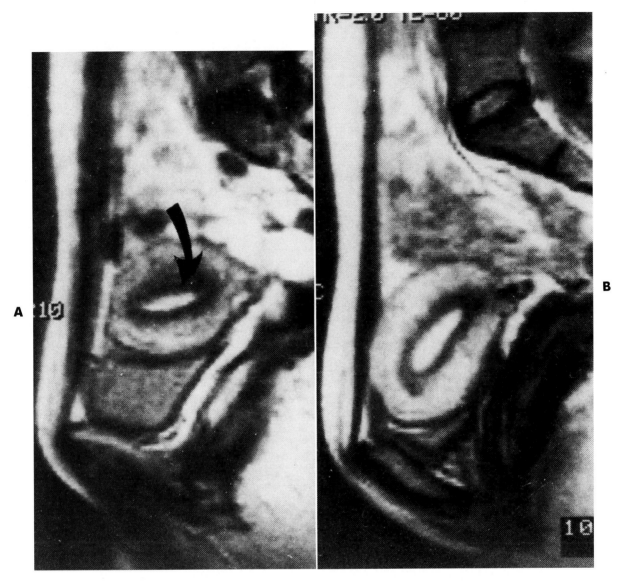

Fig. 22-5. Temporal changes in uterus of a woman of reproductive age. **A,** Sagittal MR image (spin echo, TR 2000/TE 60) obtained during early proliferative phase of the menstrual cycle shows high signal intensity endometrium surrounded by low signal intensity junctional zone *(arrow)*, which clearly separates it from myometrium. **B,** Sagittal MR image (spin echo, TR 2000/TE 60) of same uterus obtained during midsecretory phase of the menstrual cycle shows that widths of the cyclic endometrium and myometrium have increased. Myometrium now has higher signal intensity. (From Demas B, Hricak H, Jaffe RB: *Radiology* 159:123-126, 1986.)

picted: a central zone of high signal intensity, representing cervical epithelium; mucosa surrounded by a low signal intensity stripe, representing stromal tissue; and an outer zone of intermediate signal intensity.[9,10] The length of the cervix is best depicted on sagittal images. The position of the internal and external os are depicted well by MRI (Fig. 22-6).

Although the cervix can be imaged well by transpelvic sonography in many pregnant women, the examination requires a full bladder, which alters the normal cervical morphology. Distension of the bladder causes apposition of the lower uterine walls and elongation of the cervix, obscuring the position of the internal os. This results in errors of judgment regarding cervical incompetence and placenta previa.[10] Because of the risk of hemorrhage, transvaginal sonography is limited when placenta previa is suspected. Using MRI, these problems are avoided, since bladder distension is not required.

Vessels

With the spin-echo (SE) technique, blood flow velocities greater than 10 cm/sec do not demonstrate a signal in

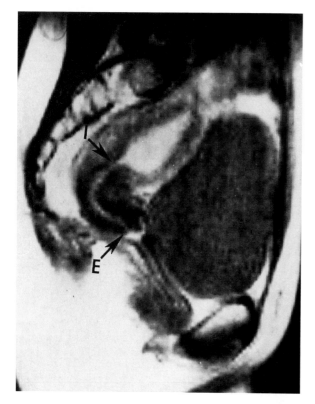

Fig. 22-6. Sagittal MR image of normal 9-week pregnant patient demonstrates elongation of the cervix. *I,* internal os; *E,* external os. (From McCarthy SM, et al: *Radiology* 154:421-425, 1985.)

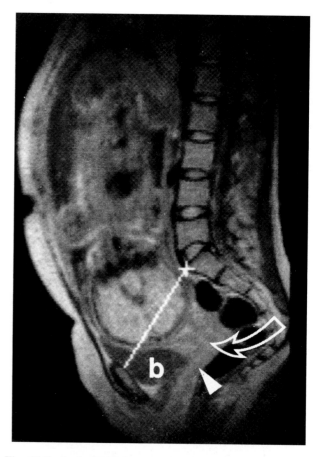

Fig. 22-7. Sagittal MR image at midline shows fetus in vertex presentation with fetal head imaged coronally and maternal pelvis imaged sagittally. Electronic cursor measures distance between inner cortex of symphysis pubis and sacral promontory (±), the anteroposterior pelvic inlet diameter. Maternal cervix *(arrow),* vagina *(arrowhead),* and urinary bladder *(b)* are visualized well. Bony fetal calvaria has low signal intensity and is covered by scalp fat of high signal intensity. (From Stark DD, et al: *AJR* 144:947-950, 1985.)

MRI.[13] As the velocity of flow decreases, the signal increases. The more intense the signal, the slower the flow.

Venous congestion occurs in late pregnancy. The maternal pelvic veins may be two to three times the size of their arterial counterparts and may exhibit high signal intensity, particularly on the second echo. The inferior vena cava may be greatly compressed or not visible. Multiple venous channels, not seen in nonpregnant patients, are noted. Ovarian veins are visible and enlarged.[10] During pregnancy, venous stasis may result in pedal edema, varicose veins, and pulmonary embolization, the second leading cause of maternal death. In the future, MRI may be used to quantitate and monitor the degree of pelvic and abdominal venous stasis.

Pelvis

MRI dimensions for pelvimetry are reliable, with measurement errors caused by the instrument being less than 1% in the sagittal and transverse planes using the SE technique. Sagittal images centered 5 cm below the maternal umbilicus identify the anteroposterior pelvic inlet diameter and demonstrate the presentation and lie of the fetus (Fig. 22-7). Transverse slices centered 5 cm above the symphysis pubis include one section through the widest transverse inlet diameter. A more caudal section through the ischial

spines gives the midpelvis diameter (Fig. 22-8). Patients are positioned supine for the whole examination, which takes approximately 18 minutes.[14] Delineation of maternal pelvic dimensions is unaffected by uterine or fetal motion. Cortical bone is sharply defined as a low signal intensity line on all SE images.

MRI is a completely noninvasive technique for evaluating fetal and pelvic proportions and provides more soft tissue information than radiographic techniques. Plain film pelvimetry has the disadvantages of heavy exposure of the mother and fetus to ionizing radiation and geometric distortion caused by magnification. CT pelvimetry provides soft tissue information at the expense of radiographic exposure, but more careful patient centering is required than with MRI.

Pelvimetry is of value particularly in breech presentations, since evidence of cephalopelvic disproportion or un-

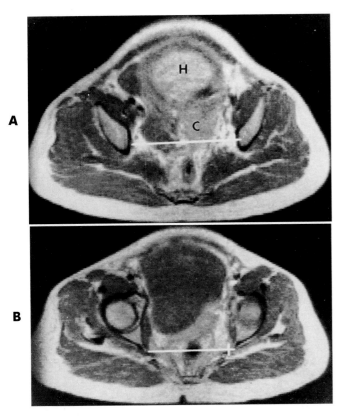

A

B

Fig. 22-8. A, Transverse MRI at pelvic inlet. Vertex of fetal head *(H)* and part of cervix *(C)* are identified. Transverse inlet diameter is measured at its widest point. **B,** Transverse MRI at midpelvis. Measurement of transverse (bispinous) midpelvis diameter is shown. (From Stark DD, et al: *AJR* 144:947-950, 1985.)

favorable pelvic configuration can support a clinical decision to perform a cesarean delivery.

PLACENTAL ABNORMALITIES

For technical reasons, placental abnormalities such as placenta previa and abruptio placenta are sometimes poorly depicted by sonography. MRI offers superb delineation of the cervix during pregnancy and demonstrates the relationship of the cervix to the placenta. Since MRI does not require filling of the bladder, the cervical-placental relationship is depicted well.[8]

Abruptio placentae

Normally the placenta and uterine wall are effaced during pregnancy. If an acute hemorrhage has occurred, separating the uterus from the placenta, the hemorrhage has medium signal intensity on T1WI, which is typically less than the signal intensity of the placenta or uterine wall. A subacute hemorrhage has high signal intensity relative to that of the placenta and uterus on T1WI. Coronal, sagittal, or transverse planes may be required to demonstrate abruptio placentae, depending on the position of the placenta.

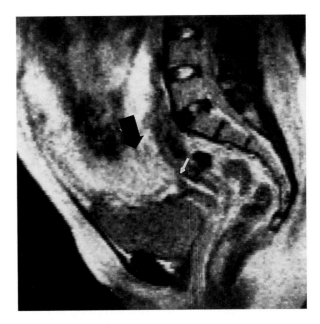

Fig. 22-9. Sagittal MR image (TR 2.0, TE 28) demonstrates that location of the internal os *(small arrow)* relative to placenta previa *(large arrow)* is readily discerned.

Placenta previa

The relationship of the inferior extent of the placenta to the internal cervical os is superbly delineated with MRI (Fig. 22-9). Bladder filling is not required, thus avoiding distortion of the anatomy and providing more accuracy in distinguishing marginal from complete placenta previa. The relationship of the placenta and the cervical os is rendered best by sagittal images.

INTRAUTERINE GROWTH RETARDATION

Intrauterine growth retardation (IUGR) significantly increases perinatal morbidity and mortality and is associated with long-term neurologic impairment. Therefore, early detection is needed to improve perinatal management. Sonography currently is the most useful test for diagnosing IUGR. However, the ability of sonography to separate normal and growth-retarded fetuses is hampered by the normal variation in body size and by uncertainty of gestational age in patients evaluated only in the third trimester. Oligohydramnios also limits the sonographic examination and obscures the boundaries between fetal soft tissues, placenta, and uterus.

The characteristic high amplitude MRI signal of fat allows clear delineation of subcutaneous and intraabdominal adipose tissue.[16] Amniotic fluid and skeletal muscle have long T1 relaxation times. Differentiation of fluid and muscle from fat tissue is best obtained with a T1-weighted sequence such as a short TR (0.5 sec) spin-echo technique.[15]

Preliminary studies show that subcutaneous scalp and facial fat are easily demonstrated by MRI, whereas fat in the extremities and trunk are not visualized well. This is

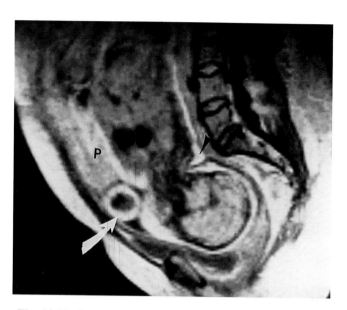

Fig. 22-10. Large amount of subcutaneous fat is in macrosomic fetus of a diabetic mother. Upper extremity *(arrow)*, shoulder *(arrowhead)*, and anterior placenta *(P)* are shown. Oligohydramnios is present; a small amount of amniotic fluid *(dark)* surrounds the upper extremity. (From Stark DD, et al: *Radiology* 155:425-427, 1985.)

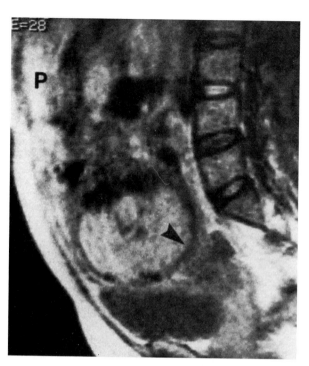

Fig. 22-11. MRI shows absent subcutaneous fat. Infant is determined to have IUGR by sonography, birthweight, and clinical criteria. Bony calvaria *(arrowhead)* is immediately adjacent to the internal cervical os without intervening subcutaneous fat. *P,* anterior placenta. (From Stark DD, et al: *Radiology* 155:425-427, 1985.)

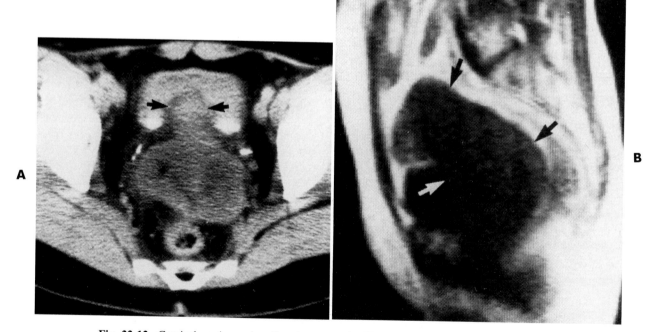

Fig. 22-12. Cervical carcinoma invading the uterus. **A,** CT scan shows enlargement of uterus and prominent lobulation of the anterior border *(arrows)*. Decreased attenuation inside the uterine mass represents necrosis. **B,** Sagittal MRI (SE; TR, 250, TE 30) shows enlargement of uterus *(arrows)*. MRI defines edges of the bowel and bone in relation to enlarged uterus. (From Butler H, et al: *AJR* 143:1263, 1984.)

perhaps because of the greater variability in the size of these fat deposits.[15] Also, although the range of normal percentages of body fat in normal infants is large, it is still possible to discern a difference among healthy infants, infants of diabetic mothers, and infants with growth retardation (Figs. 22-10 and 22-11).[16] With further clinical and investigational experience, MRI may help distinguish small babies suffering from IUGR from babies who are small but otherwise normal. MRI may also enhance the understanding of the metabolic consequences of IUGR.

PATHOLOGIC CONDITIONS OF THE CERVIX
Cervical incompetence

As mentioned previously, a distended urinary bladder, which is required for sonography, acts as a mass that alters normal cervical morphology and may disguise pathologic conditions. Distension of the bladder compresses and elongates the cervix. Thus, an abnormally shortened, incompetent cervix may appear normal. Membranes and amniotic fluid also invaginate into the cervical canal because of the opened internal os. The distended bladder expresses this fluid and obscures the sign.[10] MRI does not require any bladder filling and thus avoids these problems.

Cervical malignancies

Carcinoma of the cervix is the second most common gynecologic cancer. The prognosis falls steeply from stage I to stage IV disease with 5-year survival rates of 90% for those with stage I disease and approximately 15% for those with stage IV disease.[17]

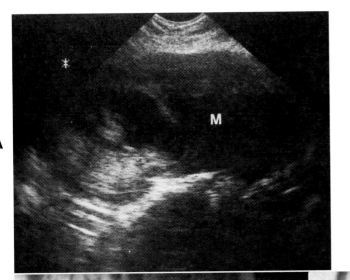

A

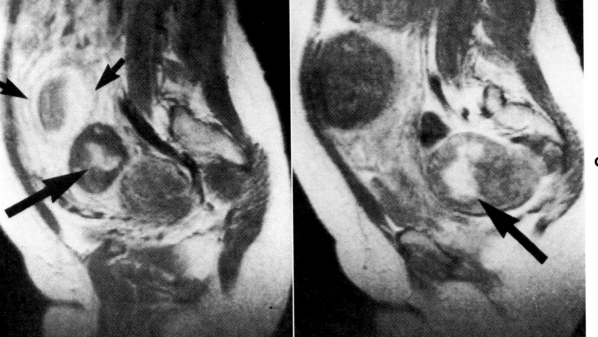

B

C

Fig. 22-13. Multiple leiomyomas (surgically proven) in a patient. **A,** Transverse ultrasound scan shows large mass *(M)* arising from left side of the uterus. Its full extent could not be determined. **B** and **C,** Parasagittal SE MR images (TR 2000, TE 30) identify 10 low signal intensity uterine leiomyomas (not all are shown). Some contained high signal intensity regions *(large arrows),* which represent areas of degeneration. Small arrows point to gestational sac. (From Weinreb JC, et al: *Radiology* 159:715-720, 1986.)

Accuracy in staging is important, since staging determines the type of treatment offered to patients. Clinical assessment of parametrial involvement, spread to the pelvic sidewall, and metastasis to regional lymph nodes is difficult and may result in staging errors.[17-19]

Until recently, CT was the only imaging technique available for directly assessing parametrial and pelvic sidewall involvement. Although reported accuracy rates of MRI staging vary, it has been used with promising results. On T2WI a cervical neoplasm has high signal intensity that is distinguishable from normal cervical tissue. On T1WI a cervical neoplasm is isointense with the normal cervical tissue, and only gross parametrial extension causing contour abnormalities can be visualized. Sagittal views are most helpful in assessing tumor extension into the bladder, body of the uterus, or vagina (Fig. 22-12). Parametrial extension is diagnosed by the asymmetric appearance of the parametrium or by abnormal tumor intensity extending into the parametrial region.[9,17] With invasion of the full thickness of the stroma, microscopic parametrial spread cannot be excluded. The presence of paraaortic or common iliac lymphadenopathy indicates the need to consider extended-field radiotherapy. (See Chapter 21 for further discussion of cervical carcinoma.) MRI is the imaging technique of choice to evaluate a pregnant woman with carcinoma of the cervix. Determination of appropriate management of the delivery is expedited by knowledge of the extent of the disease and the distortion of pelvic anatomy.

PELVIC MASSES

The identification of a pelvic mass in a pregnant patient presents a difficult diagnostic challenge. Ultrasound has been the technique of choice for assessment because of the lack of ionizing radiation. However, ultrasound may be difficult to perform in some patients because of a large gravid uterus, overlying bowel gas, or obesity. Even when a mass is identified, its origin and extent may be difficult to determine. Its lack of ionizing radiation, multiplanar imaging capabilities, and ability to clearly depict uterine anatomy make MRI a useful alternative for patients in whom sonography is limited or for whom a precise anatomic determination is critical.

Leiomyoma is the most common uterine neoplasm. MRI provides a more accurate assessment than sonography of the number, size, and precise location of leiomyomas.[11,21] Also, the relationship of these masses to the fetus and vagina are more apparent on MRI.[21] This occasionally helps in determining the best route of delivery or in evaluating the necessity for myomectomy. Leiomyomas have a uniform low signal intensity on T1WI and T2WI. Degenerative leiomyomas demonstrate heterogeneous signal intensity on T2WI (Fig. 22-13).

The origin of ovarian masses is more clearly depicted with MRI because of the direct multiplanar imaging capa-

bility. Simple ovarian cysts appear as well-circumscribed, homogeneous masses with almost imperceptible walls. Cysts have low signal intensity on T1WI and high signal intensity on T2WI. MRI cannot distinguish between the solid component of hemorrhage and malignant lesions, nor can it differentiate old hemorrhage from fat.

MRI with fat suppression and gadopentetate dimeglumine contrast agent is helpful in distinguishing neoplastic from hemorrhagic masses. The use of contrast agents in obstetrics, although not an indication approved by the Food and Drug Administration (FDA), should be considered on an individual basis.

REFERENCES

1. Averette HE et al: Staging of cervical cancer, *Clin Obstet Gynecol* 18:215-232, 1975.
2. Chervenak FA et al: Outcome of fetal ventriculomegaly, *Lancet* 2:179-181, 1984.
3. Cobby M, Browning J, Jones A, et al: Magnetic resonance imaging, computed tomography and endosonography in the local staging of carcinoma of the cervix, *Br J Radiol* 63:673-679, 1990.
4. Deans HE, Smith FW. Lloyd DJ, et al: Fetal fat measurement by magnetic resonance imaging, *Br J Radiol* 62:603-607, 1989.
5. Demas B, Hricak H, Jaffe RB: Uterine MR imaging: effects of hormonal stimulation, *Radiology* 159:123-126, 1986.
6. Dinh DH, Wright RM, Hanigan WC: The use of magnetic resonance imaging for the diagnosis of fetal intracranial anomalies, *Childs Nerv Syst* 6(4):212-215, 1990.
7. Gelman SR et al: Fetal movements and ultrasound: effects of intravenous glucose administration, *Am J Obstet Gynecol* 137:459-461, 1980.
8. Hallman M, Teramo K: Measurement of the lecithin/sphingomyelin ratio and phosphatidylglycerol in amniotic fluid: an accurate method of the assessment of fetal lung maturity, *Br J Obstet Gynaecol* 88:806-813, 1981.
9. Hanigan WC et al: Medical imaging of fetal ventriculomegaly, *J Neurosurg* 64:575-580, 1986.
10. Hill MC, Lande IM, Larsen JW: Prenatal diagnosis of fetal anomalies using ultrasound and MRI, *Radiol Clin North Am* 26(2):287-306, 1988.
11. Hricak H: MRI of the female pelvis: a review, *AJR* 146(6):1115-1122, 1986.
12. Kaufman L et al: Evaluation of NMR imaging for detection and quantitation of obstruction in vessels, *Invest Radiol* 17:554-560, 1982.
13. Laggasse LD et al: Results and complications of operative staging in cervical cancer: experience of the Gynecologic Oncology Group, *Gynecol Oncol* 9:90-98, 1980.
14. Mattison DR et al: Magnetic resonance imaging: a noninvasive tool for fetal and placental physiology, *Radiol Reprod* 38:39-49, 1988.
15. McCarthy SM, Filly RA, Stark DD, et al: Obstetrical magnetic resonance imaging: fetal anatomy, *Radiology* 154:427-432, 1985.
16. McCarthy SM, Stark DD, Filly RA, et al: Obstetrical magnetic resonance imaging: maternal anatomy, *Radiology* 154:421-425, 1985.
17. Miller FC, Skiba H, Klapholz H: The effect of maternal blood sugar levels in fetal activity, *Obstet Gynecol* 52:662-665, 1978.
18. Minors DS, Waterhouse JM: The effect of maternal posture, meals, and time of day on fetal movements, *Br J Obstet Gynaecol* 86:717-723, 1979.
19. Patrick J et al: Human fetal breathing movements and gross fetal body movements at 34 to 35 weeks of gestation, *Am J Obstet Gynecol* 130:693-699, 1978.

20. Possmayer F: The perinatal lung. In Jones C, ed: *The biochemical development of the fetus and neonate,* Amsterdam, 1982, Elsevier Biomedical.

21. Powell MC et al: Magnetic resonance imaging (MRI) in obstetrics, *Br J Obstet Gynaecol* 95:38-46, 1988.

22. Sadovsky E, Polishuk WZ: Fetal movements in utero: nature, assessment, prognostic value, timing of delivery, *Obstet Gynecol* 50:49-55, 1977.

23. Stark DD, McCarthy SM, Filly RA, et al: Intrauterine growth retardation: evaluation by magnetic resonance, *Radiology* 155:425-427, 1985.

24. Stark DD, McCarthy SM, Filly RA, et al: Pelvimetry by magnetic resonance imaging, *AJR* 144:947-950, 1985.

25. Tomá P, Lucigrai G, Dodero P, et al: Prenatal detection of an abdominal mass by MR imaging performed while the fetus is immobolized with pancuronium bromide, *AJR* 154:1049-1050, 1990.

26. Weinreb JC, Lowe T, Cohen JM, et al: Human fetal anatomy: MR imaging, *Radiology* 157:715-720, 1985.

27. Weinreb JC, Brown CE, Lowe TW, et al: Pelvic masses in pregnant patients: MR and US imaging, *Radiology* 159:717-724, 1986.

Chapter 23

MALE PELVIS

Gladys M. Torres

Magnetic resonance imaging (MRI) has emerged as an important imaging modality in the evaluation of the male pelvis. During the last few years its role in pelvic imaging has grown. Among the features that make MRI suitable for studying the pelvis are the relative freedom from respiratory motion artifacts and the superb natural soft tissue contrast resolution provided by abundant pelvic fat. The capacity to produce images in multiple planes makes MRI ideal for evaluation of complex anatomic features and for assessment of local tumor spread. These properties makes MRI an ideal imaging modality for evaluating of prostatic carcinoma.

COMPARISON OF CT AND MRI

Although computed tomography (CT) has superior spatial resolution, it has less contrast resolution than MRI.[1] Another disadvantage of CT is that significant image degradation occurs when reformatting to coronal or sagittal planes is attempted. CT is limited in the evaluation of the pelvis after surgery because surgical clips create streak artifacts; in addition, beam hardening, usually from adjacent bone, degrades CT images. Surgical clips produce no significant artifacts on MRI. CT uses ionizing radiation and usually intravenous (IV) contrast agents. MRI uses no ionizing radiation and shows superb soft tissue contrast resolution without the use of IV contrast agents.

The limitations of MRI are relatively few for imaging the pelvis; however gastrointestinal MRI contrast agents, lower examination cost, and reduced examination time would be helpful.

TECHNIQUES

MRI of the pelvis requires no special bowel preparation other than no oral intake within 3 hours of the study. Administration of 400 ml of barium through the rectum improves delineation of the colon. Three cups of barium given orally over a period of about 1 hour improve small bowel delineation and reduce artifacts from bowel contents. Patients are scanned in the supine position with an abdominal compression belt and a respiratory compensation transducer applied.

The pelvis is evaluated with a body coil, simple surface coils, Helmholtz coil or endorectal coil. The Helmholtz coil is designed for imaging small anatomic areas with limited motion and is well-suited for evaluation of the prostate gland.[38] Because of the enhanced signal-to-noise ratio (SRN) of the Helmholz coil, the images obtained have superior anatomic detail. The limited field of view of this coil limits the size of the organ that can be evaluated and makes precise patient positioning important. The endorectal coil consists of a surface coil mounted in the inner surface of a balloon and an outer concave-shaped balloon on its anterior border. The main advantage of endorectal coils is better imaging of the prostatic capsule and seminal vesicles and identification of the neurovascular bundle.[9,42] Endorectal coils have improved resolution and SNR, providing increased conspicuity of prostatic lesions.

The basic pulse technique for the pelvis is T1-weighted

(i.e., weighted to the spin-lattice or longitudinal relaxation time [T1]) spin-echo (SE) sequence with a repetition time (TR) of 400 to 600 msec and echo time (TE) 15 to 20 msec. This sequence is performed in the coronal and axial planes. A matrix of 256 × 192 pixels, slice thickness of 5 to 10 mm, and three excitations are used. The coronal series serves as a localizer for the axial images. T1-weighted images (T1WI) are useful for definition of normal pelvic anatomy, for assessment of tumor extension into the pelvic fat, and for detection of lymphadenopathy.

Axial T2-weighted images (T2WI) (weighted to the spin-spin or transverse relaxation time [T2]) are done using a TR of 2000 to 2700 msec and TE of 20 to 80 msec. A T2-weighted sequence is essential because diseases and internal zonal anatomy of the prostate gland and muscular bladder wall are better demonstrated than with T1WI.[19] Sagittal T2-weighted sequences also are done if the patient has a history of pelvic masses or rectal masses. Gradient echo is performed to demonstrate flow within the vessels. A breath-hold gradient-echo sequence reduces motion artifacts and improves imaging quality. Multiple 10 mm axial views are taken to cover the entire region of interest.

ANATOMY
Prostate gland and seminal vesicles

Understanding the prostatic anatomy and the surrounding structures is important in evaluating prostatic pathologic conditions. MR demonstrates the different zonal anatomies described by McNeal and colleagues in the mid-1960s.[30,31,33] They divided the prostate gland into three distinct areas: anterior, central, and (true) glandular. The anterior region is composed of fibromuscular stroma. The central or inner portion is a combination of the smooth muscle of the internal sphincter, the transitional zone, and the periurethral glandular tissue. The glandular region (peripheral) is composed of central and peripheral zones. The central zone extends from the base of the gland to the level of the verumontanum and posterior to the urethra to surround the ejaculatory ducts. It occupies about 20% of the gland in young men, and it atrophies with age, usually being replaced with benign prostatic hypertrophy.[13] The peripheral zone composes the lateral margins of the prostate gland and is posterior to the central zone and inferior prostatic urethra. It occupies nearly 75% of the glandular tissue and is the site of origin of most prostatic carcinomas.

On T1WI the normal prostate gland has intermediate signal intensity without differentiation of the zonal anatomy (Fig. 23-1).[16] T1-weighted sequences demonstrate the periprostatic fat, which appears as a thin structure with relatively high signal intensity. The periprostatic venous plexus is identified as serpiginous structures anteriorly and laterally to the gland in the periprostatic fat at the apex and at the posterolateral aspect of the prostate-bladder-base junction. On gradient-echo images in which flow compensation techniques are used, the serpiginous structures have high signal intensity.

The zonal anatomy of the prostate gland is better demonstrated with T2-weighted pulsing sequences.[24,40] The peripheral zone appears higher in signal intensity, perhaps because it has more water content and glandular stroma, less protein, or less fibrous stroma than the central zone. The central zone appears hypointense because of its shorter T2 relaxation time. This is explained by the compact arrangement of the muscle fiber bundles in this region.[16] The zonal anatomy is best seen on axial and coronal images (Fig. 23-2).

The prostatic urethra has a higher signal intensity on T2WI and is surrounded by the lower signal intensity of the urethral mucosa (Fig. 23-3).[16] Anterior to the urethra, the area of fibromuscular stroma appears as a low signal intensity region that is best seen on sagittal views.

The prostatic capsule is not always identified. On T2WI (in the cases in which it can be identified), the prostatic capsule appears as a thin rim of low signal intensity at the periphery of the gland.[36] The prostate gland is distinguishable from adjacent structures by the capsule or by the periprostatic fatty tissue. The Denonvilliers' fascia is a low intensity line separating the rectum from the prostate gland on sagittal or axial views of T2WI.[14]

The adjacent seminal vesicles are seen superior to the prostate gland as intermediate signal intensity (isointense or slightly hyperintense to skeletal muscle) structures on T1WI. On T2WI the signal intensity is higher, similar to that of fat or urine (Fig. 23-4).[13,43]

Testes and scrotum

The normal testis is an ovoid structure of homogeneous signal intensity on both T1- and T2-weighted SE sequences. On T1-weighted sequences it has an intermediate signal intensity slightly hyperintense to water and hypointense to fat (Fig. 23-5, A). On T2WI the testis has high signal intensity and is isointense or hyperintense to fat (Fig. 23-5, B). The testis is surrounded by a thin layer of low signal intensity, which is the fibrous tunica albuginea. The tunica vaginalis invests the testicle completely, except for the bare area where the testis is anchored to the scrotal wall. It has two layers that can be separated by a small amount of water, which is hyperintense on T2WI. Along the bare area the tunica albuginea invaginates the testes to form the low intensity mediastinum testis.[1,28]

The epididymis is an area of inhomogeneous intermediate signal intensity equal to or less than that of the normal testes on T1WI and hypointense to the testes on T2WI. The scrotal wall fat is identified sometimes as an area of high signal intensity and the dartos muscle as a thin layer of low to intermediate intensity. The spermatic cord appears as a tubular structure of low signal intensity, projecting from the posterosuperior aspect of the testes. Tortuous serpiginous structures within the spermatic cord represent the pampiniform plexus. Areas of high signal intensity within the cord on T2WI represent phase shift from slow blood flow in the venous plexus.[1,28]

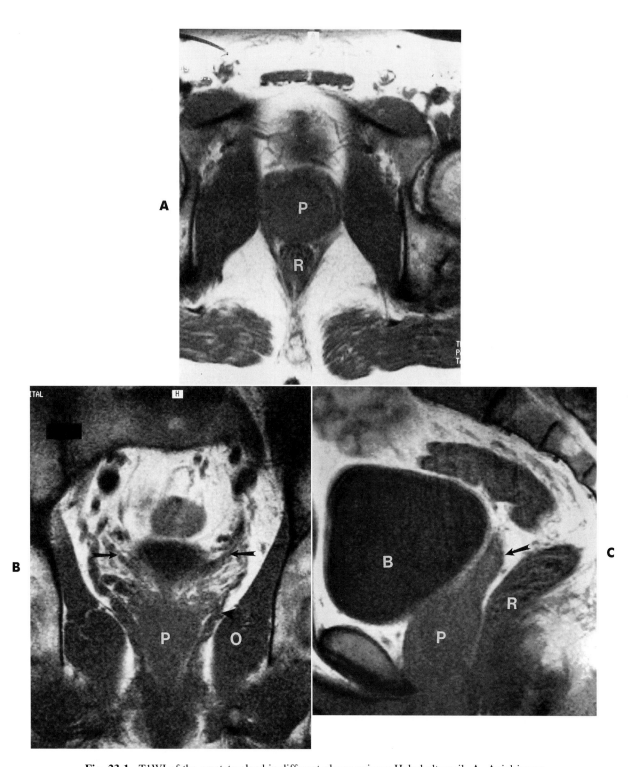

Fig. 23-1. T1WI of the prostate gland in different planes using a Helmholtz coil. **A,** Axial image shows normal prostate gland *(P)* with intermediate signal intensity similar to that of muscle. Rectum *(R)* lies posterior to prostate gland. **B,** Coronal image shows periprostatic venous plexus *(arrowhead)* superior and lateral to the gland *(P)*. Both ureters *(arrows)* are well-demonstrated. Obturator internus muscle *(O)* has intermediate signal intensity. *C,* Sagittal view demonstrates plane between the bladder *(B)*, rectum *(R)*, and prostate gland *(P)*. Seminal vesicles have intermediate signal intensity *(arrow)*.

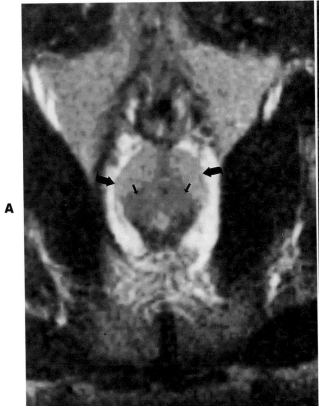

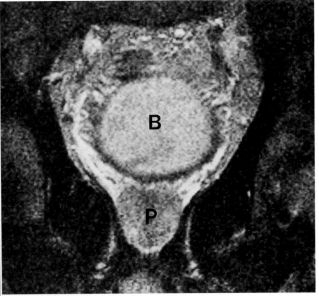

Fig. 23-2. Axial and coronal T2WI of a normal prostate. **A,** Axial image demonstrates prostate gland with higher signal intensity than that of muscle. Prostatic zonal anatomy is shown, with peripheral zone (between *large curved arrows*) having higher signal intensity than central zone (between *small arrows*). **B,** Coronal view shows increased signal intensity of the prostate gland *(P)* and bladder *(B)* superior to it.

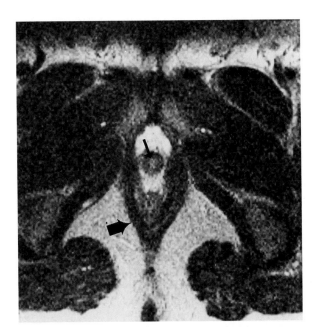

Fig. 23-3. Axial T2-weighted image demonstrates urethra *(black arrow)*, which has high signal intensity and is surrounded by the lower signal intensity of the urethral mucosa. *Solid arrow,* Levator ani muscle.

PATHOLOGIC CONDITIONS
Prostate gland

Benign prostatic hypertrophy. Benign prostatic hypertrophy (BPH) and prostatic carcinoma are frequent pathologic conditions in older men.[35] Several studies have been done attempting to differentiate between BPH and prostate carcinoma using MRI.[7,20,26,41] Currently, whether this determination is possible with MRI is controversial. Initial studies suggested that the two lesions had different signal intensities, but recent reports state that MRI cannot distinguish between BPH and carcinoma on the basis of their relative signal intensities.[6,15,18,37,46] Diffuse inhomogeneity of the prostate gland is a nonspecific indicator of glandular abnormality, not a distinguishing sign between BPH and carcinoma.

BPH is a benign process that involves the central transitional zone of the gland. The transitional zone enlarges and compresses the peripheral zone. The gland develops inhomogeneous signal intensity, with hypo-, hyper-, or isointense nodules, particularly on the T2WI.[15,26] A rim of low signal intensity between the hypertrophic central zone and the peripheral zone is sometimes visible on T2WI. This finding is not visible on T1WI.

Carcinoma. On T2WI, prostatic cancer appears in the peripheral zone as focal areas of low signal intensity that

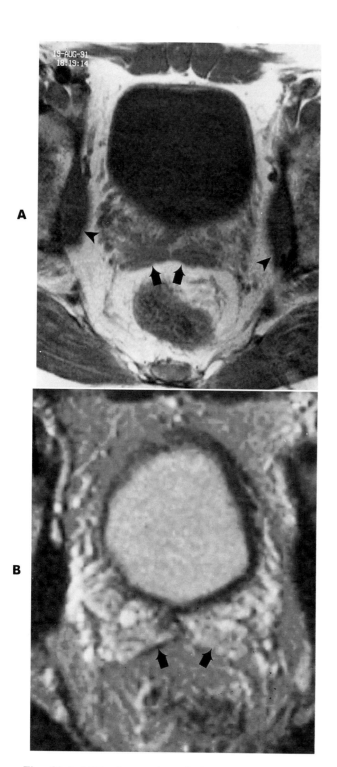

Fig. 23-4. MRI of normal seminal vesicles. **A,** Axial T1-weighted image shows intermediate signal intensity of the seminal vesicles *(solid arrows),* which is similar to that of muscle *(arrowheads).* **B,** Axial T2-weighted image demonstrates high signal intensity of the normal seminal vesicles *(arrows).*

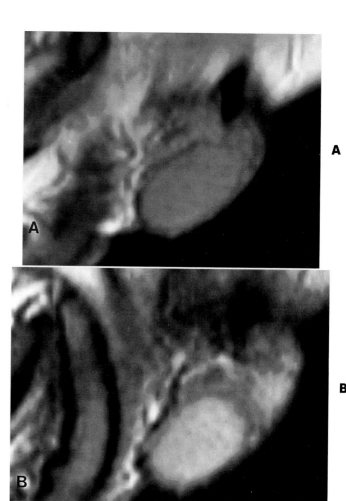

Fig. 23-5. Sagittal T1-weighted imge (**A**) and T2-weighted image (**B**) of the testis show that it has intermediate signal intensity on **A** and increased signal intensity on **B.**

disrupt the normal high signal intensity of the glandular tissue. Other benign processes, such as fibrosis, atrophy, scar, smooth muscle hypertrophy, and chronic prostatitis, may have the same appearance and may mimic carcinoma (Fig. 23-6).[40] On T1WI, tumor cannot be identified, because it has the same signal intensity as the normal glandular tissue. Prostatic cancer is unifocal, multifocal, or diffuse. When it is diffuse, prostatic cancer is difficult to identify, for there is relatively homogeneous, decreased signal intensity in the entire peripheral zone.

The role of MRI in the evaluation of prostatic carcinoma is in the staging of the disease.[5,6,17] Staging is crucial, since treatment selection depends on the extent of disease. Stages A and B and minimal Stage C carcinomas are treated surgically. Patients with more advanced Stage C and D carcinomas are treated with radiation therapy or with orchiectomy and hormones.[4,33]

Correlation has been made between Gleason's tumor grade, tumor volume, and clinical stage (with special em-

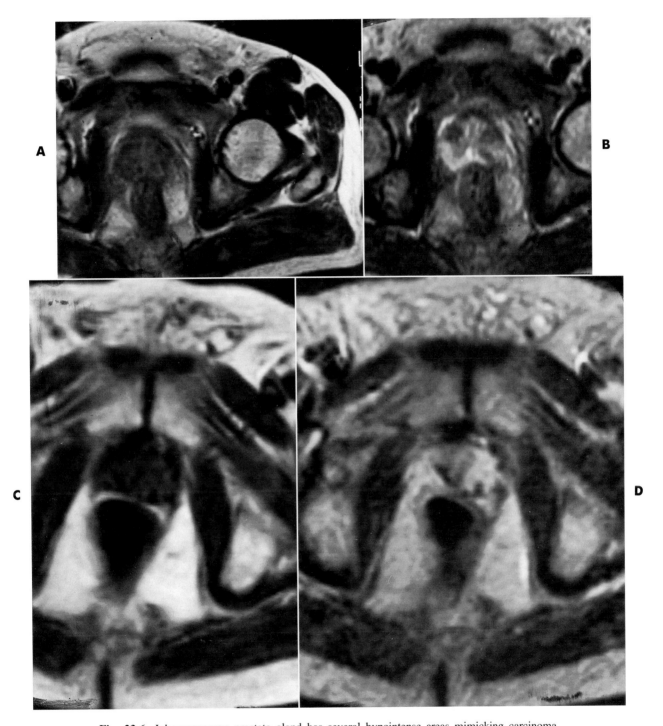

Fig. 23-6. Inhomogeneous prostate gland has several hypointense areas mimicking carcinoma. Axial T1-weighted image **(A)** and T2-weighted image **(B)** show patient with prostatic tuberculosis. Axial T1-weighted image **(C)** and axial T2-weighted image **(D)** show patient with prostatic calcifications.

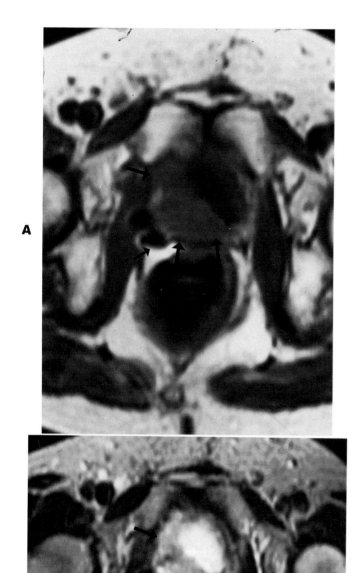

A

B

Fig. 23-7. Male patient with history of prostatic carcinoma. **A,** Axial T1-weighted image shows extracapsular tumor extension with involvement of the bladder wall *(large arrows)*. *Small arrow,* Clip artifact. **B,** T2-weighted image of same area shows tumor extending to the bladder wall *(large arrows).*

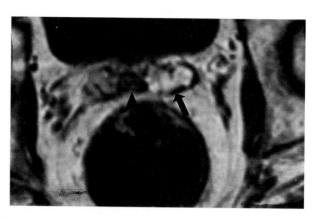

Fig. 23-8. Axial T1-weighted image of the seminal vesicles of patient with prostatic carcinoma demonstrates hemorrhage within left seminal vesicle *(large arrow)* caused by tumor extension *(arrowhead).*

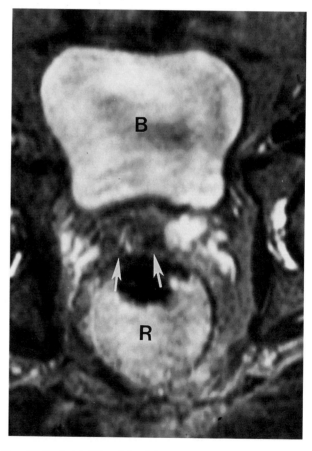

Fig. 23-9. Axial T2-weighted image demonstrates hypointense tumor extending to fluid-filled hyperintense seminal vesicles *(arrows)*. *B,* Bladder; *R,* rectum.

phasis on the extent of capsular invasion, metastasis to the seminal vesicles, and lymphadenopathy) and the malignant potential of prostatic carcinoma.[12,45] Tumor volume assessment with MRI is limited, since contrast between the hypointense tumor and hyperintense peripheral zone allows only the extent of tumor in the peripheral zone to be estimated. The degree of invasion to the central zone cannot be assessed, because frequently BPH, which has signal characteristics similar to neoplasm, is also present in these patients.[31] Tumor volume determination for multifocal carcinoma appearing in more than one zone is difficult.

Detection of capsular invasion is important in the evaluation of tumor aggressiveness. Extension to the periprostatic fat usually occurs in the dorsolateral area of the neurovascular bundle. This may be seen in T1WI as disruption of the periprostatic fat. Identification of the prostatic capsule is considered to be a good landmark for distinguishing between Stage B and C disease. Unfortunately, this is not a consistent finding, because the capsule is not consistently visualized, even in normal patients (Figs. 23-6 and 23-7).[6]

MRI has improved the detection of seminal vesicle invasion (Fig. 23-8), which is identified on T2WI as hypointense solid material replacing the normally hyperintense fluid-filled seminal vesicles (Fig. 23-9). Asymmetry of the seminal vesicles is demonstrated well on axial views. The differential diagnosis of abnormal hypointensity in the seminal vesicles includes alcoholism, orchiectomy, radiation therapy, and advanced age (greater than 75 years).[10]

The detection of lymphadenopathy remains difficult with MRI and CT because detection depends on node size rather than signal characteristics. Neither MRI nor CT detects nodal microinvasion or distinguishes benign enlarged nodes from those infiltrated with tumor. The main advantage of MRI is its ability to differentiate vessels from lymph nodes (Fig. 23-10).[6]

Although the accuracy of MRI staging of prostatic carcinoma is debatable, ranging from 70% to 90%, at present it is the most accurate technique.[5,6,17,25] Compared to CT and ultrasound, MRI is superior for depiction of the local extent of disease and for evaluation of lymphadenopathy.

Sarcoma. Prostatic sarcomas arise from smooth or striated muscle. Rhabdomyosarcoma is the most common form in children and adolescents. It presents as a very large mass that tends to expand toward the bladder and metastasize to lymph nodes (Fig. 23-11). Multiplanar MRI is valuable in the determination of the origin of the tumor and for evaluation of extension to adjacent structures. Sometimes a well-defined pseudocapsule is identified.[3]

Primary malignant fibrous histiocytoma occurs infrequently in the prostate gland and paratesticular region in adults. Their MRI signal intensity typically is low on T1WI and high on T2WI.

Testes and scrotum

The capability of ultrasound in the evaluation of testicular and intratesticular lesions and in the depiction of scrotal anatomy is well-known.[47] MRI is emerging as an alternative imaging modality for the evaluation of scrotal diseases because of its excellent rendering of anatomic detail of the scrotum and inguinal region.[8,27] On T2WI, normal testes have increased signal intensity that provides excellent background for the detection of intratesticular abnormalities.

Primary tumors. Primary tumors originate from germ or stromal cells. The germ cell tumors are grouped as seminomatous and nonseminomatous or as having mixed elements. Nonseminomatous tumors include embryonal cell

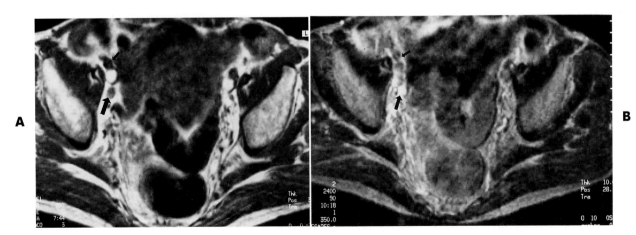

Fig. 23-10. Lymphadenopathy remains difficult to be detect. Main advantage of MR is the ability to differentiate vessels *(small arrow)* from lymph nodes *(large arrow).* **A,** On T1-weighted image, lymph nodes have intermediate signal intensity. **B,** T2-weighted image shows increase in signal intensity of the lymph node. Note rectosigmoid outlined with barium.

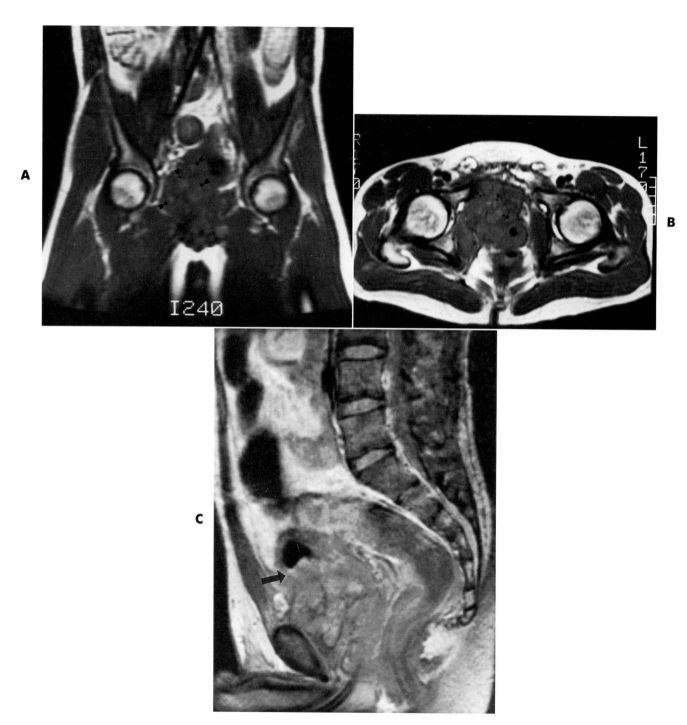

Fig. 23-11. Coronal **(A)** and axial **(B)** T1WI show patient with prostatic rhabdomyosarcoma. Note a large tumor with inhomogeneous signal intensity and some focal areas of increased signal intensity representing hemorrhage *(small arrows)*. Sagittal T2-weighted image **(C)** shows increase in tumor signal intensity and extension to the bladder wall *(arrow)*.

carcinoma, teratocarcinoma, teratomas, and choriocarcinomas.[34]

On MRI, testicular tumors typically have inhomogeneous signal intensity, less than or equal to that of the normal testis on T1WI and much lower on T2WI. The size, margins, and extension of the tumor are well-demonstrated by MRI because the normal tunica albuginea and epididymis are depicted well (Fig. 23-12).[2] Tumor extension to the tunica albuginea produces high intensity discontinuities in the normally low intensity layer that can no longer be followed continuously around the testis. Nonseminomatous tumors have inhomogeneous signal intensity and have areas of low and high signal intensity on T1WI and T2WI because of hemorrhage in various stages and necrosis within the tumor (Fig. 23-13). Seminomas have more homogeneous signal intensity, being isointense or hypointense to normal testes on T1WI and markedly hypointense to normal testicular tissue on T2WI (Fig. 23-14).[22]

Intratesticular abnormalities. Epididymitis is the most common intrascrotal infection. On MRI, it appears as focal or diffuse enlargement of the epididymis with isointensity or hyperintensity on T2WI (Fig. 23-15).[2] Acute epididymitis is sometimes associated with increased vascularity of the testis and with sympathetic hydroceles. MRI characteristics of chronic epididymitis are epididymal enlargement and hypointensity in contrast to the normal testis.

MRI is not selective in the differentiation of benign and malignant intratesticular lesions, since their signal characteristics frequently overlap. Orchitis usually occurs as a direct extension of infection from the epididymis. On MRI, it appears as testicular enlargement with lower signal intensity than normal on T1WI.

Acute scrotal trauma is evaluated accurately with MRI, because the integrity of the tunica albuginea and the extent of intratesticular hematoma can be assessed. On T1WI and T2WI after trauma, the testes are inhomogeneous, with some areas of increased and decreased signal intensity, depending on the age of the blood products.[2]

Testicular torsion occurs usually in the teens and twenties, and emergency surgery is necessary to save the testis. A characteristic MRI finding is reduced or absent vascularity in the spermatic cord of the affected side. Other findings include direct demonstration of the twisted testicular cord, which produces a spiral or whirlpool pattern. This twisted stalk is hypointense at the point of torsion. The epididymis is enlarged, with areas of swelling and hemorrhage. In the subacute phase the affected testis is smaller than the contralateral testis, has decreased signal intensity, and is inhomogeneous on T2WI. When the torsion is remote, the testis is small and hypointense on T2WI.[48]

Extratesticular abnormalities. MRI selectively differentiates intra- and extratesticular lesions. The most com-

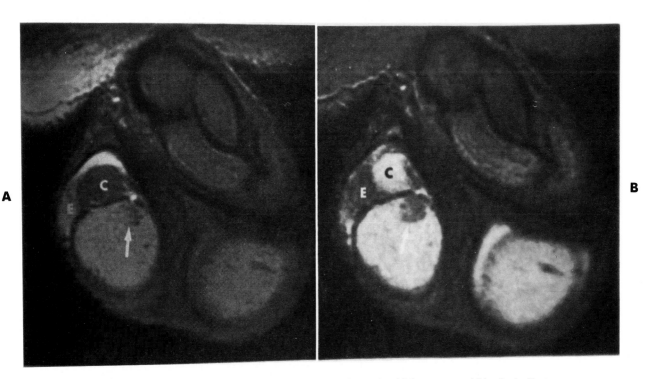

Fig. 23-12. Mildly inhomogeneous testicular tumor *(arrow)*, which was proved histologically to be a Leydig's cell tumor, is better seen on T2-weighted image (**B**) than on proton-density image (**A**). Epididymal cyst *(C)* within normal epididymal head *(E)* has MR characteristics of water. (From Baker LL et al: *Radiology* 163:93-98, 1987.)

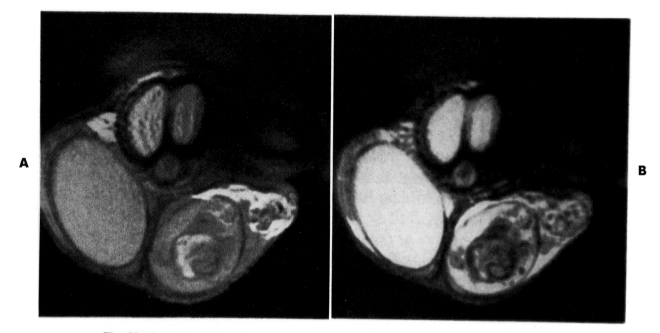

Fig. 23-13. Multinodular embryonal cell carcinoma of left testis. **A,** Proton-density MR image (TR 2000, TE 20) shows heterogeneous signals. **B,** T2-weighted image (TR 2000, TE 70), the second echo of **A,** shows further increase in signal heterogeneity compared with normal testicular tissue of ipsilateral and contralateral testes. (From Johnson JO, Mattrey RF, Phillipson J: *AJR* 154:539-543, 1990.)

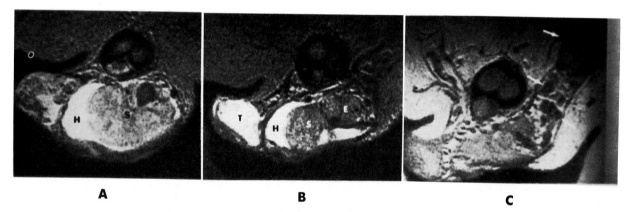

Fig. 23-14. A, Seminoma of left testis *(S)* is inhomogeneous on T2-weighted image. *H,* hydrocele. **B,** Epididymal involvement *(E)* and decreased signal intensity of affected testis relative to normal testis *(T)* and hydrocele *(H)* are evident. **C,** Multiple tumor nodules in the spermatic cord *(arrows)* are easily seen. (From Baker LL et al: *Radiology* 163:93-98, 1987.)

mon extra-testicular lesions are epididymitis, spermatocele, hydrocele, and varicocele.

Spermatoceles occur in the head of the epididymis. They may be single or multiloculated cysts containing fluid, spermatozoa, and sediment (composed of lymphocytes, fat globules, and cellular debris). The signal intensity varies according to the composition of the lesion.

Simple hydroceles are an accumulation of fluid between the layers of the tunica vaginalis. The signal intensity of a hydrocele is homogeneous and similar to that of water on all pulse sequences.

Patients with varicoceles have prominence of the spermatic canal and the intrascrotal spermatic cord. The spermatic cord contains numerous serpiginous structures with increased signal caused by phase shift artifacts from slow blood flow on T1WI and T2WI.[2]

Less commonly seen are scrotal lipomas. These have characteristic hyperintensity on T1WI (Fig. 23-16).

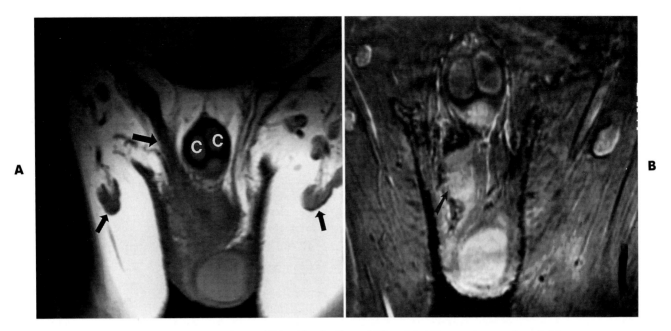

Fig. 23-15. Right tuberculous epididymitis. **A,** Coronal T1-weighted image shows enlarged right spermatic cord *(large arrow)* with multiple serpentine vessels, indicating increased vascularity. Multiple bilateral inguinal enlarged lymph nodes are seen *(small arrows)*. *CC,* Corpora cavernosa. **B,** Coronal T2-weighted image of same area shows increased signal intensity of the enlarged spermatic cord and inflamed epididymis *(arrow)*.

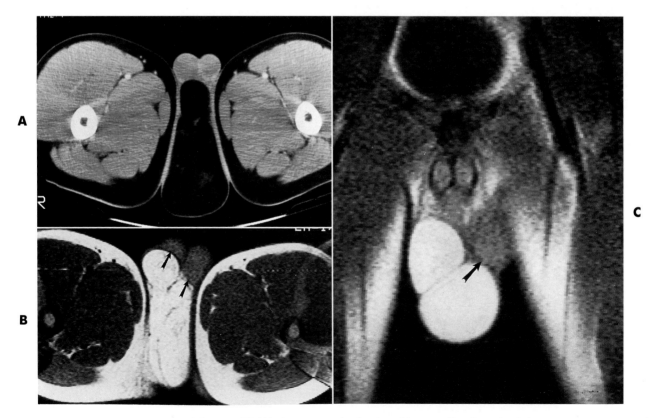

Fig. 23-16. Scrotal lipoma. CT **(A)** shows mass the density of fat extending through whole scrotum. Axial **(B)** and coronal **(C)** T1WI show bilobed hyperintense mass displacing normal testes *(arrows)* anteriorly.

Undescended testis. MRI has a role in the evaluation of the nonpalpable undescended testis. The absence of a testis in the scrotum may be from agenesis, ectopia, or incomplete descent of the testis from the abdomen.[11,12,23,49,50] It is important to localize the testis, because the patients have increased risk of infertility and malignant degeneration. Precise localization of the undescended testis is mandatory for the planning of the surgical approach.

Ultrasound is helpful for the localization of the incompletely descended testis in the inguinal region but not for detection of an intraabdominal testis. CT also is sensitive for detection of an intraabdominal testis but is less selective in distinguishing the testis from adjacent structures.[49]

The sensitivity of MRI for localization of an undescended testis ranges from 80% to 90%.[11,23,49,50] Like

scrotal testes, undescended testes are hypointense on T1WI and hyperintense on T2WI. Atrophic testes may have low signal intensity on T2WI (Fig. 23-17).[23] This characteristic allows the evaluation of the functional status of the testis.

Some of the limitations of MRI in the evaluation of these patients are related to patient movement (long scan times) and lack of an optimal gastrointestinal contrast agent. An intraabdominal testis also may be similar in intensity to adjacent small bowel loops.

In general, although MRI has high sensitivity for undescended testes, the modality is not sensitive enough to completely exclude the condition. Thus if no testis is positively identified in the abdomen, the patient should have surgical exploration.

SUMMARY

MRI clearly has a role in the evaluation of certain pathologic conditions in the male pelvis. It is considered to be a primary tool for the staging of some pelvic malignancies and a problem-solving technique in other cases. The multiplanar imaging capability of MRI depicts exquisite anatomic detail of the pelvis, inguinal region, and scrotum. The major limitations of MRI in the male pelvis are cost, limited availability in some areas, and lack of specificity for some pathologic conditions.

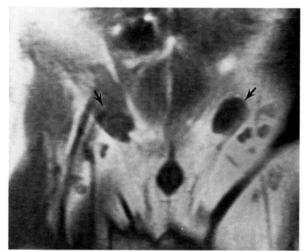

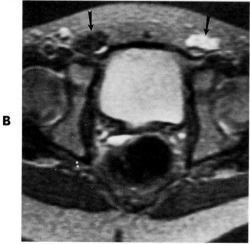

Fig. 23-17. MRI of 2-year-old child with bilateral nonpalpable testes. **A,** In coronal image (TR 600, TE 20) bilateral inguinal testes *(arrows)* are visualized well. **B,** In axial image (TR 1700, TE 80) right testis remains hypointense to fat *(arrow)*, and left testis is hyperintense *(arrow)*. (From Kier R et al: *Radiology* 169:429-433, 1987.)

REFERENCES

1. Baker LL, Hajek PC, Burkhard TK, et al: MR imaging of the scrotum: normal anatomy, *Radiology* 163:89-92, 1987.
2. Baker LL, Hajek PC, Burkhard TK, et al: MR imaging of the scrotum: pathologic conditions, *Radiology* 163:93-98, 1987.
3. Bartolozzi C, Selli C, Olmastroni M, et al: Rhabdomyosarcoma of the prostate: MR findings, *AJR* 150:1333-1334, 1988.
4. Bartsch G et al: Incidental carcinoma of the prostate: grading and tumor volume in relation to survival rate, *World J Urol* 1:24-28, 1983.
5. Bezzi M, Kressel HY, Allen KS, et al: Prostatic carcinoma: staging with MR imaging at 1.5 T, *Radiology* 169:339-346, 1988.
6. Biondetti PR, Lee JKT, Ling D, et al: Clinical Stage B prostate carcinoma: staging with MR imaging, *Radiology* 162:435-329, 1987.
7. Carroll BA, Gross DM: High frequency scrotal sonography, *AJR* 140:511-515, 1983.
8. Carroll CL, Somme FG, McNeal JE, et al: The abnormal prostate: MR imaging at 1.5 T with histopathologic correlation, *Radiology* 163:521-525, 1987.
9. Carswell H: Support grows for MR in staging of prostate, *Diagn Imag* pp 85-93, March 1991.
10. Edson SB, Hricak H, Change YCF: MR imaging of the seminal vesicles (abstract). *Radiology* 165(P):59, 1987.
11. Friedland GW, Chang P: The role of imaging in the management of the impalpable undescended testes, *AJR* 151:1107-1111, 1988.
12. Fritzsche PJ: Male pelvis. In *Syllabus: a categorical course in diagnostic radiology—MR imaging,* Oak Brook, Ill, 1988, Radiological Society of North America, pp 149-154.
13. Fritzsche PJ, Hricak H, Kogan BA, et al: Undescended testis: value of MR imaging, *Radiology* 164:169-173, 1987.
14. Heiken JP, Lee JK: MR imaging of the pelvis, *Radiology* 166:11-16, 1988.
15. Hricak H et al: Anatomy and pathology of the male pelvis by magnetic resonance imaging, *AJR* 141:1101-1110, 1983.

16. Hricak H et al: Magnetic resonance imaging of the female pelvis: initial experience, *AJR* 141:1119-1128, 1983.

17. Hricak H, Dooms GC, McNeal JE, et al: MR imaging of the prostate gland: normal anatomy, *AJR* 148:51-58, 1987.

18. Hricak H, Dooms GC, Jeffrey RB, et al: Prostatic carcinoma: staging by clinical assessment, CT, and MR imaging, *Radiology* 162:331-336, 1987.

19. Hricak H et al: Imaging prostatic carcinoma, *Radiology* 169:569-571, 1988.

20. Hruban RH, Zerhouni EA, Dagher AP, et al: Morphologic basis of the MR imaging of benign prostatic hyperplasia, *J Comput Assist Tomogr* 11(6):1035-1041, 1987.

21. Javitt MCF, Lovecchio JL, Stein HL: Imaging strategies for MRI of the pelvis, *Radiol Clin North Am* 26:633-649, 1988.

22. Johnson JO, Mattrey RF, Phillipson J: Differentiation of seminomatous from nonseminomatous testicular tumors with MR imaging, *AJR* 154:539-543, 1990.

23. Kier R, McCarthy S, Rosenfield AT, et al: Nonpalpable testes in young boys: evaluation with MR imaging, *Radiology* 169:429-433, 1988.

24. Koslin DB, Kenney PJ, Koehler RE, et al: Magnetic resonance imaging of the internal anatomy of the prostate gland, *Invest Radiol* 22:947-953, 1987.

25. Lee KJT, Heiken JP, Ling D, et al: Magnetic resonance imaging of abdominal and pelvic lymphadenopathy, *Radiology* 153:181-188, 1984.

26. Leopold GR, Woo VL, Scheible FW, et al: High resolution ultrasonography of scrotal pathology, *Radiology* 131:719-722, 1979.

27. Ling D, Lee JKT, Heiken JP, et al: Prostatic carcinoma and benign prostatic hyperplasia: inability of MR imaging to distinguish between the two diseases, *Radiology* 158:103-107, 1986.

28. Mattrey RF: MRI of the scrotum, *Semin Ultrasound CT MR* 12:95-108, 1991.

29. McNeal JE: Regional morphology and pathology of the prostate, *Am J Clin Pathol* 49:347-357, 1968.

30. McNeal JE: Normal anatomy of the prostate and changes in benign prostatic hypertrophy and carcinoma, *Semin Ultrasound CT MR* 9:329-334, 1988.

31. McNeal JE et al: The prostate gland: morphology and pathobiology. In Stamey TA, ed: *Monographs in urology,* vol 4, Princeton, NJ, 1983, Custom Publishing Services.

32. McNeal JE et al: The prostate gland: morphology and pathobiology. In Stamey TA, ed: *1983 monographs in urology,* vol 4, Research Triangle Park, NC, 1983, Burroughs Wellcome.

33. McNeal JE et al: Patterns of progression in prostate cancer, *Lancet* 1:60-63, 1986.

34. Morrison AS, Cole P, Maclure KM: Epidemiology of urogenital cancers. In Javadpour N, ed: *Principles and management of urologic cancer,* ed 2, Baltimore, 1983, Williams and Wilkins.

35. Morse MJ, Whitmore WF: Neoplasms of the testis. In Walsh PC et al, ed: *Campbell's urology,* Philadelphia, 1986, WB Saunders.

36. Phillips ME, Kressel HY, Spritzer CE, et al: Normal prostate and adjacent structures: MR imaging at 1.5 T, *Radiology* 164:381-385, 1987.

37. Poon PY, McCallum RW, Henkelman MM, et al: Magnetic resonance imaging of the prostate, *Radiology* 154:143-149, 1985.

38. Reiman TH, Heiken JD, Totty WG, et al: Clinical MR imaging with a Helmholtz-type surface coil, *Radiology* 169:564-566, 1988.

39. Rholl KS, Lee JKT, Ling D, et al: MR imaging of the scrotum with a high-resolution surface coil, *Radiology* 163:99-103, 1987.

40. Rifkin M: *MR Syllabus: MR imaging of the prostate gland,* Oak Brooke, Ill, 1989, Radiological Society of America, pp. 175-182.

41. Schiebler ML, Tomaszewski JE, Bezzi M, et al: Prostatic carcinoma and benign prostatic hyperplasia: correlation of high-resolution MR and histopathologic findings, *Radiology* 172:131-137, 1989.

42. Schnall MD, Lenkinski RE, Pollack HM, et al: Prostate: MR imaging with endorectal surface coil, *Radiology* 172:570-574, 1989.

43. Secaf E, Nuruddin RN, Hricak H, et al: MR imaging of the seminal vesicle, *AJR* 156:989-994, 1991.

44. Seidenwurm D, Smathers RL, Lo RK, et al: Testes and scrotum: MR imaging at 1.5 T, *Radiology* 164:393-398, 1987.

45. Stamey TA et al: Morphometric and clinical studies on 68 consecutive radical prostatectomies, *J Urol* 139:1235-1241 1988.

46. Stey JH, Smith FW: Nuclear magnetic resonance of the prostate, *Br J Urol* 54:726-728, 1982.

47. Thurnher S, Hricak H, Carroll PR, et al: Imaging the testis: comparison between MR imaging and US, *Radiology* 167:631-636, 1988.

48. Trambert MA, Mattrey RF, Levine D, et al: Subacute scrotal pain: evaluation of torsion versus epididymitis with MR imaging, *Radiology* 175:53-56, 1990.

49. Troughton AH, Waring J, Longstaff A, et al: The role of magnetic resonance imaging in the investigation of undescended testes, *Clin Radiol* 41:178-181, 1990.

50. Zobel BB et al: Magnetic resonance imaging in the localization of undescended abdominal testes, *Eur Urol* 17:145-148, 1990.

Chapter 24

BLADDER

Cynthia L. Janus
David S. Mendelson

A variety of imaging modalities have been used to evaluate the urinary bladder. Urography is limited in demonstrating anatomic detail and is inadequate for staging bladder tumors. Ultrasound and computed tomography (CT) allow for more detailed evaluation, especially of the surrounding pelvic structures.[14,17,22,30] However, these modalities also have some limitations in resolution and cannot always differentiate tumors from blood clots adherent to the bladder wall or from asymmetric bladder wall hypertrophy and trabeculation. Most importantly, these modalities have also proved inadequate in determining the depth of tumor invasion in bladder carcinoma.

The superior contrast resolution and multiplanar imaging capability of magnetic resonance imaging (MRI) make this newer imaging technique well-suited to demonstrate pathologic conditions of the urinary bladder. Advantages include virtual lack of artifacts from respiratory motion in the pelvis and the ability to obtain good quality images of the bladder and its surrounding structures without intravenous (IV) contrast agents. For these reasons, MRI has been investigated and shows great promise as a means of more precisely defining abnormalities of the urinary bladder and more accurately staging bladder cancer.[1,4,26]

TECHNIQUE

Imaging protocols for evaluating the bladder generally consist of T1-weighted (TR 300 to 500 msec, TE 15 to 35 msec) and T2-weighted (TR 1500 to 2500 msec, TE 90 to 120 msec) spin-echo (SE) sequences in the axial plane (Figs. 24-1 and 24-2). Section thickness should be 1 cm or less, with 1 mm gaps. Additional T1- or T2-weighted sequences in the sagittal or coronal plane, depending on the site of the pathologic condition, generally are also performed (Figs. 24-3 and 24-4). When MRI is utilized for staging bladder neoplasms, the T1-weighted sequences are best for detecting the presence of lymphadenopathy and for delineating the extension of the primary tumor into the surrounding fat, whereas T2-weighted images (T2WI) are optimal in distinguishing the wall of the bladder from its urine content. The urinary bladder should be at least half full before beginning the examination, so that the bladder wall is adequately visualized.

ANATOMY

On T1-weighted images (T1WI) the urinary bladder demonstrates low signal intensity because of the extremely long T1 of urine (Figs. 24-1 and 24-3). It is difficult to differentiate the bladder wall from the urine content. On T2-weighted sequences, this distinction is possible because of the high signal intensity of urine (long T2) and low signal intensity of the bladder wall (short T2), which is approximately 2 mm thick[4,20] (Fig. 24-2).

When the bladder is evaluated, it is important to be cognizant of the chemical shift artifact, which is seen at

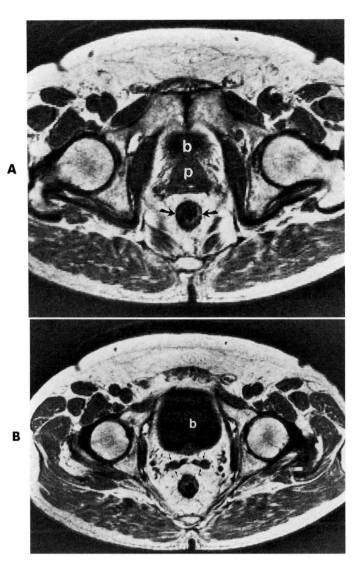

Fig. 24-1. A, T1-weighted axial image at level of the base of the urinary bladder *(b)* shows prostate gland *(p)* and rectum *(between arrows)*. Urine in the bladder is low in signal intensity because of the long T1 of urine. Wall of the bladder is barely perceptible. **B,** Axial T1-weighted image of the urinary bladder *(b)* is from a more cephalad level. Seminal vesicles *(between small arrows)* are easily delineated from surrounding pelvic fat.

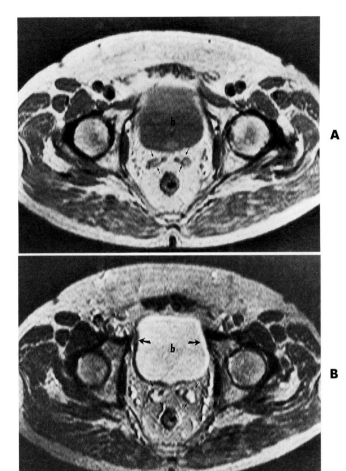

Fig. 24-2. A, Signal intensity of the urine-filled bladder and seminal vesicles increases on proton density-weighted image. Seminal vesicles are between the small arrows. *b,* Urinary bladder. **B,** With more T2 weighting, signal intensity of the urine in the bladder *(b)* and the seminal vesicles (between *small arrows*) further increases. Bladder wall becomes distinct from urine because of its lower signal intensity. Chemical shift artifact on this T2-weighted image is a dark band along the lateral wall of the bladder and bright band along the opposite wall *(thick curved arrows).*

the interface of the bladder and perivesical fat in the direction of the frequency encoding gradient.[2] The location of this artifact depends on the imaging plane. Thus on transverse views, it is manifested as a dark band along the lateral bladder wall on one side and a bright band along the opposite wall (Figs. 24-2, *B* and 24-5, *A*). On sagittal views, the superior and inferior walls of the bladder demonstrate the artifact, assuming the direction of the frequency encoding gradient is unchanged (Fig. 24-5, *B*). The chemical shift artifact is more pronounced at higher field strengths, and its significance is that it either simu-

lates or obscures pathologic conditions of the bladder. The dark band should not be misinterpreted as a normal bladder wall. This artifact is overcome by imaging in another plane or by rotating the direction of the frequency encoding gradient.[11]

HYPERTROPHY AND INFLAMMATION

Congenital and acquired abnormalities of the bladder shape and structure are readily displayed by MRI, particularly with its ability to image in multiple planes (Fig. 24-6). Two common benign pathologic conditions of the bladder wall are hypertrophy and inflammation. The appear-

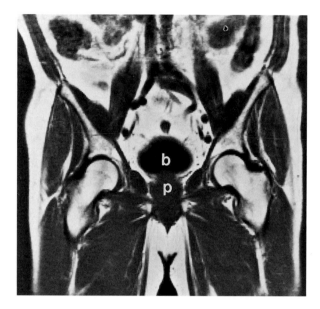

Fig. 24-3. T1-weighted image of the urinary bladder *(b)* in the coronal plane is at the level of the prostate gland *(p)*.

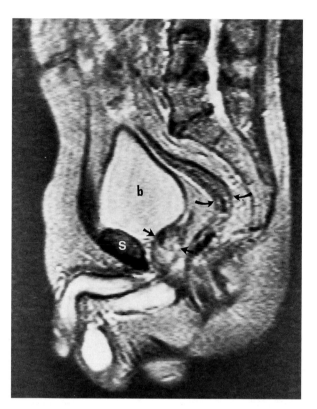

Fig. 24-4. Sagittal T2-weighted view of the urinary bladder helps demonstrate the anterior and posterior walls of the bladder and surrounding pelvic structures. Prostate gland is between the straight arrows. Curved arrows point to rectum. *b,* Urinary bladder; *s,* symphysis pubis.

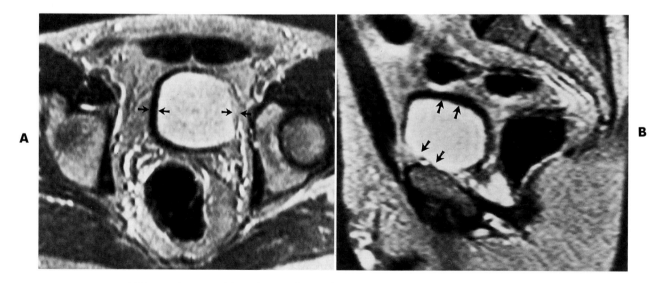

Fig. 24-5. A, On T2-weighted image of the urinary bladder in the axial plane, chemical shift artifact is represented by dark band along the lateral wall and bright band along the opposite lateral wall *(between arrows).* **B,** On T2-weighted image in the sagittal plane, chemical shift artifact appears as dark and light bands along the superior and inferior aspects of the urinary bladder, respectively *(arrows).*

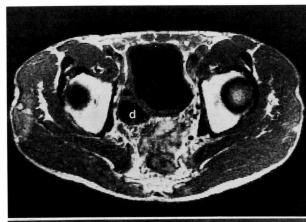

A

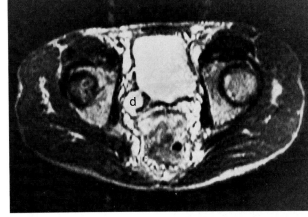

B

Fig. 24-6. A diverticulum *(d)* is seen at posterolateral aspect of the urinary bladder on T1-weighted image **(A)** and T2-weighted image **(B)**. Pelvic vessels are depicted as serpiginous, low signal intensity structures on **A** and demonstrate high signal intensity on **B**.

ance of these two abnormalities on MRI was studied by Fisher, Hricak, and Crooks[8] in 1985 by a retrospective analysis of 50 patients. Thirty of these patients had no history of genitourinary tract disease and were undergoing MRI examinations of the pelvis for unrelated reasons. This group included 10 men and 20 women, and ages of the patients ranged from 27 to 63 years. In 10 other patients, all of whom were men 57 to 75 years of age, hypertrophy of the bladder wall was secondary to prostatic enlargement. Congestion of the trigonum was present in seven additional patients; six of these cases were related to bladder outlet obstruction, and one case occurred following transurethral prostatic resection. Bladder wall inflammation was present in two patients with cystitis after radiation therapy and in one patient following surgery. The diagnosis of bladder wall hypertrophy was confirmed by cystoscopy in the 10 patients. Congestion of the base of the bladder was verified at cystoscopy in six patients and by cystectomy in the remaining patient.

In hypertrophy of the urinary bladder wall, such as that associated with bladder outlet obstruction, the signal inten-

sity of the hypertrophic wall is similar to that of the normal bladder wall (Fig. 24-7). This is differentiable from edema or inflammation of the bladder wall, both of which have high signal intensities on T2WI.[8,20] However, the signal intensities of bladder wall inflammation and edema overlap those seen with bladder neoplasms, which also demonstrate increased signal intensities on T2-weighted imaging sequences.[4,9,20]

CARCINOMA

Primary tumors of the bladder wall (transitional-cell carcinoma) are generally detected by MRI if they are larger than 1 to 2 cm in diameter. The T1 and T2 relaxation times of bladder tumors, although less than those of urine, are relatively long.[4] Bladder wall neoplasms are usually best demonstrated on T1WI, since the signal intensity of the tumor is greater than that of urine but less than that of fat.[4,26] With more T2 weighting the signal intensity of bladder tumors has been found to increase above that of urine on the first echo and become similar to or slightly lower than that of urine on the second echo.[4] The normal low intensity bladder wall may be interrupted on these images by the high signal intensity tumor.

Staging

Various classifications have been proposed for staging carcinoma of the urinary bladder.[12,21,24] The most well-known staging systems are the TNM (tumor-node-metastasis) classification (Table 24-1) and the modified Jewett-Strong-Marshall System (Table 24-2).

Accurate staging of carcinoma of the urinary bladder is of utmost importance in order to plan the appropriate treat-

Table 24-1. TNM classification of bladder carcinoma

Staging	Criteria
TIS	Carcinoma in situ
Ta	Papillary noninvasive carcinoma
T1	Infiltration of the lamina propria
T2	Extension to the superficial muscle layer
T3A	Extension to the deep muscle layer
T3B	Infiltration of the perivesical fat
T4A	Invasion of neighboring structures (prostate gland, uterus, or vagina)
T4B	Invasion of pelvic or abdominal wall
N0	No regional lymph node metastases
N1	Solitary homolateral regional (internal or external iliac) lymph node metastasis
N2	Contralateral, bilateral, or multiple regional lymph node metastases
N3	Fixed regional lymph node metastases
N4	Juxtaregional (common iliac, inguinal, or aortic lymph node metastases)
Mo	No distant metastases
M1	Distant metastases present

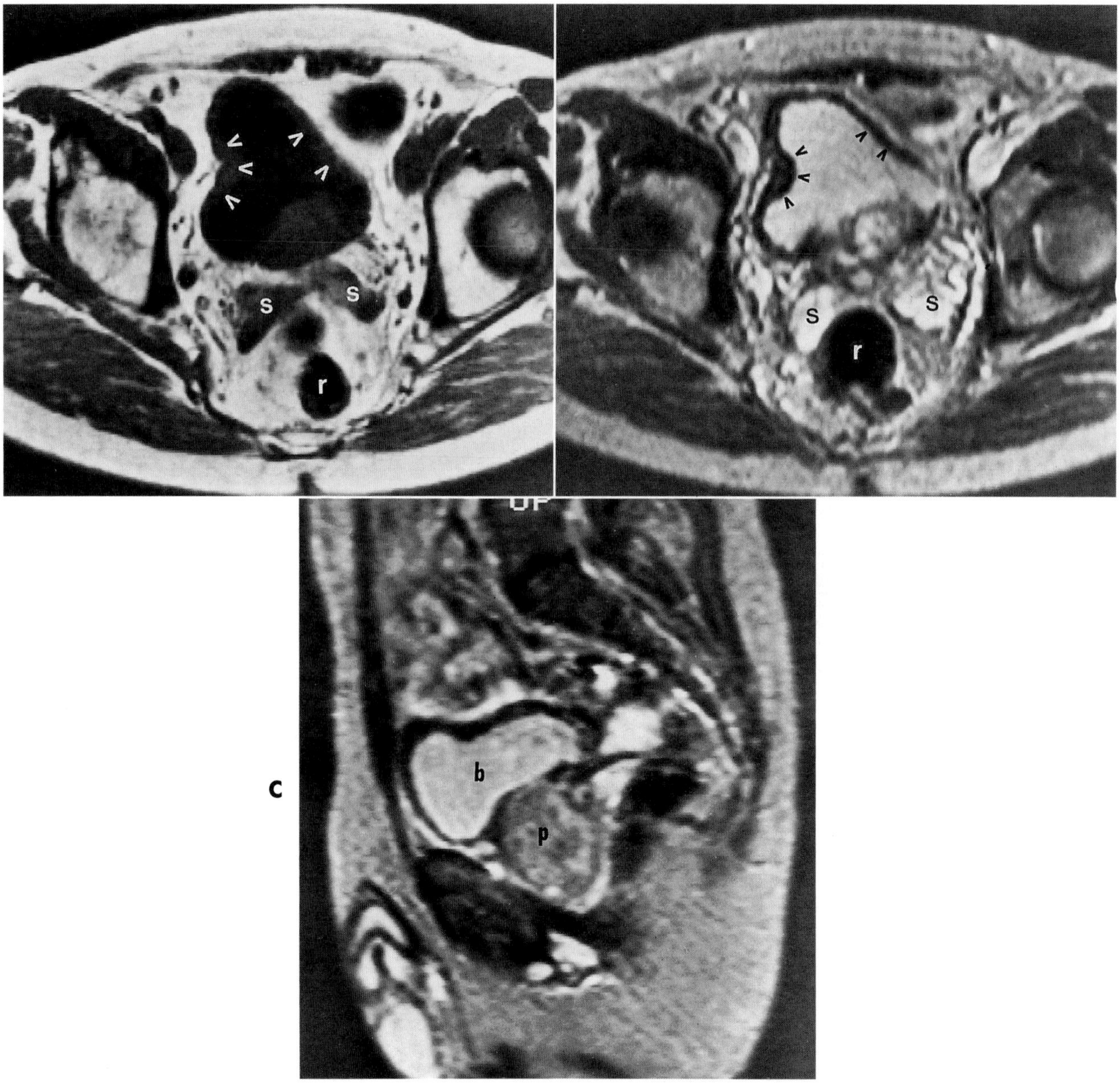

Fig. 24-7. Bladder wall is thickened in this patient with benign prostatic hyperplasia. **A,** On T1-weighted axial view, thickened bladder wall has moderate signal intensity. **B,** On corresponding T2-weighted axial view, thickened, low signal intensity bladder wall is more easily distinguished. **C,** T2-weighted view in the sagittal plane shows enlarged prostate gland, which has heterogeneous signal intensity and contains many small nodules of low and high signal intensity. Arrows (>) point to portions of thickened bladder wall. *s,* Seminal vesicles; *r,* rectum; *p,* prostate gland.

Table 24-2. Modified Jewett-Strong-Marshall system

Staging	Criteria
0	Confined to the mucosa
A	Infiltration of the submucosa
B1	Infiltration of the superficial muscle
B2	Infiltration of the deep muscle
C	Perivesical infiltration—involvement of the perivesical fat or even the capsule of adjacent organs but no farther
D1	Involvement of adjacent organs and pelvic lymph nodes
D2	Distant metastases or nodes above bifurcation

ment protocol.[15,25,28] Treatment of carcinoma in situ and T1 lesions (involvement of the mucosa or submucosa) consists of fulguration or transurethral resection. Patients with low-grade T2 lesions in which there is involvement of the superficial muscle layer are often treated with segmental cystectomy, whereas the treatment of choice for patients with Stage 3A and 3B neoplasms (deep muscle invasion or perivesical fat involvement) is radical cystectomy. Stage 4 lesions, with involvement of the perivesical organs and rectum, are commonly treated with palliative radiation therapy with an ileal loop.[4,20]

Conventional methods of staging include bimanual examination under anesthesia, urography, cystoscopy, and transurethral resection, and they have not proved to be reliable.[1,28,30] Errors in clinical staging increase as the tumor becomes more invasive. Determination of deep muscle invasion and detection of lymphadenopathy are particular problem areas.[1]

MRI staging

Carcinoma of the urinary bladder is considered superficial (Stage T2 or less) if the low signal intensity line of the bladder wall underlying the tumor is intact.[4] MRI cannot differentiate Stage TIS, T1, and T2 neoplasms. The inability to discriminate Stage T2 lesions is an important clinical limitation, because patients with the lesions are treated differently than those with lower stage tumors.

Deep muscle invasion by bladder carcinoma (Stage T3A) can be demonstrated. This is seen on T2-weighted sequences as focal disruption of the normal low signal intensity line by high signal intensity in the region underlying the tumor (Fig. 24-8). This sign was originally interpreted by Bryan et al.[3] to indicate spread to the perivesical fat, but other investigators have found that it represents deep muscle invasion.[4] A problem area regarding bladder wall invasion involves the region of the periurethral glands, since the bladder wall normally appears interrupted at this level.

Extension of bladder carcinoma into the perivesical fat (Stage T3B) is visualized as a soft tissue mass with signal

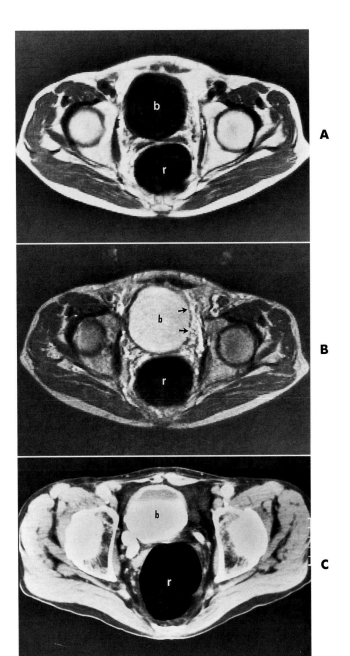

Fig. 24-8. A, T1-weighted axial image shows patient with carcinoma of the urinary bladder. *b,* Urinary bladder; *r,* rectum. **B,** T2-weighted axial view reveals interruption of low signal intensity bladder wall at anterior and left lateral aspects *(arrows),* representing deep muscle invasion. *b,* Urinary bladder; *r,* rectum. **C,** Corresponding CT scan fails to provide any information regarding depth or site of bladder wall invasion. *b,* Urinary bladder; *r,* rectum.

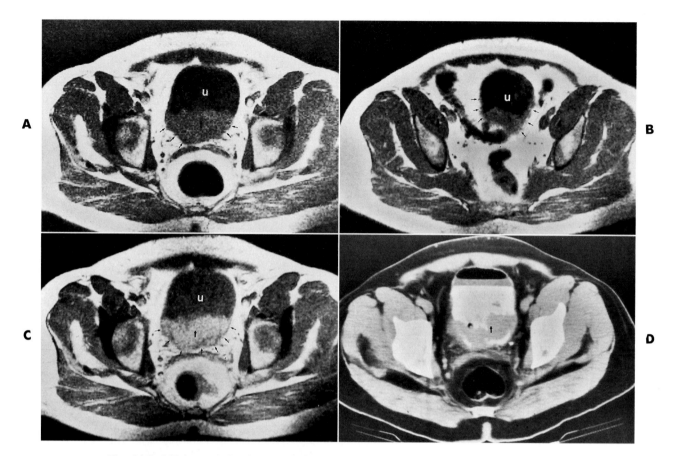

Fig. 24-9. MR images of patient with large bulky tumor of the bladder are shown. T1-weighted axial images through the mid portion (**A**) and upper part (**B**) of the urinary bladder demonstrate irregularity in bladder contour at site of the mass and irregular, low signal intensity areas extending into the perivesical fat. **C,** Signal intensity of urine and tumor increase on this proton-density image. **D,** CT scan also shows irregular extension of the bladder tumor into perivesical fat. Air in the superior aspect of the bladder was introduced when patient was catheterized. Small arrows point to areas of irregularity of the bladder wall. *t,* Bladder tumor; *u,* urine content of bladder.

intensity similar to that of the primary tumor (Figs. 24-9 and 24-10). Stage T4A lesions are depicted as masses with signal intensities similar to that of the primary tumor that extend into adjacent organs. These stages may be easier to visualize on T1WI, because the tumor may be less intense than the bright fat (Fig. 24-11). Since there is often some degree of indistinctness between the base of the bladder and the prostate gland or urethra, the radiologist should exercise caution in cases of tumors close to the bladder cervix, where extension to the prostate gland or periurethral glands can be missed.[4]

Lymph node metastasis is suspected when the short axis of a lymph node is 10 mm or more in the transverse plane[4] (Fig. 24-12). MRI has proved more reliable than CT in differentiating an enlarged lymph node from a small blood vessel. As is the case with CT, lymph node enlargement from benign causes cannot be distinguished reliably from malignant involvement of the node. In 1985, Dooms et

al.[7] reported the results of excision of normal and malignant lymph nodes from seven patients in whom T1 and T2 relaxation times were analyzed in vitro by MR spectroscopy. T1 and T2 relaxation times of the lymph nodes were also obtained from MRI examinations in 86 other patients. Measurements of T1 and T2 relaxation times and relative

Fig. 24-10. T1-weighted coronal (**A**), sagittal (**B**), and axial (**C**) images of patient with bladder carcinoma are shown. Tumor is seen along the superior and anterior aspects of the bladder and extends deeply into surrounding fat. It is higher in signal intensity than urine. The multiplanar imaging capability of MRI is invaluable in assessing the full extent of tumor involvement. On T2-weighted image in the sagittal (**D**) and axial (**E**) planes, tumor is lower in signal intensity than urine in the bladder. (**F**) Extension of the tumor into perivesical fat is well-demonstrated on CT scan, but this modality is limited to imaging in the axial plane. Arrows point to areas of tumor extension into surrounding fat. *u,* Urine; *t,* bladder tumor.

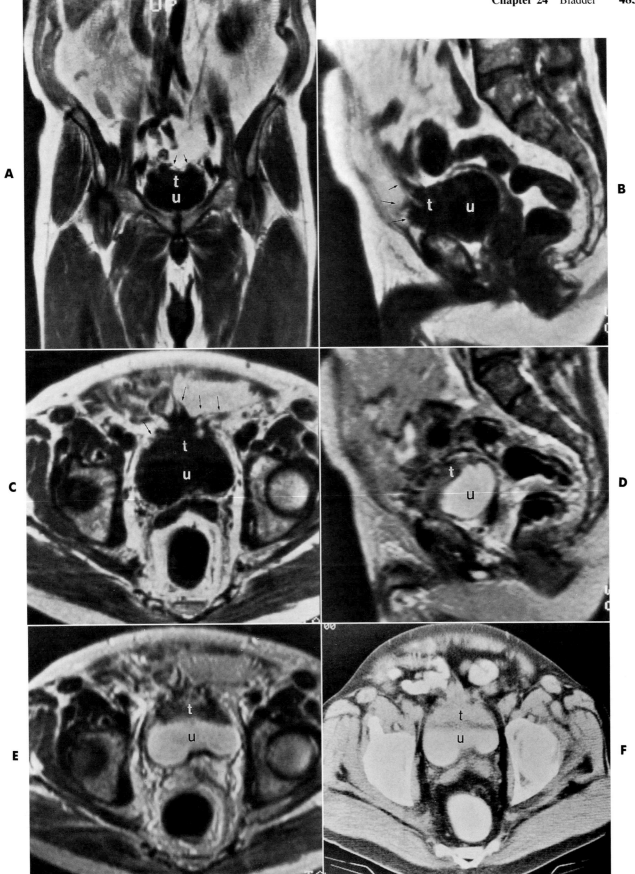

Fig. 24-10. For legend see opposite page.

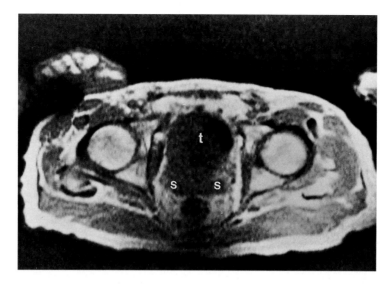

Fig. 24-11. Tumor extends to the right seminal vesicle in this patient with large bladder carcinoma. This is manifested by loss of the fat plane between the bladder and seminal vesicle. *t,* Bladder tumor; *s,* seminal vesicle.

spin density overlapped in those patients with malignant lymph nodes, nodes involved with granulomatous processes, and nonspecific lymphadenopathy. Dooms demonstrated that MRI and CT are comparable in demonstrating lymph nodes greater than 13 to 15 mm in size. MRI showed these nodes better because of its excellent soft tissue contrast resolution and clearly distinguished lymph nodes from normal fat, musculature, and vasculature. A normal-sized lymph node replaced by tumor is not necessarily recognizable as abnormal by either modality.[20]

Comparison of MRI and CT staging

Investigations have been undertaken to evaluate and compare the accuracy of CT and MRI for staging carcinoma of the bladder. Even early studies have shown that MRI is highly accurate in staging bladder cancer.

In 1985, Fisher, Hricak, and Tanagho,[9] evaluated a group of patients all of whom except one had lesions that were Stage T3B or above. Using the TNM classification, they showed that MRI correctly staged 86% of the cases.

In a study by Amendola et al.[1] in 1986, 11 patients with transitional cell carcinoma of the urinary bladder underwent MRI at 0.35 T and findings in 10 of the cases were compared with the results of CT. The patients subsequently underwent radical cystectomy and pelvic lymph node dissection. Accuracy of MRI for staging was 64% using the TNM classification and 73% using the Jewett-Strong-Marshall System in comparison to a 40% accuracy for CT. Delineation of tumor invasion of the perivesical fat, prostate gland, and seminal vesicles was improved with MRI. Direct sagittal and coronal imaging contributed to improved anatomic detail, particularly in tumors of the bladder base and dome. The group concluded that MRI ap-

peared to be highly promising for staging local extravesical tumor extension of bladder cancer.

The following year, Bryan et al.[3] did a comparative study of MRI and CT in 13 patients with bladder cancer. They reported that neither modality was capable of determining the depth of invasion of the bladder wall in the absence of extravesical spread. MRI accurately showed the presence or absence of tumor spread outside the bladder in 10 of 13 patients (77%). Two patients were understaged, whereas one patient was overstaged. CT correctly staged 9 of 13 patients (69%). Three patients were understaged and one was overstaged.

Rholl et al.[26] studied 23 patients with 25 bladder neoplasms. The examinations were evaluated retrospectively and compared with CT scan results and findings at pathologic examination. The group concluded that MRI showed promise in staging neoplasms of the bladder. They found MRI to be at least as accurate as CT in demonstrating extravesical tumor invasion and to have the additional advantage of being able to assess the depth of bladder wall involvement.

In 1988, Buy et al.[4] reported on 40 patients with carcinoma of the bladder who underwent preoperative MRI examinations before total cystectomy with enterocystoplasty and pelvic node dissection. There was extension through the deep muscle in 20 of the patients; diagnostic sensitivity and specificity of MRI were 95%. Invasion of the perivesical fat occurred in 18 of the 40 patients. This was demonstrated by MRI with a sensitivity of 66% and a specificity of 100%. In determining invasion of adjacent organs, which was present in 9 of the 40 patients, sensitivity was 44% and specificity was 96%. MRI correctly staged bladder tumors in 60% (24 out of 40) of the patients according

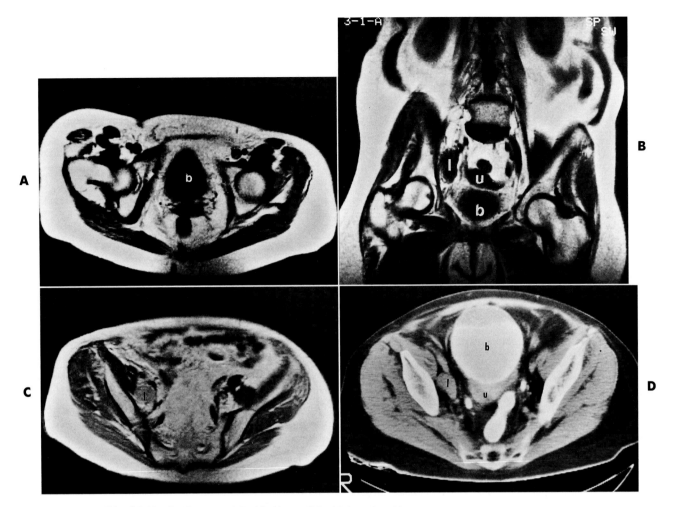

Fig. 24-12. A, Contour of the bladder wall is thickened and irregular, with streaky infiltration of perivesical fat in this patient with bladder carcinoma. **B,** Lymph node enlargement *(arrows)* is seen in the right side of the pelvis on coronal T1-weighted image. *b,* Urinary bladder; *u,* uterus; *l,* lymphadenopathy. **C,** On proton-density (intermediate weighting) MR axial image, enlarged lymph node is easily distinguished from adjacent vascular structures and muscle. With more T2 weighting (not shown), signal intensity of the involved lymph node increased further. This may be seen with tumor involvement and acute inflammatory change. *l,* Lymph node. **D,** CT scan in this patient shows enlarged lymph node. CT criteria of lymphadenopathy depend on size of the node. *b,* Urinary bladder; *u,* uterus; *l,* lymphadenopathy.

to the TNM staging classification. Tumor involvement was overestimated in 7% (3 out of 40) of the patients and underestimated in 32.5% (13 out of 40) of the cases. The researchers concluded that MRI is accurate in identification of lymphadenopathy and deep muscle invasion. It proved to be at least as useful as CT in evaluating perivesical extension of tumors. MRI was better than CT in diagnosing invasion of adjacent organs.

In 1982, Vock et al.[30] determined that it was extremely difficult to correctly identify stages of bladder tumor lower than T3 or B2 with CT. Mucosal, submucosal, and deep muscle invasion could not be distinguished from one another. Amendola et al.[1] reported similar limitations for MRI in 1986. Both modalities were found to be very accu-

rate in diagnosing infiltration of the perivesical fat (Stage T3 or C). MRI was superior in diagnosing seminal vesicle involvement. Fewer false positives were recorded. MRI also was slightly better than CT in demonstrating involvement of the prostate gland. CT and MRI missed metastatic deposits in normal-sized lymph nodes.

Husband et al.[11] in 1989 compared the results of MRI and CT in 30 patients with histologically proven bladder cancer. MRI accurately diagnosed the presence or absence of extravesical spread of tumor in 22 patients (accuracy 73%, sensitivity 82%, specificity 62%), whereas CT proved accurate in 24 patients (accuracy 80%, sensitivity 94%, specificity 62%). Two of the MRI examinations were not of diagnostic quality. Each modality yielded five false-positive studies and one false-negative study in the diagnosis of extravesical spread. Disruption of the low signal intensity line representing the bladder wall was seen in 22 patients, and 18 of these had deep muscle invasion. In six of the patients the bladder wall was intact, and none of these patients had evidence of deep muscle invasion. In this study CT was slightly better than MRI in demonstrating tumor invasion beyond the bladder wall. However, the authors point out that if the two nondiagnostic MRI studies are excluded, there is no significant difference between the two modalities in the ability to show extravesical tumor spread. The results of this study again demonstrate the ability of MRI to distinguish Stage T3A tumors from superficial lesions. None of the patients with deep muscle invasion demonstrated an intact bladder wall. However, there was apparent disruption of the bladder wall in four patients with histologically proven Stage T2 tumors. In seven patients, a continuous or interrupted double black line was apparent at the site of the tumor. This finding, not previously described, was postulated by the authors to represent tumor or edema extending within the layers of the bladder wall, coupled with a susceptibility effect caused by local inhomogeneity at the tumor-urine and tumor-perivesical fat interfaces.[11]

As Husband et al.[11] point out in their report, comparative studies of two modalities are subject to a variety of variables. These include the type of equipment and imaging techniques used, the experience of the radiologist with the modality, and the method of patient selection. For example, fast scanning with automated table movement during IV administration of contrast medium improves delineation of the tumor on CT examinations.

CT has been a valuable modality with which to stage bladder cancer, and accuracy rates have been reported to range from 64% to 92%.[14,17,22] However, CT has important limitations, because it cannot distinguish among the early stages of cancer in which the tumor is confined to the bladder wall,[13] and because it poorly demonstrates minimal extravesical spread and early invasion of adjacent organs.[27]

Postsurgical changes and some benign abnormalities may cause diagnostic difficulties. In a study of 77 patients with bladder carcinoma, Vock et al.[30] showed the overall accuracy of CT for estimation of local tumor extension to be 81%. In patients with previous bladder surgery or radiation therapy, perivesical tumor extension was overestimated in approximately one half of the cases. They reported that cystitis, trabeculation of the bladder wall related to outflow obstruction, and other benign conditions may lead to overestimation of tumor extent. Similar conclusions were drawn by Sager et al.,[27] who reported that perivesical extension of tumors found at histopathologic examination was demonstrated by CT in all of the 11 patients studied. There were seven false positives in diagnosing perivesical spread by CT. Three of these patients had

perivesical fibrosis. In all seven patients the suspicious perivesical findings were adjacent to the area of present or previous changes in the bladder wall, for example, at a biopsy site. Edema and fibrosis of the bladder wall in patients who have already undergone radiation therapy cannot be distinguished with certainty from tumor.

Some of the limitations of CT are also shared by MRI, such as the inability to distinguish among the earliest stages of bladder carcinoma. The problems of overstaging caused by edema or fibrosis are also not necessarily eliminated by MRI. It has been shown that MRI and CT are comparable in the ability to detect retroperitoneal and pelvic lymphadenopathy.[19] Both modalities rely on the size of the lymph nodes to diagnose pathologic conditions, and neither reliably distinguishes among the causes of lymph node enlargement.[6] However, an advantage of MRI is its ability to differentiate lymph nodes from vascular structures without the use of IV contrast agents. Although the use of MRI may not be appropriate for screening because of its longer imaging times, it is helpful in selected cases in which CT findings are indeterminate. In cases of advanced bladder carcinoma, however, MRI has no particular advantage over CT.[11] CT is in fact probably preferable, because it evaluates abdominal adenopathy, and its shorter examination time is an advantage for those patients who may have a small bladder capacity.[11]

OTHER MALIGNANT TUMORS

In addition to primary carcinoma of the urinary bladder, MRI also demonstrates other bladder masses. Pheochromocytomas may occur in the bladder, and this location accounts for 1% of these tumors. The MR (magnetic resonance) appearance of these lesions has been described.[10,31] In these reports, the masses were easily identified on T1WI images and were isointense with nearby muscle in one patient. The tumors became brighter on T2WI. MR was useful in estimating depth of invasion, as evidenced by disruption of the bladder wall in one patient. In the proper clinical setting, MR is useful in identifying an intravesical pheochromocytoma.

Bladder lymphoma is also identifiable with MRI.[13] The signal characteristics of the bladder wall lesion are similar to those of the involved lymph nodes. Again, on T1WI the lesion is easily separated from the low signal intensity urine. On T2WI the tumor and nodes have intermediate signal strength.

Clearly, MR can be used to identify bladder masses other than transitional cell carcinoma. As in other anatomic regions, MRI characteristics of a variety of lesions appears to overlap. In specific clinical settings such as the localization of pheochromocytoma, MR characterization may be of particular benefit.

Secondary involvement of the bladder by adjacent pelvic tumors is also readily demonstrated by MRI. Generally, the high signal intensity fat plane between the bladder and adjacent tumor is lost, as is the low signal intensity line representing the bladder wall.

FUTURE TRENDS

The use of IV contrast material with newer and faster imaging sequences and specially designed surface coils promises to improve the delineation of pathologic conditions of the bladder.

In an early study (1984), Carr et al.[5] performed MRI examinations at 0.15 T on 20 patients, including one case of transitional cell carcinoma, before and after IV administration of gadopentetate dimeglumine. On short TR/TE imaging sequences the bladder wall appeared thickened and showed slight enhancement. The urine initially displayed low signal intensity, but 25 minutes after administration of 0.005 mmol gadopentetate dimeglumine per kilogram of body weight, signal intensity increased. An additional injection of 0.095 mmol of gadopentetate dimeglumine per kilogram of body weight resulted in lower signal intensity, but which was still greater than the original signal.

In 1988, Simon and Szumowski[29] evaluated the use of chemical shift imaging in combination with paramagnetic contrast material. In contrast to conventional enhanced studies in which high signal intensity lesions become similar to the high signal intensity of adjacent fat, the predominant high signal intensity in the images provided by this method result from paramagnetic relaxation enhancement. Using this technique in which the signal from fat is suppressed, contrast agent administration may improve demonstration of tumor margins.

In 1989, Neuerburg[23] studied 48 patients with neoplasms of the urinary bladder before and after IV administration of gadopentetate dimeglumine using SE sequences with short repetition and echo times. The signal intensity of the tumor increased significantly, with an average rise in signal intensity of 120% for the tumor-fat ratio (tumor-marrow ratio, 105%; tumor-muscle ratio, 85%). The signal intensity of the tumor reached a peak within 120 seconds and remained on a plateau for up to 45 minutes. Necrotic portions of the tumor were visible only on the contrast-enhanced images.

Another significant advance may be the development of surface coils for more detailed evaluation of bladder and perivesical abnormalities.

Barentsz et al.[2] (1988) described a wraparound double surface coil that provided a significant improvement in spatial resolution compared with images obtained with the body coil. The field of view was sufficiently large so that the pelvis and abdomen could be studied with one sequence. The improvement in signal-to-noise ratio resulted in a greater staging accuracy of 79% with the double surface coil, compared to 54% with the body coil.

In another area of research, Klutke et al.[16] performed a preliminary investigation of MRI in the evaluation of stress incontinence. Their results were encouraging in that they found that the pertinent urethral, paraurethral, and bladder neck anatomy were well demonstrated. The abnormal position of the urethra and ureteropelvic ligaments was well-demonstrated in patients with stress incontinence. The authors emphasized that the superior delineation of the urethra on MRI as compared to sonography and CT suggests that this modality has great promise in this type of evaluation.

Other related studies have utilized gradient echo techniques to perform dynamic studies of the pelvis.[18,32] Prolapse of pelvic structures, including cystocele, has been imaged in this fashion.[32] Normal and abnormal migration of the organs can be demonstrated. Dynamic studies of the rectum and its support musculature and ligaments have been performed in this fashion. These preliminary studies suggest that dynamic techniques may be developed to evaluate a variety of urodynamic problems.

SUMMARY

In conclusion, it is evident that the urinary bladder is visualized well on MRI. The most significant clinical implication is the ability of MRI to delineate bladder tumor. Reports have shown that it is quite accurate in staging bladder carcinoma, particularly in demonstrating the depth of bladder wall invasion and tumor extent into the perivesical fat and adjacent organs. It differentiates lymphadenopathy from vascular structures without the use of IV contrast agents. The superior contrast resolution and multiplanar imaging capabilities of MRI allow better resolution of the bladder base and dome.

MRI does share some of the same limitations as CT, such as the inability to definitively diagnose tumor in normal-sized lymph nodes and the lack of differentiation among the causes of lymph node enlargement.

Currently, MRI is used when findings on CT are equivocal. However, the use of specially designed surface coils, faster imaging sequences, and even IV contrast media may expand the use of MRI in the diagnosis of bladder abnormalities and the staging of bladder cancer.

REFERENCES

1. Amendola MA, Glazer GM, Grossman HB, et al: Staging of bladder carcinoma: MR-CT-surgical correlation, *AJR* 146:1179-1183, 1986.
2. Barentsz JO, Lemmens JAM, Ruijs SHJ, et al: Carcinoma of the urinary bladder: MR imaging with a double surface coil, *AJR* 151:107-112, 1988.
3. Bryan PJ, Butler HE, LiPuma JP, et al: CT and MR imaging in staging bladder neoplasms, *J Comput Assist Tomogr* 11:96-101, 1987.
4. Buy J-N, Moss AA, Guinet C, et al: MR staging of bladder carcinoma: correlation with pathologic findings, *Radiology* 169:695-700, 1988.
5. Carr DH, Brown J, Bydder GM, et al: Gadolinium DTPA as a contrast agent in MRI: initial clinical experience in 20 patients, *AJR* 143:215-244, 1984.
6. Dooms GC, Hricak H, Crooks LE, et al: Magnetic resonance imaging of the lymph nodes: comparison with CT, *Radiology* 153:719-728, 1984.

7. Dooms GC, Hricak H, Moseley ME, et al: Characterization of lymphadenopathy by magnetic resonance relaxation times: preliminary results, *Radiology* 155:691-697, 1985.

8. Fisher MR, Hricak H, Crooks LE: Urinary bladder MR imaging. I. Normal and benign conditions, *Radiology* 157:467-470, 1985.

9. Fisher MR, Hricak H, Tanagho EA: Urinary bladder MR imaging. II. Neoplasm, *Radiology* 157:471-477, 1985.

10. Heyman J et al: Bladder pheochromocytoma: evaluation with magnetic resonance imaging, *J Urol* 141:1424-1426, 1989.

11. Husband JES, Olliff JFC, Williams MP, et al: Bladder cancer: staging with CT and MR imaging, *Radiology* 173:435-440, 1989.

12. Jewett HJ, Strong GH: Infiltrating carcinoma of the bladder: relation of depth of penetration of the bladder wall to incidence of local extension and metastases, *J Urol* 55:366-372, 1966.

13. Johnson AJ, Dixon CM, Negendank W: Bladder lymphoma: diagnosis and documentation of response by magnetic resonance imaging, *J Urol* 142:1318-1320, 1989.

14. Kellett MJ et al: Computed tomography as an adjunct to bimanual examination for staging bladder tumors, *Br J Urol* 52:101-106, 1980.

15. Kenny GM, Hardner GJ, Murphy GP: Clinical staging of bladder tumors, *J Urol* 104:720-723, 1970.

16. Klutke C et al: The anatomy of stress incontinence: magnetic resonance imaging of the female bladder neck and urethra, *J Urol* 143:563-566, 1990.

17. Koss JC, Arger PH, Coleman BG, et al: CT staging of bladder carcinoma, *AJR* 137:359-362, 1981.

18. Kruyt RH, Delemarre JBVM, Doorubos J, et al: Normal anorectum: dynamic MR imaging anatomy, *Radiology* 179:159-163, 1991.

19. Lee JKT, Heiken JP, Ling D, et al: Magnetic resonance imaging of abdominal and pelvic lymphadenopathy, *Radiology* 153:181-188, 1984.

20. Lee JKT, Rholl KS: MRI of the bladder and prostate, *AJR* 147:732-736, 1986.

21. Marshall VF: The relation of preoperative estimate of the pathologic demonstration of the extent of vesical neoplasms, *J Urol* 68:714-723, 1952.

22. Morgan CL, Calkins RF, Cavalcanti EJ: Computed tomography in the evaluation, staging and therapy of carcinoma of the bladder and prostate, *Radiology* 140:751-761,1981.

23. Neuerburg JM: Urinary bladder neoplasms: evaluation with contrast-enhanced MR imaging, *Radiology* 172:739-743, 1989.

24. Prout GR Jr: Bladder carcinoma and a TNM system of classification, *J Urol* 117:583-590, 1977.

25. Richie JP, Skinner DG, Kaufman JJ: Carcinoma of the bladder: treatment by radical cystectomy, *J Surg Res* 18:271-275, 1975.

26. Rholl KS, Lee JKT, Heiken JP, et al: Primary bladder carinoma: evaluation with MR imaging, *Radiology* 163:117-121, 1987.

27. Sager EM, Talle K, Fossa S, et al: The role of CT in demonstrating perivesical tumor growth in the preoperative staging of carcinoma of the urinary bladder, *Radiology* 146:443-446, 1983.

28. Schmidt JD, Weinstein SH: Pitfalls in clinical staging of bladder tumors, *Urol Clin North Am* 3:107-127, 1976.

29. Simon JH, Szumowski J: Paramagnetic contrast-enhanced chemical shift imaging: a new approach to improved lesion detection on contrast-enhanced MR imaging, *Radiology* 169(P):339, 1988 (abstract).

30. Vock P et al: Computed tomography in staging of carcinoma of the bladder, *Br J Urol* 54:158-163, 1982.

31. Warshawsky R, Bow SN, Waldbaum RS, et al: Bladder pheochromocytoma with MR correlation, *J Comput Assist Tomogr* 13:714-716, 1989.

32. Yang A, Mostwin JL, Rosenshein NB, et al: Pelvic floor descent in women: dynamic evaluation with fast MR imaging and cinematic display, *Radiology* 179:25-33, 1991.

Appendix A

PATIENT PREPARATION FOR ABDOMINAL MRI

Mary Ellen Bentham

Patient preparation for MRI imaging begins at the time the appointment is made by the referring physician. Patients are prescreened and given instructions, which include the location and a map of the MRI center, and they are questioned concerning metallic implants and are given guidelines for being NPO before the examination.

The more information that is available to the patient before their arrival at the MRI center, the more likely the patient will be able to comply with the unusual nature of the MRI exam. A variety of literature available to MRI departments is distributed to the referring physicians for their patients. Appointment confirmation and screening for metallic implants and other contraindications for MRI is done 2 to 3 days before the scheduled appointment. Arrangements for pre-MRI exam of the orbits for patients with histories of having metal in the eyes may be made so as not to interfere with the MRI schedule. Patients with implants or devices that may not be MR compatible have time to obtain more information about these devices. Patients with histories of claustrophobia may bring medication to take after their arrival and before the exam. Before abdominal scans, special instructions are given to patients regarding their eating habits. These patients are asked not to eat or drink anything for 3 hours before they arrive.

PATIENT ARRIVAL

When the patients arrive at the MRI center, they are screened by a technologist and the exam is explained in detail. Any questions they may have are answered. A patient that is well-prepared and knowledgeable knows what to expect and is able to follow the technologist's instructions. A relaxed patient breaths normally, which minimizes breathing and motion artifacts. This speeds up the exam process for the patient and gives them a feeling of participation in their diagnosis and ultimate treatment. The utilization of scan time improves without the need for repeat sequences and scans.

PROTOCOLING CONTRAST MEDIA

Protocols for MRI exams are prepared before the patient arrives at the MRI facility. This information is provided by the radiologist and is based on the reasons for the MRI exam and the information the clinician hopes to obtain from the exam. Protocols provide the technologist with the information necessary to prepare the patient properly. Information about the type of contrast agent to be given, the number of imaging sequences and their approximate duration, and the specific area of interest allows the technologist to instruct the patient as to what to expect and to position the patient properly in the scanner.

ORAL CONTRAST MEDIA

Patients who are to receive oral contrast agents are instructed to arrive at the center 1 hour before the scheduled exam time. A barium suspension oral contrast agent is not given if it is known that the patient is also scheduled for a CAT scan or an angiogram. Patients diagnosed with liver metastasis, lymphadenopathy or lymphoma, pancreatic disease, or diseases involving the renal vein do take oral contrast agents. The first of three 8 oz cups of contrast agent is given 1 hour before the time the patient is to be placed in the scanner. The second cup is given 30 minutes later. Just before the patient goes to the scan room, half of the third cup is given. The last of the contrast agent is given as the patient gets on the table and is instructed to lie on the right side for 5 minutes. The patient is then positioned with abdominal compression to minimize breathing motion.

RECTAL FLUSH

Patients requiring rectal contrast agents are prepared in the scan room. Protective padding is placed on the table under the patient. An enema bag is filled with approximately 400 cc of contrast agent. A straight enema tip is inserted and contrast agent is administered until the patient feels slightly full, but not to the point of discomfort. The enema tip is removed and the patient is positioned with compression over the upper abdomen. The rectal flush is used in patients for scans of masses, adenopathy, and the prostate gland.

FEMALE PELVIS

Female patients having MRI exams of the pelvis are asked to insert a tampon into the vagina. This better opacifies the vaginal area for the radiologist.

INTRAVENOUS CONTRAST MEDIA

An intravenous (IV) contrast agent is indicated in a few patients in whom characterization of liver lesions or renal tumors is necessary. Dynamic studies of the liver have increased with the development of faster scanning techniques. Intravenous catheters are placed and a solution of sodium chloride is administered to give access for the intravenous contrast agent. This is done before the patient is placed in the scan room so that the room may be used by others. Before the contrast agent is given, scans are obtained and the area of interest is localized. The contrast agent may then be injected through the open line without moving the patient and delaying the scan time.

AFTERCARE

Aftercare instructions are given to each patient who has received an oral contrast agent for MRI. The patient is informed about what to expect after drinking the barium suspension liquids and what to do in the event that they should experience any problems following the MRI exam. The instructions also concern their resuming regular eating habits, drinking plenty of fluids for the next 8 hours, and consulting their doctor if prolonged constipation occurs.

CONCLUSION

Patient education and preparation assures better patient compliance before and during the MRI procedure. Patients have a more pleasant experience and are more willing to help the techologists and doctor obtain a better exam. This not only improves image quality but also improves utilization of the MRI facility.

Appendix B

PROTOCOLS FOR ABDOMINAL MRI

W. Dean Bidgood, Jr.
Richard W. Briggs
Pablo R. Ros

See opposite page.

Sequences 1, 2, and 3 are common to all examinations:

SEQUENCE #	PLANE	WEIGHT	THICKNESS	NOTES:
1	Cor	T1W	8mm	
2	Ax	T1W	8-10mm	Use 5-8mm if "thin sections"
3	Ax	T2W	8-10mm	are indicated for the region.

Additional sequences and region-specific technique modifications are listed below:

ADRENAL Mass

Use thin sections and no gap for the initial axial sequences. Sagittal sections may also be necessary to separate the adrenal from the liver.

4	Ax	T1W FS	5-8mm	

FEMALE PELVIS Ovaries

Use thin sections and no gap for the initial axial sequences. Administer rectal contrast. Rectangular FOV can be used to compensate for increased NEX in sequence 4.

4	Cor	T2W	5-8mm	

FEMALE PELVIS Uterus

Use thin sections for the initial axial sequences. Administer rectal contrast.

4	Sag	T2W	8mm	
5	Sag	T1W	8mm	

KIDNEY Carcinoma (Staging)

4	Ax	GRE	5mm	For blood products
5	Ax	MRA	Thin	Renal veins and IVC

KIDNEY Mass (Characterization)

Match slice thickness to the size of the mass.

4	Ax	T1W FS	5-8mm	
5	Sag	T1W FS	5-8mm	

LIVER Hemangioma

If possible, perform a dynamic series of images at a single slice position, following administration of i.v. gadolinium for sequence 5. Use oral contrast agent if the lesion is small or if bowel artifact is likely. Reverse the phase-encoding and frequency readout axes if necessary.

4	Ax	T2W	10mm	Extended TE
5	Ax	T1W	8mm	With gadolium

LIVER Metastasis or Mass

Use oral contrast agent when screening for metastases and when characterizing a known mass, if bowel artifacts are likely (i.e. in the left lobe or caudal right lobe).

4	Ax	GRE	10mm	

MALE OR FEMALE PELVIS Bladder, Rectum, or Mass

Administer rectal contrast agent.

4	Sag	T1W	5-8mm	
5	Sag	T2W	5-8mm	

MALE PELVIS Prostate

Administer rectal contrast agent. Do thin section axial T1W and Sagittal T2W instead of basic sequences 2 and 3.

1	Cor	T1W	8mm	
2	Ax	T1W	5-8mm	
3	Sag	T2W	5-8mm	
4	Sag	T1W FS	5-8mm	With gadolinium
5	Ax	T1W FS	5-8mm	With gadolinium

PANCREAS Mass

Administer oral contrast agent.

4	Ax	T1W FS	8mm	With gadolinium
5	Ax-Oblique	T1W FS	8mm	With gadolinium

VESSELS Thrombus or Tumor

4	Ax	GRE	10mm	FS beneficial
5	Ax/Cor	MRA	Thin	Or GRE with flow comp

DEFINITIONS: Ax = Axial, Cor = Coronal, Sag = Sagittal, FS = Fat suppression, GRE = Gradient-recalled echo.

INDEX